DISEASE & DRUG CONSULT

Cardiovascular Disorders

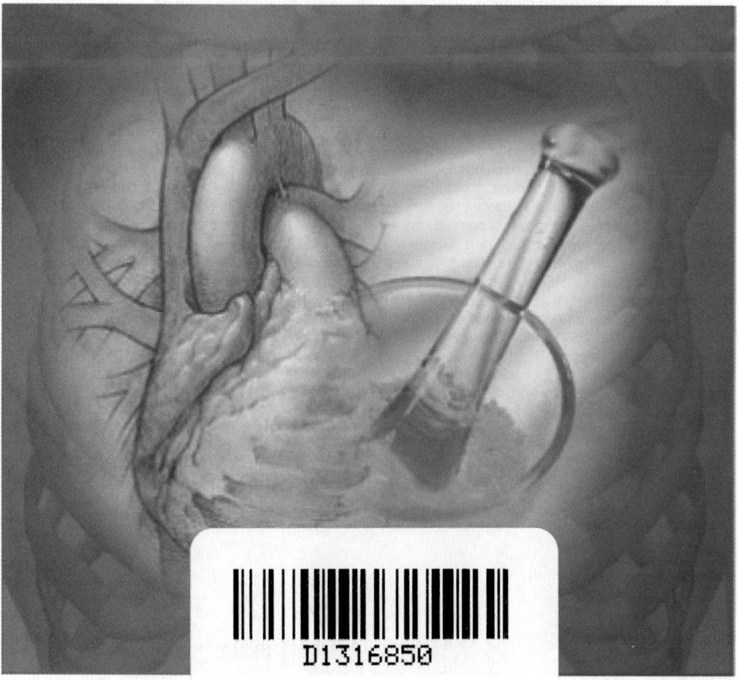

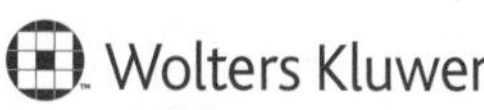

Wolters Kluwer Health | Lippincott Williams & Wilkins

Philadelphia • Baltimore • New York • London
Buenos Aires • Hong Kong • Sydney • Tokyo

Staff

Executive Publisher
Judith A. Schilling McCann, RN, MSN

Clinical Director
Joan M. Robinson, RN, MSN

Art Director
Elaine Kasmer

Editorial Project Manager
Deborah Grandinetti

Clinical Project Manager
Kathryn Henry, RN, BSN, CCRC

Editor
Catherine Harold

Clinical Editor
Lisa Morris Bonsall, RN, MSN, CRNP

Copy Editor
Amy Furman, Linda Hager

Designer
Joe Clark

Associate Manufacturing Manager
Beth Welsh

Editorial Assistants
Karen J. Kirk, Linda K. Ruhf

Production Project Manager
Cynthia Rudy

The clinical procedures described and recommended in this publication are based on research and consultation with nursing, medical, pharmaceutical, and legal authorities. To the best of our knowledge, these procedures reflect currently accepted practice; nevertheless, they can't be considered absolute and universal recommendations. For individual application, all recommendations must be considered in light of the patient's clinical condition and, before the administration of new or infrequently used drugs, in light of the latest package-insert information. The authors and publisher disclaim responsibility for adverse effects resulting directly or indirectly from the suggested procedures, from undetected errors, or from the reader's misunderstanding of the text.

 Printed in China. For information, write Lippincott Williams & Wilkins, 323 Norristown Road, Suite 200, Ambler, PA 19002-2758.

DDCCD010209

Library of Congress Cataloging-in-Publication Data

Disease & drug consult. Cardiovascular disorders.
p. ; cm.
Includes bibliographical references and index.
ISBN 978-1-60547-049-8 (alk. paper)
1. Heart—Diseases—Nursing—Handbooks, manuals, etc. 2. Cardiovascular agents—Handbooks, manuals, etc. I. Lippincott Williams & Wilkins. II. Title: Disease and drug consult. Cardiovascular disorders. III. Title: Cardiovascular disorders.
[DNLM: 1. Cardiovascular Diseases—nursing—Handbooks. 2. Cardiovascular Diseases—drug therapy—Handbooks. 3. Drug Therapy—methods—Handbooks. WY 49 D6105 2009]

RC674.D57 2009
616.1'20231—dc22 2008045630

RRS0811

Contents

Contributors and consultants

Nancy Blake, RN, MN, CCRN, CNAA-BC
Director, Critical Care Services and Education
Children's Hospital
Los Angeles, CA

Karen Crisfulla, MSN, CCRN
Clinical Nurse Specialist
Hospital of the University of Pennsylvania
Philadelphia, PA

Kathleen M. Hill, RN, MSN, CCNS-CSC
Clinical Nurse Specialist, Cardiovascular Intensive Care Units
Cleveland Clinic
Cleveland, OH

Theresa M. Leonard, RN, BSN, CCRN
Unit Educator, Invasive Cardiology
Stony Brook University Medical Center
Stony Brook, NY

Debra K. Moser, RN, DNSc, FAAN
Professor and Gill Endowed Chair of Nursing
University of Kentucky College of Nursing
Lexington, KY

Cheryl L. Rader, RN, BSN, CCRN-CSC
RN IV
Saint Luke's Hospital of Kansas City
Kansas City, MO

Nancy M. Richards, RN, MSN, CCRN, CCNS
Cardiovascular Surgery Clinical Nurse Specialist
Saint Luke's Hospital, Mid America Heart Institute
Kansas City, MO

Part 1

Disorders

Abdominal aneurysm

An aneurysm is an abnormal dilation in an arterial wall. In the abdomen, dilation typically occurs in the aorta between the renal arteries and iliac branches. The dangers of abdominal aneurysm are twofold: dissection, in which the artery's lining tears and blood leaks into the arterial wall, and rupture, in which the aneurysm breaks open, resulting in profuse bleeding. Rupture is a common complication in larger aneurysms.

CAUSES AND INCIDENCE

Abdominal aortic aneurysms (AAAs) result from atherosclerosis, hypertension, congenital weakening, cystic medial necrosis, trauma, syphilis, and other infections. Smoking is a prominent risk factor. In children, abdominal aneurysm can result from blunt abdominal injury or Marfan syndrome.

These aneurysms develop slowly. First, a focal weakness in the muscular layer of the aorta (tunica media), caused by degenerative changes, allows the inner layer (tunica intima) and outer layer (tunica adventitia) to stretch outward. Blood pressure in the aorta continues to weaken the vessel walls and enlarge the aneurysm.

Nearly all AAAs are fusiform, which means that the arterial walls balloon on all sides. A fusiform aneurysm develops when the arterial wall weakens around its circumference, creating a spindle shape. The resulting sac fills with necrotic debris and thrombi.

Abdominal aneurysm is four times more common in men than in women and usually occurs in whites ages 40 to 70. Less than half of people with a ruptured AAA aneurysm survive.

SIGNS AND SYMPTOMS

Although abdominal aneurysms usually produce no symptoms, they typically (unless the patient is obese) produce a pulsating mass in the periumbilical area and a systolic bruit over the aorta. The patient may feel some tenderness on deep palpation.

A large aneurysm may produce symptoms that mimic renal calculi, lumbar disk disease, and duodenal compression. Unless embolization occurs, abdominal aneurysms rarely cause reduced peripheral pulses or claudication.

Lumbar pain that radiates to the flank and groin stems from pressure on the lumbar nerves and may signify enlargement and imminent rupture. A rare symptom is unrelenting testicular pain.

If an aneurysm ruptures into the peritoneal cavity, it will cause severe, persistent abdominal and back pain, mimicking renal or ureteral colic. Signs and symptoms of hemorrhage—such as weakness, sweating, tachycardia, and hypotension—may be subtle because rupture into the retroperitoneal space produces a tamponade effect that prevents continued hemorrhage. Patients with such rupture may remain stable for hours before shock and death occur, although 20% die immediately.

COMPLICATIONS

- Rupture
- Dissection
- Hemorrhage
- Shock
- Obstruction of blood flow to other organs
- Embolization to a peripheral artery

DIAGNOSIS

Because abdominal aneurysms seldom produce symptoms, they're commonly detected accidentally during an X-ray or a routine physical examination. Several tests can confirm a suspected abdominal aneurysm.

- Serial ultrasonography can accurately determine the aneurysm's size, shape, and location.
- Anteroposterior and lateral X-rays of the abdomen can detect aortic calcification, which outlines the mass, at least 75% of the time.
- Aortography shows the condition of vessels proximal and distal to the aneurysm and the aneurysm's extent, but it may underestimate the aneurysm's diameter because it shows only the flow channel and not the surrounding clot.
- Computed tomography scanning is used to diagnose and size the aneurysm.
- Magnetic resonance imaging can be used as an alternative to aortography.

TREATMENT

Usually, abdominal aneurysm requires resection of the aneurysm and replacement of the damaged aortic section with a Dacron graft. (See *Abdominal aneurysms: Before and after surgery,* and *Endovascular grafting for repair of an AAA,* page 6.) If the aneurysm is small and asymptomatic, surgery may be delayed and the aneurysm followed and allowed to expand to a size at which the risk from the aneurysm exceeds the risk of the surgery. However, small aneurysms may also rupture. Surgical repair is recommended for symptomatic patients and for patients with aneurysms greater than 2″ (5 cm) in diameter.

Stenting is also a treatment option. It can be performed without an abdominal incision by introducing the catheters through arteries in the groin. However, not all patients with AAAs are candidates for this treatment.

Regular physical examination and ultrasound checks are needed to detect enlargement, which may forewarn rupture. Large aneurysms or those that produce symptoms pose a significant risk of rupture and need immediate repair. In patients with

ABDOMINAL ANEURYSMS: BEFORE AND AFTER SURGERY

During surgery, a prosthetic graft replaces or encloses the weakened area.

Before surgery

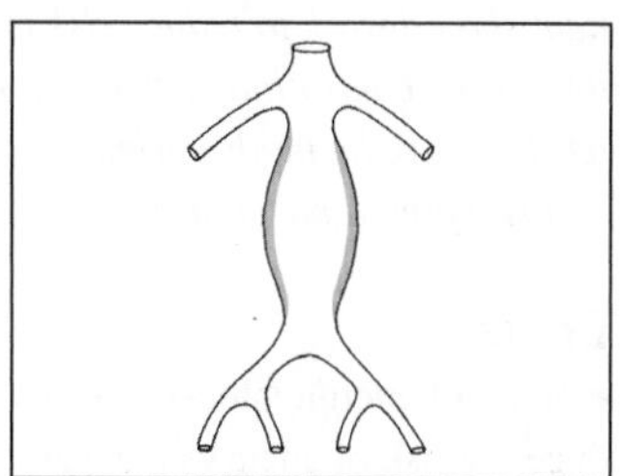

Aneurysm below renal arteries and above bifurcation

After surgery

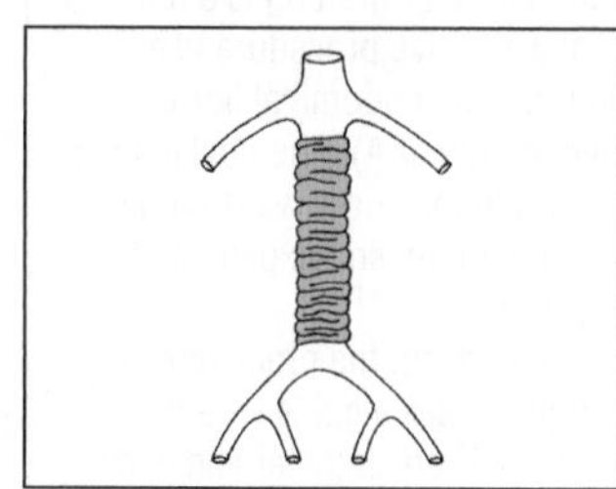

The prosthesis extends distal to the renal arteries to above the aortic bifurcation.

Before surgery

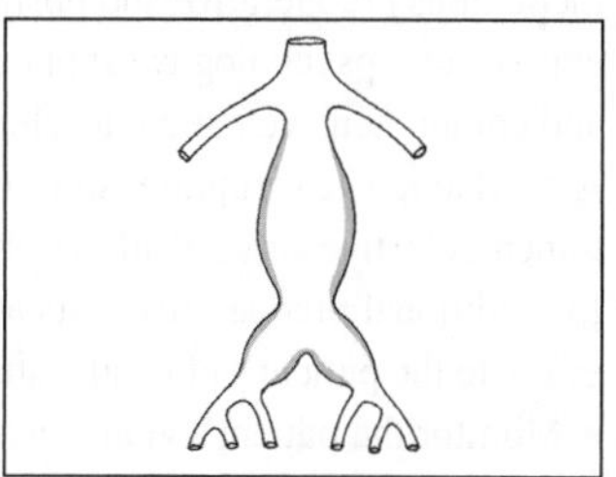

Aneurysm below renal arteries involving the iliac branches

After surgery

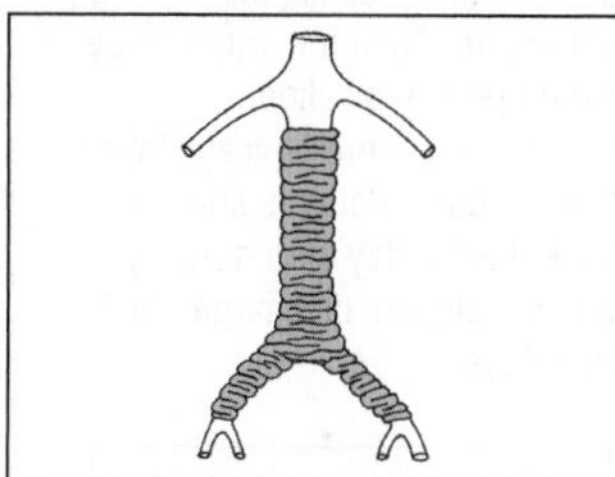

The prosthesis extends to the common femoral arteries.

Before surgery

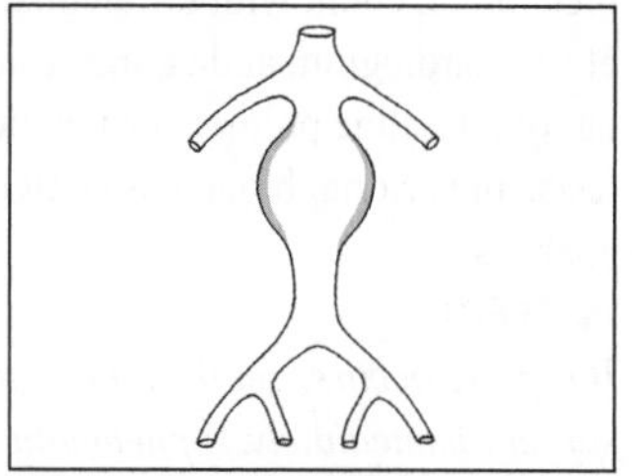

Small aneurysm in patient with poor distal runoff (poor risk)

After surgery

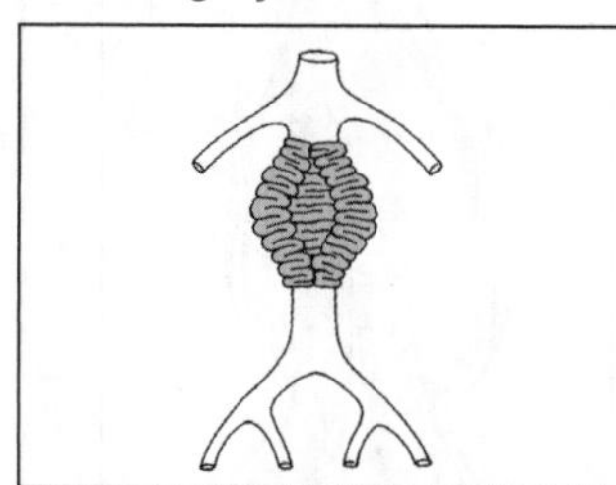

The external prosthesis encircles the aneurysm and is held in place with sutures.

ENDOVASCULAR GRAFTING FOR REPAIR OF AN AAA

Endovascular grafting is a minimally invasive procedure used to repair an abdominal aortic aneurysm (AAA). The goal is to reinforce the aortic walls so the aneurysm doesn't expand and rupture.

To perform the procedure, a surgeon uses a guide wire to insert a delivery catheter and compressed graft through a small incision in the patient's femoral or iliac artery. Under fluoroscopic guidance, the surgeon advances the catheter into the patient's aorta until it reaches the aneurysm. Then the graft can be fixed open by a balloon.

The procedure typically takes 2 to 3 hours. Patients should walk the 1st day after surgery and usually are discharged in 1 to 3 days.

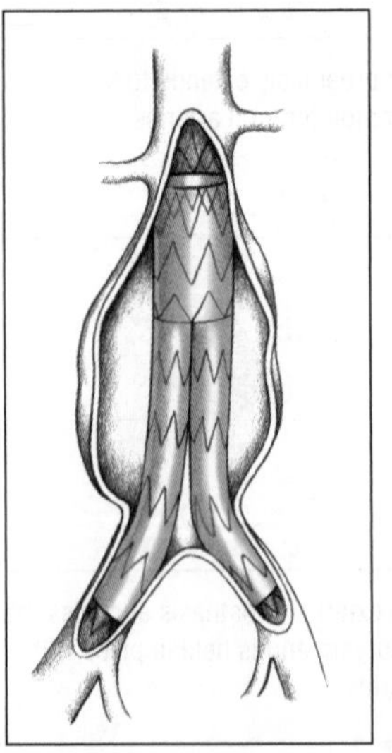

poor distal runoff, external grafting may be done.

PREVENTION

To help prevent an abdominal aneurysm from rupturing, the patient should work to reduce risk factors, as by controlling hypercholesterolemia, reducing hypertension, and stopping tobacco use.

Drugs

- Beta-adrenergic blockers to reduce the risk of aneurysm expansion and rupture

SPECIAL CONSIDERATIONS

Abdominal aneurysm requires meticulous preoperative and postoperative care, psychological support, and comprehensive patient teaching. After diagnosis, if rupture isn't imminent, elective surgery allows time for additional preoperative tests to evaluate the patient's clinical status.

- Monitor the patient's vital signs, and type and crossmatch his blood.
- Obtain renal function tests (blood urea nitrogen, creatinine, and electrolyte levels), blood samples (complete blood count with differential), electrocardiogram and cardiac evaluation, baseline pulmonary function tests, and arterial blood gas (ABG) analysis.

ALERT

If rupture occurs, get the patient to surgery immediately. A pneumatic antishock garment may be used during transport. Surgery allows direct compression of the aorta to control hemorrhage. Large amounts of blood may be needed during the resuscitative period to replace lost blood. Renal failure from ischemia is a major postoperative complication, and the patient may need hemodialysis.

- Before elective surgery, weigh the patient, insert an indwelling urinary catheter and an I.V. line, and assist with insertion of an arterial line and pulmonary artery catheter to monitor fluid and hemodynamic balance. Give prophylactic antibiotics.
- Explain the surgical procedure and the expected postoperative care in the intensive care unit (ICU) for patients undergoing complex abdominal surgery (I.V. lines, end tracheal [ET] and nasogastric [NG] intubation, and mechanical ventilation).
- After surgery, in the ICU, closely monitor the patient's vital signs, intake and hourly output, peripheral pulses, neurologic status (level of consciousness, pupil size, and sensation in arms and legs), and ABG values. Assess the depth, rate, and character of respirations and breath sounds at least every hour.
- Watch for signs of bleeding (increased pulse and respiratory rates and hypotension) and back pain, which may indicate that the graft is tearing. Check abdominal dressings for excessive bleeding or drainage. Be alert for increased temperature and other signs of infection. After NG intubation for intestinal decompression, irrigate the tube often to ensure patency. Record the amount and type of drainage.
- Suction the ET tube often. If the patient can breathe unassisted and has good breath sounds and adequate ABG values, tidal volume, and vital capacity 24 hours after surgery, he will be extubated and will need oxygen by mask.
- Weigh the patient daily to evaluate fluid balance.
- Help the patient walk as soon as he's able (typically the 2nd day after surgery).
- Provide psychological support for the patient and his family. Help ease their fears about the ICU, the threat of impending rupture, and surgery by providing appropriate explanations and answering all questions.

Aortic insufficiency

In aortic insufficiency (also called *aortic regurgitation*), the aortic valve weakens or balloons, which prevents it from closing tightly. This allows blood to flow backward from the aorta into the left ventricle.

CAUSES AND INCIDENCE

This disorder may be associated with Marfan syndrome, ankylosing spondylitis, or a ventricular septal defect, even after surgical closure. (See *Types of valvular heart disease,* page 8.) It also may result from rheumatic fever, syphilis, hypertension, endocarditis, trauma, or congenital abnormalities of the aortic valve (such as a bicuspid valve). Degenerative changes in aging can also lead to aortic insufficiency. In

(*Text continues on page 12*)

TYPES OF VALVULAR HEART DISEASE

Causes and incidence	Signs and symptoms	Diagnostic measures
Aortic insufficiency		
▪ Results from rheumatic fever, syphilis, hypertension, or endocarditis or may be idiopathic ▪ Most common in males ▪ Associated with Marfan syndrome ▪ Associated with ventricular septal defect, even after surgical closure	▪ Dyspnea, cough, fatigue, palpitations, angina, syncope ▪ Pulmonary venous congestion, heart failure, pulmonary edema (left-sided heart failure), "pulsating" nail beds ▪ Rapidly rising and collapsing pulses (pulsus biferiens), cardiac arrhythmias, wide pulse pressure in severe insufficiency ▪ *Auscultation:* reveals S_3 and diastolic blowing murmur at left sternal border ▪ Palpation and visualization of apical impulse in chronic disease	▪ *Cardiac catheterization:* reduced arterial diastolic pressures, aortic insufficiency, other valvular abnormalities, increased left ventricular end-diastolic pressure ▪ *X-ray:* left ventricular enlargement, pulmonary vein congestion ▪ *Echocardiography:* left ventricular enlargement, changes in mitral valve movement (indirect indication of aortic valve disease), mitral thickening ▪ *Electrocardiography (ECG):* sinus tachycardia, left ventricular hypertrophy, and left atrial hypertrophy in severe disease
Aortic stenosis		
▪ Results from congenital aortic bicuspid valve (associated with coarctation of the aorta), congenital stenosis of valve cusps, rheumatic fever, or atherosclerosis in elderly patients ▪ Most common in males	▪ Dyspnea on exertion, paroxysmal nocturnal dyspnea, fatigue, syncope, angina, palpitations ▪ Pulmonary venous congestion, heart failure, pulmonary edema ▪ Diminished carotid pulses, decreased cardiac output, cardiac arrhythmias, possible pulsus alternans ▪ *Auscultation:* reveals systolic murmur at base or in carotids, possible S_4	▪ *Cardiac catheterization:* pressure gradient across valve (indicating obstruction), increased left ventricular end-diastolic pressures ▪ *X-ray:* valvular calcification, left ventricular enlargement, pulmonary venous congestion ▪ *Echocardiography:* thickened aortic valve and left ventricular wall ▪ *ECG:* left ventricular hypertrophy

TYPES OF VALVULAR HEART DISEASE *(continued)*

Causes and incidence	Signs and symptoms	Diagnostic measures
Mitral insufficiency		
▪ Results from rheumatic fever, hypertrophic cardiomyopathy, mitral valve prolapse, myocardial infarction, severe left-sided heart failure, or ruptured chordae tendineae ▪ Associated with other congenital anomalies, such as transposition of the great arteries ▪ Rare in children without other congenital anomalies	▪ Orthopnea, dyspnea, fatigue, angina, palpitations ▪ Peripheral edema, jugular vein distention, hepatomegaly (right-sided heart failure) ▪ Tachycardia, crackles, pulmonary edema ▪ *Auscultation:* holosystolic murmur at apex, split S_2 (possible), S_3	▪ *Cardiac catheterization:* mitral insufficiency with increased left ventricular end-diastolic volume and pressure, increased atrial pressure and pulmonary artery wedge pressure (PAWP), decreased cardiac output ▪ *X-ray:* left atrial and ventricular enlargement, pulmonary venous congestion ▪ *Echocardiography:* abnormal valve leaflet motion, left atrial enlargement ▪ *ECG:* left atrial and ventricular hypertrophy, sinus tachycardia, atrial fibrillation
Mitral stenosis		
▪ Most commonly results from rheumatic fever ▪ Most common in females ▪ May be associated with other congenital anomalies	▪ Dyspnea on exertion, paroxysmal nocturnal dyspnea, orthopnea, weakness, fatigue, palpitations ▪ Peripheral edema, jugular venous distention (JVD), ascites, hepatomegaly (right-sided heart failure in severe pulmonary hypertension) ▪ Crackles, cardiac arrhythmias (atrial fibrillation), signs of systemic emboli ▪ *Auscultation:* loud S_1 or opening snap and diastolic murmur at apex	▪ *Cardiac catheterization:* diastolic pressure gradient across valve, elevated left atrial pressure, PAWP greater than 15 mm Hg with severe pulmonary hypertension and pulmonary artery pressure, elevated right-sided heart pressure, decreased cardiac output, abnormal contraction of left ventricle ▪ *X-ray:* left atrial and ventricular enlargement, enlarged pulmonary arteries, mitral valve calcification

(continued)

TYPES OF VALVULAR HEART DISEASE *(continued)*

Causes and incidence	Signs and symptoms	Diagnostic measures
Mitral stenosis (*continued*)		▪ *Echocardiography:* thickened mitral valve leaflets, left atrial enlargement ▪ *ECG:* left atrial hypertrophy, atrial fibrillation, right ventricular hypertrophy, right-axis deviation
Mitral valve prolapse syndrome		
▪ Cause unknown (researchers speculate that metabolic or neuroendocrine factors cause constellation of signs and symptoms) ▪ Most commonly affects young women but may occur in both sexes and in all age-groups	▪ May produce no signs ▪ Chest pain, palpitations, headache, fatigue, exercise intolerance, dyspnea, lightheadedness, syncope, mood swings, anxiety, panic attacks ▪ *Auscultation:* typically reveals mobile, midsystolic click, with or without mid to late systolic murmur	▪ *Two-dimensional echocardiography:* prolapse of mitral valve leaflets into left atrium ▪ *Color-flow Doppler studies:* mitral insufficiency ▪ *Resting ECG:* ST-segment changes, biphasic or inverted T waves in leads II, III, AV_F ▪ *Exercise ECG:* evaluates chest pain and arrhythmias
Pulmonic insufficiency		
▪ May be congenital or may result from pulmonary hypertension ▪ Rarely, may result from prolonged use of pressure monitoring catheter in the pulmonary artery	▪ Dyspnea, weakness, fatigue, chest pain ▪ Peripheral edema, JVD, hepatomegaly (right-sided heart failure) ▪ *Auscultation:* reveals diastolic murmur in pulmonic area	▪ *Cardiac catheterization:* pulmonic insufficiency, increased right ventricular pressure, associated cardiac defects ▪ *X-ray:* right ventricular and pulmonary arterial enlargement ▪ *ECG:* right ventricular or right atrial enlargement
Pulmonic stenosis		
▪ Results from congenital stenosis of valve cusp or rheumatic heart disease (infrequent)	▪ May be asymptomatic or symptomatic, with dyspnea on exertion, fatigue, chest pain, syncope	▪ *Cardiac catheterization:* increased right ventricular pressure, decreased pulmonary artery pressure

TYPES OF VALVULAR HEART DISEASE *(continued)*

Causes and incidence	Signs and symptoms	Diagnostic measures
Pulmonic stenosis (*continued*) ▪ Associated with other congenital heart defects such as tetralogy of Fallot	▪ May lead to peripheral edema, JVD, hepatomegaly (right-sided heart failure) ▪ *Auscultation:* reveals systolic murmur at left sternal border, split S_2 with delayed or absent pulmonic component	▪ *ECG:* possible right ventricular hypertrophy, right-axis deviation, right atrial hypertrophy, atrial fibrillation
Tricuspid insufficiency ▪ Results from right-sided heart failure, rheumatic fever and, rarely, trauma and endocarditis ▪ Associated with congenital disorders ▪ Associated with I.V. drug abuse and infective endocarditis manifesting as tricuspid valve disease	▪ Dyspnea and fatigue ▪ May lead to peripheral edema, JVD, hepatomegaly, and ascites (right-sided heart failure) ▪ *Auscultation:* reveals possible S_3 and systolic murmur at lower left sternal border that increases with inspiration	▪ *Right-sided cardiac catheterization:* high atrial pressure, tricuspid insufficiency, decreased or normal cardiac output ▪ *X-ray:* right atrial dilation, right ventricular enlargement ▪ *Echocardiography:* systolic prolapse of tricuspid valve, right atrial enlargement ▪ *ECG:* right atrial or right ventricular hypertrophy, atrial fibrillation
Tricuspid stenosis ▪ Results from rheumatic fever ▪ May be congenital ▪ Associated with mitral or aortic valve disease ▪ Most common in women	▪ May be symptomatic with dyspnea, fatigue, syncope ▪ Possible peripheral edema, JVD, hepatomegaly, and ascites (right-sided heart failure) ▪ *Auscultation:* reveals diastolic murmur at lower left sternal border that increases with inspiration	▪ *Cardiac catheterization:* increased pressure gradient across valve, increased right atrial pressure, decreased cardiac output ▪ *X-ray:* right atrial enlargement ▪ *Echocardiography:* leaflet abnormality, right atrial enlargement ▪ *ECG:* right atrial hypertrophy, right or left ventricular hypertrophy, atrial fibrillation

some patients, the condition may be idiopathic.

Because of the weakened valve, blood flows back into the left ventricle during diastole when pressure in the aorta is greater than the pressure in the left ventricle. This causes fluid overload in the ventricle, which then dilates and hypertrophies. The excess volume leads to fluid overload in the left atrium and, finally, the pulmonary system. Left-sided heart failure and pulmonary edema eventually result.

Aortic insufficiency by itself occurs most commonly among males. When it occurs with mitral valve disease, however, it's more common among females.

SIGNS AND SYMPTOMS

A patient with aortic insufficiency may have dyspnea, cough, fatigue, palpitations, angina, and syncope. Dyspnea may occur with exertion, or it may be paroxysmal nocturnal dyspnea with diaphoresis, orthopnea, and cough.

Inspection commonly reveals pulmonary venous congestion, pulmonary edema from left-sided heart failure, and pulsating nail beds (Quincke's sign). Quincke's sign is evident by alternating flushing and paling of the nail root when pressure is applied at the nail tip. Other signs include rapidly rising and collapsing pulses (pulsus biferiens), cardiac arrhythmias, and widened pulse pressure. In chronic disease, palpation and visualization of the apical impulse is possible.

Auscultation may reveal an S_3, occasionally an S_4, and a loud systolic ejection sound.

A high-pitched, blowing, decrescendo diastolic murmur may be heard at the left sternal border, third intercostal space. Use the diaphragm of your stethoscope with the patient sitting up, leaning forward, and holding his breath in forced expiration. (See *Identifying the murmur of aortic insufficiency.*) A grade 5 or 6 midsystolic ejection murmur may be heard at the base of the heart; it typically is higher pitched, shorter, and less rasping than the murmur of aortic stenosis. Another murmur that may occur is a soft, low-pitched, rumbling, mid-diastolic or presystolic bruit (Austin Flint murmur); it's best heard at the base of the heart.

COMPLICATIONS

- Left-sided heart failure
- Fatal pulmonary edema
- Myocardial ischemia

IDENTIFYING THE MURMUR OF AORTIC INSUFFICIENCY

In aortic insufficiency, you'll hear a high-pitched, blowing decrescendo murmur that radiates from the aortic valve area to the left sternal border.

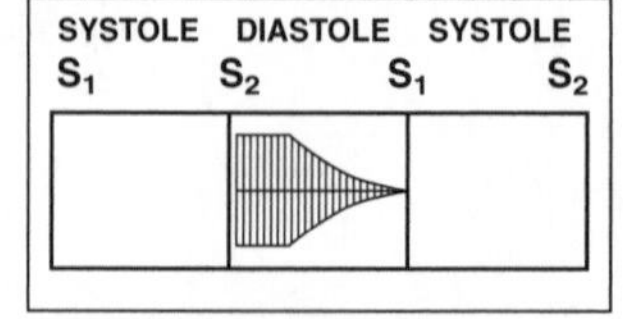

DIAGNOSIS

- Cardiac catheterization shows reduced arterial diastolic pressures, aortic insufficiency, other valvular abnormalities, and increased left ventricular end-diastolic pressure.
- Chest X-rays show left ventricular enlargement and pulmonary vein congestion.
- Echocardiography reveals left ventricular enlargement, dilation of the aortic annulus and left atrium, and thickening of the aortic valve. It also reveals a rapid, high-frequency fluttering of the anterior mitral leaflet caused by the impact of aortic insufficiency.
- Electrocardiography shows sinus tachycardia, left ventricular hypertrophy, and left atrial hypertrophy in patients with severe disease. ST-segment depressions and T-wave inversions appear in leads I, aVL, V_5, and V_6 and indicate left ventricular strain.

TREATMENT

Valve replacement is the treatment of choice and should be performed before significant ventricular dysfunction occurs. This may be impossible, however, because signs and symptoms seldom occur until after myocardial dysfunction develops. A low-sodium diet is recommended and, for acute episodes, supplemental oxygen may be needed. Patients with symptomatic aortic regurgitation may need aortic valve replacement as definitive treatment.

Drugs

- Angiotensin-converting enzyme inhibitors, diuretics, and vasodilators to treat left-sided heart failure

SPECIAL CONSIDERATIONS

- If the patient needs bed rest, stress its importance. Help with bathing if needed. Provide a bedside commode; it will put less stress on the patient's heart than using a bedpan. Offer the patient diversionary, physically undemanding activities.
- Alternate periods of activity with periods of rest to prevent extreme fatigue and dyspnea.
- To reduce anxiety, let the patient express his concerns about the effects of activity restrictions on his responsibilities and routines. Reassure him that the restrictions are temporary.
- Keep the patient's legs elevated while he sits in a chair to improve venous return to the heart.
- Place the patient in an upright position to relieve dyspnea, if needed, and give oxygen to prevent tissue hypoxia.
- Keep the patient on a low-sodium diet. Consult a dietitian to make sure the patient receives foods that he enjoys and that keep the diet restrictions.
- Watch for evidence of heart failure, pulmonary edema, and adverse reactions to drug therapy.

Aortic stenosis

Aortic stenosis is a narrowing or obstruction of the aortic valve. Because the valve doesn't open properly, blood flow from the left ventricle to the aorta is blocked. The obstruction may occur at the level of the valve or above or below the valve.

CAUSES AND INCIDENCE

Aortic stenosis may result from a congenital bicuspid aortic valve, congenital stenosis of valve cusps, rheumatic fever or, in elderly patients, atherosclerosis and calcification.

When the aortic valve narrows, the left ventricle exerts increased pressure to drive blood through the opening. Resistance to the ejection of blood increases pressure in the left ventricle, forcing more blood through the steno tic valve during systole. The added workload increases oxygen demand. Diminished cardiac output reduces coronary artery perfusion, causes ischemia of the left ventricle, and leads to heart failure.

Signs and symptoms of aortic stenosis may not appear until the patient reaches age 50 to 70, even though the lesion has been present since childhood. Incidence increases with age, and aortic stenosis is the most significant valvular lesion in elderly people. About 80% of patients with aortic stenosis are male.

SIGNS AND SYMPTOMS

Even with severe aortic stenosis (narrowing to about one-third of the normal opening), the patient may have no symptoms. If they occur, they may include exertional dyspnea, fatigue, exertional syncope, angina, and palpitations. Left-sided heart failure can cause orthopnea and paroxysmal nocturnal dyspnea. Signs of aortic stenosis may include pulmonary venous congestion, heart failure, pulmonary edema, diminished carotid pulses, decreased cardiac output, cardiac arrhythmias, and pulsus alternans.

Auscultation may reveal an early systolic ejection murmur in children and adolescents who have noncalcified valves. The murmur begins shortly after S_1 and increases in intensity, peaking toward the middle of the ejection period. It diminishes just before the aortic valve closes. (See *Identifying the murmur of aortic stenosis*.) The murmur is low-pitched, rough, and rasping and is loudest at the base at the second intercostal space. In patients with stenosis, the murmur is at least grade 3 or 4. It disappears when the valve calcifies. A split S_2 develops as aortic stenosis becomes more severe. An S_4 reflects left ventricular hypertrophy and may be heard at the apex in patients with severe aortic stenosis.

COMPLICATIONS

- Angina
- Syncope
- Left-sided heart failure
- Sudden cardiac death

IDENTIFYING THE MURMUR OF AORTIC STENOSIS

In aortic stenosis, you'll hear a low-pitched, harsh crescendo-decrescendo murmur that radiates from the aortic valve area to the carotid artery.

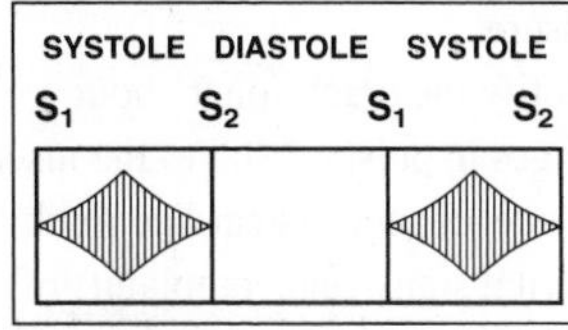

DIAGNOSIS

- Echocardiography is the recommended test to evaluate the severity of aortic stenosis. It will show a thickened aortic valve and left ventricular wall and, possibly, mitral valve stenosis.
- Cardiac catheterization reveals the pressure gradient across the valve (indicating the severity of the obstruction), increased left ventricular end-diastolic pressures (indicating left ventricular function), and the location of the left ventricular outflow obstruction. Catheterization is indicated when there's a discrepancy between echocardiography results and the patient's clinical presentation.
- Chest X-rays show valvular calcification, left ventricular enlargement, pulmonary vein congestion and, in later stages, left atrial, pulmonary artery, right atrial, and right ventricular enlargement.
- Electrocardiography reveals left ventricular hypertrophy. In advanced stages, the patient has ST-segment depression and T-wave inversion in standard leads I and aVL and in the left precordial leads. Up to 10% of patients have atrioventricular and intraventricular conduction defects.

TREATMENT

For the patient with no symptoms, no specific treatment is needed for aortic stenosis. Aortic valve replacement (AVR) is recommended for a symptomatic patient with severe aortic stenosis. If a patient has aortic stenosis and also needs coronary artery bypass surgery, the valve replacement and bypass should be done together.

Patients may be surgical candidates if their aortic stenosis progresses rapidly or causes an abnormal response to exercise. Percutaneous balloon valvotomy, in which a balloon is passed across the stenotic valve and inflated to enlarge the opening, may be used in children or young adults. This procedure could delay the need for AVR. In older adults, valvotomy could be considered for palliation. Valvotomy also may be used in an unstable high-risk patient until the patient is stable enough for definitive surgery.

Drugs

- Antihypertensives to manage hypertension

- Drugs to treat elevated lipids in patients with atherosclerosis
- Diuretics and digoxin (Lanoxin) to treat heart failure

SPECIAL CONSIDERATIONS

- If the patient needs bed rest, stress its importance. Help with bathing, if needed. Provide a bedside commode; it will put less stress on the patient's heart than using a bedpan. Offer the patient diversionary, physically undemanding activities.
- Alternate periods of activity with periods of rest to prevent extreme fatigue and dyspnea.
- To reduce anxiety, let the patient express his concerns about the effects of activity restrictions on his responsibilities and routines. Reassure him that the restrictions are temporary.
- Keep the patient's legs elevated while he sits in a chair to improve venous return to the heart.
- Place the patient in an upright position to relieve dyspnea, if needed, and give oxygen to prevent tissue hypoxia.
- Keep the patient on a low-sodium diet. Consult a dietitian to make sure the patient receives foods that he enjoys and that keep the diet restrictions.
- Watch for evidence of heart failure, pulmonary edema, and adverse reactions to drug therapy.
- Let the patient express his fears and concerns about the disorder, its impact on his life, and any upcoming surgery. Reassure him as needed.
- After cardiac catheterization, apply firm pressure to the catheter insertion site, usually in the groin. Check the site every 15 minutes for at least 6 hours for signs of bleeding. If the site bleeds, remove the pressure dressing and apply firm pressure.
- Notify the practitioner about changes in pulses distal to the insertion site, changes in cardiac rhythm and vital signs, and complaints of chest pain.
- If the patient has surgery, watch for hypotension, arrhythmias, and thrombus formation. Monitor his vital signs, arterial blood gas levels, intake and output, daily weight measurements, blood chemistry results, chest X-rays, and pulmonary artery catheter readings.

Atrial septal defect

A congenital defect that increases pulmonary blood flow, an atrial septal defect (ASD) is an opening between the left and right atria that shunts blood between the chambers. (See *Types of atrial septal defects*.)

CAUSES AND INCIDENCE

The cause of ASD is unknown. Blood shunts from left to right because left atrial pressure is slightly higher than right atrial pressure, a difference that forces large amounts of blood through the defect. The left-to-right shunt results

TYPES OF ATRIAL SEPTAL DEFECTS

Of the three types of atrial septal defect, ostium secundum is the most common. It occurs in the region of the fossa ovalis and occasionally extends inferiorly, close to the vena cava.

The sinus venosus defect occurs in the superior-posterior portion of the atrial septum, sometimes extends into the vena cava, and is almost always associated with abnormal drainage of pulmonary veins into the right atrium.

The ostium primum defect occurs in the inferior portion of the septum primum and usually is associated with atrioventricular valve abnormalities (cleft mitral valve) and conduction defects.

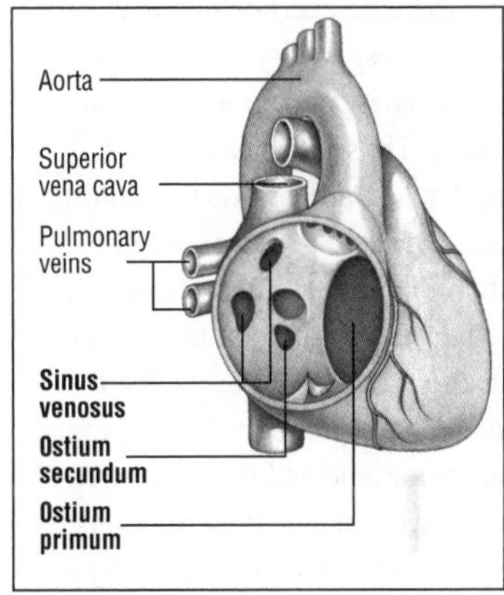

in right-heart volume overload, which affects the right atrium, right ventricle, and pulmonary arteries. Eventually, the right atrium enlarges and the right ventricle dilates to accommodate the increased blood volume.

If pulmonary artery hypertension develops because of the shunt (rare in children), increased pulmonary vascular resistance and right ventricular hypertrophy will follow. In some adults, irreversible (fixed) pulmonary artery hypertension causes reversal of the shunt direction, which results in unoxygenated blood entering the systemic circulation, causing cyanosis.

ASD occurs in 4 of every 100,000 people. Symptoms usually develop before age 30. When no other congenital defect exists, the patient—especially a child—may be asymptomatic.

ASD accounts for about 10% of congenital heart defects and appears almost twice as often in females as in males, with a strong familial tendency. Although ASD usually is a benign defect during infancy and childhood, delayed development of symptoms and complications makes it one of the most common congenital heart defects diagnosed in adults. The prognosis is excellent in asymptomatic patients but poor in those with cyanosis caused by large, untreated defects.

SIGNS AND SYMPTOMS

ASD commonly goes undetected in preschoolers. Such children may complain about feeling tired only after extreme exertion and may have frequent respiratory tract infections but otherwise appear normal and healthy. Those with large shunts may have retarded growth. Children with ASD seldom develop heart failure, pulmonary hypertension, infective endocarditis, or other complications. However, as adults, they usually have pronounced symptoms, such as fatigue and dyspnea on exertion. Commonly, the symptoms severely limit activity, especially in patients older than age 40.

In children, auscultation reveals an early systolic to midsystolic murmur, superficial in quality, at the second or third left intercostal space. In patients with large shunts resulting from increased tricuspid valve flow, a low-pitched diastolic murmur occurs at the lower left sternal border and is more pronounced on inspiration. Although the murmur's intensity is a rough indicator of the size of the left-to-right shunt, its low pitch sometimes makes it difficult to hear and, if the pressure gradient is relatively low, a murmur may not be detectable. Other signs include a fixed, widely split S_2 (caused by delayed closure of the pulmonic valve) and a systolic click or late systolic murmur at the apex (caused by mitral valve prolapse, which occasionally affects older children with ASD).

In older patients with large, uncorrected defects and fixed pulmonary artery hypertension, auscultation reveals an accentuated S_2. A pulmonary ejection click and an audible S_4 may also be present. Clubbing and cyanosis become evident; syncope and hemoptysis may occur with severe pulmonary vascular disease.

COMPLICATIONS

- Physical underdevelopment
- Unoxygenated blood in systemic circulation
- Right and left ventricular hypertrophy
- Atrial arrhythmias
- Heart failure
- Emboli
- Respiratory tract infections
- Mitral valve prolapse

DIAGNOSIS

A history of increasing fatigue and characteristic physical features suggest ASD. The following findings confirm it.

- Chest X-ray shows an enlarged right atrium and right ventricle, a prominent pulmonary artery, and increased pulmonary vascular markings.
- Electrocardiography may be normal but usually shows right axis deviation, prolonged PR interval, varying degrees of right bundle-branch block, right ventricular hypertrophy, atrial fibrillation (particularly in severe cases after age 30) and, in ostium primum defect, left axis deviation.

• Echocardiography measures right ventricular enlargement, may locate the defect, and shows volume overload in the right side of the heart. (Other causes of right ventricular enlargement must be ruled out.)
• Two-dimensional echocardiography with color Doppler flow, contrast echocardiography, or both have supplanted cardiac catheterization as the confirming tests for ASD.
• Cardiac catheterization is used if inconsistencies exist in the clinical data or if significant pulmonary hypertension is suspected.

TREATMENT

Surgical repair is advised for all patients with uncomplicated ASD and significant left-to-right shunting. Ideally, this is performed when the patient is between ages 2 and 4. Surgery shouldn't be performed on patients with small defects and minor left-to-right shunts. Because ASD seldom causes complications in infants and toddlers, surgery can be delayed until they reach preschool or early school age. A large defect may need immediate surgical closure with sutures or a patch graft.

Some patients may benefit from a procedure known as catheter closure or transcatheter closure of the ASD. In this procedure, the surgeon introduces wires or catheters through a small incision in the groin, advances them into the heart, and places a closure device across the ASD.

Drugs

• Prophylactic antibiotics before dental procedures to reduce the risk of infective endocarditis (immediately after surgery for an ASD)

SPECIAL CONSIDERATIONS

• Before cardiac catheterization, explain pretest and posttest procedures to the child and her caregivers. If possible, use drawings or other visual aids to explain it to the child.
• As needed, teach the patient about prophylactic antibiotics to prevent infective endocarditis. They may be needed before dental or other invasive procedures.
• If surgery is scheduled, teach the child and her parents about the intensive care unit, and introduce them to the staff. Show caregivers where they can wait during surgery. Explain postoperative procedures, tubes, dressings, and monitoring equipment.
• After surgery, closely monitor the patient's vital signs, central venous and intra-arterial pressures, and intake and output. Watch for atrial arrhythmias, which may remain uncorrected.

B

Buerger's disease

Also called *thromboangiitis obliterans,* Buerger's disease is an inflammatory, nonatheromatous occlusive condition that causes segmental lesions and thrombus formation in small and medium-sized arteries and sometimes veins. As a result, blood flow decreases in affected vessels. This disorder may produce ulceration and, eventually, gangrene.

CAUSES AND INCIDENCE

Buerger's disease is caused by vasculitis, an inflammation of blood vessels. Polymorphonuclear leukocytes infiltrate the vessel walls, and thrombi develop in the vascular lumen. As the disease progresses, mononuclear cells, fibroblasts, and giant cells replace the neutrophils. In later stages, perivascular fibrosis and recanalization occur.

This disorder affects the legs more commonly than the arms. Cerebral, visceral, and coronary vessels also may be affected.

Buerger's disease occurs in 6 of every 10,000 people and is most common among men ages 20 to 40 with a history of smoking or chewing tobacco. Affected people also may have a history of Raynaud's disease or autoimmune disease.

SIGNS AND SYMPTOMS

Buerger's disease typically produces intermittent claudication of the instep that's worsened by exercise and relieved by rest. In low temperature, the feet initially become cold, cyanotic, and numb; later, they redden, become hot, and tingle. Occasionally, Buerger's disease affects the hands and may cause painful fingertip ulcerations, severe digital ischemia, trophic nail changes, and gangrene. Other signs and symptoms may include impaired peripheral pulses, migratory superficial thrombophlebitis and, in later stages, ulceration, muscle atrophy, and gangrene.

COMPLICATIONS

- Gangrene
- Muscle atrophy
- Ulceration
- Painful fingertip ulcerations if the hands are affected

DIAGNOSIS

Patient history and physical examination strongly suggest Buerger's disease. Supportive diagnostic tests include:

- Doppler ultrasonography to detect diminished circulation in peripheral vessels
- Plethysmography to help detect decreased circulation in peripheral vessels

• Angiography or arteriography to locate lesions and rule out atherosclerosis.

TREATMENT

The main goals of treatment are to relieve symptoms and prevent complications. It may include an exercise program that uses gravity to fill and drain the blood vessels or, in severe disease, a lumbar sympathectomy to increase blood supply to the skin. Amputation may be needed for ulcers that don't heal, intractable pain, or gangrene.

Drugs

• Aspirin and vasodilators to improve blood flow

SPECIAL CONSIDERATIONS

• If the patient smokes or uses another form of tobacco, urge him to stop. Explain that treatment will be more effective and his symptoms may disappear if he stops using tobacco. If needed, refer him to a self-help group to stop smoking.
• Warn the patient to avoid precipitating factors, such as emotional stress, exposure to extreme temperatures, and trauma.
• Teach the patient proper foot care, especially the need for wearing well-fitting shoes and cotton or wool socks. Show him how to inspect his feet daily for cuts, abrasions, and evidence of skin breakdown, such as redness and soreness. Remind him to seek medical attention at once after any injury.
• If the patient has ulcers and gangrene, enforce bed rest and use a padded footboard or bed cradle to avoid pressure from bed linens. Protect the patient's feet with soft padding. Wash them gently with mild soap and tepid water, rinse thoroughly, and pat dry with a soft towel.
• Provide emotional support and, if needed, refer the patient for psychological counseling to help him cope with the effects of his chronic disease. If he has had an amputation, assess his rehabilitation needs, especially regarding changes in body image. Refer him for physical therapy, occupational therapy, and social services, as needed.

C

Cardiac arrhythmias

In cardiac arrhythmias (sometimes called *cardiac dysrhythmias*), abnormal electrical conduction or automaticity alters the normal heart rate and rhythm. (See *Comparing normal and abnormal conduction*.) Arrhythmias vary in severity. Some are mild, asymptomatic, and need no treatment, such as sinus arrhythmia, in which the heart rate increases and decreases with respiration. Others are catastrophic, such as ventricular fibrillation, which requires immediate resuscitation.

Usually, arrhythmias are classified as ventricular or supraventricular based on their origin. Their effect on cardiac output and blood pressure, partly influenced by site of origin, determines their clinical significance.

CAUSES AND INCIDENCE

Arrhythmias have many causes. (See *Types of cardiac arrhythmias,* page 25.) For instance, they may result from enhanced automaticity, reentry, escape beats, or abnormal electrical conduction. They may be congenital. They may be caused by myocardial ischemia, myocardial infarction (MI), or organic heart disease. Sometimes an arrhythmia results from drug ingestion (cocaine, amphetamines, caffeine, beta-adrenergic blockers, psychotropics, sympathomimetics), drug toxicity, or degeneration of the conductive tissue needed to maintain a normal heart rhythm (sick sinus syndrome). Other causes include:

- acid-base imbalances
- cellular hypoxia
- congenital defects
- connective tissue disorders
- emotional stress
- hypertrophy of the heart muscle.

People with imbalances of blood chemistries and those with a history of cardiac conditions (coronary artery disease or heart valve disorders) are at increased risk for arrhythmias.

SIGNS AND SYMPTOMS

Depending on the arrhythmia, the patient may have any number of signs and symptoms, including:

- palpitations
- light-headedness
- altered level of consciousness (LOC)
- dizziness
- chest pain
- shortness of breath
- changes in pulse patterns
- paleness
- cold and clammy extremities
- reduced urine output.

COMPARING NORMAL AND ABNORMAL CONDUCTION

Normal cardiac conduction originates in the sinoatrial (SA) node, the heart's pacemaker, as shown below. When the impulse leaves the SA node, it travels through the atria along Bachmann's bundle and the internodal pathways to the atrioventricular (AV) node. It then moves down the bundle of His, along the bundle branches and, finally, down the Purkinje fibers to the ventricles.

Abnormal cardiac conduction

The normal conduction cycle may be disrupted by altered automaticity, reentry, or conduction disturbances, leading to cardiac arrhythmias.

Altered automaticity

The result of partial depolarization, altered automaticity may increase the intrinsic rate of the SA node or latent pacemakers, or it may induce ectopic pacemakers to reach threshold and depolarize.

Automaticity may be altered by drugs, such as epinephrine, atropine, and digoxin (Lanoxin), and by such conditions as acidosis, alkalosis, hypoxia, myocardial infarction (MI), hypokalemia, and hypocalcemia. Examples of arrhythmias caused by altered automaticity include atrial fibrillation and flutter; supraventricular tachycardia; premature atrial, junctional, and ventricular complexes; ventricular tachycardia and fibrillation; and accelerated idioventricular and junctional rhythms.

Reentry

In reentry, ischemia or a deformity creates an abnormal circuit in the conductive fibers. The flow of current is blocked in one direction in the circuit, but the descending impulse can travel in the other direction. By the time the impulse completes the circuit, the previously depolarized tissue in the circuit is no longer refractory to stimulation, allowing reentry of the impulse and repetition of this cycle.

A different reentry mechanism may occur when a congenital accessory pathway links the atria and

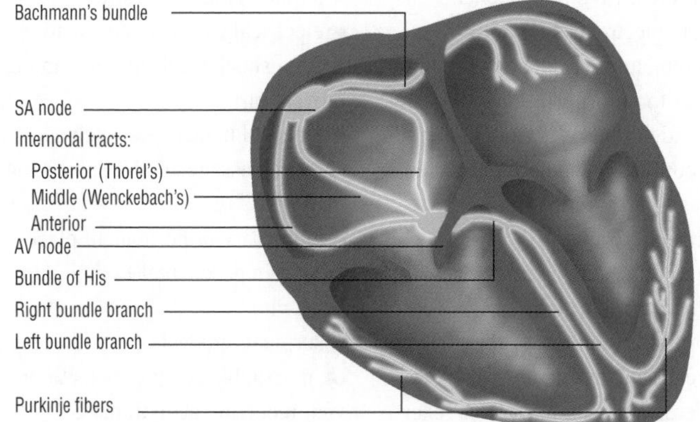

(continued)

COMPARING NORMAL AND ABNORMAL CONDUCTION *(continued)*

ventricles outside the AV junction, as in Wolff-Parkinson-White syndrome.

Conditions that increase the likelihood of reentry include hyperkalemia, myocardial ischemia, and the use of certain antiarrhythmics. Reentry may cause such arrhythmias as paroxysmal supraventricular tachycardia; premature atrial, junctional, and ventricular complexes; and ventricular tachycardia.

Conduction disturbances

Conduction disturbances occur when impulses are conducted too quickly or too slowly. Possible causes include trauma, drug toxicity, myocardial ischemia, MI, and electrolyte abnormalities. The AV blocks occur as a result of conduction disturbances.

If cerebral circulation is severely impaired, the patient may have syncope.

COMPLICATIONS

- Impaired cardiac output
- Sudden cardiac death
- MI
- Heart failure
- Thromboembolism

DIAGNOSIS

- Diagnosis is made by tests that reveal the arrhythmia, such as 12-lead electrocardiography.
- Ambulatory cardiac monitoring (Holter monitoring), echocardiography, and coronary angiography also may confirm or rule out suspected causes of arrhythmias and help determine treatment.
- Laboratory testing may reveal electrolyte abnormalities, acid-base abnormalities, or drug toxicities that may cause arrhythmias.
- Exercise testing may detect exercise-induced arrhythmias.
- Electrophysiologic testing identifies the mechanism of an arrhythmia and the location of accessory pathways. It also allows assessment of the effects of antiarrhythmics, radiofrequency ablation, and implanted cardioverter-defibrillators.

TREATMENT

Effective treatment aims to return pacer function to the sinus node, return the ventricular rate to normal, regain atrioventricular synchrony, and maintain normal sinus rhythm. Treatment may include:

- antiarrhythmic therapy
- electrical cardioversion with precordial shock (defibrillation and cardioversion)
- physical maneuvers, such as carotid massage and Valsalva's maneuver
- temporary or permanent placement of a pacemaker to maintain heart rate
- surgical removal or cryotherapy of an irritable ectopic focus to prevent recurring arrhythmias.

(*Text continues on page 36.*)

TYPES OF CARDIAC ARRHYTHMIAS

This table outlines the features, causes, and treatment of many common cardiac arrhythmias. If possible, compare a normal electrocardiogram strip with the rhythm strips included here. As a reminder, characteristics of a normal rhythm include:

- ventricular and atrial rates of 60 to 100 beats/minute
- regular and uniform QRS complexes and P waves
- PR interval of 0.12 to 0.2 second
- QRS duration of less than 0.12 second
- identical atrial and ventricular rates, with a constant PR interval.

Arrhythmia and features	Causes	Treatment
Sinus arrhythmia 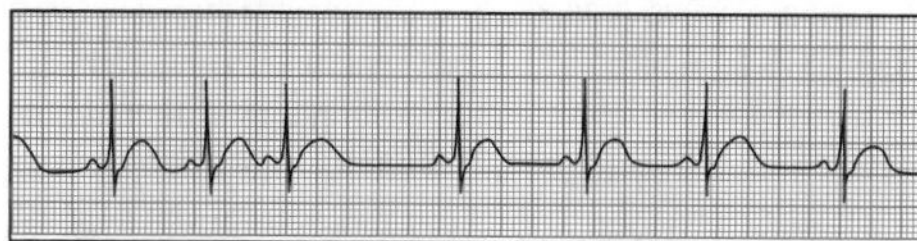		
■ Irregular atrial and ventricular rhythms ■ Normal P wave preceding each QRS complex	■ In athletes, children, and the elderly, a normal variation of normal sinus rhythm ■ Also seen in digoxin (Lanoxin) toxicity and inferior myocardial infarction (MI)	■ Atropine if rate decreases below 40 beats/minute and if patient is symptomatic (hypotension, for example)
Sinus tachycardia 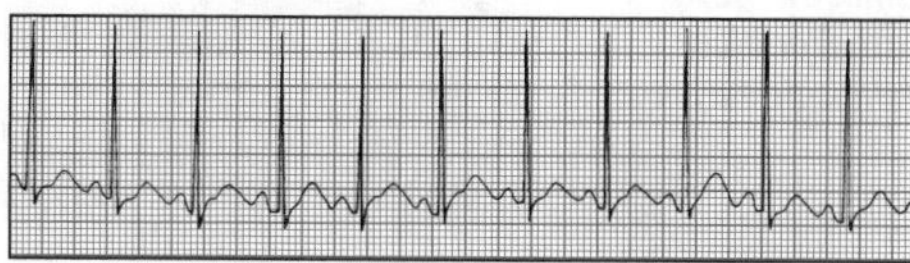		
■ Atrial and ventricular rhythms regular ■ Rate greater than 100 beats/minute; rarely, greater than 160 beats/minute ■ Normal P wave preceding each QRS complex	■ Normal physiologic response to fever, exercise, anxiety, pain, dehydration; also may accompany shock, left-sided heart failure, cardiac tamponade, hyperthyroidism, anemia, hypovolemia, pulmonary embolism, anterior MI ■ Also may occur with atropine, epinephrine, isoproterenol (Isuprel), quinidine, caffeine, alcohol, and nicotine use	■ Correction of underlying cause ■ Beta-adrenergic blockers or calcium channel blockers for symptomatic patients

(continued)

TYPES OF CARDIAC ARRHYTHMIAS *(continued)*

Arrhythmia and features	Causes	Treatment
Sinus bradycardia 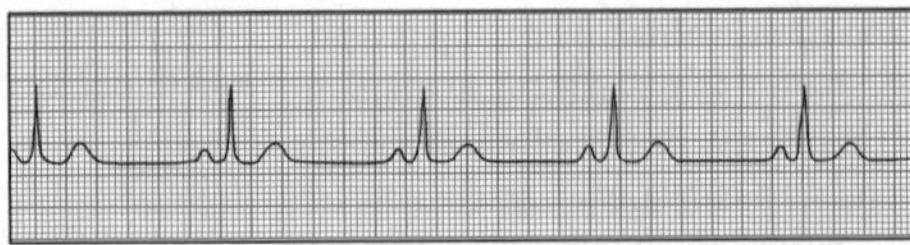		
▪ Regular atrial and ventricular rhythms ▪ Rate less than 60 beats/minute ▪ Normal P wave preceding each QRS complex	▪ Normal in a well-conditioned heart, as in an athlete ▪ Increased intracranial pressure; increased vagal tone from straining during defecation, vomiting, intubation, mechanical ventilation; sick sinus syndrome; hypothyroidism; inferior MI ▪ Also may occur with anticholinesterase, beta-adrenergic blocker, digoxin, and morphine use	▪ For low cardiac output, dizziness, weakness, altered level of consciousness, or low blood pressure, follow advanced cardiac life support (ACLS) protocol for giving atropine ▪ Temporary pacemaker; may need evaluation for permanent pacemaker in the future
Sinoatrial (SA) arrest or block (sinus arrest) 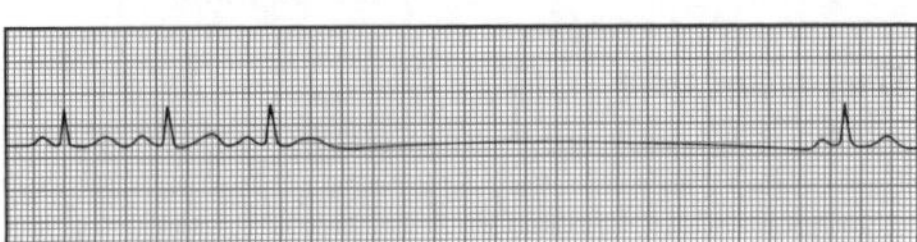		
▪ Atrial and ventricular rhythms normal except for missing complex ▪ Normal P wave preceding each QRS complex ▪ Pause not equal to a multiple of the previous sinus rhythm	▪ Acute infection ▪ Coronary artery disease (CAD), degenerative heart disease, acute inferior MI ▪ Vagal stimulation, Valsalva's maneuver, carotid sinus massage ▪ Digoxin, quinidine, or salicylate toxicity ▪ Pesticide poisoning ▪ Pharyngeal irritation from endotracheal (ET) intubation ▪ Sick sinus syndrome	▪ Treat symptoms with atropine I.V. ▪ Temporary pacemaker, with possible permanent pacemaker for repeated episodes

TYPES OF CARDIAC ARRHYTHMIAS *(continued)*

Arrhythmia and features	Causes	Treatment
Wandering atrial pacemaker 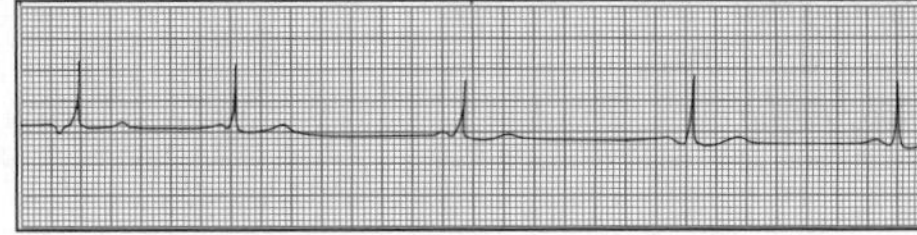		
▪ Atrial and ventricular rhythms vary slightly ▪ Irregular PR interval ▪ P waves irregular with changing configuration, indicating that they aren't all from SA node or single atrial focus; may appear after the QRS complex ▪ QRS complexes of uniform shape but irregular rhythm	▪ Rheumatic carditis from inflammation in SA node ▪ Digoxin toxicity ▪ Sick sinus syndrome	▪ No treatment if patient is asymptomatic ▪ Treatment of underlying cause if patient is symptomatic
Premature atrial contraction (PAC) 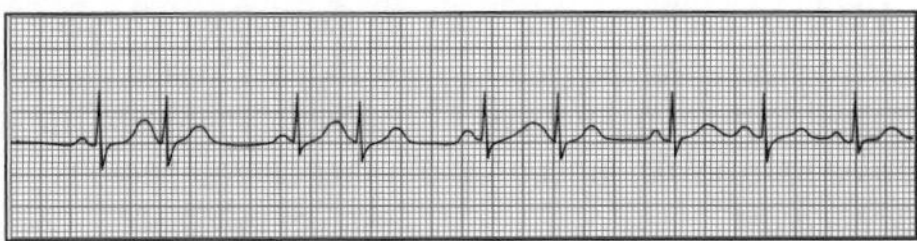		
▪ Premature, abnormal-looking P waves that differ in configuration from normal P waves ▪ QRS complexes after P waves, except in very early or blocked PACs ▪ P wave commonly buried in or identifiable in the preceding T wave	▪ Coronary or valvular heart disease, atrial ischemia, coronary atherosclerosis, heart failure, acute respiratory failure, chronic obstructive pulmonary disease (COPD), electrolyte imbalance, and hypoxia ▪ Digoxin toxicity; use of aminophylline (Phyllocontin), adrenergics, or caffeine ▪ Anxiety	▪ Usually no treatment ▪ Treatment of underlying cause if patient is symptomatic

(continued)

TYPES OF CARDIAC ARRHYTHMIAS *(continued)*

Arrhythmia and features	Causes	Treatment
Paroxysmal supraventricular tachycardia 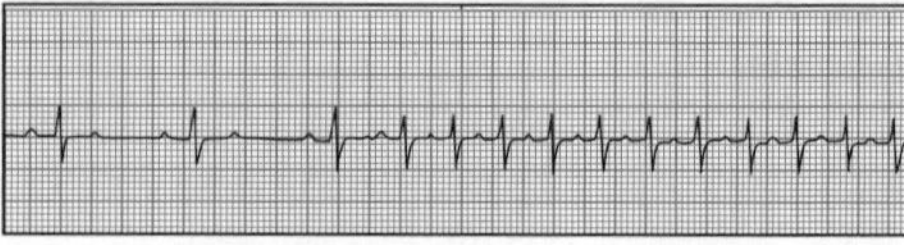		
▪ Atrial and ventricular rhythms regular ▪ Heart rate greater than 160 beats/minute; rarely exceeds 250 beats/minute ▪ P waves regular but aberrant; difficult to differentiate from preceding T wave ▪ P wave preceding each QRS complex ▪ Sudden onset and termination of arrhythmia ▪ With normal P wave, called *paroxysmal atrial tachycardia;* without normal P wave, *called paroxysmal junctional tachycardia*	▪ Intrinsic abnormality of atrioventricular (AV) conduction system ▪ Physical or psychological stress, hypoxia, hypokalemia, cardiomyopathy, congenital heart disease, MI, valvular disease, Wolff-Parkinson-White syndrome, cor pulmonale, hyperthyroidism, and systemic hypertension ▪ Digoxin toxicity; use of caffeine, marijuana, or other central nervous system stimulant	▪ Immediate cardioversion if patient is unstable ▪ Vagal stimulation, Valsalva's maneuver, carotid sinus massage if patient is stable ▪ Adenosine (Adenocard) by rapid I.V. bolus injection to rapidly convert arrhythmia ▪ Calcium channel blockers or beta-adrenergic blockers. ▪ If QRS is wide, the patient may require amiodarone (Cordarone) and synchronized cardioversion.

TYPES OF CARDIAC ARRHYTHMIAS *(continued)*

Arrhythmia and features	Causes	Treatment
Atrial flutter 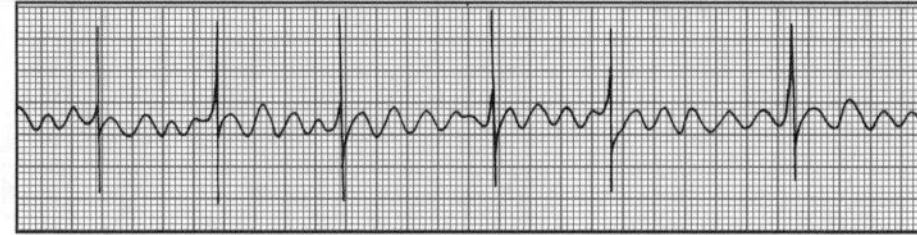		
▪ Atrial rhythm regular and 250 to 400 beats/minute ▪ Ventricular rate variable, depending on degree of AV block (usually 60 to 100 beats/minute) ▪ Sawtooth P wave configuration possible (F waves) ▪ QRS complexes of uniform shape but usually irregular rate	▪ Heart failure, tricuspid or mitral valve disease, pulmonary embolism, cor pulmonale, inferior MI, and carditis ▪ Digoxin toxicity	▪ Immediate cardioversion if patient is unstable with a ventricular rate greater than 150 beats/minute ▪ Calcium channel blockers, beta-adrenergic blockers, or antiarrhythmics if patient is stable ▪ Anticoagulation therapy may be needed
Atrial fibrillation 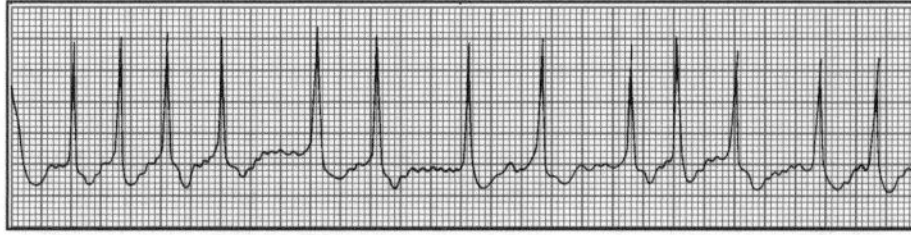		
▪ Atrial rhythm grossly irregular; rate greater than 400 beats/minute ▪ Ventricular rhythm grossly irregular ▪ QRS complexes of uniform configuration and duration ▪ PR interval indiscernible ▪ No P waves or P waves that appear as erratic, irregular, baseline fibrillatory waves	▪ Heart failure, COPD, thyrotoxicosis, constrictive pericarditis, ischemic heart disease, sepsis, pulmonary embolus, rheumatic heart disease, hypertension, mitral stenosis, atrial irritation, complication of coronary bypass or valve replacement surgery	▪ Immediate cardioversion if patient is unstable with a ventricular rate greater than 150 beats/minute ▪ Calcium channel blockers, beta-adrenergic blockers, digoxin, procainamide (Pronestyl), quinidine, ibutilide (Corvert), or amiodarone if patient is stable ▪ Anticoagulation to prevent emboli ▪ Possible dual-chamber atrial pacing, implantable atrial pacemaker, or surgical maze procedure

(continued)

TYPES OF CARDIAC ARRHYTHMIAS *(continued)*

Arrhythmia and features	Causes	Treatment
Junctional rhythm 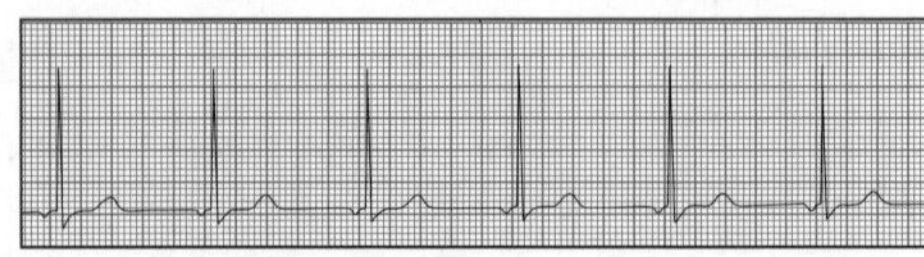		
■ Atrial and ventricular rhythms regular ■ Atrial rate 40 to 60 beats/minute ■ Ventricular rate usually 40 to 60 beats/minute (60 to 100 beats/minute in accelerated junctional rhythm) ■ P waves preceding, hidden in (absent), or after QRS complex; usually inverted if visible ■ PR interval (when present) less than 0.12 second ■ QRS complex configuration and duration normal, except in aberrant conduction	■ Inferior wall MI or ischemia, hypoxia, vagal stimulation, sick sinus syndrome ■ Acute rheumatic fever ■ Valve surgery ■ Digoxin toxicity	■ Correction of underlying cause ■ Atropine for symptomatic slow rate ■ Pacemaker insertion if patient is refractory to drugs ■ Discontinuation of digoxin if appropriate
Premature junctional contraction 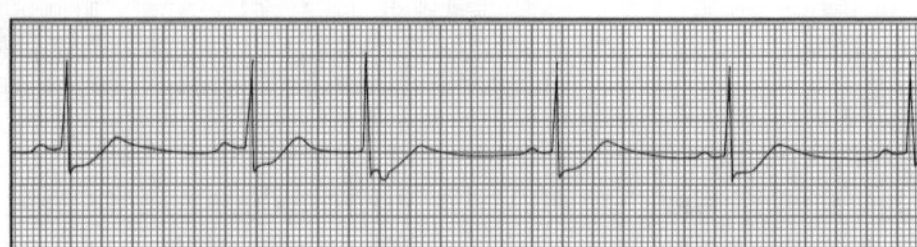		
■ Atrial and ventricular rhythms irregular ■ P waves inverted; may precede, be hidden within, or follow QRS complex ■ PR interval less than 0.12 second if P wave precedes QRS complex ■ QRS complex configuration and duration normal	■ MI or ischemia ■ Digoxin toxicity and excessive caffeine or amphetamine use	■ Correction of underlying cause ■ Discontinuation of digoxin if appropriate

TYPES OF CARDIAC ARRHYTHMIAS *(continued)*

Arrhythmia and features	Causes	Treatment
Junctional tachycardia 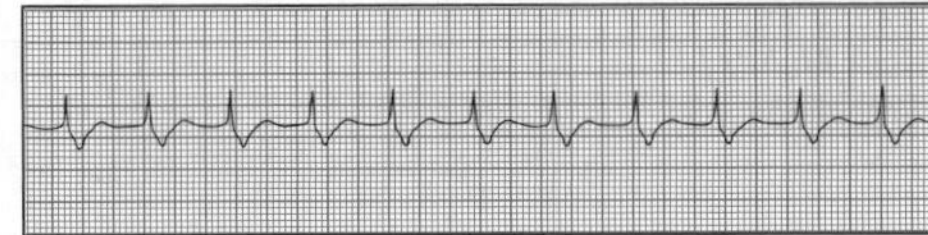		
■ Atrial rate greater than 100 beats/minute ■ P wave possibly absent, hidden in QRS complex, or preceding T wave ■ Ventricular rate greater than 100 beats/minute ■ P wave inverted ■ QRS complex configuration and duration normal ■ Onset of rhythm commonly sudden, occurring in bursts	■ Myocarditis, cardiomyopathy, inferior MI or ischemia, acute rheumatic fever, complication of valve replacement surgery ■ Digoxin toxicity	■ Cardioversion if ventricular rate is greater than 150 or if patient is symptomatic ■ Amiodarone, beta-adrenergic blockers, or calcium channel blockers if patient is stable ■ Discontinuation of digoxin if appropriate
First-degree AV block 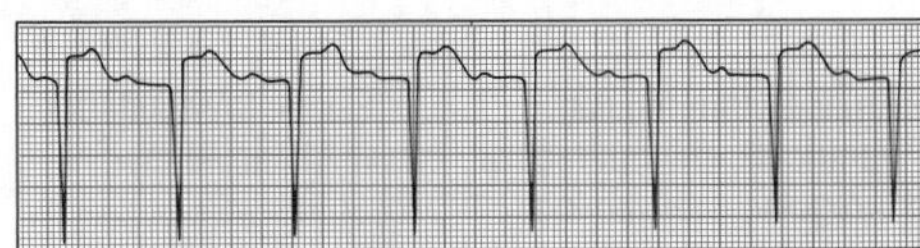		
■ Atrial and ventricular rhythms regular ■ PR interval greater than 0.2 second ■ P wave preceding each QRS complex ■ QRS complex normal	■ Inferior wall MI or ischemia, hypothyroidism, hypokalemia, hyperkalemia ■ Digoxin toxicity; use of quinidine, procainamide, beta-adrenergic blockers, calcium channel blockers, or amiodarone	■ Correction of underlying cause ■ Possibly atropine if PR interval exceeds 0.26 second and symptomatic bradycardia develops ■ Cautious use of digoxin, calcium channel blockers, and beta-adrenergic blockers

(continued)

TYPES OF CARDIAC ARRHYTHMIAS *(continued)*

Arrhythmia and features	Causes	Treatment
Second-degree AV block Mobitz I (Wenckebach's) 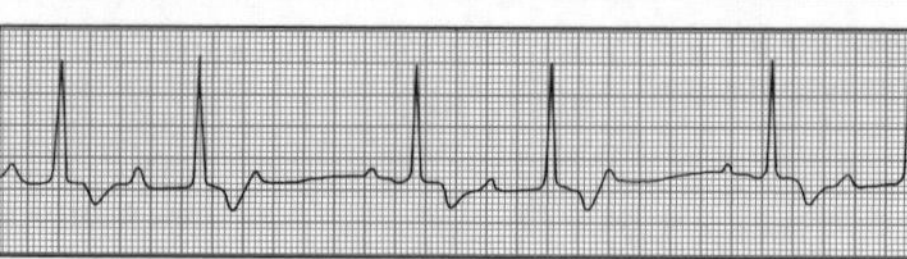		
▪ Atrial rhythm regular ▪ Ventricular rhythm irregular ▪ Atrial rate exceeds ventricular rate ▪ PR interval progressively, but only slightly, longer with each cycle until QRS complex disappears (dropped beat); PR interval shorter after dropped beat	▪ Inferior wall MI, cardiac surgery, acute rheumatic fever, vagal stimulation ▪ Digoxin toxicity; use of propranolol (Inderal), quinidine, or procainamide	▪ Treatment of underlying cause ▪ Atropine or temporary pacemaker for symptomatic bradycardia ▪ Discontinuation of digoxin if appropriate
Second-degree AV block Mobitz II 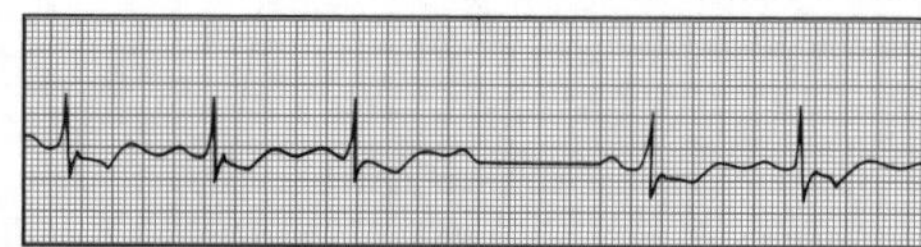		
▪ Atrial rhythm regular ▪ Ventricular rhythm regular or irregular, with varying degree of block ▪ P–P interval constant ▪ QRS complexes periodically absent	▪ Severe CAD, anterior wall MI, acute myocarditis ▪ Digoxin toxicity	▪ Atropine, epinephrine, and dopamine for symptomatic bradycardia ▪ Temporary or permanent pacemaker for symptomatic bradycardia ▪ Discontinuation of digoxin if appropriate

TYPES OF CARDIAC ARRHYTHMIAS *(continued)*

Arrhythmia and features	Causes	Treatment
Third-degree AV block (complete heart block) 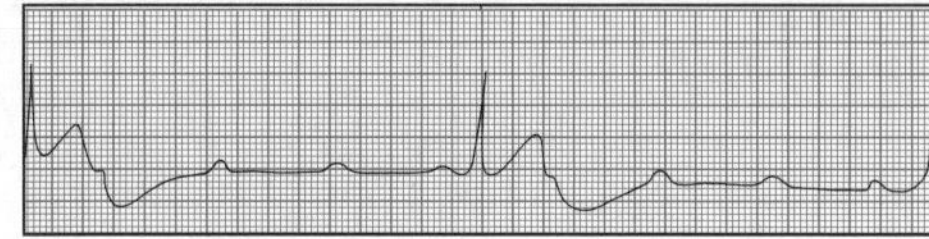		
▪ Atrial rhythm regular ▪ Ventricular rhythm regular and rate slower than atrial rate ▪ No relation between P waves and QRS complexes ▪ No constant PR interval ▪ QRS interval normal (nodal pacemaker) or wide and bizarre (ventricular pacemaker)	▪ Inferior or anterior wall MI, congenital abnormality, rheumatic fever, hypoxia, postoperative complication of mitral valve replacement, Lev's disease (fibrosis and calcification that spreads from cardiac structures to conductive tissue), Lenegre's disease (conductive tissue fibrosis) ▪ Digoxin toxicity	▪ Atropine, epinephrine, and dopamine for symptomatic bradycardia ▪ Temporary or permanent pacemaker for symptomatic bradycardia
Premature ventricular contraction (PVC) 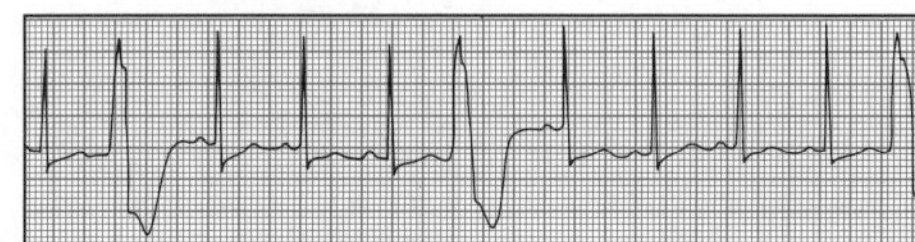		
▪ Atrial rhythm regular ▪ Ventricular rhythm irregular ▪ QRS complex premature, usually followed by a complete compensatory pause ▪ QRS complex wide and distorted, usually exceeding 0.14 second ▪ Premature QRS complexes occurring singly, in pairs, or in threes; alternating with normal beats; focus from one or more sites ▪ Ominous when clustered, multifocal, with R wave on T pattern	▪ Heart failure; old or acute myocardial ischemia, infarction, or contusion; myocardial irritation by ventricular catheter, such as a pacemaker; hypercapnia; hypokalemia; hypocalcemia ▪ Drug toxicity (cardiac glycosides, aminophylline, tricyclic antidepressants, beta-adrenergic blockers [or dopamine]) ▪ Caffeine, tobacco, or alcohol use ▪ Psychological stress, anxiety, pain, exercise	▪ If warranted, procainamide, lidocaine, or amiodarone I.V. ▪ Treatment of underlying cause ▪ Discontinuation of drug causing toxicity ▪ Potassium chloride I.V. if PVC induced by hypokalemia ▪ Magnesium sulfate I.V. if PVC induced by hypomagnesemia

(continued)

TYPES OF CARDIAC ARRHYTHMIAS *(continued)*

Arrhythmia and features	Causes	Treatment
Ventricular tachycardia (VT) 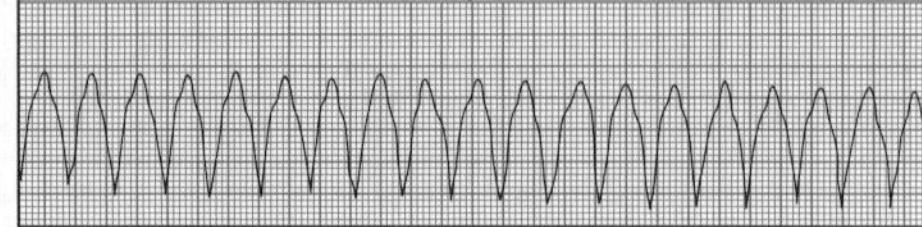		
▪ Ventricular rate 140 to 220 beats/minute, regular or irregular ▪ QRS complexes wide, bizarre, and independent of P waves ▪ P waves not discernible ▪ May start and stop suddenly	▪ Myocardial ischemia, infarction, or aneurysm; CAD; rheumatic heart disease; mitral valve prolapse; heart failure; cardiomyopathy; ventricular catheters; hypokalemia; hypercalcemia; pulmonary embolism ▪ Digoxin, procainamide, epinephrine, or quinidine toxicity ▪ Anxiety	▪ *Pulseless:* Cardiopulmonary resuscitation (CPR); ACLS protocol for defibrillation, ET intubation, and administration of epinephrine or vasopressin followed by amiodarone or lidocaine; if ineffective, possibly magnesium sulfate ▪ *With pulse:* If hemodynamically stable, ACLS protocol for administration of amiodarone; if ineffective, synchronized cardioversion

TYPES OF CARDIAC ARRHYTHMIAS *(continued)*

Arrhythmia and features	Causes	Treatment
Ventricular fibrillation 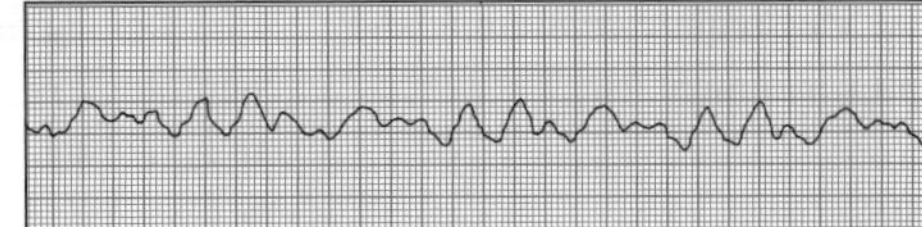		
▪ Ventricular rhythm and rate rapid and chaotic ▪ QRS complexes wide and irregular ▪ No visible P waves	▪ Myocardial ischemia or infarction, R-on-T phenomenon, untreated VT, hypokalemia, hyperkalemia, hypercalcemia, alkalosis, electric shock, hypothermia ▪ Digoxin, epinephrine, or quinidine toxicity	▪ *Pulseless:* CPR; ACLS protocol for defibrillation, ET intubation, and administration of epinephrine or vasopressin, lidocaine, or amiodarone; if ineffective, possibly magnesium sulfate
Asystole 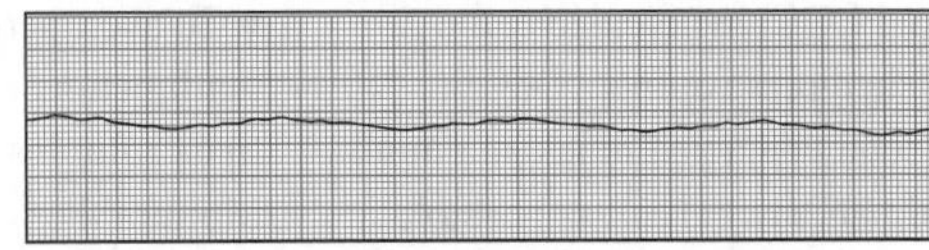		
▪ No atrial or ventricular rate or rhythm ▪ No discernible P waves, QRS complexes, or T waves	▪ Myocardial ischemia or infarction, aortic valve disease, heart failure, hypoxemia, hypokalemia, severe acidosis, electric shock, ventricular arrhythmias, AV block, pulmonary embolism, heart rupture, cardiac tamponade, hyperkalemia, electromechanical dissociation ▪ Cocaine overdose	▪ CPR; ACLS protocol for ET intubation, transcutaneous pacing, and administration of epinephrine or vasopressin; possible atropine

Arrhythmias also may respond to treatment of an underlying disorder such as correcting hypoxia. However, those associated with heart disease may require continuing and complex treatment.

Drugs

- Consult specific treatment guidelines for each arrhythmia.

SPECIAL CONSIDERATIONS

- Assess an unmonitored patient for rhythm disturbances.
- If the patient's pulse is abnormally rapid, slow, or irregular, watch for signs of hypoperfusion, such as altered LOC, hypotension, and diminished urine output.
- Document arrhythmias in a monitored patient, and assess possible causes and effects.
- When life-threatening arrhythmias develop, rapidly assess the patient's LOC, respirations, and pulse.
- Start cardiopulmonary resuscitation if indicated.
- Evaluate the patient for altered cardiac output resulting from arrhythmias.
- Give medications as ordered and prepare to assist with medical procedures, such as cardioversion, if indicated.
- Look for predisposing factors (such as fluid and electrolyte imbalance) and signs of drug toxicity, especially with digoxin (Lanoxin). If you suspect drug toxicity, report the signs immediately and withhold the next dose.
- To prevent arrhythmias in a postoperative cardiac patient, provide adequate oxygen and reduce the heart's workload while carefully maintaining the patient's metabolic, neurologic, respiratory, and hemodynamic status.
- Consider sedation for transcutaneous pacing if appropriate.
- To avoid temporary pacemaker malfunction, install a fresh battery before each insertion. Carefully secure the external catheter wires and the pacemaker box. Assess the threshold daily. Watch closely for premature contractions, a sign of myocardial irritation.
- To avert permanent pacemaker malfunction, restrict the patient's activity after insertion as appropriate. Monitor the pulse rate regularly, and watch for signs of decreased cardiac output.
- If the patient has a permanent pacemaker, warn about environmental hazards, as indicated by the pacemaker manufacturer. Although hazards may not present a problem, in doubtful situations, 24-hour Holter monitoring may be helpful. Tell the patient to report lightheadedness or syncope, and stress the need for regular checkups.
- Compare the patient's cardiac status (pulse, blood pressure, and cardiac output) with the cardiac rhythm before and after treatments.
- Maintain adequate oxygenation; normal fluid, acid-base, and electrolyte balance (especially potassium, magnesium, and calcium); and normal drug levels.

Cardiac tamponade

In cardiac tamponade, a rapid, unchecked rise in intrapericardial pressure compresses the heart, impairs diastolic filling, and reduces cardiac output. The rise in pressure usually results from blood or fluid accumulation in the pericardial sac. Even a small amount of fluid (50 to 100 ml) can cause a serious tamponade if it accumulates rapidly.

Prognosis depends on the rate of fluid accumulation. If it accumulates rapidly, this condition requires emergency lifesaving measures to prevent death. A slow accumulation and rise in pressure, as with growth of a malignant tumor, may not produce immediate symptoms because the fibrous wall of the pericardial sac can gradually stretch to accommodate as much as 1 to 2 qt (1 to 2 L) of fluid.

CAUSES AND INCIDENCE

In cardiac tamponade, progressive accumulation of fluid in the pericardial sac compresses the heart chambers, obstructs blood flow into the ventricles, and reduces the amount of blood that can be pumped out of the heart with each contraction. (See *Understanding cardiac tamponade,* page 38.)

Each time the ventricles contract, more fluid accumulates in the pericardial sac. This further limits the amount of blood that can fill the ventricular chambers—especially the left ventricle—during the next cardiac cycle.

The amount of fluid needed to cause cardiac tamponade varies greatly; it may be as little as 50 ml if fluid accumulates rapidly or more than 2 L if fluid accumulates slowly and the pericardium stretches to adapt.

Increased intrapericardial pressure and cardiac tamponade may be idiopathic (Dressler's syndrome) or may result from:

- effusion (in cancer, bacterial infections, tuberculosis and, rarely, acute rheumatic fever)
- hemorrhage from trauma (such as gunshot or stab wounds to the chest and perforation by catheter during cardiac or central venous catheterization or postcardiac surgery)
- hemorrhage from nontraumatic causes (such as rupture of the heart or great vessels or anticoagulant therapy in a patient with pericarditis)
- acute myocardial infarction
- end-stage lung cancer
- heart tumors
- radiation therapy
- hypothyroidism
- connective tissue disorders (such as rheumatoid arthritis, systemic lupus erythematosus, rheumatic fever, vasculitis, and scleroderma)
- viral or postirradiation pericarditis
- uremia.

Cardiac tamponade occurs in 2 of every 10,000 people.

UNDERSTANDING CARDIAC TAMPONADE

The pericardial sac is a multi-layered membrane that surrounds and protects the heart, as shown in the first illustration below. The *fibrous pericardium* is the tough outermost membrane. The *visceral pericardium* is the innermost layer. It clings to the heart and is also known as the *epicardial layer of the heart.* Between these two layers lies the *parietal pericardium.* Together, the visceral and parietal layers are known as the *serous membrane.*

The pericardial space—between the visceral and parietal layers—contains 10 to 30 ml of pericardial fluid that lubricates the layers of the sac and minimizes friction when the heart contracts.

NORMAL HEART AND PERICARDIUM

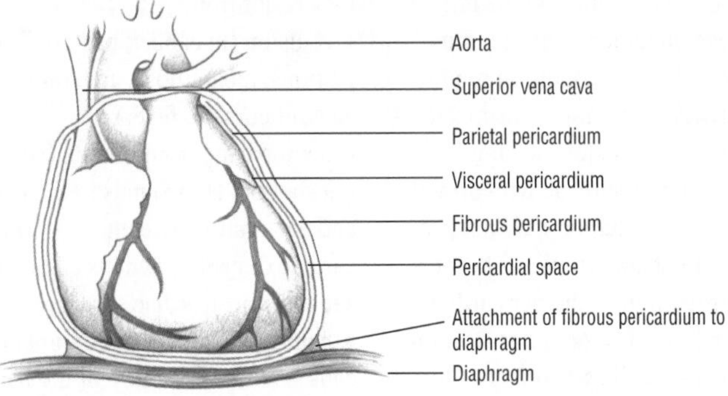

In cardiac tamponade, blood or fluid fills the pericardial space, compressing the heart chambers, increasing intracardiac pressure, and obstructing venous return, as shown in the second illustration below. As blood flow into the ventricles falls, so does cardiac output. Without prompt treatment, low cardiac output can be fatal.

CARDIAC TAMPONADE

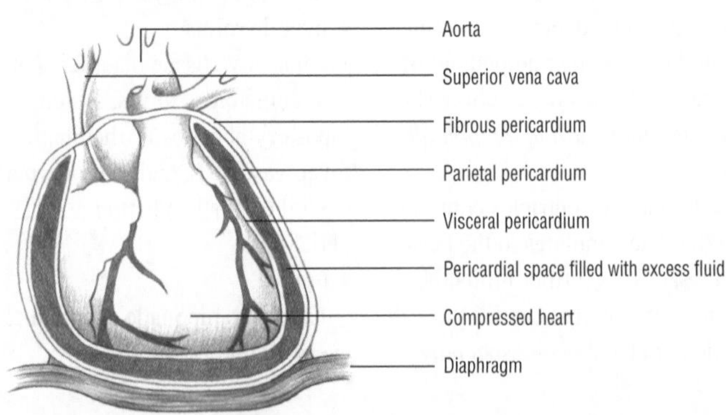

SIGNS AND SYMPTOMS

Typically, cardiac tamponade produces:

- increased venous pressure with jugular vein distention
- reduced arterial blood pressure
- muffled heart sounds on auscultation
- pulsus paradoxus (an abnormal inspiratory drop in systemic blood pressure greater than 15 mm Hg).

The absence of a preexisting pericardial friction rub may suggest an increase in fluid in the pericardial space.

These classic symptoms reflect the failure of physiologic compensatory mechanisms to override the effects of rapidly rising pericardial pressure, which limits diastolic filling of the ventricles and reduces stroke volume to a critically low level.

Generally, ventricular end-systolic volume may drop because of inadequate preload. The increasing pericardial pressure is transmitted equally across the heart cavities, producing a matching rise in intracardiac pressure, especially atrial and end-diastolic ventricular pressures.

Cardiac tamponade may also cause dyspnea, diaphoresis, pallor or cyanosis, anxiety, tachycardia, narrow pulse pressure, restlessness, and hepatomegaly, but the lung fields are clear. The patient typically sits upright and leans forward.

COMPLICATIONS

- Cardiogenic shock
- Death

DIAGNOSIS

- Chest X-ray shows a slightly widened mediastinum and cardiomegaly. The cardiac silhouette may have a goblet shape.
- Electrocardiography is rarely diagnostic but is useful in ruling out other cardiac disorders. It may reveal changes produced by acute pericarditis.
- Pulmonary artery catheterization detects increased right atrial pressure, right ventricular diastolic pressure, and central venous pressure (CVP).
- Echocardiography, computed tomography scan, or magnetic resonance imaging shows pericardial effusion with signs of right ventricular and atrial compression.

TREATMENT

The goal of treatment is to relieve intrapericardial pressure and cardiac compression by removing accumulated blood or fluid. Pericardiocentesis (needle aspiration of the pericardial cavity) or surgical creation of an opening (pericardiectomy or pericardial window) dramatically improves systemic arterial pressure and cardiac output with aspiration of as little as 25 ml of fluid. Such treatment requires continuous hemodynamic and electrocardiogram (ECG) monitoring in the intensive care unit.

In traumatic injury, treatment may include blood transfusion or a thoracotomy to drain accumulating fluid or to repair bleeding sites. Resection of part or all of the pericardium to allow full communication with the pleura may be needed if repeated pericardiocentesis fails to prevent recurrence.

Drugs

- Supplemental oxygen to improve oxygenation
- Trial volume loading with crystalloids, such as I.V. normal saline solution, to maintain systolic blood pressure
- An inotropic drug, such as isoproterenol (Isuprel) or dopamine, to improve myocardial contractility until fluid in the pericardial sac can be removed
- The heparin antagonist protamine sulfate to stop bleeding, in heparin-induced tamponade
- Vitamin K to stop bleeding, in warfarin (Coumadin)-induced tamponade

SPECIAL CONSIDERATIONS

If the patient needs pericardiocentesis:

- Explain the procedure to him. Keep a pericardial aspiration needle attached to a 50-ml syringe by a three-way stopcock, an ECG machine, and an emergency cart with a defibrillator at the bedside. Make sure the equipment is turned on and ready for immediate use. Position him at a 45- to 60-degree angle. Connect the precordial ECG lead to the hub of the aspiration needle with an alligator clamp and connecting wire, and assist with fluid aspiration. When the needle touches the myocardium, you'll see an ST-segment elevation or premature ventricular contractions.
- Monitor blood pressure and CVP during and after pericardiocentesis. Infuse I.V. solutions, as prescribed, to maintain blood pressure. Watch for a decrease in CVP and a concomitant rise in blood pressure, which indicate relief of cardiac compression.

If the patient needs thoracotomy:

- Explain the procedure to him. Tell him what to expect postoperatively (chest tubes, drainage bottles, and oxygen administration). Teach him how to turn, deep breathe, and cough.
- Give antibiotics, protamine sulfate, or vitamin K, as appropriate.
- Postoperatively, monitor critical parameters, such as vital signs and arterial blood gas values, and assess heart and breath sounds. Give pain medication as ordered. Maintain the chest drainage system, and stay alert for complications, such as hemorrhage and arrhythmias.

Cardiogenic shock

Sometimes called *pump failure,* cardiogenic shock is a condition of diminished cardiac output that severely impairs tissue perfusion. It reflects severe heart failure and occurs as a serious complication in 5% to 10% of patients hospitalized with acute myocardial infarction (MI). Historically, mortality in cardiogenic shock had been 80% to 90%; however, recent studies indicate that the rate has dropped to 56% to 67%

because of the use of thrombolytics, improved interventional procedures, and better therapies.

CAUSES AND INCIDENCE

Cardiogenic shock can result from any condition that causes significant left ventricular dysfunction with reduced cardiac output, such as MI (most common), myocardial ischemia (particularly with existing left ventricular dysfunction), papillary muscle dysfunction, or end-stage cardiomyopathy.

Other causes of cardiogenic shock include:

- arrhythmias
- heart failure
- pericardial tamponade
- pulmonary embolism
- tension pneumothorax.

Regardless of the underlying cause, left ventricular dysfunction sets into motion a series of compensatory mechanisms that attempt to increase cardiac output and, in turn, maintain vital organ function. (See *What happens in cardiogenic shock,* page 42.) As cardiac output falls in left ventricular dysfunction, aortic and carotid baroreceptors initiate sympathetic nervous responses, which increase heart rate, left ventricular filling pressure, and peripheral resistance to flow, to enhance venous return to the heart. These compensatory responses initially stabilize the patient but later cause deterioration with rising oxygen demands of the already compromised myocardium. These events comprise a vicious circle of low cardiac output, sympathetic compensation, myocardial ischemia, and even lower cardiac output.

There are three basic stages common to all types of shock: compensatory, progressive, and irreversible, or refractory, stages.

Compensatory stage

When arterial pressure and tissue perfusion decline, compensatory mechanisms are activated to maintain perfusion to the heart and brain. As baroreceptors in the carotid sinus and aortic arch sense a decrease in blood pressure, epinephrine and norepinephrine are secreted to increase peripheral resistance, blood pressure, and myocardial contractility. Reduced blood flow to the kidneys activates the renin-angiotensin-aldosterone system, causing vasoconstriction and sodium and water retention, leading to increased blood volume and venous return. As a result of these compensatory mechanisms, cardiac output and tissue perfusion are maintained.

Progressive stage

The progressive stage of shock begins as compensatory mechanisms fail to maintain cardiac output. Tissues become hypoxic because of poor perfusion. As cells switch to anaerobic metabolism, lactic acid builds up, producing metabolic acidosis. This acidotic state depresses myocardial function. Tissue hypoxia also promotes release of endothelial mediators, which produce vasodilation and endothelial abnormalities,

WHAT HAPPENS IN CARDIOGENIC SHOCK

If a patient's left ventricle can't maintain adequate cardiac output, he develops cardiogenic shock. Compensatory mechanisms increase his heart rate, strengthen myocardial contractions, promote sodium and water retention, and cause selective vasoconstriction. However, these mechanisms increase myocardial workload and oxygen consumption, which reduces the heart's ability to pump blood, especially if the patient has myocardial ischemia. Consequently, blood backs up, resulting in pulmonary edema. Eventually, as shown in the flowchart, cardiac output falls and multisystem organ failure develops as compensatory mechanisms fail to maintain perfusion.

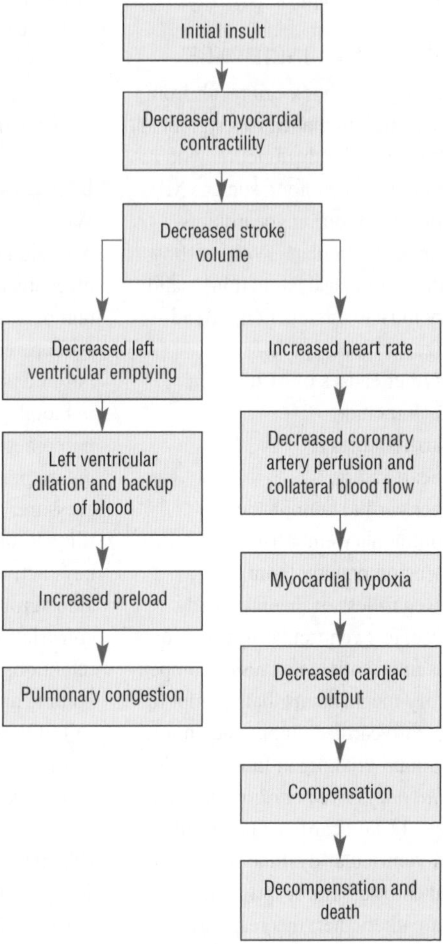

leading to venous pooling and increased capillary permeability. Sluggish blood flow increases the risk of disseminated intravascular coagulation.

Irreversible (refractory) stage

As the shock syndrome progresses, permanent organ damage occurs as compensatory mechanisms can no longer maintain cardiac output. Reduced perfusion damages cell membranes, lysosomal enzymes are released, and energy stores are depleted, possibly leading to cell death. As cells use anaerobic metabolism, lactic acid accumulates, increasing capillary permeability and the movement of fluid out of the vascular space. This loss of intravascular fluid further contributes to hypotension. Perfusion to the coronary arteries is reduced, causing myocardial depression and a further reduction in cardiac output. Eventually, circulatory and respiratory failure occur. Death is inevitable.

Incidence of cardiogenic shock is higher in men than in women because of their higher incidence of coronary artery disease. However, among people with MI, women have a higher incidence of cardiogenic shock than men.

SIGNS AND SYMPTOMS

Cardiogenic shock produces signs of poor tissue perfusion:

- cold, pale, clammy skin
- decreased systolic blood pressure to 30 mm Hg below baseline, or a sustained reading below 80 mm Hg not attributable to medication
- tachycardia
- rapid, shallow respirations
- oliguria (less than 20 ml/hour)
- restlessness
- mental confusion and obtundation
- narrowing pulse pressure
- cyanosis.

Although many of these clinical features also occur in heart failure and other shock syndromes, they're usually more profound in cardiogenic shock.

COMPLICATIONS

- Multisystem organ failure
- Death

DIAGNOSIS

- Auscultation may detect S3 and S4 heart sounds, faint heart sounds, and possibly a holosystolic murmur if shock results from rupture of the ventricular septum or papillary muscles.
- Pulmonary artery pressure (PAP) monitoring may show increased PAP and increased pulmonary artery wedge pressure (PAWP), reflecting a rise in left ventricular end-diastolic pressure (preload) and increased resistance to left ventricular emptying (afterload) due to ineffective pumping and increased peripheral vascular resistance. Cardiac output is decreased. (See *Understanding hemodynamic monitoring,* page 44.)
- Invasive arterial pressure monitoring may indicate hypotension from impaired ventricular ejection.
- Arterial blood gas (ABG) analysis may show metabolic acidosis and hypoxia.
- Electrocardiography may show possible evidence of acute MI, ischemia, or ventricular aneurysm.
- Echocardiography can determine left ventricular function and reveal valvular abnormalities.
- Enzyme testing may show elevated creatine kinase, lactate dehydrogenase, aspartate aminotransferase, and alanine aminotransferase levels, which point to MI or ischemia and suggest heart failure or shock.

UNDERSTANDING HEMODYNAMIC MONITORING

Hemodynamic monitoring provides information on intracardiac pressures and cardiac output, as outlined in this table. To understand intracardiac pressures, picture the cardiovascular system as a continuous loop with constantly changing pressure gradients that keep the blood moving.

Measurement	Normal values	Implications of abnormal values
Right atrial pressure (RAP) or central venous pressure RAP reflects right atrial (right-sided) function and end-diastolic pressure.	1 to 6 mm Hg (1.34 to 8 cm H_2O)*	▪ Elevated value suggests right-sided heart failure, volume overload, tricuspid valve stenosis or regurgitation, constrictive pericarditis, pulmonary hypertension, cardiac tamponade, or right ventricular infarction. ▪ Low value suggests reduced circulating blood volume.
Right ventricular pressure Right ventricular systolic pressure normally equals pulmonary artery systolic pressure. Right ventricular end-diastolic pressure, which equals RAP, reflects right ventricular function.	*Systolic:* 15 to 25 mm Hg *Diastolic:* 0 to 8 mm Hg	▪ Elevated value suggests mitral stenosis or insufficiency, pulmonary disease, hypoxemia, constrictive pericarditis, chronic heart failure, atrial and ventricular septal defects, and patent ductus arteriosus.
Pulmonary artery pressure Pulmonary artery systolic pressure reflects right ventricular function and pulmonary circulation pressures. Pulmonary artery diastolic pressure reflects left ventricular pressures, specifically left ventricular end-diastolic pressure.	*Systolic:* 15 to 25 mm Hg *Diastolic:* 8 to 15 mm Hg *Mean:* 10 to 20 mm Hg	▪ Elevated value suggests left-sided heart failure, increased pulmonary blood flow (left or right shunting, as in atrial or ventricular septal defects), mitral stenosis or insufficiency, or any condition causing increased pulmonary arteriolar resistance.

UNDERSTANDING HEMODYNAMIC MONITORING *(continued)*

Measurement	Normal values	Implications of abnormal values
Pulmonary artery wedge pressure (PAWP) PAWP reflects left atrial and left ventricular pressures unless the patient has mitral stenosis. Changes in PAWP reflect changes in left ventricular filling pressure. The heart momentarily relaxes during diastole as it fills with blood from the pulmonary veins; this permits the pulmonary vasculature, left atrium, and left ventricle to act as a single chamber.	*Mean:* 6 to 12 mm Hg	■ Elevated value suggests left-sided heart failure, mitral stenosis or insufficiency, and pericardial tamponade. ■ Low value suggests hypovolemia.
Left atrial pressure Left atrial pressure reflects left ventricular end-diastolic pressure in patients without mitral valve disease.	6 to 12 mm Hg	
Cardiac output Cardiac output is the amount of blood ejected by the heart each minute. Adjusting the cardiac output to the patient's size yields a measurement called the cardiac index.	4 to 8 L Varies with patient's weight, height, and body surface area	

*To convert Hg mm to cm H_2O, multiply mm Hg by 1.34.

Troponin I, troponin T, and isoenzyme values may confirm acute MI.

Additional tests can be used to diagnose other conditions that may lead to pump dysfunction and failure, such as cardiac arrhythmias, cardiac tamponade, papillary muscle infarction or rupture, ventricular septal rupture, pulmonary emboli, venous pooling (associated with vasodilators and continuous intermittent positive-pressure breathing), and hypovolemia.

TREATMENT

The aim of treatment is to enhance cardiovascular status by increasing cardiac output, improving myocardial perfusion, and decreasing cardiac workload with combinations of various cardiovascular drugs and mechanical-assist techniques. Myocardial reperfusion can be accomplished by percutaneous transluminal coronary angioplasty, stents, thrombolytic therapy, or bypass grafting.

The intra-aortic balloon pump (IABP) is a mechanical-assist device used to improve coronary artery perfusion and decrease cardiac workload. (See *Understanding the IABP*.) The inflatable balloon pump is percutaneously or surgically inserted through the femoral artery into the descending thoracic aorta. The balloon inflates during diastole to increase coronary artery perfusion pressure and deflates before systole (before the aortic valve opens) to reduce resistance to ejection (afterload) and reduce cardiac workload. Improved ventricular ejection, which significantly improves cardiac output, and a subsequent vasodilation in the peripheral vasculature lead to lower preload volume.

When drug and IABP therapy fail, the patient may require a ventricular assist device. This device (which may be either temporary or permanent) diverts systemic blood flow from a diseased ventricle into a centrifugal pump. It assists the heart's pumping action rather than replacing it. Heart transplantation may be considered when other medical and surgical therapeutic measures fail.

Drugs

- Inotropic drugs, such as dopamine, dobutamine, and epinephrine, to increase heart contractility and cardiac output
- Phosphodiesterase inhibitors, such as inamrinone (Amrinone) and milrinone (Primacor), to increase heart contractility, decrease preload, and decrease afterload
- Diuretics to reduce preload if the patient has fluid volume overload
- Thrombolytic therapy to restore coronary artery blood flow if cardiogenic shock is due to an acute MI

SPECIAL CONSIDERATIONS

- At the first sign of cardiogenic shock, check the patient's blood pressure and heart rate. If the patient is hypotensive or is having trouble breathing, ensure a patent I.V. line and a patent airway, and provide oxygen to promote tissue oxygenation. Notify the practitioner immediately.
- Monitor ABG values to measure oxygenation and detect acidosis from poor tissue perfusion. Increase oxygen delivery, as indicated. Check the complete blood count and electrolyte levels.
- After diagnosis, monitor cardiac rhythm continuously and assess skin color, temperature, and other vital signs often. Watch for a drop in

UNDERSTANDING THE IABP

An intra-aortic balloon pump (IABP) consists of a polyurethane balloon attached to an external pump via a large-lumen catheter. The balloon is inserted percutaneously through the femoral artery and positioned in the descending aorta just distal to the left subclavian artery and above the renal arteries.

Push…

This external pump works in precise counterpoint to the left ventricle, inflating the balloon with helium early in diastole and deflating it just before systole. As the balloon inflates, it forces blood toward the aortic valve, thereby raising pressure in the aortic root and augmenting diastolic pressure to improve coronary perfusion. It also improves peripheral circulation by forcing blood through the brachiocephalic, common carotid, and subclavian arteries arising from the aortic trunk.

…and pull

The balloon deflates rapidly at the end of diastole, creating a vacuum in the aorta. This reduces aortic volume and pressure, thereby decreasing the resistance to left ventricular ejection (afterload). This decreased workload, in turn, reduces the heart's oxygen requirements and, combined with improved myocardial perfusion, helps reduce or prevent myocardial ischemia.

DIASTOLE

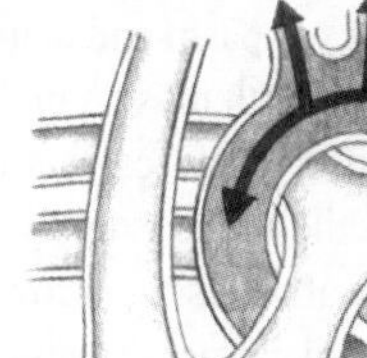

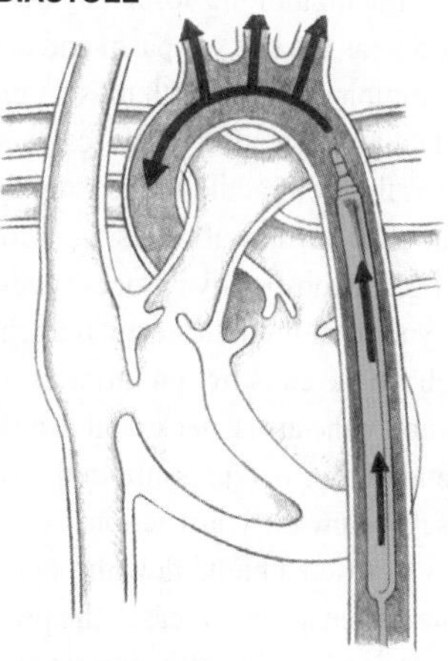

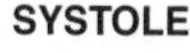

SYSTOLE

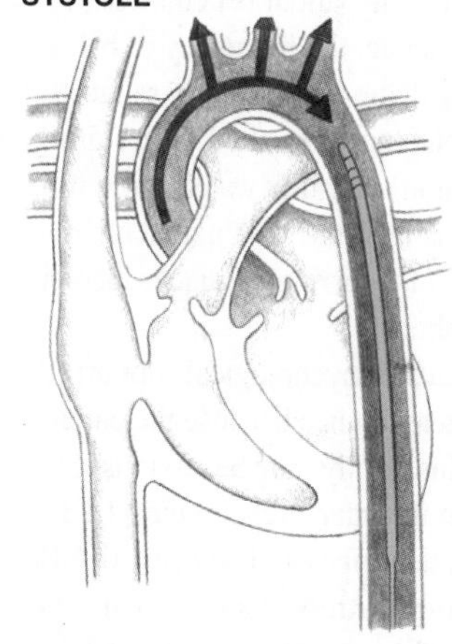

systolic blood pressure to less than 80 mm Hg (usually compromising cardiac output further). Report hypotension immediately.

- An indwelling urinary catheter may be inserted to measure urine output. Notify the practitioner if output drops below 30 ml/hour.

- Using a pulmonary artery catheter, closely monitor PAP, PAWP, and cardiac output. A high PAWP indicates heart failure and should be reported.
- When a patient has an IABP, reposition him often and perform passive range-of-motion exercises to prevent skin breakdown. However, don't flex the patient's "ballooned" leg at the hip because doing so may displace or fracture the catheter. Assess pedal pulses and skin temperature and color to ensure adequate circulation to the leg. Check the dressing on the insertion site often for bleeding, and change it according to facility protocol. Also, check the site for hematoma or signs of infection, and culture any drainage.
- After the patient is hemodynamically stable, the frequency of balloon inflation is gradually reduced to wean him from the IABP. During weaning, carefully watch for monitor changes, chest pain, and other signs of recurring cardiac ischemia and shock.
- Provide psychological support and reassurance because the patient and his family may be anxious about the intensive care unit, IABP, and other tubes and devices. To ease emotional stress, plan your care to allow frequent rest periods, and provide as much privacy as possible.

Coarctation of the aorta

Coarctation is a narrowing of the aorta, usually just below the left subclavian artery, near the site where the ligamentum arteriosum (the remnant of the ductus arteriosus, a fetal blood vessel) joins the pulmonary artery to the aorta. Coarctation may occur with aortic valve stenosis (usually of a bicuspid aortic valve) and with severe cases of hypoplasia of the aortic arch, patent ductus arteriosus (PDA), and ventricular septal defect. In general, the prognosis for coarctation of the aorta depends on the severity of associated cardiac anomalies; the prognosis for isolated coarctation is good if corrective surgery is performed before this condition induces severe systemic hypertension or degenerative changes in the aorta.

CAUSES AND INCIDENCE

Coarctation of the aorta may develop as a result of spasm and constriction of the smooth muscle in the ductus arteriosus as it closes. Possibly, this contractile tissue extends into the aortic wall, causing narrowing. The obstructive process causes hypertension in the aortic branches above the constriction (arteries that supply the arms, neck, and head) and diminished pressure in the vessels below the constriction.

Restricted blood flow through the narrowed aorta increases the pressure load on the left ventricle and causes dilation of the proximal aorta and ventricular hypertrophy. Untreated, this condition may lead to left-sided heart failure and, rarely, cerebral hemorrhage and aortic rupture. If ventricular septal defect accompanies coarctation, blood shunts left to right, straining the right side of the heart. This leads to pulmonary hypertension and, eventually, right-sided heart hypertrophy and failure. (See *Understanding coarctation of the aorta.*) As oxygenated blood leaves the left ventricle, a portion travels through the arteries that branch off the aorta proximal to the coarctation. If a PDA is present, the rest of the blood travels through the coarctation, mixes with deoxygenated blood from the PDA, and travels to the legs. If the PDA is closed, the legs and lower portion of the body must rely solely on the blood that gets through the coarctation.

Coarctation of the aorta occurs in 1 of every 10,000 people and is usually diagnosed in children or adults younger than age 40. It accounts for about 7% of all congenital heart defects in children and is twice as common in males as in females. When it occurs in females, it's commonly associated with Turner's syndrome, a chromosomal disorder that causes ovarian dysgenesis.

UNDERSTANDING COARCTATION OF THE AORTA

Fetal circulation normally includes three shunts that bypass the fetus's liver and lungs. One shunt, shown below, is called the *ductus arteriosus*; it connects the pulmonary artery with the aorta.

Because the fetus receives its oxygen supply from the maternal placenta, most of the blood entering the main pulmonary artery bypasses the lungs and flows directly into the aorta through the ductus arteriosus.

After birth, when the neonate's lungs must function on their own, the ductus arteriosus closes, and the right ventricular output enters the left ventricle through the pulmonary capillaries, as it does in normal adult circulation.

If the ductus arteriosus closes improperly, an abnormal constriction known as *coarctation* may result. By restricting blood flow, the constriction increases pressure in the left ventricle so much that it may fail, causing increased end-diastolic and pulmonary artery pressures, pulmonary edema, low output and, possibly, sudden circulatory collapse. Restricted flow also dilates the proximal aorta and causes ventricular hypertrophy.

To compensate for the increased pressure, collateral circulation may develop, circumventing the narrowed aorta.

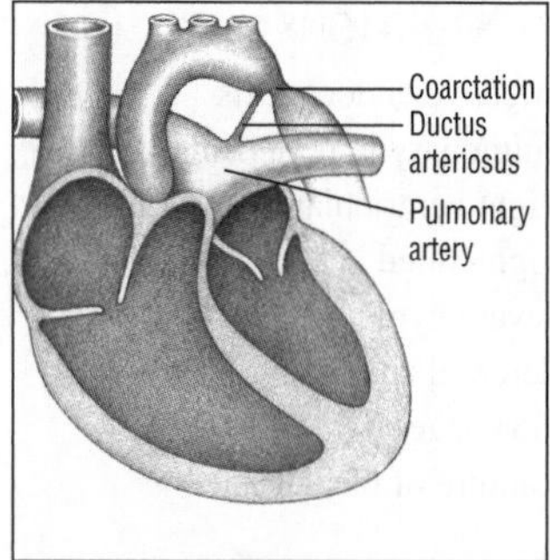

SIGNS AND SYMPTOMS

Clinical features vary with age. During the 1st year after birth, when aortic coarctation may cause heart failure, the infant displays tachypnea, dyspnea, pulmonary edema, pallor, tachycardia, failure to thrive, cardiomegaly, and hepatomegaly. In most cases, heart sounds are normal unless a coexisting cardiac defect is present. Femoral pulses are absent or diminished.

If coarctation is asymptomatic in infancy, it usually remains so throughout adolescence, as collateral circulation develops to bypass the narrowed segment. During adolescence, this defect may produce dyspnea, claudication, headaches, epistaxis, and hypertension in the upper extremities despite collateral circulation. It commonly causes resting systolic hypertension and wide pulse pressure; high diastolic pressure readings are the same in both the arms and legs. Coarctation may also produce a visible aortic pulsation in the suprasternal notch, a continuous systolic murmur, an accentuated S_2, and an S_4.

COMPLICATIONS

- Infective endocarditis
- Pulmonary hypertension
- Right ventricular hypertrophy
- Right-sided heart failure
- Severe hypertension
- Cerebral aneurysms and hemorrhage
- Rupture of the aorta

DIAGNOSIS

The cardinal signs of coarctation of the aorta are resting systolic hypertension, absent or diminished femoral pulses, and wide pulse pressure.

The following tests support the diagnosis:

- Chest X-ray may show left ventricular hypertrophy, heart failure, a wide ascending and descending aorta, and notching of the undersurfaces of the ribs due to extensive collateral circulation.
- Electrocardiography may eventually reveal left ventricular hypertrophy.
- Echocardiography may show increased left ventricular muscle thickness, coexisting aortic valve abnormalities, and the coarctation site.
- Doppler ultrasound and cardiac catheterization evaluate collateral circulation and measure pressure in the right and left ventricles and in the ascending and descending aortas (on both sides of the obstruction).
- Aortography locates the site and extent of coarctation.
- Magnetic resonance imaging can identify the site and extent of coarctation as well as the involvement of adjacent vessels.

TREATMENT

For an infant with heart failure caused by coarctation of the aorta, treatment includes medical management with digoxin (Lanoxin), diuretics, oxygen, and sedatives. If medical management fails, surgery may be needed.

The child's condition usually determines the timing of surgery. Signs of heart failure or hypertension may call for early surgery. If signs don't appear, surgery usually occurs during the preschool years.

Before the operation, the child may need endocarditis prophylaxis or, if he's older and has previously undetected coarctation, antihypertensive therapy. During surgery, the surgeon uses a flap of the left subclavian artery to reconstruct an unobstructed aorta.

Balloon therapy may be indicated for some patients as an alternative to surgical repair. It uses a technique similar to that used to open the coronary arteries, but is performed on the aorta.

Drugs

- Digoxin, a diuretic, oxygen, and a sedative in infants with heart failure
- Prostaglandin infusion to keep the ductus open
- Antibiotic prophylaxis against infective endocarditis before and after surgery
- Antihypertensive therapy for children with previous undetected coarctation until surgery

SPECIAL CONSIDERATIONS

- Palpate leg pulses in neonates and at well-baby visits to detect absent or diminished pulses.
- When coarctation in an infant requires rapid digitalization, monitor his vital signs closely and watch for digoxin toxicity (poor feeding and vomiting).
- Balance intake and output carefully, especially if the infant is receiving diuretics with fluid restriction.
- Because the infant may not be able to maintain proper body temperature, regulate environmental temperature with an overbed warmer if needed.
- Monitor blood glucose level to detect possible hypoglycemia, which may occur as glycogen stores are depleted.
- Offer caregivers emotional support and an explanation of the disorder. Also explain diagnostic procedures, surgery, and drug therapy. Tell caregivers what to expect postoperatively.
- For an older child, assess blood pressure in his limbs regularly, explain any exercise restrictions, stress the need to take medications properly and to watch for adverse effects, and teach him about tests and other procedures.

After corrective surgery

- Monitor blood pressure closely using an intra-arterial line. Measure blood pressure in the arms and legs. Monitor intake and output.
- If the patient develops hypertension and needs nitroprusside (Nitropress) or trimethaphan, give the drug as ordered by continuous I.V. infusion, using an infusion pump. Watch for severe hypotension, and regulate the dosage carefully.

- Provide pain relief, and encourage a gradual increase in activity.
- Promote adequate respiratory function through turning, coughing, and deep breathing.
- Watch for abdominal pain or rigidity and signs of GI or urinary bleeding.
- If an older child needs to continue antihypertensives after surgery, teach him and his parents about them.
- Stress the importance of continued endocarditis prophylaxis.

Cor pulmonale

The World Health Organization defines chronic cor pulmonale as "hypertrophy of the right ventricle resulting from diseases affecting the function or the structure of the lungs, except when these pulmonary alterations are the result of diseases that primarily affect the left side of the heart or of congenital heart disease." Invariably, cor pulmonale follows a disorder of the lungs, pulmonary vessels, chest wall, or respiratory control center. For instance, chronic obstructive pulmonary disease (COPD) produces pulmonary hypertension, which leads to right ventricular hypertrophy and right-sided heart failure. Because cor pulmonale typically occurs late during the course of COPD and other irreversible diseases, the prognosis is generally poor.

CAUSES AND INCIDENCE

About 85% of patients with cor pulmonale have COPD, and 25% of patients with COPD eventually develop cor pulmonale.

Other respiratory disorders that produce cor pulmonale include:

- obstructive lung diseases, such as bronchiectasis and cystic fibrosis
- restrictive lung diseases, such as pneumoconiosis, interstitial pneumonitis, scleroderma, and sarcoidosis
- loss of lung tissue after extensive lung surgery
- congenital cardiac shunts such as a ventricular septal defect
- pulmonary vascular diseases, such as recurrent thromboembolism, primary pulmonary hypertension, schistosomiasis, and pulmonary vasculitis
- respiratory insufficiency without pulmonary disease, as in chest wall disorders such as kyphoscoliosis, neuromuscular incompetence from muscular dystrophy and amyotrophic lateral sclerosis, polymyositis, and spinal cord lesions above C6
- obesity hypoventilation syndrome (pickwickian syndrome) and upper airway obstruction
- living at high altitudes (chronic mountain sickness).

Pulmonary capillary destruction and pulmonary vasoconstriction (usually secondary to hypoxia) reduce the area of the pulmonary vascular bed. Thus, pulmonary vascular resistance is increased, causing pulmonary hypertension. To compensate for the extra work needed to force blood through the lungs, the right ventricle dilates and hypertrophies. In response to low oxygen content, the bone marrow produces more red blood cells (RBCs), causing erythrocytosis. When hematocrit exceeds 55%, blood viscosity increases, which further aggravates pulmonary hypertension and increases the hemodynamic load on the right ventricle. Right-sided heart failure is the result. (See *Cor pulmonale: An overview.*)

In COPD, increased airway obstruction makes airflow worse. The resulting hypoxia and hypercarbia can have vasodilatory effects on systemic arterioles. However, hypoxia increases pulmonary vasoconstriction. The liver becomes palpable and tender because it's engorged and displaced downward by the low diaphragm. Hepatojugular reflux may occur.

Compensatory mechanisms begin to fail, and larger amounts of blood remain in the right ventricle at the end of diastole, causing ventricular dilation. Increasing intrathoracic pressures impede venous return and raise pressure within the jugular vein. Peripheral edema can occur, and right ventricular hypertrophy increases progressively. The main pulmonary arteries enlarge, pulmonary hypertension increases, and heart failure occurs.

Cor pulmonale accounts for about 25% of all types of heart failure. It's most common in areas of the world where the incidence of cigarette smoking and COPD is high; cor pulmonale affects middle-aged to elderly men more often than women, but the incidence in women is increasing. In children, cor pulmonale may be a complication of cystic fibrosis, hemosiderosis, upper airway obstruction, scleroderma, extensive bronchiectasis, neurologic diseases affecting respiratory

COR PULMONALE: AN OVERVIEW

Cor pulmonale may be caused by restrictive pulmonary disorders (such as fibrosis or obesity), obstructive disorders (such as bronchitis), or primary vascular disorders (such as recurrent pulmonary emboli). However, they all share this common pathway.

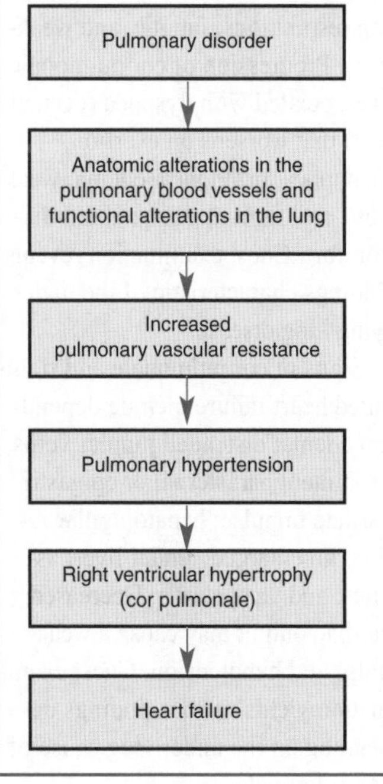

muscles, or abnormalities of the respiratory control center.

SIGNS AND SYMPTOMS

As long as the heart can compensate for increased pulmonary vascular resistance, clinical features reflect the underlying disorder and occur mostly in the respiratory system. They include chronic productive cough, exertional dyspnea, wheezing respirations, fatigue, and weakness. Progression of cor pulmonale is associated with dyspnea (even at rest) that worsens on exertion, tachypnea, orthopnea, edema, weakness, and right upper quadrant discomfort. Chest examination reveals findings characteristic of the underlying lung disease.

Signs of cor pulmonale and right-sided heart failure include dependent edema; distended jugular veins; prominent parasternal or epigastric cardiac impulse; hepatojugular reflux; an enlarged, tender liver; ascites; and tachycardia. Decreased cardiac output may cause a weak pulse and hypotension. Chest examination yields various findings depending on the underlying cause of cor pulmonale.

In COPD, auscultation reveals wheezing, rhonchi, and diminished breath sounds. When the disease is secondary to upper airway obstruction or damage to central nervous system respiratory centers, chest findings may be normal, except for a right ventricular lift, gallop rhythm, and loud pulmonic component of S_2. Tricuspid insufficiency produces a pansystolic murmur heard at the lower left sternal border; its intensity increases on inspiration, distinguishing it from a murmur due to mitral valve disease. A right ventricular early murmur that increases on inspiration can be heard at the left sternal border or over the epigastrium. A systolic pulmonic ejection click may also be heard. Alterations in the patient's level of consciousness may occur.

COMPLICATIONS

- Right- and left-sided heart failure
- Hepatomegaly
- Edema
- Ascites
- Pleural effusions
- Thromboembolism

DIAGNOSIS

- Pulmonary artery pressure (PAP) measurements show increased right ventricular and pulmonary artery pressures, stemming from increased pulmonary vascular resistance. Right ventricular systolic and pulmonary artery systolic pressures exceeds 30 mm Hg. Pulmonary artery diastolic pressure exceeds 15 mm Hg.
- Echocardiography or angiography indicates right ventricular enlargement; echocardiography can estimate PAP while also ruling out structural and congenital lesions.
- Chest X-ray shows large central pulmonary arteries and suggests right ventricular enlargement by rightward enlargement of the heart's silhouette on an anterior chest film.

- Arterial blood gas (ABG) analysis shows decreased partial pressure of arterial oxygen, typically to less than 70 mm Hg and usually no more than 90 mm Hg on room air.
- Electrocardiography commonly shows arrhythmias, such as premature atrial and ventricular contractions and atrial fibrillation during severe hypoxia; it also may show right bundle-branch block, right axis deviation, prominent P waves and inverted T waves in right precordial leads, and right ventricular hypertrophy.
- Pulmonary function tests show results consistent with the underlying pulmonary disease.
- Hematocrit typically exceeds 50%.

TREATMENT

Treatment of cor pulmonale aims to reduce hypoxemia, increase the patient's exercise tolerance and, when possible, correct the underlying condition. In addition to drug therapy, treatment includes bed rest, a low-sodium diet, and restricted fluid intake. Phlebotomy may be used to reduce the RBC count. Treatment may vary with the underlying cause. For example, a tracheotomy may be needed if the patient has an upper airway obstruction. In acute disease, the patient may need mechanical ventilation to reduce the workload of breathing.

Drugs

- Cardiac glycosides (digoxin [Lanoxin]) to increase the strength of myocardial contractions
- Antibiotics (with culture and sensitivity of a sputum sample) if the patient has a respiratory infection
- Potent pulmonary artery vasodilators, such as diazoxide, nitroprusside (Nitropress), hydralazine, angiotensin-converting enzyme inhibitors, calcium channel blockers, or prostaglandin to reduce primary pulmonary hypertension
- Continuous administration of low concentrations of oxygen to decrease pulmonary hypertension, polycythemia, and tachypnea
- Diuretics, such as furosemide (Lasix), to reduce edema
- Anticoagulants to reduce the risk of thromboembolism
- Corticosteroids to treat vasculitis or an underlying immune disorder

SPECIAL CONSIDERATIONS

- Plan the diet carefully with the patient and staff dietitian. Because the patient may lack energy and tire easily when eating, provide small, frequent feedings rather than three heavy meals.
- Prevent fluid retention by limiting the patient's fluid intake to 1 to 2 qt (1 to 2 L) daily and providing a low-sodium diet.
- Monitor the serum potassium level closely if the patient is receiving diuretics. Low serum potassium level can increase the risk of arrhythmias associated with cardiac glycosides.
- Watch the patient for evidence of digoxin toxicity, such as anorexia, nausea, vomiting, and halos around visual images and color perception

shifts. Monitor the patient for cardiac arrhythmias. Teach him to check his radial pulse before taking digoxin or any cardiac glycoside. Instruct him to notify the practitioner if his pulse rate changes.

- Reposition bedridden patients often to prevent atelectasis.
- Provide meticulous respiratory care, including oxygen therapy and, for a patient with COPD, pursed-lip breathing exercises. Periodically measure ABG levels and watch for signs of respiratory failure, such as changes in pulse rate, labored respirations, changes in mental status, and increased fatigue after exertion.

Before discharge

- Make sure that the patient understands the need to maintain a low-sodium diet, weigh himself daily, and watch for increased edema. Teach him to detect edema by pressing the skin over a shin with one finger, holding it for a second or two, and then checking for a finger impression. Increased weight, increased edema, and respiratory difficulty should be reported to the health care provider.
- Instruct the patient to plan for frequent rest periods and to do breathing exercises regularly.
- If the patient needs supplemental oxygen therapy at home, refer him to an agency that can help obtain the required equipment and, as needed, arrange for follow-up examinations.
- If the patient is on anticoagulant therapy, stress the need to watch for bleeding (epistaxis, hematuria, bruising) and to report it. Also urge him to return for periodic laboratory tests to monitor partial thromboplastin time, fibrinogen level, platelet count, hematocrit, hemoglobin level, and prothrombin time.
- Because pulmonary infection commonly worsens COPD and cor pulmonale, tell the patient to watch for and immediately report early signs of infection, such as increased sputum production, a change in sputum color, increased coughing or wheezing, chest pain, fever, and tightness in the chest. Tell the patient to avoid crowds and people with respiratory tract infections, especially during the flu season. The patient should receive pneumococcal and annual influenza vaccines.
- Warn the patient to avoid substances that may depress the ventilatory drive, such as sedatives and alcohol.

Coronary artery disease

Coronary artery disease (CAD) occurs when arteries that supply blood to the heart muscle are narrowed by the development of plaque in the vessel lumens. The result is reduced coronary blood flow and reduced oxygen and nutrients to myocardial tissue. This reduction in blood flow can also lead to coronary syndrome (angina or myocardial infarction [MI]).

CAUSES AND INCIDENCE

Atherosclerosis is the usual cause of CAD. In this form of arteriosclerosis, fatty, fibrous plaques, possibly including calcium deposits, narrow coronary artery lumens, reduce the volume of blood that can flow through them, and lead to myocardial ischemia. (See *Atherosclerotic plaque development.*)

As atherosclerosis progresses, luminal narrowing is accompanied by vascular changes that impair the ability of the diseased vessel to dilate. This causes a precarious balance between myocardial oxygen supply and demand, threatening the myocardium beyond the lesion. When oxygen demand exceeds what the diseased vessel can supply, localized myocardial ischemia results.

Myocardial cells become ischemic within 10 seconds of a coronary artery occlusion. Transient ischemia causes reversible changes at the cellular and tissue levels, depressing myocardial function. Untreated, this can lead to tissue injury or necrosis. Within several minutes, oxygen deprivation forces the myocardium to shift from aerobic to anaerobic metabolism, leading to an accumulation of lactic acid and reduced cellular pH.

The combination of hypoxia, reduced energy availability, and acidosis rapidly impairs left ventricular function. The strength of contractions in the affected myocardial region is reduced as the fibers shorten inadequately. Moreover, wall motion is abnormal in the ischemic area, resulting in less blood being ejected from the heart with each contraction. Restoring blood flow through

ATHEROSCLEROTIC PLAQUE DEVELOPMENT

The coronary arteries are made up of three layers: intima (the innermost layer), media (the middle layer), and adventitia (the outermost layer).

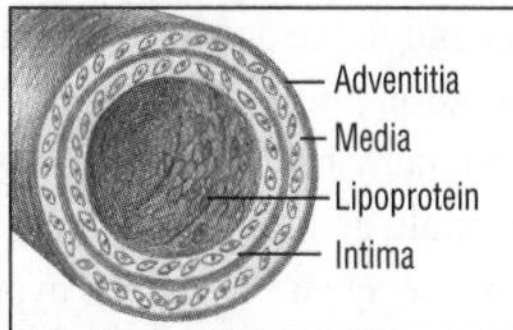

With damage to the vessel, a fatty streak begins to build up on the intimal layer.

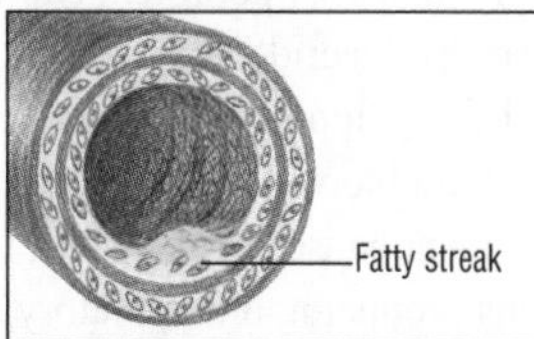

Fibrous plaque and lipids progressively narrow the lumen and impede blood flow to the myocardium.

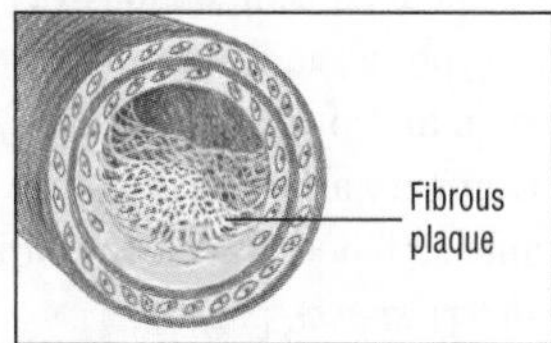

The plaque continues to grow and, in advanced stages, may become a complicated calcified lesion at risk of rupture.

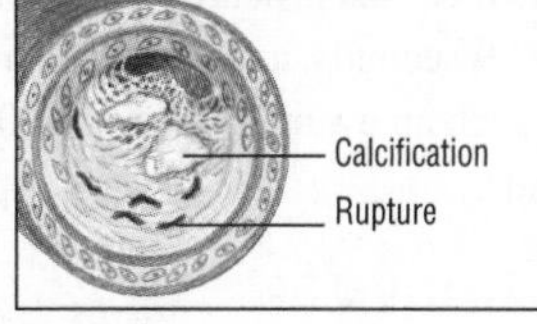

the coronary arteries restores aerobic metabolism and contractility. If blood flow isn't restored, MI results. (See *Patient-teaching aid: Coronary artery disease*.)

Atherosclerosis usually develops in high-flow, high-pressure arteries, such as those in the heart, brain, and kidneys and in the aorta, especially at bifurcation points. It has been linked to many risk factors: family history, male gender, age (increased risk in those age 65 or older), hypertension, obesity, smoking, diabetes mellitus, stress, sedentary lifestyle, high serum cholesterol (particularly high low-density lipoprotein cholesterol) or triglyceride levels, low high-density lipoprotein cholesterol levels, high blood homocysteine levels, menopause and, possibly, infections producing inflammatory responses in the artery walls. (See *The role of genes in CAD,* page 60.) Uncommon causes of reduced coronary artery blood flow include dissecting aneurysms, infectious vasculitis, syphilis, and congenital defects in the coronary vascular system. Coronary artery spasms may also impede blood flow. (See *Coronary artery spasm,* page 61.)

CAD is the leading cause of death in the United States. According to the American Heart Association, someone in the United States suffers a coronary heart event about every 29 seconds, and someone dies from such an event about every 60 seconds.

SIGNS AND SYMPTOMS

The classic symptom of CAD is angina, the direct result of inadequate oxygen flow to the myocardium. Especially in men, anginal pain is usually described as a burning, squeezing, or tight feeling in the substernal or precordial chest that may radiate to the left arm, neck, jaw, or shoulder blade. Typically, the patient clenches his fist over his chest or rubs his left arm when describing the pain, which may be accompanied by nausea, vomiting, fainting, sweating, and cool extremities. Anginal episodes usually follow physical exertion but may also follow emotional excitement, exposure to cold, or a large meal. Women and certain other people, such as those with diabetes, may not have typical anginal pain but may have dyspnea, fatigue, diaphoresis, or more vague symptoms.

Angina has four major forms: stable (pain is predictable in frequency and duration and can be relieved with nitrates and rest), unstable (pain increases in frequency and duration and is more easily induced), Prinzmetal's or variant (from unpredictable coronary artery spasm), and microvascular (in which impairment of vasodilator reserve causes angina-like chest pain in a patient with normal coronary arteries). Severe and prolonged anginal pain generally suggests MI, with potentially fatal arrhythmias and mechanical failure.

PATIENT-TEACHING AID: CAD

Dear Patient:

Your practitioner has determined that you have coronary artery disease (CAD). This handout will help you to understand how CAD can affect your body.

- For your heart muscle to work properly and stay healthy, it needs a constant supply of oxygen- and nutrient-filled blood. That blood is brought to the heart in blood vessels called coronary arteries, which you can see on the surface of the heart in the drawing below.
- In CAD, plaque begins to develop inside the coronary arteries. This fatty, fibrous plaque progressively narrows and blocks the arteries, reducing the amount of blood that can reach the heart muscle.
- When blood flow to the heart muscle becomes severely reduced or completely blocked, a heart attack (or myocardial infarction) may occur because the heart muscle isn't receiving enough oxygen.
- Depending on how severe it is and how long it lasts, this reduced oxygen may cause permanent damage to the muscle cells, or it may kill them. The pain of a heart attack is caused by the injury and death of heart muscle tissue.

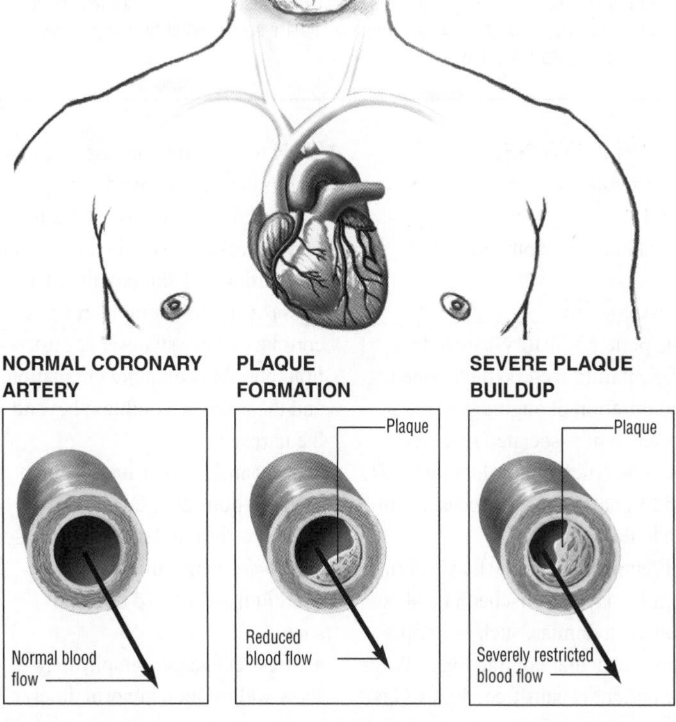

THE ROLE OF GENES IN CAD

Researchers have identified more than 250 genes that may play a role in coronary artery disease (CAD). It commonly results from the combined effects of multiple genes, making it difficult to determine the influence of specific genes on a person's risk for the disease. Here's a review of some of the best understood CAD-related genes.

- **Low-density lipoprotein (LDL) receptor.** This protein removes LDL from the bloodstream. A mutation in this gene is responsible for familial hypercholesterolemia.
- **Apolipoprotein E.** Mutations in this gene, commonly called apo E, also affect blood levels of LDL.
- **Apolipoprotein B-100.** Commonly called apo B-11, this is a component of LDL. Mutations of this gene cause LDL to stay in the blood longer than normal, leading to high LDL levels.
- **Apolipoprotein A.** This glycoprotein combines with LDL to form a particle called Lp(a); it appears as part of the plaque in blood vessels.
- **Methylenetetrahydrofolate reductase (MTHFR).** This enzyme clears homocysteine from the blood; mutations in MTHFR genes may increase homocysteine levels.
- **Cystathionine B-synthase.** Also known as CBS, this enzyme is involved in homocysteine metabolism. Mutations to CBS cause a condition known as homocystinuria, in which homocysteine levels are so high that homocysteine can be detected in urine.

COMPLICATIONS

- Arrhythmias
- MI
- Ischemic cardiomyopathy

DIAGNOSIS

The patient's history—including precipitating factors, the frequency and duration of angina, and the presence of associated risk factors—is crucial in evaluating CAD. Additional diagnostic measures include the following:

- Electrocardiogram (ECG) during angina may show ischemia and possibly arrhythmias, such as premature ventricular contractions. (When the patient is pain-free, the ECG is likely to be normal unless myocardial tissue has infarcted.)
- Treadmill or exercise stress test may provoke chest pain and signs of myocardial ischemia on the ECG.
- Coronary angiography reveals coronary artery stenosis or obstruction, possible collateral circulation, and the arteries' condition beyond the narrowing.
- Myocardial perfusion imaging with thallium-201, Cardiolite, or Myoview during treadmill exercise detects ischemic areas of the myocardium, visualized as "cold spots."
- Stress echocardiography may show wall motion abnormalities.

CORONARY ARTERY SPASM

In coronary artery spasm, a spontaneous, sustained contraction of one or more coronary arteries causes ischemia and dysfunction of the heart muscle. This disorder also causes Prinzmetal's angina and even myocardial infarction in patients with unoccluded coronary arteries. The cause of coronary artery spasm isn't known, but possible contributing factors include:

- an altered flow of calcium into the cell
- intimal hemorrhage into the medial layer of the blood vessel
- hyperventilation
- elevated catecholamine levels
- fatty buildup in vessel lumens.

Signs and symptoms

The major symptom of coronary artery spasm is angina. However, unlike classic angina, this pain commonly occurs spontaneously and may not be related to physical exertion or emotional stress. It's also more severe, usually lasts longer, and may be cyclic, typically occurring every day at the same time. Such ischemic episodes may cause arrhythmias, an altered heart rate, decreased blood pressure and, occasionally, fainting from a reduced cardiac output.

Spasm in the left coronary artery may cause mitral insufficiency, producing a loud systolic murmur and possibly pulmonary edema with dyspnea, crackles, hemoptysis, or sudden death.

Treatment

After diagnosis by coronary angiography and an electrocardiogram (ECG), the patient may receive calcium channel blockers (verapamil [Calan], nifedipine [Procardia], or diltiazem [Cardizem]) to reduce coronary artery spasm and vascular resistance and nitrates (nitroglycerin or isosorbide dinitrate [Isordil]) to relieve chest pain.

When caring for a patient with coronary artery spasm, explain all needed procedures and teach him how to take his medications safely. For calcium antagonist therapy, monitor blood pressure, pulse rate, and ECG patterns to detect arrhythmias. For nifedipine and verapamil therapy, monitor digoxin (Lanoxin) levels and check for evidence of digoxin toxicity. Because nifedipine may cause peripheral and periorbital edema, watch for fluid retention.

Because coronary artery spasm is commonly linked to atherosclerotic disease, advise the patient to stop smoking, avoid overeating, maintain a low-fat diet, use alcohol sparingly, and maintain a balance between exercise and rest.

- Electron-beam computed tomography identifies calcium within arterial plaque; the more calcium seen, the higher the likelihood of CAD.

TREATMENT

The goal of treatment in patients with angina is to either reduce myocardial oxygen demand or increase oxygen supply.

Percutaneous transluminal coronary angioplasty (PTCA) may be performed during cardiac catheterization to compress and crack atherosclerotic plaque, which may be fatty, calcific, fibrous, and thrombotic. PTCA carries a certain risk, but its morbidity is lower than that for surgery. (See *Relieving occlusions with angioplasty*.)

PTCA is indicated for patients who don't have a large myocardial area at risk. For example, patients with collateral circulation protecting large areas commonly have PTCA and stent placement. Patients with multivessel or left main lesions commonly don't unless PTCA is their only option. Extremely torturous or threadlike coronary arteries aren't amenable to percutaneous intervention. Patients with lesions that are older than 3 months or that don't produce angina symptoms also typically don't undergo PTCA.

Balloon angioplasty

Most patients first have balloon angioplasty followed by stent placement. Few patients receive a stent without angioplasty. A stent is a prosthetic, stainless steel,

RELIEVING OCCLUSIONS WITH ANGIOPLASTY

Percutaneous transluminal coronary angioplasty can be used to open an occluded coronary artery without opening the chest—an important advantage over bypass surgery. First, coronary angiography must confirm the presence and location of the arterial occlusion. Then, the practitioner threads a guide catheter through the patient's femoral artery and into the coronary artery under fluoroscopic guidance, as shown at right.

When angiography shows the guide catheter positioned at the occlusion site, the practitioner carefully inserts a smaller double-lumen balloon catheter through the guide catheter and directs the balloon through the occlusion, shown at left. A marked pressure gradient will be obvious.

The practitioner alternately inflates and deflates the balloon until an angiogram verifies successful arterial dilation, shown at right, and the pressure gradient has decreased.

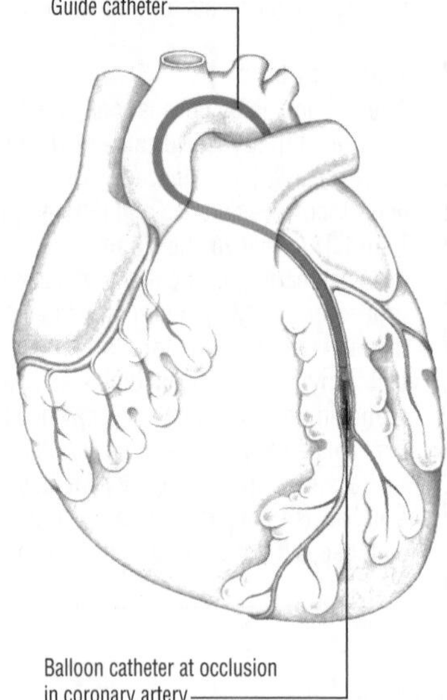

cylindrical coil that's positioned and expanded at the site of stenosis. It provides a framework to hold the artery open by securing the flaps of the tunica media against the arterial wall and by preventing elastic recoil of the stretched and reactive muscular arterial wall. The major disadvantage of angioplasty is restenosis, a result of smooth muscle cells proliferating into the artery's lumen.

Angioplasty and bare metal stent procedures result in a restenosis rate of about 25%. Angioplasty and drug-eluting stents reduce the restenosis rate to about 9%, although some controversy exists about the possible offsetting effect of late thrombosis in drug-eluting stents. Bare metal stents are prone to thrombosis until the stent is endothelialized within 1 month. Therefore, patients require antiplatelet medications, including aspirin and clopidogrel (Plavix), for the 1st month. Drug-eluting stents release the antiproliferative agents sirolimus (Rapamune) or paclitaxel (Taxol). The resultant blocking of smooth muscle cell migration into the arterial lumen also prevents the stent from becoming

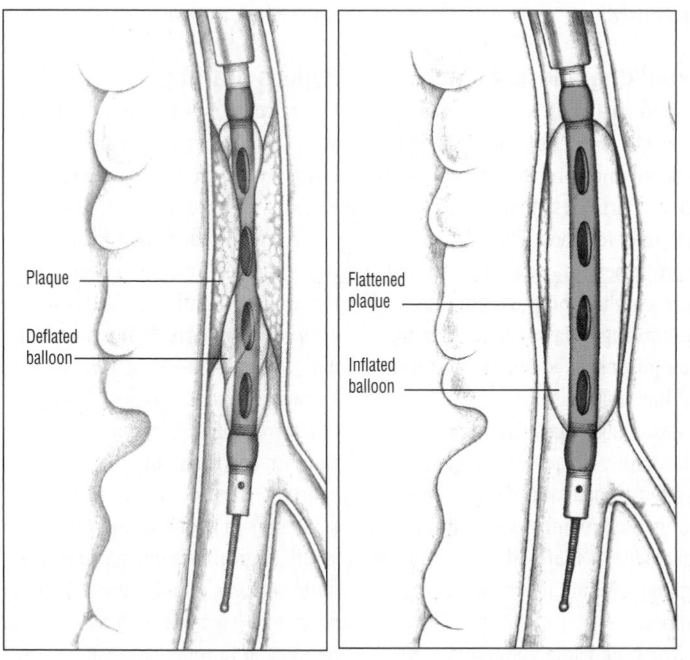

endothelialized. Antiplatelet medications are required for 1 to 3 years following the placement of drug-eluting stents. Most patients receive drug-eluting stents unless they are scheduled for surgery or have a history of nonadherence to medical regimens. Patients who can't adhere to antiplatelet therapy are at high risk for acute thrombotic occlusion of the stent, which is frequently associated with MI and death.

Coronary brachytherapy, which involves delivering beta or gamma radiation into the coronary arteries, was initially used to treat in-stent restenosis. However, insertion of drug-eluting stents into restenosed bare metal stents has become routine. Therefore, brachytherapy is rarely used.

Debulking interventions

Rotational and directional atherectomy and laser angioplasty are types of debulking coronary interventions that comprise less than 3% of coronary interventions. They show no improvement in restenosis rate and have a higher complication rate than balloon angioplasty alone. If used, their purpose is to prepare the arterial lumen for a stent.

Laser angioplasty vaporizes atherosclerotic plaque with an excimer or a hot-tipped laser device. This tool is used mainly to pass through a tight stenosis that will accommodate a guide wire but not an angioplasty balloon.

Rotational atherectomy is used mainly to pulverize calcific plaque using a diamond-chip, studded burr that rotates at high speed. Directional atherectomy shaves plaque and removes it from the artery, allowing for histologic examination. It's best used for short, eccentric lesions.

Transmyocardial revascularization lasers channel into the myocardium so blood can flow from the left ventricular cavity into the myocardium. This was initially performed surgically, from epicardium to endocardium, and later percutaneously, from endocardium to partially through the myocardial wall thickness. It's indicated for patients who are refractory to medical treatment and not surgical candidates. Although it doesn't improve myocardial performance or survival, it may reduce angina.

Bypass grafting

Unprotected multivessel or left main stenosis may require coronary artery bypass grafting (CABG). Patients with blockages in just one or two easily reached arteries may be candidates for a less invasive alternative to traditional CABG surgery called minimally invasive coronary artery bypass surgery, also known as *keyhole surgery.* Instead of sawing open the patient's sternum and spreading the ribs apart, the surgeon makes several small cuts in the torso and inserts small surgical instruments and fiber-optic cameras into the chest. This procedure has a shorter recovery period and fewer postoperative complications.

Drugs

- Nitrates, such as nitroglycerin (given sublingually, orally, transdermally, or topically in ointment form), to decrease preload by dilating coronary arteries and improving blood supply to the heart
- Glycoprotein IIb-IIIa inhibitors and antithrombin drugs to reduce the risk of blood clots
- Beta-adrenergic blockers to lower oxygen demand by decreasing heart rate and cardiac contractility
- Calcium channel blockers to relax the coronary arteries and all systemic arteries, reducing the heart's workload
- Angiotensin-converting enzyme inhibitors to lower preload and afterload
- Diuretics or other drugs to lower blood pressure
- Antiplatelet drugs to minimize platelet aggregation and the risk of coronary occlusion
- Antilipemics to reduce serum cholesterol or triglyceride levels

SPECIAL CONSIDERATIONS

- During angina, monitor the patient's blood pressure and heart rate. Raise the head of the bed to 45 degrees to reduce preload, and give oxygen via nasal cannula to increase myocardial oxygen supply. Take an ECG during anginal episodes and before giving nitroglycerin or other nitrates. Record the duration of pain, the amount of medication needed to relieve it, and accompanying symptoms.
- Keep nitroglycerin available for immediate use. Tell the patient to call immediately whenever he feels chest, arm, or neck pain.
- Before cardiac catheterization, explain the procedure to the patient. Make sure he knows why it's needed, understands the risks, and realizes that it may indicate a need for surgery. Identify allergies, especially to shellfish, iodine, or lidocaine, and premedicate with steroids as indicated.
- After catheterization, review the expected course of treatment with the patient and his family. Maintain complete bed rest, with the head of the bed at no more than 30 degrees for 6 hours after the catheterization. Discourage isometric activities, such as straining, coughing, or laughing, which may jeopardize hemostasis at the femoral access site. Monitor the catheter site for bleeding. Also, check for distal pulses. To counter the dye's diuretic effect, make sure the patient drinks plenty of fluids. Assess the potassium level. Observe for and treat possible contrast dye reactions.
- If the patient is scheduled for surgery, explain the procedure to him and his family. Give them a tour of the intensive care unit and introduce them to the staff.
- After surgery, monitor blood pressure, intake and output, breath sounds, chest tube drainage, and ECG, watching for signs of ischemia and arrhythmias. Be alert for sudden fluid shifts during rewarming, causing hypotension;

PREVENTION

PREVENTING CAD

Because coronary artery disease (CAD) is so widespread, prevention is of great importance. Encourage the patient to restrict calories (if obese) and salt, saturated fats, and cholesterol. This alone will minimize the risk, especially when supplemented with regular exercise. Also, urge the patient to stop smoking and to reduce stress.

Other preventive actions to encourage include:

- control of hypertension with diet, exercise, and stress reduction
- control of elevated serum cholesterol or triglyceride levels with diet, exercise, and antilipemics
- measures to minimize platelet aggregation and the danger of blood clots using aspirin or other antiplatelet drugs.

administer volume expanders quickly. When the intravascular volume is stable, monitor for adventitious breath sounds, follow intake and output, and administer diuretics as ordered to avoid pulmonary edema. Also, observe for and treat chest pain and possible dye reactions. Give vigorous chest physiotherapy and guide the patient in removal of secretions through deep breathing, coughing, and expectoration of mucus.

- Before discharge, stress the need to follow the prescribed drug regimen (antihypertensives, nitrates, antiplatelets, and antilipemics, for example), exercise program, and diet. (See *Preventing CAD*.) Encourage regular, moderate exercise. If needed, refer the patient to a self-help program to stop smoking.

D

Dilated cardiomyopathy

Dilated cardiomyopathy results from extensively damaged myocardial muscle fibers. This disorder interferes with myocardial metabolism and grossly dilates all four chambers of the heart, giving the heart a globular shape. In this disorder, hypertrophy may be present. Dilated cardiomyopathy leads to intractable heart failure, arrhythmias, and emboli. Because this disease isn't usually diagnosed until it's in the advanced stages, the patient's prognosis typically is poor.

CAUSES AND INCIDENCE

The cause of most cardiomyopathies is unknown. (See *Comparing cardiomyopathies,* page 68.) Occasionally, dilated cardiomyopathy results from myocardial destruction by toxic, infectious, or metabolic agents, such as certain viruses, endocrine and electrolyte disorders, and nutritional deficiencies.

Other causes include muscle disorders (myasthenia gravis, progressive muscular dystrophy, and myotonic dystrophy), infiltrative disorders (hemochromatosis and amyloidosis), and sarcoidosis. Cardiomyopathy also may be a complication of alcoholism. In such cases, it may improve with abstinence from alcohol but recurs when the patient resumes drinking.

How viruses induce cardiomyopathy is unclear, but researchers suspect a link between viral myocarditis and subsequent dilated cardiomyopathy, especially after infection with poliovirus, coxsackievirus B, influenza virus, or human immunodeficiency virus.

Metabolic cardiomyopathies are related to endocrine and electrolyte disorders and nutritional deficiencies. Thus, dilated cardiomyopathy may develop in patients with hyperthyroidism, pheochromocytoma, beriberi (thiamine deficiency), kwashiorkor (protein deficiency), or eating disorders. Cardiomyopathy may also result from rheumatic fever, especially among children with myocarditis.

Antepartum or postpartum cardiomyopathy may develop during the last trimester or within months after delivery. Its cause is unknown, but usually it occurs in multiparous women older than age 30, particularly those with malnutrition or preeclampsia. In these patients, cardiomegaly and heart failure may reverse with treatment, allowing a subsequent normal pregnancy. If cardiomegaly persists despite treatment, the prognosis is poor.

COMPARING CARDIOMYOPATHIES

Cardiomyopathies include various structural or functional abnormalities of the ventricles. They're grouped into three main pathophysiologic types—dilated, hypertrophic, and restrictive. These conditions may lead to heart failure by impairing myocardial structure and function.

Normal heart	Dilated cardiomyopathy
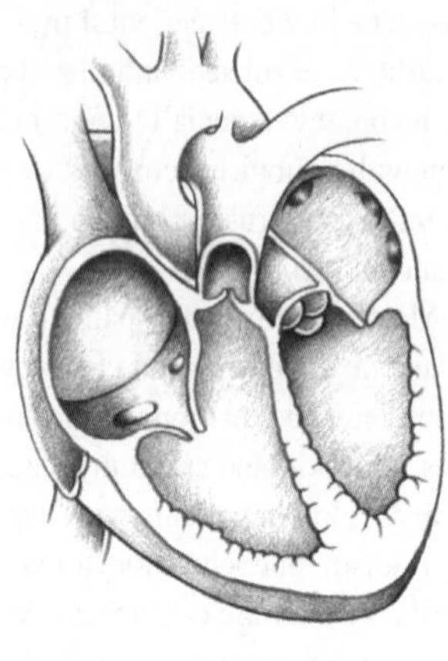	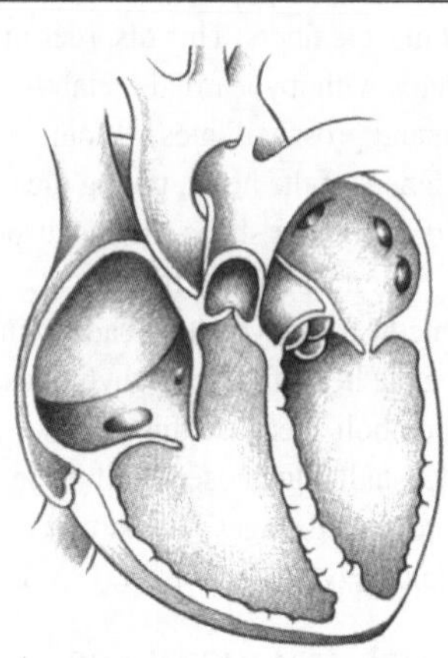
Ventricles	■ Greatly increased chamber size ■ Thinning of left ventricular muscle
Atrial chamber size	■ Increased
Myocardial mass	■ Increased
Ventricular inflow resistance	■ Normal
Contractility	■ Decreased
Possible causes	■ Cardiotoxic effects of drugs or alcohol ■ Chemotherapy ■ Drug hypersensitivity ■ Hypertension ■ Ischemic heart disease ■ Peripartum syndrome related to preeclampsia ■ Valvular disease ■ Viral or bacterial infection

Hypertrophic cardiomyopathy	Restrictive cardiomyopathy
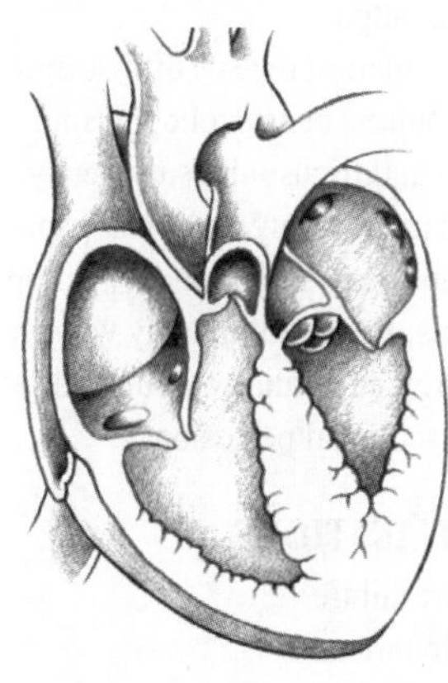	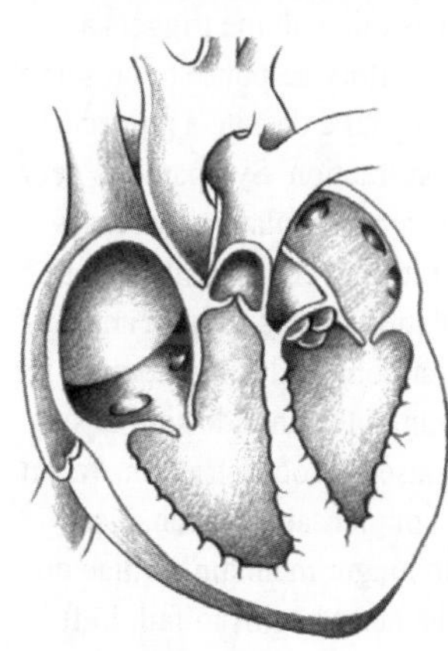
■ Normal right and decreased left chamber size ■ Left ventricular hypertrophy ■ Thickened interventricular septum (hypertrophic obstructive cardiomyopathy [HOCM])	■ Decreased ventricular chamber size ■ Left ventricular hypertrophy
■ Increased on left	■ Increased
■ Increased	■ Normal
■ Increased	■ Increased
■ Increased or decreased	■ Decreased
■ Autosomal dominant trait (HOCM) ■ Hypertension ■ Obstructive valvular disease ■ Thyroid disease	■ Amyloidosis ■ Hemochromatosis ■ Infiltrative neoplastic disease ■ Sarcoidosis

Regardless of the cause, extensive damage to myocardial muscle fibers decreases contractility in the left ventricle. As systolic function declines, stroke volume, ejection fraction, and cardiac output fall. As end-diastolic volumes rise, pulmonary congestion may occur. The elevated end-diastolic volume triggers a compensatory response to preserve stroke volume despite a reduced ejection fraction. Sympathetic nervous system stimulation increases heart rate and contractility. Renal stimulation causes sodium and water retention. And stimulation of the renin-angiotensin-aldosterone system causes vasoconstriction. When these compensatory mechanisms can no longer maintain cardiac output, the heart begins to fail. Left ventricular dilation occurs as venous return and systemic vascular resistance rise. Eventually, the atria also dilate as more work is required to pump blood into the ventricles. Blood pooling in the ventricles increases the risk of emboli.

Dilated cardiomyopathy occurs in 2 of every 100 people and affects all ages and sexes. It's most common in adult men.

SIGNS AND SYMPTOMS

In dilated cardiomyopathy, the heart ejects blood less efficiently than normal. Consequently, a large volume of blood remains in the left ventricle after systole, causing signs of heart failure—both left-sided (shortness of breath, orthopnea, dyspnea on exertion, paroxysmal nocturnal dyspnea, fatigue, dry cough at night) and right-sided (edema, liver engorgement, jugular vein distention).

Dilated cardiomyopathy also produces peripheral cyanosis and sinus tachycardia or atrial fibrillation at rest in some patients because of low cardiac output.

Auscultation reveals diffuse apical impulses, pansystolic murmur (mitral and tricuspid insufficiency from cardiomegaly and weak papillary muscles), and S_3 and S_4 gallop rhythms. Renal failure may worsen as decreased cardiac output leads to decreased renal perfusion.

COMPLICATIONS

- Heart failure
- Arrhythmias
- Emboli
- Ventricular arrhythmias
- Syncope
- Sudden death

DIAGNOSIS

No single test confirms dilated cardiomyopathy. Diagnosis requires elimination of other possible causes of heart failure and arrhythmias. (See *Comparing diagnostic tests in cardiomyopathy,* page 72.)

- An electrocardiogram (ECG) and angiography rule out ischemic heart disease; ECG also may show biventricular hypertrophy, sinus tachycardia, atrial enlargement and, in 20% of patients, atrial fibrillation and bundle-branch block.
- Chest X-ray shows cardiomegaly—usually affecting all

heart chambers—and may show pulmonary congestion, pleural or pericardial effusion, or pulmonary venous hypertension.

- Chest computed tomography scan or echocardiography identifies left ventricular thrombi, global hypokinesia, and the degree of left ventricular dilation.
- Nuclear heart scans, such as multiple-gated acquisition scanning and ventriculography, show heart enlargement, lung congestion, heart failure, and decreased movement or functioning of the heart.

TREATMENT

Therapeutic goals include correcting the underlying causes, improving the heart's pumping ability, reducing cardiac work, and improving cardiac output.

- Cardiomyoplasty, in which the latissimus dorsi muscle is wrapped around the ventricles, helps the ventricle pump blood effectively.
- A cardiomyostimulator can deliver bursts of electrical impulses during systole to contract the muscle.
- An implantable cardioverter-defibrillator may be used to treat ventricular arrhythmias and for prophylaxis (because of the high risk of sudden death in patients with New York Heart Association [NYHA] class III or IV heart failure).
- Cardioversion may be used to convert atrial fibrillation to sinus rhythm.
- Pacemaker insertion can correct arrhythmias.
- A biventricular pacemaker can provide cardiac resynchronization if symptoms continue despite optimal drug therapy, the patient has NYHA class III or IV heart failure, the QRS complex is 0.13 second or longer, or the ejection fraction is 35% or less.
- Revascularization, such as coronary artery bypass graft surgery, may be used if dilated cardiomyopathy is caused by ischemia.
- Valve repair or replacement may be needed if dilated cardiomyopathy is from valve dysfunction.
- Heart transplantation may be used if the patient is unresponsive to medical therapy.
- Lifestyle modifications are necessary, such as smoking cessation; a low-fat, low-sodium diet; physical activity; and abstinence from alcohol.

Drugs

- Angiotensin-converting enzyme (ACE) inhibitors, as first-line therapy, to reduce afterload through vasodilation
- Diuretics taken with an ACE inhibitor to reduce fluid retention
- Digoxin (Lanoxin), if the patient doesn't respond to ACE inhibitor and diuretic therapy, to improve myocardial contractility
- Hydralazine (Apresazide) and isosorbide dinitrate (Isordil) in combination to produce vasodilation
- Beta-adrenergic blockers if the patient has NYHA class II or class III heart failure (see *Classifying heart failure,* page 74)

COMPARING DIAGNOSTIC TESTS IN CARDIOMYOPATHY

The main forms of cardiomyopathy each have unique diagnostic test findings, as shown here.

	Electrocardiography	Echocardiography
Dilated cardiomyopathy	▪ Biventricular hypertrophy ▪ Sinus tachycardia ▪ Atrial enlargement ▪ Atrial and ventricular arrhythmias ▪ Bundle-branch block ▪ ST-segment and T-wave abnormalities	▪ Left ventricular thrombi ▪ Global hypokinesia ▪ Enlarged atria ▪ Left ventricular dilation ▪ Valvular abnormalities (possibly)
Hypertrophic cardiomyopathy	▪ Left ventricular hypertrophy ▪ ST-segment and T-wave abnormalities ▪ Left anterior hemiblock ▪ Q waves in precordial and inferior leads ▪ Ventricular arrhythmias ▪ Atrial fibrillation (possibly)	▪ Symmetrical thickening of the left ventricular wall and intraventricular septum ▪ Left atrial dilation
Hypertrophic obstructive cardiomyopathy	▪ Left ventricular hypertrophy with QRS complexes tallest across midprecordium ▪ ST-segment and T-wave abnormalities ▪ Left-axis deviation ▪ Left atrial abnormality ▪ Supraventricular tachycardia ▪ Ventricular tachycardia	▪ Asymmetrical septal hypertrophy ▪ Anterior movement of the anterior mitral leaflet during systole ▪ Early termination of left ventricular ejection that worsens with dobutamine or nitrate provocation ▪ Mitral insufficiency ▪ Atrial dilation
Restrictive cardiomyopathy	▪ Low voltage ▪ Hypertrophy ▪ Atrioventricular conduction defects ▪ Arrhythmias	▪ Increased left ventricular muscle mass ▪ Normal or reduced left ventricular cavity size ▪ Decreased systolic function ▪ Rules out constrictive pericarditis

Chest X-ray	Cardiac catheterization	Radionuclide studies
▪ Cardiomegaly ▪ Pulmonary congestion ▪ Pulmonary venous hypertension ▪ Pleural or pericardial effusions	▪ Elevated left atrial and left ventricular end-diastolic pressures ▪ Left ventricular enlargement ▪ Mitral and tricuspid incompetence ▪ May identify coronary artery disease as cause	▪ Left ventricular dilation and hypokinesia ▪ Reduced ejection fraction
▪ Cardiomegaly	▪ Elevated ventricular end-diastolic pressure ▪ Mitral insufficiency, hyperdynamic systolic function, and aortic valve pressure gradient if aortic valve is stenotic (possibly)	▪ Reduced left ventricular volume ▪ Increased muscle mass ▪ Ischemia
▪ Normal or mild cardiomegaly	▪ Asymmetrical septal hypertrophy ▪ Early termination of systole with decreased ejection fraction ▪ Outflow tract pressure gradient increasing from apex to just below aortic valve ▪ Mitral insufficiency	▪ Reduced left ventricular volume ▪ Increased septal muscle mass ▪ Septal ischemia
▪ Cardiomegaly ▪ Pericardial effusion ▪ Pulmonary congestion	▪ Reduced systolic function and myocardial infiltration ▪ Increased left ventricular end-diastolic pressure ▪ Rules out constrictive pericarditis	▪ Left ventricular hypertrophy with restricted ventricular filling and reduced ejection fraction

CLASSIFYING HEART FAILURE

The New York Heart Association classification is a standard gauge of heart failure severity based on physical limitations.

Class I: Minimal

- No limitations
- Ordinary physical activity causes no undue fatigue, dyspnea, palpitations, or angina.

Class II: Mild

- Slightly limited physical activity
- Comfortable at rest
- Ordinary physical activity causes fatigue, palpitations, dyspnea, or angina.

Class III: Moderate

- Markedly limited physical activity
- Comfortable at rest
- Less than ordinary activity produces symptoms.

Class IV: Severe

- Unable to perform physical activity without discomfort
- Angina or symptoms of cardiac inefficiency may develop at rest.

- Antiarrhythmics, such as amiodarone (Cordarone), used cautiously to control arrhythmias
- Anticoagulants (controversial) to reduce the risk of emboli

SPECIAL CONSIDERATIONS

In a patient with acute failure:

- Watch for evidence of progressive failure (increasing crackles and dyspnea and increased jugular vein distention) and compromised renal perfusion (oliguria, elevated blood urea nitrogen and creatinine levels, and electrolyte imbalances). Weigh the patient daily.
- If the patient is receiving vasodilators, check his blood pressure and heart rate. If he becomes hypotensive, stop the infusion and give fluids or positive inotropes as ordered.
- If the patient is receiving diuretics, watch for signs of resolving congestion (decreased crackles and dyspnea) or too vigorous diuresis (orthostatic hypotension). Check serum potassium and magnesium levels for hypokalemia and hypomagnesemia, especially if therapy includes digoxin.
- Therapeutic restrictions and an uncertain prognosis usually cause profound anxiety and depression. Offer support, and let the patient express his feelings. Be flexible with visiting hours.
- Before discharge, teach the patient about his illness and its treatment. Emphasize the need to avoid alcohol and smoking, to restrict sodium intake, to watch for weight gain (a gain of 3 lb [1.4 kg] over 1 to 2 days indicates fluid accumulation), and to take digoxin as prescribed and watch for adverse effects (anorexia, nausea, vomiting, yellow vision).
- Encourage family members to learn cardiopulmonary resuscitation.

Disseminated intravascular coagulation

Disseminated intravascular coagulation (DIC) is a life-threatening complication of diseases and conditions that accelerate clotting, causing small blood vessel occlusion, organ necrosis, depletion of circulating clotting factors and platelets, and activation of the fibrinolytic system. This, in turn, can provoke severe hemorrhage. (See *Three mechanisms of DIC,* page 76.)

Clotting in the microcirculation usually affects the kidneys and limbs but may occur in the brain, lungs, pituitary and adrenal glands, and GI mucosa. Other conditions, such as vitamin K deficiency, hepatic disease, and anticoagulant therapy, may cause a similar hemorrhage.

DIC, also called *consumption coagulopathy* or *defibrination syndrome,* usually is an acute condition, but it may be chronic in cancer patients. The prognosis depends on early detection and treatment, the severity of the hemorrhage, and treatment of the underlying disease or condition.

CAUSES AND INCIDENCE

DIC may result from:

- infection, such as gram-negative or gram-positive septicemia; viral, fungal, or rickettsial infection; or protozoal infection
- obstetric complications, such as abruptio placentae, amniotic fluid embolism, a retained dead fetus, septic abortion, or eclampsia
- neoplastic disease, such as acute leukemia, metastatic carcinoma, or aplastic anemia
- disorders that produce necrosis, such as extensive burns and trauma, brain tissue destruction, transplant rejection, or hepatic necrosis
- other factors, such as heatstroke, shock, poisonous snakebite, cirrhosis, fat embolism, incompatible blood transfusion, cardiac arrest, surgery that requires cardiopulmonary bypass, giant hemangioma, severe venous thrombosis, or purpura fulminans.

It isn't clear why such disorders lead to DIC, nor is it certain that they lead to it through a common mechanism. In many patients, DIC is triggered by entry of a foreign protein into the circulation and vascular endothelial injury. Regardless of how DIC begins, the typical accelerated clotting results in generalized activation of prothrombin and a consequent excess of thrombin. Excess thrombin converts fibrinogen to fibrin, producing fibrin clots in the microcirculation. This process consumes large amounts of coagulation factors (especially fibrinogen, prothrombin, platelets, factor V, and factor VIII), causing hypofibrinogenemia, hypoprothrombinemia, thrombocytopenia, and deficiencies of factors V and VIII. Circulating thrombin activates the fibrinolytic system, which lyses fibrin clots into fibrin degradation products (FDPs). The hemorrhage that occurs may

THREE MECHANISMS OF DIC

Disseminated intravascular coagulation (DIC) may develop by three different mechanisms, as outlined here. In all mechanisms, accelerated clotting usually results in excess thrombin, which leads to fibrinolysis, formation of excess fibrin and fibrin degradation products (FDPs) and activation of fibrin-stabilizing factor (factor XIII); consumption of platelet and clotting factors; and, eventually, hemorrhage.

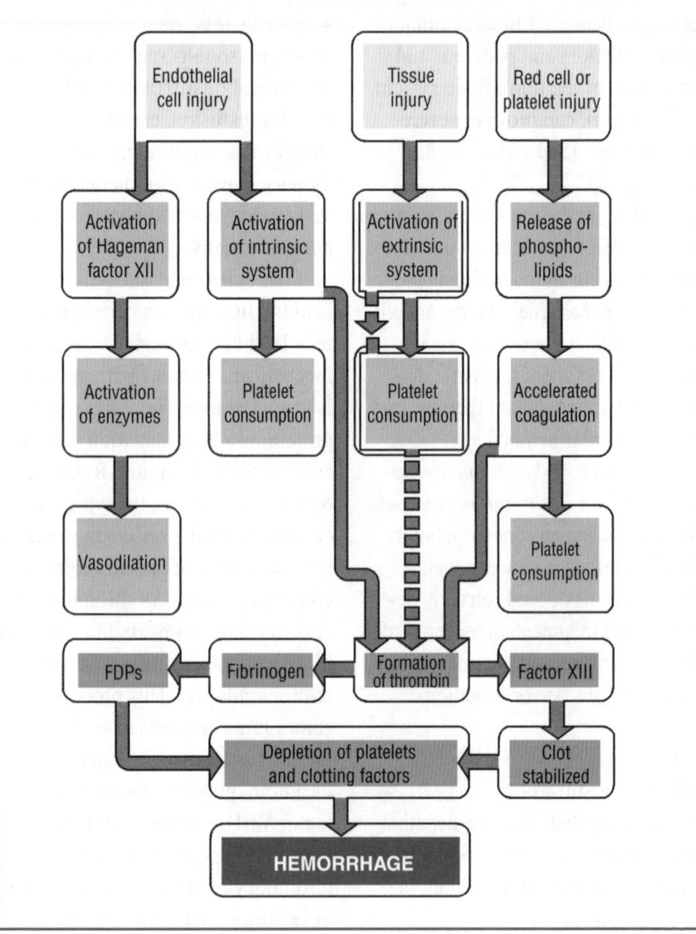

result largely from the anticoagulant activity of FDPs as well as depletion of plasma coagulation factors.

SIGNS AND SYMPTOMS

The most significant feature of DIC is abnormal bleeding with no history of a serious hemorrhagic disorder. Principal signs of such bleeding include cutaneous oozing, petechiae, ecchymoses, and hematomas caused by bleeding into the skin. Bleeding from surgical or I.V. sites and from the GI tract are equally significant signs, as are acrocyanosis (cyanosis of the limbs) and signs of acute tubular necrosis. Related signs, symptoms, and other effects include nausea, vomiting, dyspnea, oliguria, seizures, coma, shock, major organ failure, confusion, epistaxis, hemoptysis, and severe muscle, back, abdominal, and chest pain.

COMPLICATIONS

- Acute tubular necrosis
- Ischemia of the legs, arms, or organs
- Severe bleeding
- Shock
- Multiple organ failure
- Stroke
- Death

DIAGNOSIS

Abnormal bleeding in the absence of a known hematologic disorder suggests DIC, but may be late in the pathophysiologic process. Initial laboratory findings reflect coagulation factor deficiencies, including:

- decreased platelet count (less than 100,000/mm^3)
- decreased fibrinogen level (less than 150 mg/dl).

As the excessive clotting breaks down, hemorrhagic diathesis occurs, and test results reflect coagulation abnormalities, such as:

- prolonged prothrombin time (more than 15 seconds)
- prolonged partial thromboplastin time (more than 60 seconds)
- increased FDPs (commonly more than 45 mcg/ml).

Other supportive data include positive fibrin monomers, decreased levels of factors V and VIII, fragmentation of red blood cells (RBCs), and a decreased hemoglobin (Hb) level (less than 10 g/dl). Assessment of renal status reveals reduced urine output (less than 30 ml/hour) and elevated blood urea nitrogen (more than 25 mg/dl) and serum creatinine (more than 1.3 mg/dl) levels.

A positive D-dimer test (less than 1:8 dilution and decreased levels of factors V and VIII) is specific for DIC. Confirming the diagnosis may be difficult because many of these test results also occur in other disorders (primary fibrinolysis, for example).

TREATMENT

Successful management of DIC requires prompt recognition and adequate treatment of the underlying disorder. Treatment may be supportive when the underlying disorder is self-limiting or highly specific. If the patient isn't bleeding, supportive care alone may reverse DIC. However, bleeding may require delivery of blood, fresh frozen plasma, platelets, or packed RBCs to

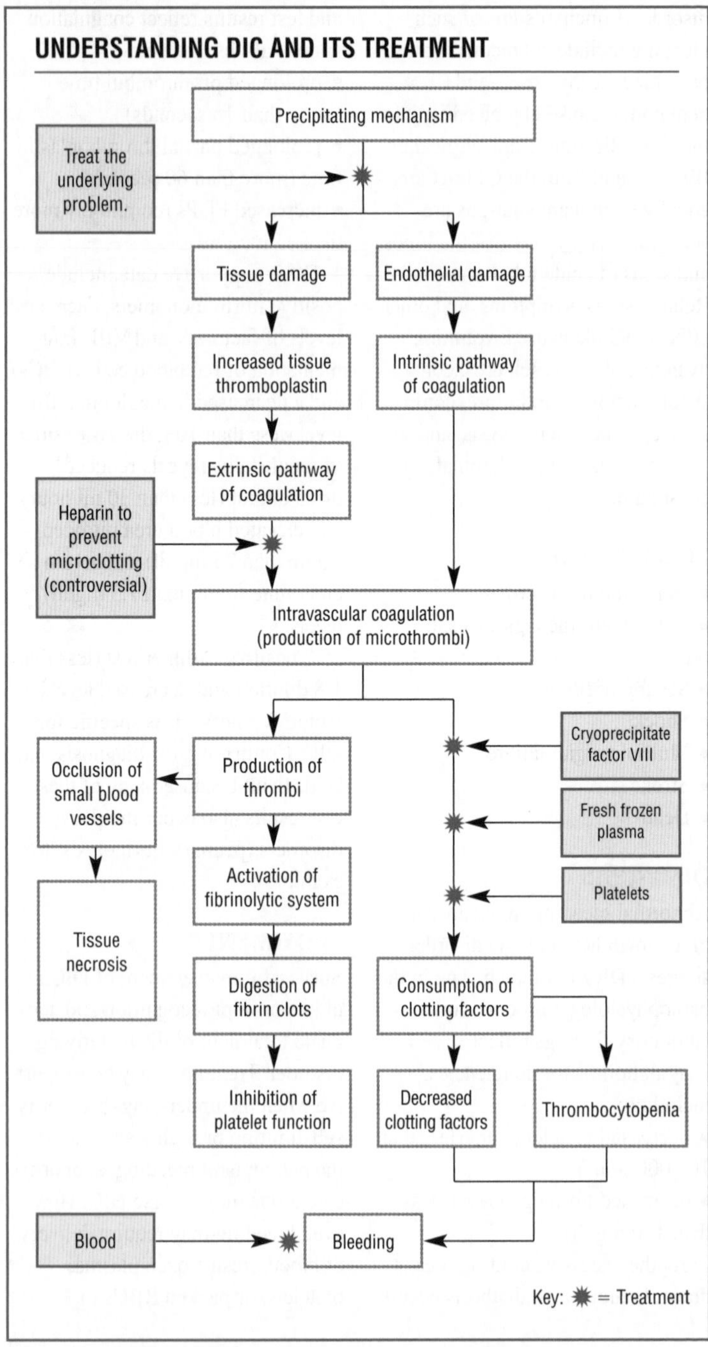
UNDERSTANDING DIC AND ITS TREATMENT
Precipitating mechanism
Treat the underlying problem.
Tissue damage
Endothelial damage
Increased tissue thromboplastin
Intrinsic pathway of coagulation
Extrinsic pathway of coagulation
Heparin to prevent microclotting (controversial)
Intravascular coagulation (production of microthrombi)
Cryoprecipitate factor VIII
Occlusion of small blood vessels
Production of thrombi
Fresh frozen plasma
Activation of fibrinolytic system
Platelets
Tissue necrosis
Digestion of fibrin clots
Consumption of clotting factors
Inhibition of platelet function
Decreased clotting factors
Thrombocytopenia
Blood
Bleeding
Key: = Treatment

support hemostasis. Cryoprecipitates also may be used if fibrinogen is significantly decreased. (See *Understanding DIC and its treatment*.)

Drugs

- Heparin in early stages to prevent microclotting and as a last resort in hemorrhage (controversial in acute DIC after sepsis)

SPECIAL CONSIDERATIONS

Patient care must focus on early recognition of abnormal bleeding, prompt treatment of the underlying disorders, and prevention of further bleeding.

- To avoid dislodging clots and causing fresh bleeding, don't scrub bleeding areas. Use pressure, cold compresses, and topical hemostatic agents to control bleeding.
- To prevent injury, enforce complete bed rest during bleeding episodes. If the patient is agitated, pad the side rails.
- Monitor intake and output hourly in acute DIC, especially when giving blood products. Watch for transfusion reactions and evidence of fluid overload. To measure the amount of blood lost, weigh dressings and linen, and record drainage. Weigh the patient daily, particularly if he has renal involvement.
- Monitor the results of serial blood studies (particularly hematocrit, Hb level, and coagulation times).
- Explain all diagnostic tests and procedures. Allow time for questions.
- Inform the patient's family of his progress. Prepare them for his appearance (I.V. lines, nasogastric tubes, bruises, dried blood). Provide emotional support for the patient and his family. As needed, enlist the aid of a social worker, chaplain, and other members of the health care team in providing such support.

E

Endocarditis

Endocarditis (also known as *infective* or *bacterial endocarditis*) is a bacterial or fungal infection of the endocardium, heart valves, or cardiac prosthesis. Untreated, endocarditis usually is fatal. With proper treatment, 70% of patients recover. The prognosis is worst when endocarditis involves a prosthetic valve or when it causes severe valve damage, leading to insufficiency and heart failure.

CAUSES AND INCIDENCE

At one time, rheumatic heart disease was the leading risk factor for endocarditis. Nowadays, however, most cases of endocarditis occur in I.V. drug abusers, patients with prosthetic heart valves, and those with mitral valve prolapse (especially men with systolic murmurs). Other predisposing conditions include coarctation of the aorta, tetralogy of Fallot, subaortic and valvular aortic stenosis, ventricular septal defects, pulmonary stenosis, Marfan syndrome, degenerative heart disease (especially calcific aortic stenosis) and, rarely, a syphilitic aortic valve. Some patients with endocarditis have no underlying heart disease.

Infecting organisms differ among these groups. In patients with native valve endocarditis who aren't I.V. drug abusers, causative organisms usually include—in order of frequency—streptococci (especially *Streptococcus viridans*), staphylococci, and enterococci. Although many other bacteria may cause the disorder, fungal causes are rare in this group. The mitral valve is usually involved, followed by the aortic valve.

In patients who are I.V. drug abusers, *Staphylococcus aureus* is the most common infecting organism. Less commonly, streptococci, enterococci, gram-negative bacilli, or fungi cause the disorder. The tricuspid valve is involved most often, followed by the aortic and then the mitral valve.

In patients with prosthetic valve endocarditis, early cases (those that develop within 60 days of valve insertion) are usually from staphylococcal infection. However, gram-negative aerobic organisms, fungi, streptococci, enterococci, or diphtheroids also may cause the disorder. The course is usually fulminant and fatal. Late cases (occurring after 60 days) are similar to native valve endocarditis.

Regardless of the cause, bacteremia—even transient bacteremia after dental or urogenital procedures—introduces the pathogen into the bloodstream. Fibrin and platelets aggregate on valve tissue and engulf circulating bacteria or fungi, producing vegetative growths on the heart valves, endocardial lining of a heart chamber, or endothelium of a blood vessel. (See *Degenerative changes in endocarditis*.)

Such vegetations may cover the valve surfaces, causing ulceration and necrosis. They also may extend to the chordae tendineae, leading to their rupture and subsequent valvular insufficiency. Ultimately, they may embolize to the spleen, kidneys, central nervous system (CNS), and lungs.

In the United States, endocarditis affects 2 to 4 people out of every 100,000 each year. Men are twice as likely as women to acquire this infection, and the mean age of onset is 50. Mortality rates vary with the infecting organism; death is more likely with increased age, infection of the aortic valve, heart failure and underlying heart disease, and CNS complications.

SIGNS AND SYMPTOMS

Early clinical features of endocarditis are usually nonspecific and include malaise, weakness, fatigue, weight loss, anorexia, arthralgia, night sweats, chills, valvular insufficiency and, in 90% of patients, an intermittent fever that may recur for weeks. Organisms of high pathogenicity, such as *S. aureus,* may cause a more acute onset.

DEGENERATIVE CHANGES IN ENDOCARDITIS

In endocarditis, fibrin and platelets are deposited at sites of infection, forming endocardial growths (called *vegetations*) such as those shown here.

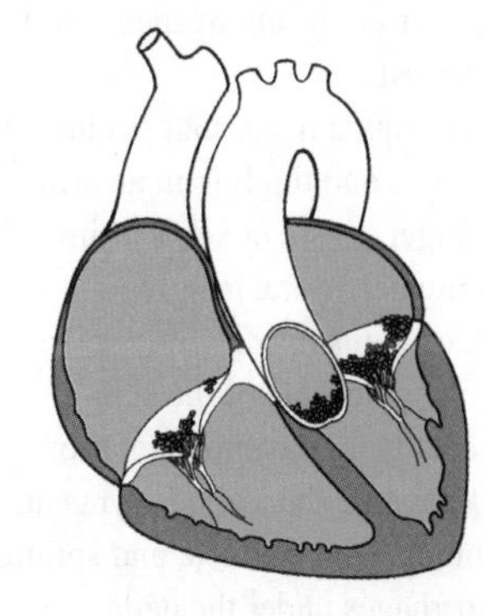

Endocarditis commonly causes a loud, regurgitant murmur typical of the underlying heart lesion. A suddenly changing murmur or the discovery of a new murmur with fever is a classic physical sign of endocarditis.

In about 30% of patients, embolization from vegetating lesions or diseased valvular tissue may produce typical features of splenic, renal, cerebral, or pulmonary infarction or of peripheral vascular occlusion:

- for splenic infarction, pain in the left upper quadrant radiating to the left shoulder and abdominal rigidity
- for renal infarction, hematuria, pyuria, flank pain, and decreased urine output

• for cerebral infarction, hemiparesis, aphasia, or other neurologic deficits
• for pulmonary infarction (most common in right-sided endocarditis, which commonly occurs among I.V. drug abusers and after cardiac surgery), cough, pleuritic pain, pleural friction rub, dyspnea, and hemoptysis
• for peripheral vascular occlusion, numbness and tingling in an arm, leg, finger, or toe or signs of impending peripheral gangrene.

Other signs may include splenomegaly; petechiae of the skin (especially on the upper anterior trunk) and the buccal, pharyngeal, or conjunctival mucosa; and splinter hemorrhages under the nails. Rarely, endocarditis produces Osler's nodes (tender, raised, subcutaneous lesions on the fingers or toes), Roth's spots (hemorrhagic areas with white centers on the retina), and Janeway lesions (purplish macules on the palms or soles).

COMPLICATIONS

• Left-sided heart failure
• Valvular stenosis or insufficiency
• Myocardial erosion
• Death
• Aortic root abscesses
• Myocardial abscesses
• Pericarditis
• Cardiac arrhythmias
• Meningitis
• Cerebral emboli
• Brain abscesses
• Septic pulmonary infarcts
• Arthritis
• Glomerulonephritis
• Acute renal failure

DIAGNOSIS

Three or more blood cultures in a 24- to 48-hour period (each from a separate venipuncture) identify the causative organism in up to 90% of patients. Blood cultures should be drawn from three different sites with 1 hour between each draw. The remaining 10% may have negative blood cultures, possibly suggesting fungal infection or infections that are difficult to diagnose, such as with *Haemophilus parainfluenzae.*

Other abnormal but nonspecific laboratory test results include:
• normal or elevated white blood cell count
• abnormal histiocytes (macrophages)
• elevated erythrocyte sedimentation rate
• normocytic, normochromic anemia (in 70% to 90% of patients)
• proteinuria and microscopic hematuria (in about 50% of patients)
• positive serum rheumatoid factor (in about 50% of patients after endocarditis is present for 3 to 6 weeks).

Echocardiography (particularly transesophageal) may identify valve damage. Electrocardiography may show atrial fibrillation and other arrhythmias that accompany valvular disease.

TREATMENT

The goal of treatment is to eradicate the infecting organism with appropriate antimicrobial therapy, which should start promptly and continue for 4 to 6 weeks. Selection of an antibiotic is based on identifying the infecting organism and on sensitivity studies. While awaiting results, or if blood cultures are negative, empiric antimicrobial therapy is based on the likely infecting organism.

Supportive treatment includes bed rest and sufficient fluid intake. Severe valvular damage, especially aortic or mitral insufficiency, may require corrective surgery if refractory heart failure develops or if an infected prosthetic valve must be replaced.

Drugs

- Antimicrobial therapy to eradicate the infecting organism. (First-line therapy usually includes penicillin and an aminoglycoside, usually gentamicin.)
- Aspirin to treat fever and aches

> **PREVENTION**
>
> **PREVENTING ENDOCARDITIS**
>
> For any patient with an increased risk of endocarditis—someone with a valvular defect, a murmur, or another predisposing factor—take these preventive steps:
>
> - Make sure the patient receives prophylactic antibiotics before dental procedures.
> - Instruct the patient to practice good hygiene, including thoroughly washing his hands, washing fruits and vegetables, and thoroughly cooking all food to avoid introducing organisms into his system.
> - Urge the patient to maintain his oral health through daily toothbrushing and flossing and having regular dental checkups.
> - Urge the patient to notify his family practitioner, his dentist, and other health care providers that he has a condition that increases his risk of endocarditis.

SPECIAL CONSIDERATIONS

- Before giving antibiotics, obtain a patient history of allergies. Give antibiotics on time to maintain consistent antibiotic blood levels.
- Watch for signs of infiltration or inflammation at the venipuncture site, possible complications of long-term I.V. drug administration. To reduce the risk of these complications, rotate venous access sites.
- Monitor the patient's renal status (blood urea nitrogen level, creatinine clearance, urine output) to check for evidence of renal emboli or drug toxicity.
- Observe the patient for evidence of heart failure, such as dyspnea, tachypnea, tachycardia, crackles, jugular vein distention, edema, and weight gain.
- Provide reassurance by teaching the patient and his family about endocarditis and the need for prolonged treatment. (See *Preventing Endocarditis.*) Tell them to watch closely for fever, anorexia, and other

signs of relapse about 2 weeks after treatment stops. Suggest quiet diversionary activities to prevent excessive physical exertion.

- Make sure susceptible patients understand the need for prophylactic antibiotics before, during, and after dental work, childbirth, and genitourinary, GI, or gynecologic procedures.
- Teach the patient how to recognize signs and symptoms of endocarditis, and tell him to notify a practitioner at once if they occur.

F-G

Femoral and popliteal aneurysms

Femoral and popliteal aneurysms (sometimes called *peripheral arterial aneurysms*) are the end result of progressive atherosclerotic changes in the medial layer of these major peripheral arteries. These aneurysms may be fusiform (spindle-shaped) or saccular (pouchlike); the fusiform type is three times more common. They may be singular or multiple segmental lesions, commonly affecting both legs, and they may accompany other arterial aneurysms in the abdominal aorta or iliac arteries. (See *Arteries of the leg,* page 86.)

CAUSES AND INCIDENCE

Femoral and popliteal aneurysms usually result from atherosclerosis and congenital weakness in the arterial wall. They also may result from trauma (blunt or penetrating), bacterial infection, or peripheral vascular reconstructive surgery (which causes "suture line" aneurysms or false aneurysms [also called *pseudoaneurysm*]).

With atherosclerotic changes, fatty, fibrous plaques narrow the lumen of the blood vessel. Narrowing of the lumen reduces the volume of blood flow, causing arterial insufficiency to the affected area.

This condition usually occurs in men older than age 50. The clinical course is usually progressive, eventually ending in thrombosis, embolization, and gangrene. Elective surgery before complications arise greatly improves the prognosis.

SIGNS AND SYMPTOMS

A popliteal aneurysm may cause pain in the popliteal space if it's large enough to compress the medial popliteal nerve. It may cause edema and venous distention below the aneurysm if it compresses the vein. Femoral and popliteal aneurysms can produce symptoms of severe ischemia in the leg or foot from acute thrombosis in the aneurysmal sac, embolization of mural thrombus fragments and, rarely, rupture. Symptoms of acute aneurysmal thrombosis include severe pain, loss of pulse and color, coldness in the affected leg or foot, and gangrene. Distal petechial hemorrhages may develop from aneurysmal emboli.

COMPLICATIONS

- Thrombosis or distal embolization
- Gangrene requiring amputation
- Rupture and bleeding (rare)

DIAGNOSIS

Diagnosis of a femoral or popliteal aneurysm usually is confirmed

ARTERIES OF THE LEG

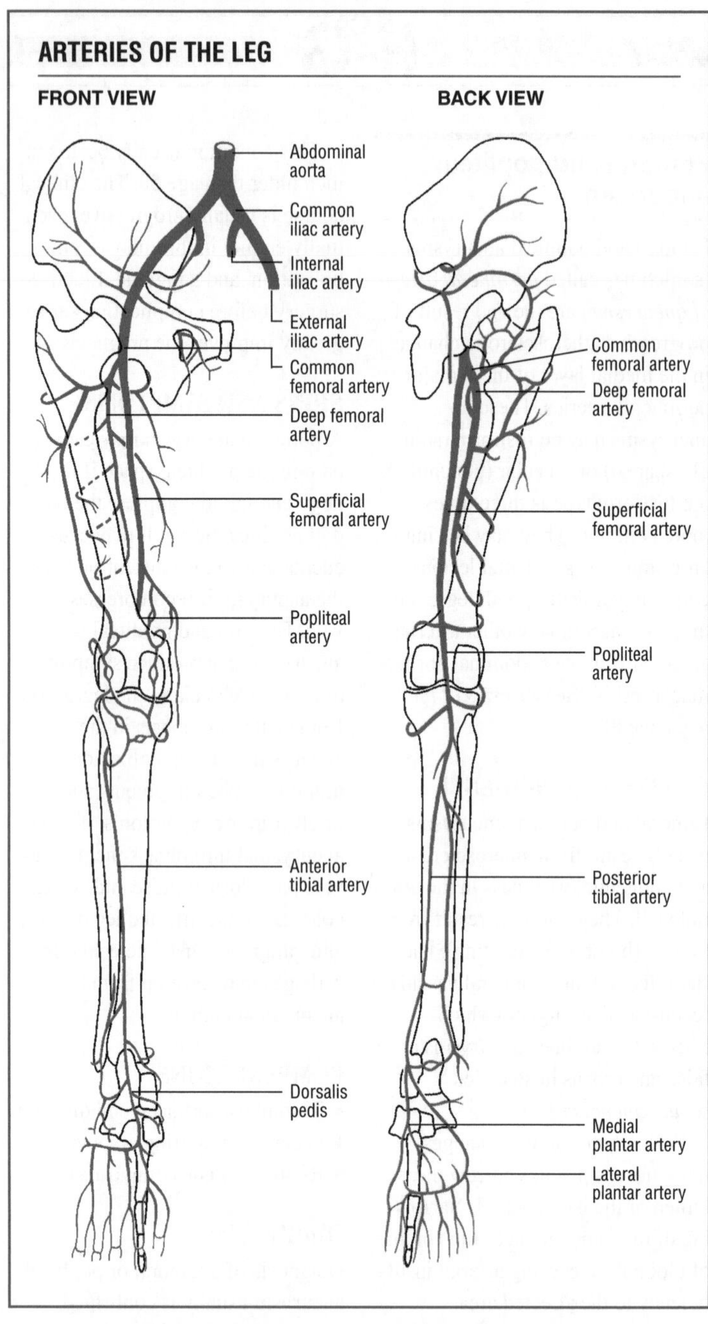
FRONT VIEW
BACK VIEW
Abdominal aorta
Common iliac artery
Internal iliac artery
External iliac artery
Common femoral artery
Deep femoral artery
Superficial femoral artery
Popliteal artery
Anterior tibial artery
Dorsalis pedis
Common femoral artery
Deep femoral artery
Superficial femoral artery
Popliteal artery
Posterior tibial artery
Medial plantar artery
Lateral plantar artery

when bilateral palpation reveals a pulsating mass above or below the inguinal ligament or within the popliteal fossa. When thrombosis has occurred, palpation reveals a firm, nonpulsating mass.

- Duplex ultrasound may be needed in doubtful situations.
- Duplex ultrasound may be helpful in determining the size and blood flow characteristics of a popliteal or femoral artery. Ultrasound can reveal the presence of mural thrombus.
- Computed tomography or magnetic resonance imaging scans also can confirm the presence of a peripheral aneurysm.

TREATMENT

Femoral and popliteal aneurysms require surgical bypass and reconstruction of the artery, usually using an autogenous saphenous vein graft or a synthetic graft. An endovascular stent graft may also be used. Arterial occlusion that causes severe ischemia and gangrene may require leg amputation.

Drugs

- Thrombolytics to dissolve clots in preparation for bypass surgery
- Prophylactic antibiotics or anticoagulants before surgery

SPECIAL CONSIDERATIONS

Before corrective surgery

- Assess and record circulatory status, noting the location and quality of peripheral pulses in the affected arm or leg.
- Administer prophylactic antibiotics or anticoagulants as ordered.
- Discuss postoperative procedures, and review the explanation of the surgery.

After arterial surgery

- Monitor the patient carefully for early evidence of thrombosis or graft occlusion (loss of pulse, decreased skin temperature and sensation, and severe pain) and infection (fever).
- Palpate distal pulses at least every hour for the first 24 hours and then as ordered. Correlate these findings with preoperative circulatory assessment. Mark the sites on the patient's skin where pulses are palpable or arterial Doppler signals are detected to facilitate repeated checks.
- Help the patient walk soon after surgery to prevent venostasis and possible thrombus formation.

Preparing for discharge

- Tell the patient to immediately report the recurrence of symptoms because the saphenous vein graft replacement can fail or another aneurysm may develop.
- Explain to a patient with a popliteal artery resection that swelling may persist for some time. If antiembolism stockings are ordered, make sure they fit properly and teach the patient how to apply them. Warn against wearing constrictive clothing.

• If the patient is receiving anticoagulants, suggest measures to prevent bleeding such as using an electric razor. Tell him to report evidence of bleeding (bleeding gums, tarry stools, easy bruising) immediately. Explain the importance of follow-up blood studies to monitor anticoagulant therapy. Warn the patient to avoid traumatic injuries, tobacco, and aspirin.

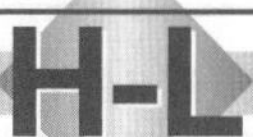

Heart failure

Heart failure is a term used to describe the heart's inability to pump enough blood to the body's tissues. This inability typically results from a complex set of interlinked causes and effects in which impaired pump performance (diminished cardiac output) leads to abnormal circulatory congestion.

Heart failure may be classified according to the side of the heart affected (left- or right-sided failure) or by the cardiac cycle involved (systolic or diastolic dysfunction). Usually, pump failure occurs in a damaged left ventricle (left-sided heart failure), but it may occur in the right ventricle (right-sided heart failure), either as a primary disorder or as a result of left-sided heart failure. Sometimes, left- and right-sided heart failure develop simultaneously. (See *What happens in heart failure,* page 90.)

Congestion of systemic venous circulation (from left-sided heart failure) may result in peripheral edema or hepatomegaly. Congestion of the pulmonary circulation (from right-sided heart failure) may cause pulmonary edema, a life-threatening emergency. Although heart failure may be acute (as a direct result of myocardial infarction [MI]), it usually is a chronic disorder associated with sodium and water retention by the kidneys. Advances in diagnostic and therapeutic techniques have greatly improved the outlook for patients with heart failure, but the prognosis still depends on the underlying cause and its response to treatment.

CAUSES AND INCIDENCE

Heart failure may be caused by a primary abnormality of the heart muscle (such as infarction), by inadequate myocardial perfusion (as from coronary artery disease), or from cardiomyopathy. (See *Causes of heart failure,* page 92.) Other causes include:

- diastolic dysfunction, preserved ejection fraction, impairment of ventricular filling by diminished relaxation or reduced compliance in hypertrophic cardiomyopathy, myocardial hypertrophy, and pericardial restriction
- mechanical disturbances in ventricular filling during diastole when there's too little blood for the ventricle to pump, as in mitral stenosis secondary to rheumatic heart disease or constrictive pericarditis and atrial fibrillation
- systolic hemodynamic disturbances, such as excessive cardiac workload due to volume overloading or pressure overload that limit the heart's pumping ability. These

WHAT HAPPENS IN HEART FAILURE

Heart failure develops when cardiac output is inadequate to meet the body's needs. You can trace the pathophysiology of heart failure using this flowchart.

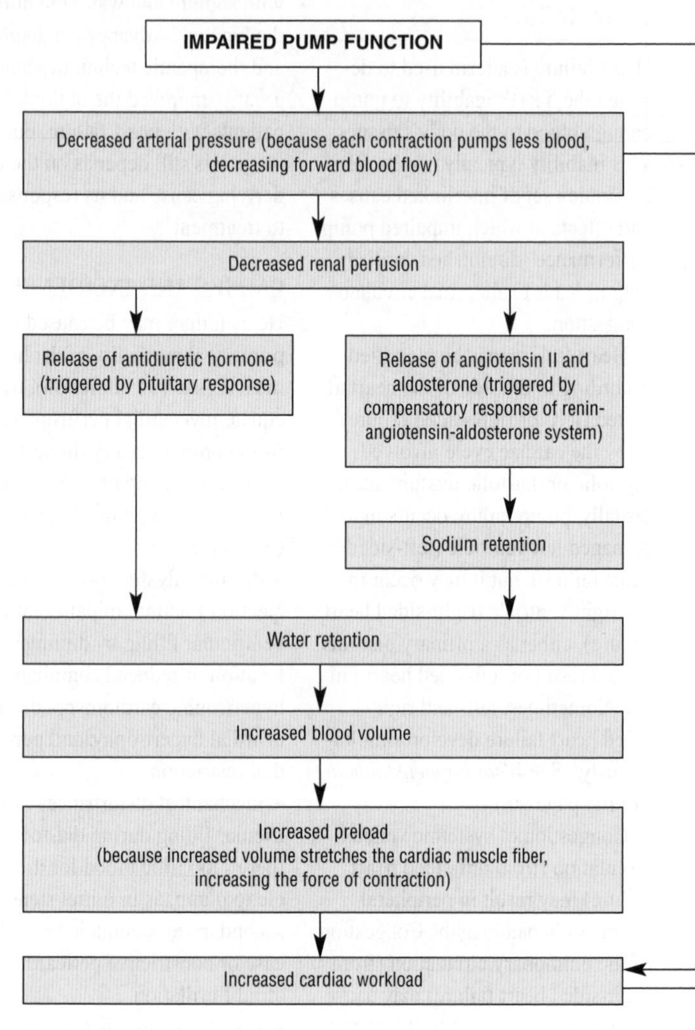

disturbances can result from mitral or aortic insufficiency, which causes volume overloading, and aortic stenosis or systemic hypertension, which result in increased resistance to ventricular emptying. (See *Left-sided and right-sided heart failure,* page 93.)

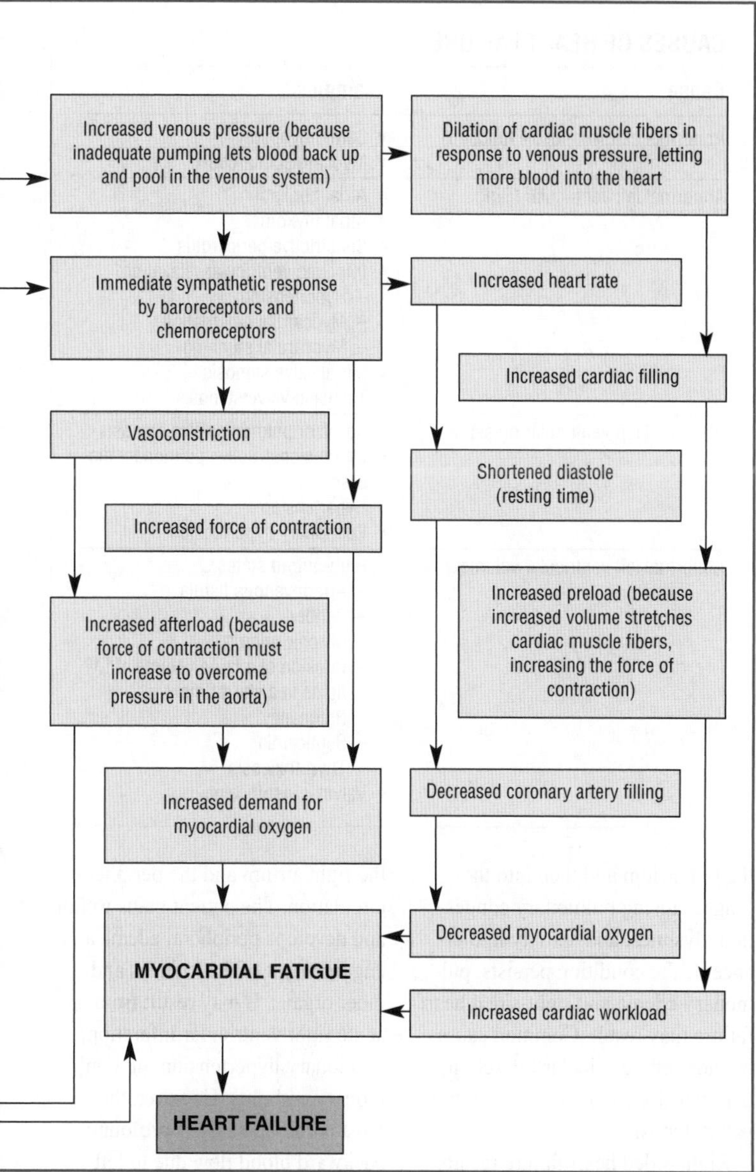

Left-sided and right-sided

Left-sided heart failure occurs as a result of ineffective left ventricular contractile function. As the pumping ability of the left ventricle fails, cardiac output falls. Blood is no longer effectively pumped out into the body and instead backs up into

CAUSES OF HEART FAILURE

Cause	Examples
Abnormal cardiac muscle function	■ Cardiomyopathy ■ Myocardial infarction
Abnormal left ventricular filling	■ Atrial fibrillation ■ Atrial myxoma ■ Constrictive pericarditis ■ Impaired ventricular relaxation: – Hypertension – Myocardial hibernation – Myocardial stunning ■ Mitral valve stenosis ■ Tricuspid valve stenosis
Abnormal left ventricular pressure	■ Aortic or pulmonic valve stenosis ■ Chronic obstructive pulmonary disease ■ Hypertension ■ Pulmonary hypertension
Abnormal left ventricular volume	■ High-output states: – Arteriovenous fistula – Beriberi – Chronic anemia – Infusion of a large volume of I.V. fluids in a short time – Pregnancy – Septicemia – Thyrotoxicosis ■ Valvular insufficiency

the left atrium and then into the lungs, causing pulmonary congestion, dyspnea, and activity intolerance. If the condition persists, pulmonary edema and right-sided heart failure may result. Common causes include left ventricular infarction, hypertension, and aortic and mitral valve stenosis.

Right-sided heart failure results from ineffective right ventricular contractile function. Consequently, blood isn't pumped effectively through the right ventricle to the lungs, causing blood to back up into the right atrium and the peripheral circulation. The patient gains weight and develops peripheral edema and engorgement of the kidneys and other organs. It may result from an acute right ventricular infarction, pulmonary hypertension, or a pulmonary embolus. However, the most common cause is profound backward blood flow due to left-sided heart failure.

Systolic and diastolic

Systolic dysfunction occurs when the left ventricle can't pump enough

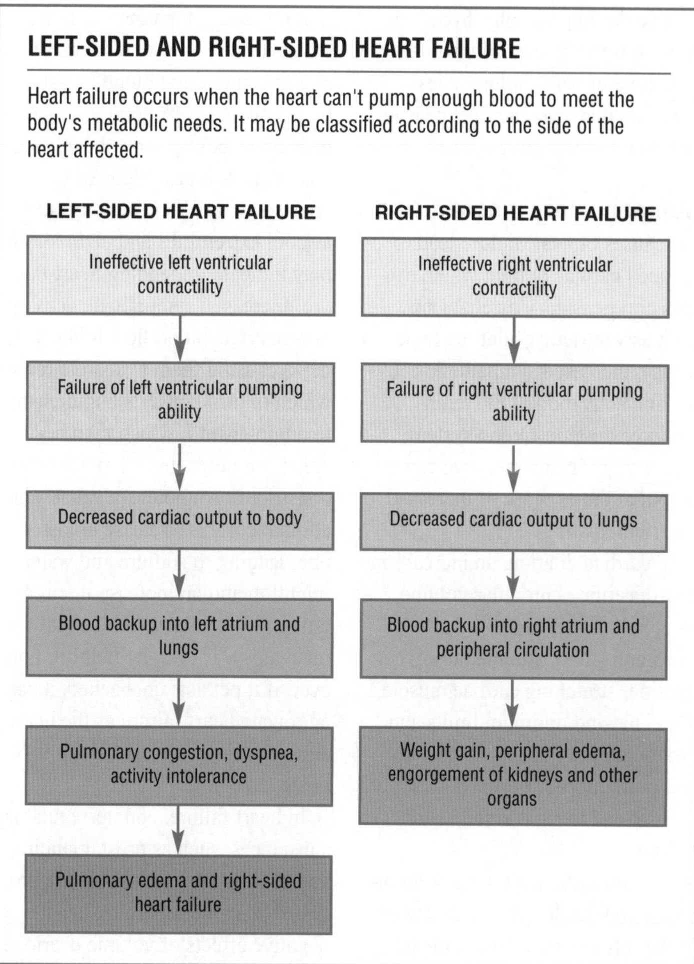

blood out to the systemic circulation during systole and the ejection fraction falls. Consequently, blood backs up into the pulmonary circulation and pressure increases in the pulmonary venous system. Cardiac output falls; weakness, fatigue, and shortness of breath may occur. Causes of systolic dysfunction include MI and dilated cardiomyopathy.

LEFT-SIDED AND RIGHT-SIDED HEART FAILURE
Heart failure occurs when the heart can't pump enough blood to meet the body's metabolic needs. It may be classified according to the side of the heart affected.
LEFT-SIDED HEART FAILURE
Ineffective left ventricular contractility
Failure of left ventricular pumping ability
Decreased cardiac output to body
Blood backup into left atrium and lungs
Pulmonary congestion, dyspnea, activity intolerance
Pulmonary edema and right-sided heart failure
RIGHT-SIDED HEART FAILURE
Ineffective right ventricular contractility
Failure of right ventricular pumping ability
Decreased cardiac output to lungs
Blood backup into right atrium and peripheral circulation
Weight gain, peripheral edema, engorgement of kidneys and other organs

Diastolic dysfunction occurs when the ability of the left ventricle to relax and fill during diastole is reduced and the stroke volume falls. Therefore, higher volumes are needed in the ventricles to maintain cardiac output. Consequently, pulmonary congestion and peripheral edema develop. Diastolic dysfunction may occur as a result of left ventricular hvpertrophy, hypertension, or restrictive cardiomyopathy. This type of heart failure is less common than systolic dysfunction, and its treatment isn't as clear.

Compensatory mechanisms

All causes of heart failure lead to reduced cardiac output, which triggers compensatory mechanisms, such as ventricular dilation, hypertrophy, increased sympathetic activity, and activation of the renin-angiotensin-aldosterone system. These mechanisms improve cardiac output at the expense of increased ventricular work.

In cardiac dilation, an increase in end-diastolic ventricular volume (preload) causes increased stroke work and stroke volume during contraction, stretching cardiac muscle fibers beyond optimum limits and producing pulmonary congestion and pulmonary hypertension, which in turn lead to right-sided heart failure.

In ventricular hypertrophy, an increase in muscle mass or diameter of the left ventricle allows the heart to pump against increased resistance (impedance) to the outflow of blood. This increased muscle mass also increases myocardial oxygen requirements. An increase in ventricular diastolic pressure necessary to fill the enlarged ventricle may compromise diastolic coronary blood flow, limiting the oxygen supply to the ventricle and causing ischemia and impaired muscle contractility.

Increased sympathetic activity occurs as a response to decreased cardiac output and blood pressure by enhancing peripheral vascular resistance, contractility, heart rate, and venous return. Signs of increased sympathetic activity, such as cool extremities and clamminess, may indicate impending heart failure. Increased sympathetic activity also restricts blood flow to the kidneys, causing them to secrete renin, which in turn converts angiotensin to angiotensin I, which then becomes angiotensin II, a potent vasoconstrictor. Angiotensin causes the adrenal cortex to release aldosterone, leading to sodium and water retention and an increase in circulating blood volume. This renal mechanism is initially helpful; however, if it persists unchecked, it can aggravate heart failure as the heart struggles to pump against the increased volume.

In heart failure, counterregulatory substances, such as prostaglandins and atrial natriuretic factor, are produced in an attempt to reduce the negative effects of volume overload and vasoconstriction caused by the compensatory mechanisms.

The kidneys release the prostaglandins prostacyclin and prostaglandin E, which are potent vasodilators. These vasodilators also act to reduce volume overload produced by the renin-angiotensin-aldosterone system by inhibiting sodium and water reabsorption by the kidneys.

Atrial natriuretic factor is a hormone secreted mainly by the atria in response to stimulation of the stretch receptors in the atria caused by excess fluid volume. B-type natriuretic factor (BNP) is secreted by the ventricles because of fluid volume overload. These natriuretic factors work to counteract the negative effects of sympathetic nervous system stimulation and the renin-angiotensin-aldosterone system by producing vasodilation and diuresis. (See *How heart failure affects the body.*)

Chronic heart failure may worsen as a result of respiratory tract infections, pulmonary embolism, stress, increased sodium or water intake, or failure to adhere to the prescribed treatment regimen.

Heart failure affects about 2 of every 100 people ages 27 to 74. It becomes more common with advancing age.

HOW HEART FAILURE AFFECTS THE BODY

This summary highlights the effects of heart failure on major body systems and the multidisciplinary care it requires.

Cardiovascular system

- In left-sided heart failure, the pumping ability of the left ventricle fails and cardiac output falls. Blood backs up into the right atrium.
- In right-sided heart failure, the right ventricle becomes stressed and hypertrophies, leading to increased conduction time and arrhythmias.

Respiratory system

- As a result of pump failure, blood backs up into the right atrium and then into the lungs, causing pulmonary congestion.

GI system

- Congestion of peripheral tissues leads to GI tract congestion and anorexia, GI distress, and weight loss.
- Liver failure may result from blood backing up into the peripheral circulation and subsequent engorgement of organs.

Renal system

- With right-sided heart failure, blood backs up into the right atrium and the peripheral circulation. The patient gains weight and develops peripheral edema and engorgement of the kidneys and other organs.

Collaborative management

Multidisciplinary care is needed to determine the underlying cause and precipitating factors of heart failure, and it may include the expertise of a respiratory therapist, dietitian, and physical therapist. If the patient has coronary artery disease, severe limitations, or repeated hospitalizations despite maximal medical treatment, he may need surgery. He also may need social services to help him transition back home after the acute situation is resolved.

SIGNS AND SYMPTOMS

Left-sided heart failure primarily produces pulmonary signs and symptoms; right-sided heart failure, primarily systemic signs and symptoms. However, heart failure commonly affects both sides of the heart.

Clinical signs of left-sided heart failure include dyspnea, orthopnea, crackles, possible wheezing, hypoxia, respiratory acidosis, cough, cyanosis or pallor, palpitations, arrhythmias, elevated blood pressure, and pulsus alternans.

Clinical signs of right-sided heart failure include dependent peripheral edema, hepatomegaly, splenomegaly, jugular vein distention, ascites, slow weight gain, arrhythmias, positive hepatojugular reflex, abdominal distention, nausea, vomiting, anorexia, weakness, fatigue, dizziness, and syncope.

COMPLICATIONS

- Pulmonary edema
- Acute renal failure
- Arrhythmias
- Multi-organ failure
- MI

DIAGNOSIS

- Electrocardiography may reflect heart strain or enlargement, ischemia, or previous MI. It may also reveal atrial enlargement, tachycardia, and extrasystoles.
- Chest X-ray shows increased pulmonary vascular markings, interstitial edema, or pleural effusion and cardiomegaly.
- Pulmonary artery pressure monitoring typically demonstrates elevated pulmonary artery and pulmonary artery wedge pressures, left ventricular end-diastolic pressure in left-sided heart failure, and elevated right atrial pressure or central venous pressure in right-sided heart failure.
- BNP is a neuro-hormone produced predominantly by the heart ventricle and is released in response to blood volume expansion or pressure overload. Blood concentrations of BNP greater than 100 pg/ml are an accurate predictor of heart failure. (See *Linking BNP levels to heart failure symptom severity*.)
- Echocardiography may demonstrate wall motion abnormalities and chamber dilation.

Other tests that may also demonstrate enlargement of the heart or decreased functioning include chest computed tomography scan, cardiac magnetic resonance imaging, or nuclear scans, such as multiple-gated acquisition scanning and radionuclide ventriculography.

TREATMENT

The goal of therapy is to improve pump function by reversing the compensatory mechanisms producing the clinical effects, underlying disorders, and precipitating factors. Lifestyle modifications should be employed to reduce symptoms of heart failure. These include:

- weight loss, if needed
- reduced sodium intake (to no more than 3 g daily)

LINKING BNP LEVELS TO HEART FAILURE SYMPTOM SEVERITY

This graph shows the level of B-type natriuretic peptide (BNP) and its correlation with symptoms of heart failure. The higher the BNP level, the more severe the symptoms.

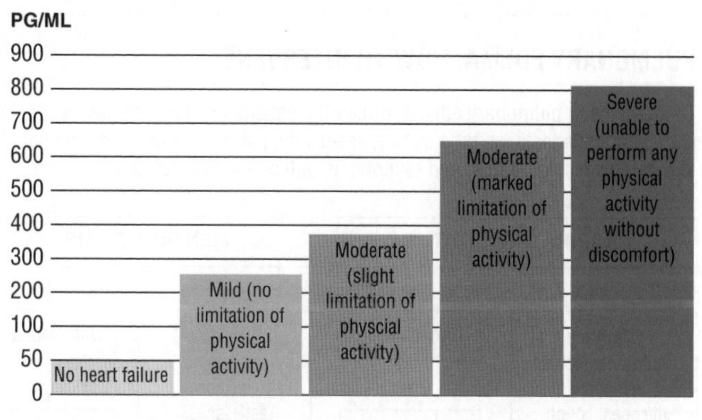

- limited alcohol intake
- reduced fat intake
- smoking cessation, if needed
- stress reduction
- an exercise program.

Other treatments may include the following.

- A biventricular pacemaker may be used to control ventricular dyssynchrony.
- Coronary artery bypass surgery or angioplasty may be needed for heart failure that results from coronary artery disease.
- Valve surgery may be used to reshape and support the mitral valve and improve cardiac functioning.
- Left ventricular remodeling surgery may be used to return the ventricle to a more normal shape and allow the heart to pump blood more efficiently. This surgical technique involves cutting a wedge about the size of a small slice of pie out of the left ventricle of an enlarged heart. The remainder of the heart is sewn together. The result is a smaller organ that can pump blood more efficiently.
- A left ventricular assist device, also known as a *bridge to transplantation,* may be used to improve the pumping ability of the heart until transplantation can be performed.
- Heart transplantation may be needed in a patient experiencing limitations or repeated hospitalizations despite aggressive medical treatment.

It's important to watch for and treat complications, which typically may include venostasis with a predisposition to thromboembolism (related mainly to prolonged bed rest), cerebral insufficiency, renal insufficiency with severe electrolyte imbalance, and pulmonary edema. (See *Pulmonary edema: How to intervene.*)

Drugs

- Angiotensin-converting enzyme (ACE) inhibitors for left ventricular

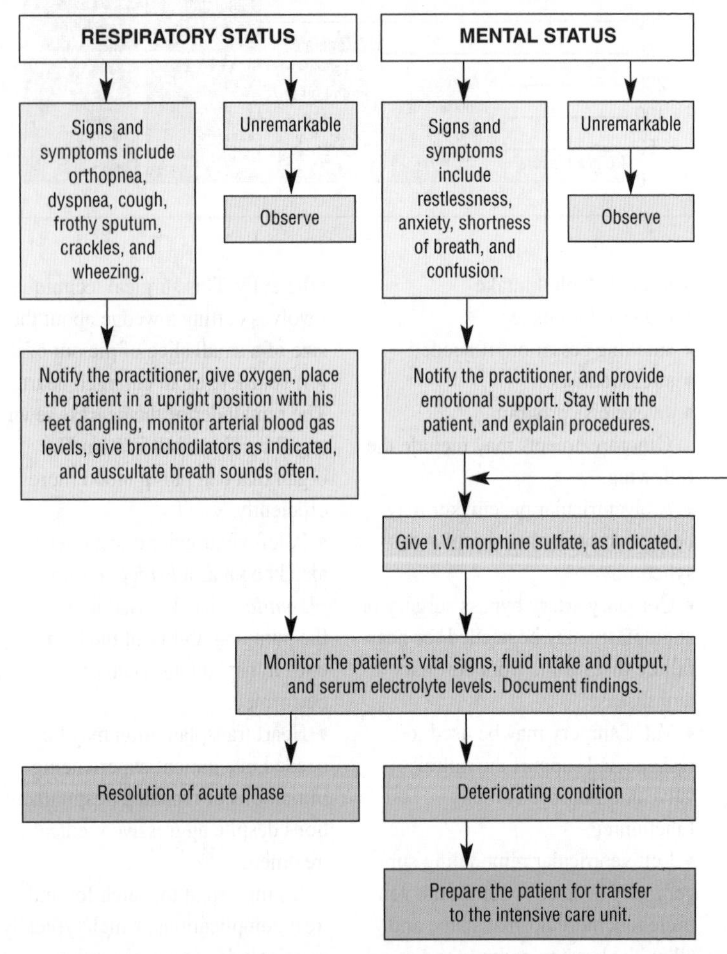
PULMONARY EDEMA: HOW TO INTERVENE
To intervene in pulmonary edema, obtain the patient's history, if possible; assist with diagnostic tests, as time allows; assess the patient's respiratory, mental, and cardiovascular status; and respond as outlined in this flowchart.
RESPIRATORY STATUS
Signs and symptoms include orthopnea, dyspnea, cough, frothy sputum, crackles, and wheezing.
Unremarkable
Observe
Notify the practitioner, give oxygen, place the patient in a upright position with his feet dangling, monitor arterial blood gas levels, give bronchodilators as indicated, and auscultate breath sounds often.
MENTAL STATUS
Signs and symptoms include restlessness, anxiety, shortness of breath, and confusion.
Unremarkable
Observe
Notify the practitioner, and provide emotional support. Stay with the patient, and explain procedures.
Give I.V. morphine sulfate, as indicated.
Monitor the patient's vital signs, fluid intake and output, and serum electrolyte levels. Document findings.
Resolution of acute phase
Deteriorating condition
Prepare the patient for transfer to the intensive care unit.

dysfunction to reduce production of angiotensin II, resulting in preload and afterload reduction

- Digoxin (Lanoxin) for heart failure caused by left ventricular systolic dysfunction to increase myocardial contractility, improve cardiac output, reduce the volume of the ventricle, and decrease ventricular stretch
- Diuretics to reduce fluid volume overload and venous return
- Beta-adrenergic blockers for New York Heart Association class II or III heart failure caused by left ventricular systolic dysfunction to prevent remodeling (Bisoprolol [Zebeta], sustained-release metoprolol [Lopressor], and carvedilol [Coreg] reduce death in patients with chronic heart failure)
- I.V. peripheral vasodilators (nitroglycerin, nitroprusside (Nitropress), or nesiritide [Natrecor]) and positive inotropic agents (dobutamine, dopamine, or milrinone [Primacor]) for acute treatment of worsening heart failure
- Nesiritide, a recombinant form of endogenous human BNP, to reduce sodium through its diuretic action
- Angiotensin II receptor blockers for patients who can't tolerate ACE inhibitors
- Aldosterone blockers to treat advanced heart failure
- Diuretics, nitrates, morphine, and oxygen to treat pulmonary edema

CARDIOVASCULAR STATUS

Signs and symptoms include hypotension; cold, clammy skin; irregular pulse; and S_3.

Unremarkable

Observe

Notify the practitioner, and give cardiopulmonary treatment as ordered: digoxin (Lanoxin), diuretics, and aminophylline. Apply rotating tourniquets as ordered.

SPECIAL CONSIDERATIONS

During acute heart failure

- Place the patient in Fowler's position and give supplemental oxygen to help him breathe more easily.
- Monitor hemodynamics using a pulmonary artery catheter. Titrate

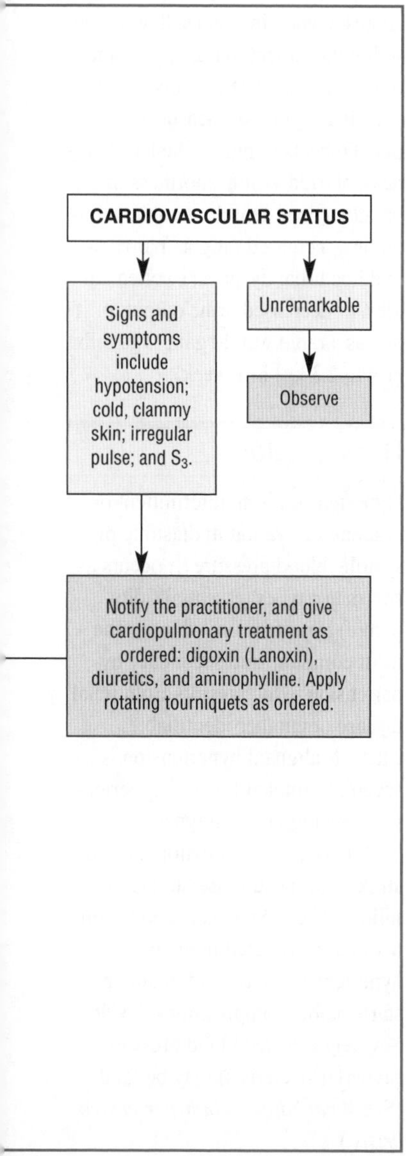

vasoactive and inotropic agents as ordered.
- Weigh the patient daily, and check for peripheral edema. Carefully monitor I.V. intake and urine output, vital signs, and mental status. Auscultate the heart for abnormal sounds (S_3 gallop) and the lungs for crackles or rhonchi. Assess for orthostatic hypotension. Report changes at once.
- Frequently monitor blood urea nitrogen, creatinine, and serum potassium, sodium, chloride, and magnesium levels.
- Make sure the patient has continuous cardiac monitoring during acute and advanced stages to identify and treat arrhythmias promptly.
- To reduce the risk of deep vein thrombosis due to vascular congestion, assist the patient with range-of-motion exercises. Enforce bed rest and apply antiembolism stockings. Check regularly for calf pain and tenderness.
- Allow adequate rest periods.

Preparing for discharge

- Advise the patient to avoid foods high in sodium, such as canned or commercially prepared foods and dairy products, to curb fluid overload.
- Encourage participation in an outpatient cardiac rehabilitation program.
- Explain that potassium lost through diuretic therapy may need to be replaced by taking a prescribed potassium supplement and eating high-potassium foods, such as bananas and apricots.
- Stress the need for regular checkups.
- Stress the importance of taking digoxin exactly as prescribed. Tell the patient to watch for and immediately report signs of toxicity, such as anorexia, vomiting, and yellow vision.
- Tell the patient to notify the practitioner promptly if his pulse is unusually irregular or measures less than 60 beats/minute; if he has dizziness, blurred vision, shortness of breath, a persistent dry cough, palpitations, increased fatigue, paroxysmal nocturnal dyspnea, swollen ankles, or decreased urine output; or if he has a rapid weight gain (3 to 5 lb [1.4 to 2.3 kg] in 1 week).

Hypertension

Hypertension is an intermittent or sustained elevation in diastolic or systolic blood pressure. It occurs as two major types: essential (idiopathic) hypertension, which is the most common, and secondary hypertension, which results from renal disease or another identifiable cause. Malignant hypertension is a severe, fulminant form of hypertension common to both types.

Hypertension is a major cause of stroke, cardiac disease, and renal failure. The prognosis is good if this disorder is detected in the prehypertension phase and treatment starts before complications develop. Severely elevated blood pressure (hypertensive crisis) may be fatal. (See *What happens in hypertensive crisis*.)

WHAT HAPPENS IN HYPERTENSIVE CRISIS

Hypertensive crisis is a severe increase in arterial blood pressure caused by a disturbance in one or more of the regulating mechanisms. If untreated, hypertensive crisis may result in renal, cardiac, or cerebral complications and, possibly, death.

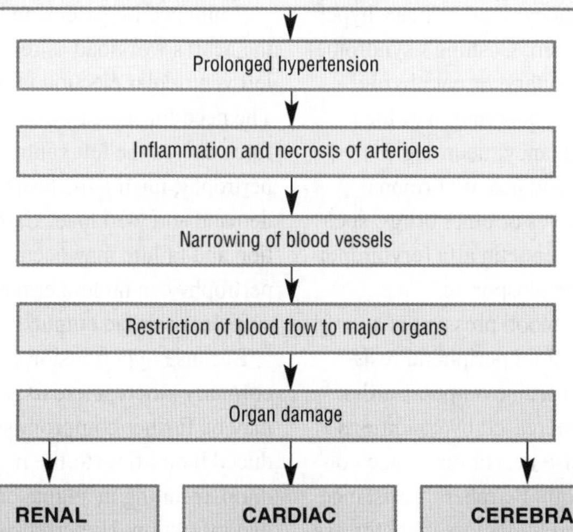

RENAL
- Decreased renal perfusion
- Progressive deterioration of nephrons
- Decreased ability to concentrate urine
- Increased serum creatinine and blood urea nitrogen levels
- Increased renal tubule permeability with protein leakage into tubules
- Renal insufficiency
- Uremia
- Renal failure

CARDIAC
- Decreased cardiac perfusion
- Coronary artery disease
- Angina or myocardial infarction
- Increased cardiac workload
- Left ventricular hypertrophy
- Heart failure

CEREBRAL
- Decreased cerebral perfusion
- Increased stress on vessel wall
- Arterial spasm
- Ischemia
- Transient ischemic attacks
- Weakening of vessel intima
- Aneurysm formation
- Intracranial hemorrhage

CAUSES AND INCIDENCE

Hypertension affects 25% of adults in the United States. If untreated, it carries a high mortality. Risk factors for hypertension include family history, race (most common in blacks), stress, obesity (especially abdominal), a diet high in saturated fats or sodium, tobacco use, sedentary lifestyle, and aging.

Secondary hypertension may result from renal vascular disease; pheochromocytoma; primary hyperaldosteronism; Cushing's syndrome; thyroid, pituitary, or parathyroid dysfunction; coarctation of the aorta; pregnancy; neurologic disorders; and use of hormonal contraceptives or other drugs, such as cocaine, epoetin alfa (erythropoietin), and cyclosporine.

Arterial blood pressure is a product of total peripheral resistance and cardiac output. Cardiac output is increased by conditions that increase heart rate, stroke volume, or both. Peripheral resistance is increased by factors that increase blood viscosity or reduce the lumen size of vessels, especially the arterioles.

Several theories help to explain the development of hypertension, including these.

- Changes in the arteriolar bed causes increased peripheral vascular resistance.
- Abnormally increased tone in the sympathetic nervous system that originates in the vasomotor system centers causes increased peripheral vascular resistance.
- Increased blood volume results from renal or hormonal dysfunction.
- An increase in arteriolar thickening caused by genetic factors leads to increased peripheral vascular resistance.
- Abnormal renin release results in the formation of angiotensin I, which constricts the arteriole and increases blood volume. (See *Understanding blood pressure regulation*.)

Prolonged hypertension increases the heart's workload as resistance to left ventricular ejection increases. The need for increased contractile force causes the left ventricle to hypertrophy, raising the heart's oxygen demand and workload. Cardiac dilation and failure may occur when hypertrophy can no longer maintain sufficient cardiac output.

Because hypertension promotes coronary atherosclerosis, the heart may be further compromised by reduced blood flow to the myocardium, resulting in angina or myocardial infarction. Hypertension also causes vascular damage, leading to accelerated atherosclerosis and target organ damage, such as retinal injury, renal failure, stroke, and aortic aneurysm and dissection.

The pathophysiology of secondary hypertension is related to the underlying disease. For example:

- The most common cause of secondary hypertension is chronic renal disease. Insult to the kidney from chronic glomerulonephritis or renal artery stenosis interferes

UNDERSTANDING BLOOD PRESSURE REGULATION

Hypertension may result from a disturbance in one of these intrinsic mechanisms.

Renin-angiotensin-aldosterone system

The renin-angiotensin-aldosterone system increases blood pressure through several related steps.

- Sodium depletion, reduced blood pressure, and dehydration stimulate renin release.
- Renin reacts with angiotensin, a liver enzyme, and converts it to angiotensin I, which increases preload and afterload.
- Angiotensin I converts to angiotensin II in the lungs; angiotensin II is a potent vasoconstrictor that targets arterioles.
- Angiotensin II increases preload and afterload by stimulating the adrenal cortex to secrete aldosterone; this increases blood volume by conserving sodium and water.

Autoregulation

When systemic blood pressure fluctuates, intrinsic mechanisms work to maintain tissue and organ perfusion by changing artery diameters. Mechanisms include stress relaxation and capillary fluid shifts.

- In stress relaxation, blood vessels dilate gradually in response to increased blood pressure, thus reducing peripheral resistance.
- In capillary fluid shift, plasma moves between vessels and extravascular spaces to maintain intravascular volume.

Sympathetic nervous system

When blood pressure drops or a person experiences stress, baroreceptors in the aortic arch and carotid sinuses decrease their inhibition of the medulla's vasomotor center. As a result, sympathetic stimulation of the heart by norepinephrine increases cardiac output by strengthening contractile force, raising the heart rate, and augmenting peripheral resistance by vasoconstriction.

Antidiuretic hormone

Release of antidiuretic hormone can regulate hypotension by increasing reabsorption of water by the kidneys. With reabsorption, blood plasma volume increases, thus raising blood pressure.

with sodium excretion, the renin-angiotensin-aldosterone system, or renal perfusion, causing blood pressure to increase.

- In Cushing's syndrome, increased cortisol levels raise blood pressure by increasing renal sodium retention, angiotensin II levels, and vascular response to norepinephrine.
- In primary aldosteronism, increased intravascular volume, altered sodium concentrations in vessel walls, or high aldosterone levels cause vasoconstriction and increased resistance.
- Pheochromocytoma is a chromaffin cell tumor of the adrenal medulla that secretes epinephrine and norepinephrine. Epinephrine increases cardiac contractility and rate, whereas norepinephrine increases peripheral vascular resistance.

SIGNS AND SYMPTOMS

By definition, a diagnosis of hypertension is based on elevated blood pressure readings on at least two consecutive occasions after an initial screening. Usually, hypertension produces no additional clinical effects, but the following signs and symptoms may occur: occipital headache (possibly worsen on rising in the morning as a result of increased intracranial pressure); nausea and vomiting; epistaxis; bruits; dizziness, confusion, and fatigue; blurry vision; nocturia; and edema.

Severely elevated blood pressure damages the intima of small vessels, resulting in fibrin accumulation in the vessels, development of local edema and, possibly, intravascular clotting. Symptoms produced by this process depend on the location of the damaged vessels:

- stroke if the brain is affected
- blindness if the retina is affected
- MI if the heart is affected
- proteinuria, edema, and eventually renal failure if the kidneys are affected.

In secondary hypertension, other signs and symptoms may be related to the cause. For example, Cushing's syndrome may cause truncal obesity and purple striae, whereas patients with pheochromocytoma may develop headache, nausea, vomiting, palpitations, pallor, and profuse perspiration.

Hypertension increases the heart's workload, causing left ventricular hypertrophy and, later, left- and right-sided heart failure and pulmonary edema.

COMPLICATIONS

- Stroke
- Coronary artery disease
- Angina
- MI
- Heart failure
- Arrhythmias
- Sudden death
- Cerebral infarction
- Hypertensive encephalopathy
- Hypertensive retinopathy
- Renal failure

DIAGNOSIS

- The patient history may show predisposing factors and help identify an underlying cause such as renal disease.
- Serial blood pressure measurements, when compared to previous readings and trends, reveal an increase in diastolic and systolic pressures. (See *Classifying blood pressure readings*.)
- Auscultation may reveal bruits over the abdominal aorta and the carotid, renal, and femoral arteries.
- Ophthalmoscopy reveals arteriovenous nicking and, in hypertensive encephalopathy, papilledema.
- In urinalysis, protein levels and red and white blood cell counts may indicate glomerulonephritis.
- In excretory urography, renal atrophy indicates chronic renal disease; one kidney more than ⅝″ (1.6 cm) shorter than the other suggests unilateral renal disease.

CLASSIFYING BLOOD PRESSURE READINGS

The National Institutes of Health, which once classified hypertension by severity (mild, moderate, severe, and very severe) now recommends a classification system based on stages: normal, pre-hypertension, and hypertension stage 1 or 2, as shown in the table below. The new system can be used for adults age 18 and older who aren't taking antihypertensives, aren't acutely ill, and don't have other health conditions, such as diabetes and kidney disease.

A patient's stage is based on an average of two or more blood pressure readings taken on separate visits after an initial screening. If systolic and diastolic pressures fall in different stages, the higher of the two pressures is used. For example, a patient whose blood pressure is 162/92 mm Hg is classified as stage 2.

For patients with target organ disease or additional risk factors, hypertension is based on more than just blood pressure readings. For example, a patient with diabetes or chronic kidney disease is considered hypertensive at a systolic pressure of 130 mm Hg or greater or a diastolic pressure of 80 mm Hg or greater. A patient with diabetes, left ventricular hypertrophy, and blood pressure of 144/98 mm Hg would be classified as "stage I hypertension with target-organ disease (left ventricular hypertrophy) and another major risk factor (diabetes)." This additional information is important to obtain a true picture of the patient's cardiovascular health.

Category	Systolic	Diastolic
Normal	Less than 120 mm Hg	Less than 80 mm Hg
Pre-hypertension	120 to 139 mm Hg	80 to 89 mm Hg
Hypertension		
Stage 1	140 to 159 mm Hg	90 to 99 mm Hg
Stage 2	160 mm Hg or higher	100 mm Hg or higher

- A serum potassium level of less than 3.5 mEq/L may indicate adrenal dysfunction (primary hyperaldosteronism).
- A blood urea nitrogen level that's normal or elevated to more than 20 mg/dl and a serum creatinine level that's normal or elevated to more than 1.5 mg/dl suggest renal disease.
- Electrocardiography may show left ventricular hypertrophy or ischemia.
- Chest X-ray may show cardiomegaly.
- Echocardiography may show left ventricular hypertrophy.

TREATMENT

The National Institutes of Health recommends the following approach for treating primary hypertension.

- Help the patient start needed lifestyle modifications, including weight reduction, moderation of alcohol intake, regular physical exercise, reduction of sodium intake, and smoking cessation.

- If the patient fails to achieve the desired blood pressure or make significant progress, continue lifestyle modifications and begin drug therapy.
- If the patient fails to achieve the desired blood pressure after starting drug therapy, continue lifestyle modifications and optimize drug dosages or add drugs until the goal blood pressure is achieved. Also, consider consultation with a hypertension specialist.

Treatment of secondary hypertension focuses on correcting the underlying cause and controlling hypertensive effects.

Typically, hypertensive emergencies require parenteral administration of a vasodilator or an adrenergic inhibitor or oral administration of a drug to rapidly reduce blood pressure, such as nifedipine (Procardia), captopril (Capoten), clonidine (Catapres), or labetalol (Trandate). The initial goal is to reduce mean arterial blood pressure by no more than 25% (within minutes to hours) and then to 160/110 mm Hg within 2 hours while avoiding excessive drops in blood pressure, which can cause renal, cerebral, or myocardial ischemia.

Examples of hypertensive emergencies include hypertensive encephalopathy, intracerebral hemorrhage, acute left-sided heart failure with pulmonary edema, stroke, and dissecting aortic aneurysm. Hypertensive emergencies also are associated with eclampsia or severe gestational hypertension, unstable angina, and acute MI.

Hypertension without accompanying symptoms or target-organ disease seldom requires emergency drug therapy.

Drugs

- For stage 1 hypertension (systolic blood pressure [SBP] 140 to 159 mm Hg, or diastolic blood pressure [DBP] 90 to 99 mm Hg) without compelling indications (heart failure, post-MI, high coronary disease risk, diabetes, chronic kidney disease, or recurrent stroke prevention), thiazide diuretics for most patients and possibly angiotensin-converting enzyme (ACE) inhibitors, beta-adrenergic blockers, calcium channel blockers, angiotensin-receptor blockers, or a combination
- For stage 2 hypertension (SBP 160 mm Hg or higher or DBP 100 mm Hg or higher) without compelling indications, a two-drug combination for most patients (usually thiazide diuretics and ACE inhibitors, angiotensin-receptor blockers, calcium channel blockers, or beta-adrenergic blockers)
- For a patient with heart failure, diuretics, beta-adrenergic blockers, ACE inhibitors, angiotensin-receptor blockers, or aldosterone antagonists
- For a patient with a high coronary disease risk, diuretics, beta-adrenergic blockers, ACE inhibitors, or calcium channel blockers

• For a patient with diabetes, diuretics, beta-adrenergic blockers, ACE inhibitors, or calcium channel blockers
• For a patient with chronic kidney disease, ACE inhibitors or angiotensin-receptor blockers
• For a patient after MI, ACE inhibitors, beta-adrenergic blockers, or aldosterone antagonists
• For recurrent stroke prevention, diuretics or ACE inhibitors
• For a hypertensive emergency, I.V. vasodilators or adrenergic inhibitors

SPECIAL CONSIDERATIONS

• To encourage adherence to antihypertensive therapy, suggest that the patient establish a daily routine for taking his medication. Warn that uncontrolled hypertension may cause stroke and heart attack. Tell him to report adverse drug effects. Also, advise him to avoid high-sodium antacids and over-the-counter cold and sinus medications, which contain harmful vasoconstrictors.
• Encourage a change in dietary habits. Help an obese patient plan a weight-reduction diet. Tell him to avoid high-sodium foods (pickles, potato chips, canned soups, and cold cuts) and table salt.
• Help the patient examine and modify his lifestyle (for example, by reducing stress and exercising regularly).
• If a patient is hospitalized with hypertension, find out if he was taking his prescribed medication. If he wasn't, ask why. If he can't afford the medication, refer him to appropriate social service agencies. Tell the patient and his family to keep a record of drugs prescribed in the past, noting especially which ones were or weren't effective. Suggest recording this information on a card so the patient can show it to his practitioner.
• When routine blood pressure screening reveals elevated pressure, first make sure the cuff size is appropriate for the patient's upper arm circumference. The cuff bladder should be 80% of the patient's upper arm. Take the pressure in both arms in lying, sitting, and standing positions. Wait 2 minutes between position changes before taking blood pressure. Ask the patient if he smoked, drank a beverage containing caffeine, or was emotionally upset before the test. Advise him to return for blood pressure testing at frequent and regular intervals.
• To help identify hypertension and prevent untreated hypertension, participate in public education programs dealing with hypertension and ways to reduce risk factors. Encourage public participation in blood pressure screening programs. Routinely screen all patients, especially those at risk (blacks and people with family histories of hypertension, stroke, or heart attack). (See *Preventing hypertension,* page 108.)

Hypertrophic cardiomyopathy

This primary disease of cardiac muscle, also called *idiopathic*

PREVENTION

PREVENTING HYPERTENSION

Some hypertension risk factors—such as family history, race, and aging—can't be changed. However, other important hypertension risks can be reduced or eliminated through lifestyle choices. To help patients prevent hypertension, offer these tips.

Maintain a healthy weight

Weight loss lowers blood pressure. Urge patients to maintain a normal weight or to lose weight if needed.

Reduce salt

Reducing salt intake can lower blood pressure in people with and without hypertension. Advise patients to limit salt intake to about 1.5 g/day.

Increase potassium

Potassium reduces blood pressure in people with and without hypertension. Tell healthy patients to eat 8 to 10 servings of fruits and vegetables daily to increase their potassium intake. Patients with kidney disease or heart failure should consult their health care provider before increasing potassium intake.

Limit alcohol intake

Alcohol consumption, especially more than two drinks daily, may increase blood pressure. Urge patients to limit consumption.

Include exercise

A sedentary lifestyle can lead to obesity and increase the risk of hypertension, myocardial infarction (MI), and stroke. Advise patients to get regular physical activity, defined by the American Heart Association as moderate to vigorous exercise for 30 to 60 minutes per day on most or all days of the week.

Manage stress

Stress can increase blood pressure, and it can lead to increased alcohol consumption, smoking, overeating, and other activities that increase the risk of hypertension, MI, and stroke. Stress management through relaxation, meditation, acupressure, biofeedback, or music therapy—even for short periods during the workday and on weekends has demonstrated the ability to help lower blood pressure.

Stop smoking

Smoking increases the risk of atherosclerosis, hypertension, MI, stroke, and other serious illnesses. Urge smokers to stop smoking and nonsmokers not to start.

Follow the DASH diet

In keeping with recommendations of the "dietary approaches to stop hypertension" study backed by the National Institutes of Health (called the *DASH diet*), encourage patients to eat mainly grains, vegetables, and fruits, with lesser amounts of low-fat dairy foods, lean meats, and nuts. Discourage consumption of fats, red meat, sweets, and sugar-containing drinks. Keep in mind, however, that the DASH diet is rich in potassium; patients with reduced kidney function should consult their health care providers before changing their diet.

hypertrophic subaortic stenosis, is characterized by hypertrophy of the left ventricle, particularly the intraventricular septum. In hypertrophic cardiomyopathy, cardiac output may be low, normal, or high, depending on whether stenosis is obstructive or nonobstructive. If cardiac output is normal or high, the disorder may go undetected for years. If output is low, it may lead to potentially fatal heart failure. The disease course varies; some patients progressively deteriorate, while others remain stable for years. (See *Comparing cardiomyopathies,* page 68.)

CAUSES AND INCIDENCE

Despite being designated as idiopathic, hypertrophic cardiomyopathy may be inherited as a non–sex-linked autosomal dominant trait in almost all cases.

In most patients, obstructive disease results from bulging inward of the intraventricular septum during systole and the movement of the anterior mitral valve leaflet into the outflow tract during systole. Forceful ejection of blood draws the anterior leaflet of the mitral valve to the intraventricular septum. This causes early closure of the outflow tract, decreasing ejection fraction. Moreover, intramural coronary arteries are abnormally small and may not be sufficient to supply the hypertrophied muscle with enough blood and oxygen to meet the increased needs of the hyperdynamic muscle. Eventually, left ventricular dysfunction, from rigidity and decreased compliance, causes pump failure.

Unlike dilated cardiomyopathy, which affects systolic function, hypertrophic cardiomyopathy primarily affects diastolic function. The hypertrophied ventricle becomes stiff, noncompliant, and unable to relax during ventricular filling. Consequently, ventricular filling is reduced and left ventricular filling pressure rises, increasing left atrial and pulmonary venous pressures and leading to venous congestion and dyspnea. Ventricular filling time is further reduced as a compensatory response to tachycardia, leading to low cardiac output. If the papillary muscles become hypertrophied and don't close completely during contraction, mitral insufficiency occurs.

The features of hypertrophic obstructive cardiomyopathy include:

- asymmetrical left ventricular hypertrophy
- hypertrophy of the intraventricular septum
- rapid, forceful contractions of the left ventricle
- impaired relaxation
- obstruction to left ventricular outflow.

This disorder affects 2 to 5 of every 1,000 people and is usually the cause of sudden death, particularly in otherwise healthy athletes.

SIGNS AND SYMPTOMS

Clinical features of the disorder may not appear until it's well advanced, when atrial dilation and possibly atrial fibrillation abruptly reduce blood flow to the left ventricle. Reduced inflow and subsequent low output may produce angina pectoris, arrhythmias, dyspnea, orthopnea, syncope, heart failure, and death. Auscultation reveals a medium-pitched systolic ejection murmur along the left sternal border and at the apex; palpation reveals a peripheral pulse with a characteristic double impulse (pulsus biferiens) and, with atrial fibrillation, an irregular pulse.

COMPLICATIONS

- Pulmonary hypertension
- Heart failure
- Ventricular arrhythmias
- Sudden death

DIAGNOSIS

No single test confirms hypertrophic cardiomyopathy. Diagnosis depends on typical clinical findings and the following test results. (See *Comparing diagnostic tests in cardiomyopathy,* page 72.)

- Echocardiography (most useful) shows increased thickness of the intraventricular septum and abnormal motion of the anterior mitral leaflet during systole, occluding left ventricular outflow in obstructive disease.
- Cardiac catheterization reveals elevated left ventricular end-diastolic pressure and, possibly, mitral insufficiency.
- Electrocardiography usually shows left ventricular hypertrophy, T-wave inversion, left anterior hemiblock, Q waves in precordial and inferior leads, ventricular arrhythmias and, possibly, atrial fibrillation.
- Auscultation confirms an early systolic murmur.

TREATMENT

Optimal control of hypertension is critical to the treatment of hypertrophic cardiomyopathy. If the aortic valve is stenotic, valve replacement may be indicated. Cardioversion may be used to treat atrial fibrillation. In the patient with hypertrophic obstructive cardiomyopathy, ablation of the atrioventricular node and implantation of a dual-chamber pacemaker may reduce the outflow gradient by altering the pattern of ventricular contractions. An implantable cardioverter-defibrillator can be inserted to treat ventricular arrhythmias. Outflow obstruction and symptoms can be relieved by ventricular myotomy or myectomy. Mitral valve replacement may be indicated to treat mitral insufficiency. A patient with intractable symptoms may need heart transplantation.

Drugs

- Beta-adrenergic blockers to slow the heart rate, reduce myocardial oxygen demands, and increase ventricular filling by relaxing the obstructing muscle, thereby increasing cardiac output
- Antiarrhythmics, such as disopyramide (Norpace) or amiodarone (Cordarone), to reduce arrhythmias
- Anticoagulation to reduce the risk of systemic embolism with atrial fibrillation

• Verapamil (Calan) or diltiazem (Cardizem) to reduce septal stiffness and elevated diastolic pressures

SPECIAL CONSIDERATIONS

• Because syncope or sudden death may follow well-tolerated exercise, warn patients against strenuous physical activity such as running.
• Give medications as prescribed.

ALERT

Avoid nitroglycerin, digoxin (Lanoxin), and diuretics because they can worsen obstruction.

• Warn the patient not to stop taking propranolol (Inderal) abruptly because doing so may increase myocardial demands. To determine the patient's tolerance for an increased dosage of propranolol, take his pulse to check for bradycardia. Also take his blood pressure while he's supine and standing. A drop in blood pressure of more than 10 mm Hg when standing may indicate orthostatic hypotension.
• Before dental work or surgery, tell the patient to discuss prophylaxis for subacute infective endocarditis with his health care provider.
• Provide psychological support. If the patient is hospitalized for a long time, be flexible with visiting hours and encourage occasional weekends away from the hospital if possible. Refer the patient for psychosocial counseling to help him and his family accept his restricted lifestyle and poor prognosis.
• If the patient is a child, have his parents arrange for him to continue his studies in the health care facility.
• Because sudden cardiac arrest is possible, urge the patient's family to learn cardiopulmonary resuscitation.

Hypovolemic shock

In hypovolemic shock, reduced intravascular blood volume causes circulatory dysfunction and inadequate tissue perfusion. Without sufficient blood or fluid replacement, hypovolemic shock syndrome may lead to irreversible cerebral and renal damage, cardiac arrest and, ultimately, death. Hypovolemic shock requires early recognition of signs and symptoms and prompt, aggressive treatment to improve the prognosis. (See *What happens in hypovolemic shock,* page 112.)

CAUSES AND INCIDENCE

Hypovolemic shock usually results from acute blood loss—about one-fifth of total volume. Such massive blood loss may result from GI bleeding, internal hemorrhage (hemothorax or hemoperitoneum), external hemorrhage (accidental or surgical trauma), or from any condition that reduces circulating intravascular plasma volume or other body fluids such as severe burns. Other underlying causes of hypovolemic shock include intestinal obstruction, peritonitis, acute pancreatitis, ascites and dehydration from excessive perspiration, severe diarrhea or protracted vomiting, diabetes insipidus, diuresis, or inadequate fluid intake.

WHAT HAPPENS IN HYPOVOLEMIC SHOCK

When loss of vascular fluid volume leads to extreme tissue hypoperfusion, the affected person has hypovolemic shock, as outlined in this flowchart. Internal fluid loss can result from hemorrhage or third-space fluid shifts. External fluid loss can result from severe bleeding, diarrhea, diuresis, or vomiting. Inadequate vascular volume leads to decreased venous return, cardiac output, and arterial pressure and activates compensatory mechanisms that work to increase vascular volume. If compensation is unsuccessful, decompensation and death may occur.

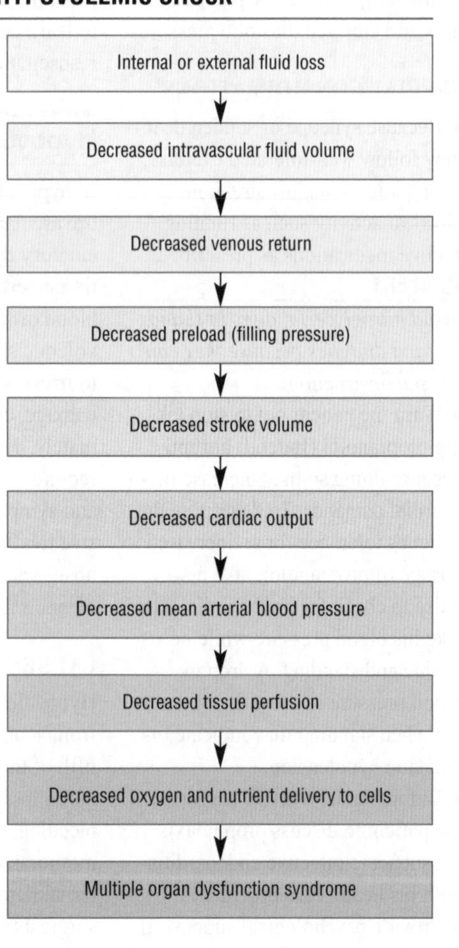

In hypovolemic shock, venous return to the heart is reduced when fluid is lost from the intravascular space through external losses or the shift of fluid from the vessels to the interstitial or intracellular spaces. This reduction in preload decreases ventricular filling, leading to a drop in stroke volume. Then cardiac output falls, causing reduced perfusion of the tissues and organs.

SIGNS AND SYMPTOMS

Hypovolemic shock produces a syndrome of hypotension, with narrowing pulse pressure; decreased sensorium; tachycardia; rapid, shallow respirations; reduced urine output (less than 25 ml/hour); and cold, pale, clammy skin. Metabolic acidosis with an accumulation of lactic acid develops as a result of tissue anoxia, as cellular metabolism shifts from aerobic to anaerobic pathways. Disseminated intravascular coagulation (DIC) can also occur with hypovolemic shock.

COMPLICATIONS

- Acute respiratory distress syndrome
- Acute tubular necrosis
- DIC
- Multiple-organ-dysfunction syndrome

DIAGNOSIS

No single symptom or diagnostic test establishes the diagnosis or severity of hypovolemic shock. Characteristic laboratory findings include:

- elevated potassium, serum lactate, and blood urea nitrogen levels
- increased urine specific gravity (more than 1.020) and urine osmolality
- decreased blood pH and partial pressure of arterial oxygen and increased partial pressure of arterial carbon dioxide.

In addition, gastroscopy, aspiration of gastric contents through a nasogastric tube, computed tomography scan, and X-rays identify internal bleeding sites; coagulation studies may detect coagulopathy from DIC. Echocardiography or right-heart catheterization can help differentiate between hypovolemic and cardiogenic shock.

TREATMENT

- Emergency treatment measures must include prompt and adequate blood and fluid replacement to restore intravascular volume and raise blood pressure. Saline solution or lactated Ringer's solution, then possibly plasma proteins (albumin) or other plasma expanders, may produce adequate volume expansion until whole blood can be matched. A rapid solution infusion system can provide these crystalloids or colloids at high flow rates. Application of a pneumatic antishock garment may be helpful. (See *Using a pneumatic antishock garment,* page 114.)
- Treatment also may include oxygen administration, identification of the bleeding site, control of bleeding by direct measures (such as application of pressure and elevation of a limb) and, possibly, surgery.

Drugs

- Fluids, such as normal saline or lactated Ringer's solution, to restore filling pressures
- Packed red blood cells in hemorrhagic shock to restore blood loss and improve the blood's oxygen-carrying capacity
- Dopamine, dobutamine, epinephrine, and norepinephrine to help increase blood pressure and cardiac output after fluid resuscitation measures

SPECIAL CONSIDERATIONS

- Management of hypovolemic shock requires prompt, aggressive supportive measures and careful

USING A PNEUMATIC ANTISHOCK GARMENT

A pneumatic antishock garment, such as the one shown here, counteracts bleeding and hypovolemia by slowing or stopping arterial bleeding; by pushing blood from the lower body to the heart, brain, and other vital organs; and by preventing blood from returning to the legs. When using an antishock garment, keep these points in mind.

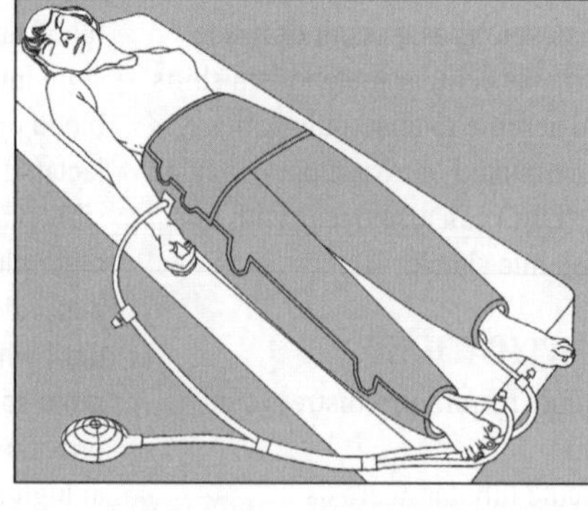

Do

- While the patient is wearing the pneumatic antishock garment, monitor her blood pressure, apical and radial pulse rates, and respirations; check her feet for pedal pulses, color, warmth, and numbness; and make sure the garment isn't too constricting.
- Remove the garment only when a practitioner is present, fluids are available for transfusion, and anesthesia and surgical teams are available. Deflate the compartments slowly, one section at a time, while monitoring the patient closely.
- To clean the garment, wash it with warm soap and water and air-dry before storing.

Don't

- Don't apply the garment if the patient shows evidence of major intrathoracic or intracranial vascular injury, compromised breathing (as in pulmonary edema), open extremity bleeding, or trauma above the application site. The garment may be used during pregnancy if the abdominal compartment isn't inflated, although some experts advise against using it during the third trimester.
- When cleaning the garment, don't autoclave it or use solvents on it.

assessment and monitoring of vital signs.

- Check for a patent airway and adequate circulation. If blood pressure and heart rate are absent, start cardiopulmonary resuscitation.
- Record blood pressure, pulse rate, peripheral pulses, respiratory rate, and other vital signs every 15 minutes and the electrocardiogram continuously. Systolic blood pressure lower than 80 mm Hg usually results in inadequate coronary artery blood flow, cardiac ischemia, arrhythmias, and further complications of low cardiac output. When blood pressure drops below 80 mm Hg, increase the oxygen flow rate and notify the practitioner immediately. A progressive drop in blood

pressure, accompanied by a thready pulse, typically signals inadequate cardiac output from reduced intravascular volume. Notify the practitioner and increase the infusion rate.

- Start I.V. lines with normal saline or lactated Ringer's solution, using a large-bore (14G) catheter, which allows easier administration of later blood transfusions.

ALERT

Don't start I.V. lines in the legs of a patient in shock who has suffered abdominal trauma because infused fluid may escape through the ruptured vessel into the abdomen.

- An indwelling urinary catheter may be inserted to measure hourly urine output. If output is less than 30 ml/hour in an adult, increase the fluid infusion rate, but watch for signs of fluid overload, such as an increase in pulmonary artery wedge pressure (PAWP). Notify the practitioner if urine output doesn't improve. An osmotic diuretic, such as mannitol (Osmitrol), may be ordered to increase renal blood flow and urine output. Determine how much fluid to give by checking blood pressure, urine output, central venous pressure (CVP), or PAWP. To increase accuracy, CVP should be measured at the level of the right atrium, using the same reference point on the chest each time.
- Draw an arterial blood sample to measure blood gas levels. Administer oxygen by face mask or airway to ensure adequate oxygenation of tissues. Adjust the oxygen flow rate to a higher or lower level, as blood gas measurements indicate.
- Draw venous blood for complete blood count and electrolyte, type and crossmatch, and coagulation studies.
- During therapy, assess skin color and temperature, and note changes. Cold, clammy skin may be a sign of continuing peripheral vascular constriction, indicating progressive shock.
- Watch for signs of impending coagulopathy (petechiae, bruising, and bleeding or oozing from gums or venipuncture sites).
- Explain procedures and their purpose. Throughout these emergency measures, provide emotional support to the patient and his family.

M-O

Metabolic syndrome

Metabolic syndrome—also called *syndrome X, insulin resistance syndrome, dysmetabolic syndrome,* and *multiple metabolic syndrome*—is a cluster of conditions characterized by abdominal obesity, high blood glucose (type 2 diabetes mellitus), insulin resistance, high blood cholesterol and triglycerides, and high blood pressure. More than 22% of people in the United States meet three or more of these criteria, raising their risk of heart disease and stroke and placing them at high risk for dying of myocardial infarction.

CAUSES AND INCIDENCE

Abdominal obesity is a strong predictor of metabolic syndrome because abdominal fat tends to be more resistant to insulin than fat in other areas. This increases the release of free fatty acids into the portal system, leading to increased apolipoprotein B, increased low-density lipoprotein (LDL), decreased high-density lipoprotein (HDL), and increased triglyceride levels. As a result, the risk of cardiovascular disease is increased.

Type 2 diabetes mellitus is a risk factor because a hallmark for metabolic syndrome is a fasting glucose level of greater than 110 mg/dl. People with diabetes develop atherosclerotic heart disease at a younger age than other people. They're also at increased risk for macrovascular disease (ischemic heart disease, stroke, and peripheral vascular disease). Diabetes is a coronary heart disease risk equivalent.

Insulin resistance and dyslipidemia are also risk factors because insulin resistance leads to hyperinsulinemia, hyperglycemia, abnormal glucose and lipid metabolism, damaged endothelium, and cardiovascular disease. Insulin is also responsible for reducing the amount of free fatty acids in the liver. However, people with insulin resistance have an increased amount of free fatty acids reaching the liver, resulting in high triglyceride and LDL levels and producing an abnormal endothelium and atherosclerosis.

High blood pressure is a risk factor because the combination of insulin resistance, hyperinsulinemia, and abdominal obesity leads to hypertension and its harmful cardiovascular effects. Moreover, insulin resistance promotes salt sensitivity in people with high blood pressure. Research also indicates that there may be a genetic predisposition to metabolic syndrome.

In normal digestion, the intestines break down food into its basic components, one of which is glucose. Glucose provides energy for cellular activity, while excess glucose is stored in cells for future use. Insulin, a hormone secreted in the pancreas, guides glucose into storage cells. However, in people with metabolic syndrome, insulin is less able to carry glucose into the cells. The body then generates excess insulin to overcome this resistance. This excess in quantity and force of insulin causes damage to the lining of the arteries, promotes fat storage deposits, and prevents fat breakdown. This series of events can lead to diabetes, blood clots, and coronary events. (See *Patient teaching aid: Metabolic syndrome,* page 118.)

SIGNS AND SYMPTOMS

Assessment commonly reveals a history of hypertension, abdominal obesity, sedentary lifestyle, poor diet, and a family history of metabolic syndrome. Physical findings include abdominal obesity (waist measurement greater than 40″ [101.6 cm] in men and 35″ [88.9 cm] in women), blood pressure of 130/85 mm Hg or higher, and a fasting blood glucose level that's 100 mg/dl or higher. The patient may feel tired, especially after eating, and may have trouble losing weight.

COMPLICATIONS

- Coronary artery disease
- Diabetes mellitus
- Hyperlipidemia
- Stroke
- Premature death

DIAGNOSIS

- Blood studies commonly indicate elevated blood glucose levels, hyperinsulinemia, and elevated serum uric acid.
- Use of lipid profile studies reveal elevated LDL levels, low HDL levels, and elevated triglycerides.
- Further diagnostic procedures are nonspecific, but may be performed to detect hypertension, diabetes, hyperlipidemia, and hyperinsulinemia.

TREATMENT

Lifestyle modification, focusing on weight reduction and exercise, is an important part of the treatment regimen. Modest weight reduction through diet and exercise considerably improves hemoglobin A1c levels, reduces insulin resistance, improves blood lipid levels, and decreases blood pressure—all elements of metabolic syndrome. Recent studies have shown that in patients with impaired glucose tolerance, losing an average of 7% of body weight reduced the risk of developing type 2 diabetes by 58%. To improve cardiovascular health, a diet rich in vegetables, fruits, whole grains, fish, and low-fat dairy products combined with regular exercise is recommended. Moreover, nutrient-dense, low-energy foods should replace low-nutrient, high-calorie foods. Meal replacements and shakes may also

PATIENT-TEACHING AID: METABOLIC SYNDROME

Dear Patient:

BRAIN
Stroke
Coronary artery disease
HEART
Diabetes
PANCREAS

Your physician has determined that you have metabolic syndrome (sometimes called *insulin resistance syndrome* or *syndrome X*). This handout will help you understand metabolic syndrome and how it can affect you.

- Although the syndrome isn't completely understood yet, it's clear that people with metabolic syndrome have an increased risk of serious health problems, including coronary artery disease, stroke, and diabetes.
- Usually, to be diagnosed with metabolic syndrome, you'll have at least three of the following: abdominal obesity (a waist measurement larger than 40 inches for men, 35 inches for women); high blood pressure (130/85 mm Hg or higher); insulin resistance, in which the body doesn't use insulin properly (fasting blood glucose level of 110 mg/dl or higher); and an abnormal cholesterol profile (an increased triglyceride level or a high-density lipoprotein level of less than 40 mg/dl in men, 50 mg/dl in women).
- The biggest risk factors for metabolic syndrome seem to be physical inactivity and overweight, although aging and genetic predisposition may be involved.
- Insulin resistance also seems central to the development of metabolic syndrome. Normally, food is absorbed into the bloodstream as glucose and other substances, and insulin released by the pancreas carries glucose out of the blood and into the cells to be used for energy. When insulin isn't working properly, glucose can't be used normally. Some of the glucose doesn't get to the cells that need it, staying instead in the bloodstream. An increased blood glucose level can lead to diabetes and organ damage.
- To reduce the risk that metabolic syndrome will lead to cardiovascular disease, stroke, or diabetes, lose weight if needed (so your body mass index is less than 25 kg/m^2), don't smoke, get at least 30 minutes of moderate exercise most days of the week, and eat a healthy diet low in saturated fat, trans fat, and cholesterol.

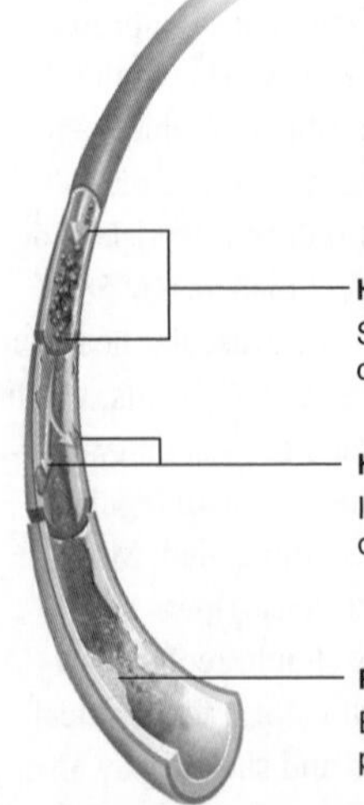
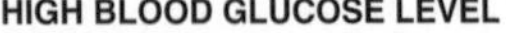
HIGH BLOOD GLUCOSE LEVEL
Sugar builds up in the bloodstream, causing damage to organs.
HIGH BLOOD PRESSURE
If untreated, high blood pressure damages the lining of the arteries.
FIBROUS PLAQUE
Elevated cholesterol levels lead to fibrous plaque deposits in the blood vessels.

THERAPEUTIC LIFESTYLE-CHANGES DIET

The therapeutic lifestyle-changes diet is low in saturated fats and cholesterol to reduce blood cholesterol levels and help prevent heart disease and its complications. This diet recommends consuming:

- less than 7% of the day's total calories as saturated fat (including trans fat)
- 25% to 35% of the day's total calories as fat
- less than 200 mg of dietary cholesterol daily
- no more than 2,400 mg of sodium daily
- just enough calories to achieve or maintain a healthy weight and cholesterol level.

Also, for most people, it recommends moderate exercise for at least 30 minutes, 3 or 4 days weekly.

If blood cholesterol isn't lowered enough by following this diet, the practitioner may recommend increasing the amount of soluble fiber in the diet or adding cholesterol-lowering foods. These include margarines and salad dressings that contain plant sterol esters or plant stanol esters. If the low-density lipoprotein level still isn't lowered enough, the patient may need a cholesterol-lowering drug.

Source: National Heart, Lung, and Blood Institute. Available at *www.nhlbi.nih.gov/chd/lifestyles.htm* and *www.nhlbi.nih.gov/cgi-bin/chd/step2intro.cgi.*

reduce risk factors for metabolic syndrome and improve weight loss. (See *Therapeutic lifestyle-changes diet.*)

A regular exercise program of moderate physical activity in addition to dietary modifications promotes weight loss, improves insulin sensitivity, and reduces blood glucose levels. According to the Surgeon General's Report on Physical Activity and Health, a person should exercise moderately for at least 30 minutes on most or all days of the week. The exercise program should be designed to improve cardiovascular conditioning, increase strength through resistance training, and improve flexibility.

Some patients may need drug treatment for metabolic syndrome in addition to changes in diet and exercise. They include:

- patients with a body mass index (BMI) of 27 kg/m^2 or greater plus other risk factors, such as diabetes, hypertension, and hyperlipidemia
- patients with a BMI of 30 kg/m^2 or greater
- patients who haven't had significant weight loss after 12 weeks.

Surgical treatment of obesity, such as through gastric bypass procedures, produces a greater degree and duration of weight loss than other therapies and improves or resolves most aspects of metabolic syndrome. Candidates for surgical intervention include patients with a BMI greater than 40 kg/m^2 or those with a BMI greater than 35 kg/m^2 and obesity-related medical conditions. Gastric bypass procedures produce permanent weight loss in most patients.

Drugs

- Orlistat (Xenical) to decrease the absorption of dietary fat by inhibiting pancreatic lipase, which is needed for fat breakdown and absorption. (When obese patients take orlistat while dieting, they achieve greater weight loss and serum glucose control than by dieting alone. Because the absorption of fat-soluble vitamins is reduced, the patient may need vitamin supplementation.)
- Sibutramine (Meridia) to inhibit the reuptake of serotonin, norepinephrine, and dopamine; increase the satiety-producing effects of serotonin; and reduce the drop in metabolic rate that commonly occurs with weight loss

SPECIAL CONSIDERATIONS

- Monitor the patient's blood pressure and blood glucose, blood cholesterol, and insulin levels.
- Because longer lifestyle modification programs tend to improve weight loss maintenance, encourage a patient with metabolic syndrome to start an exercise and weight loss program with a friend or family member. Help him explore options, and support his efforts.
- To improve compliance, schedule frequent follow-up with the patient. At each appointment, review his food diaries and exercise logs. Be positive, and promote his active participation and partnership in his treatment plan.
- A patient planning gastric bypass surgery should receive psychological and nutritional counseling before and after surgery to help with diet and lifestyle changes.

Mitral insufficiency

Mitral insufficiency—also known as *mitral regurgitation*—occurs when a damaged mitral valve allows blood from the left ventricle to flow back into the left atrium during systole. (See *Types of valvular heart disease,* page 8.)

CAUSES AND INCIDENCE

Damage to the mitral valve can result from rheumatic fever, hypertrophic cardiomyopathy, mitral valve prolapse, myocardial infarction, severe left-sided heart failure, ruptured chordae tendineae, or infective endocarditis. In older patients, mitral insufficiency may occur because the mitral annulus has become calcified. The cause is unknown, but it may be linked to a degenerative process.

Blood from the left ventricle flows back into the left atrium during systole, causing the atrium to enlarge to accommodate the backflow. As a result, the left ventricle also dilates to accommodate the increased blood volume from the atrium and to compensate for diminishing cardiac output. Ventricular hypertrophy and increased end-diastolic pressure result in increased

IDENTIFYING THE MURMUR OF MITRAL INSUFFICIENCY

Mitral insufficiency produces a high-pitched, rumbling pansystolic murmur that radiates from the mitral area to the left axillary line, as diagrammed here.

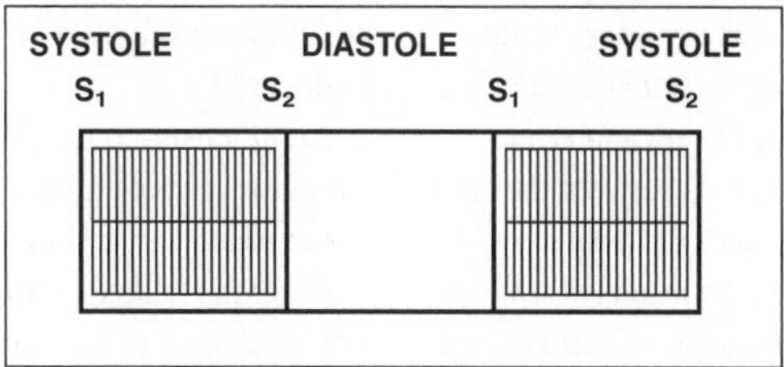

pulmonary artery pressure (PAP), eventually leading to left-sided and right-sided heart failure.

SIGNS AND SYMPTOMS

Depending on the severity of the disorder, the patient may be asymptomatic or complain of trouble breathing when lying flat, shortness of breath with exertion, fatigue, weakness, weight loss, chest pain, and palpitations. Inspection may reveal jugular vein distention with an abnormally prominent *a* wave. Peripheral edema may be present.

Auscultation may detect a soft S_1 that may be buried in the systolic murmur. A grade 3 to 6 or louder holosystolic murmur, most characteristic of mitral insufficiency, is best heard at the apex. A split S_2 and a low-pitched S_3 may also be heard. The S_3 may be followed by a short, rumbling diastolic murmur. A fourth heart sound may be heard in patients who have severe mitral insufficiency of recent onset and who are in normal sinus rhythm. (See *Identifying the murmur of mitral insufficiency*.)

Auscultation of the lungs may reveal crackles if the patient has pulmonary edema. Palpation of the chest may disclose a regular pulse rate with a sharp upstroke. A systolic thrill at the apex may be palpable. When the left atrium is markedly enlarged, it may be palpable along the sternal border late during ventricular systole. It resembles a right ventricular lift. Abdominal palpation may reveal hepatomegaly if the patient has right-sided heart failure.

COMPLICATIONS

- Ventricular hypertrophy and increased end-diastolic pressure
- Increased PAP
- Left- and right-sided heart failure
- Pulmonary edema
- Cardiovascular collapse

DIAGNOSIS

- Cardiac catheterization is used to detect mitral insufficiency with increased left ventricular end-diastolic volume and pressure, increased left atrial and pulmonary artery wedge pressures, and decreased cardiac output. Cardiac catheterization can resolve discrepancies between the clinical presentation of a patient's symptoms and the results of a noninvasive transthoracic echocardiogram. If coronary artery disease is suspected, the need for coronary artery bypass graft surgery can be determined.
- Chest X-rays show left atrial and ventricular enlargement, pulmonary vein congestion, and calcification of the mitral leaflets in patients with long-standing mitral insufficiency and stenosis.
- Echocardiography reveals abnormal motion of the valve leaflets, left atrial enlargement, and a hyperdynamic left ventricle.
- Transesophageal echocardiogram can establish the severity of mitral regurgitation and the need for surgical repair or replacement.
- Electrocardiography may show left atrial and ventricular hypertrophy, sinus tachycardia, and atrial fibrillation.

TREATMENT

The nature and severity of symptoms determine treatment for a patient with valvular heart disease. For example, he may need to restrict activities to avoid extreme fatigue and dyspnea. If the patient has severe signs and symptoms that can't be managed medically, he may need open-heart surgery with cardiopulmonary bypass for valve replacement.

Drugs

- Antibiotics to treat infective endocarditis
- Angiotensin-converting enzyme inhibitors or beta-adrenergic blockers to treat heart failure
- Digoxin (Lanoxin), calcium channel blockers, or beta-adrenergic blockers to treat arrhythmias
- Anticoagulants (warfarin [Coumadin]) to prevent thrombus formation around diseased, repaired, or replaced valves

SPECIAL CONSIDERATIONS

- Provide periods of rest between periods of activity to prevent excessive fatigue.
- To reduce anxiety, let the patient express his concerns about the effects of activity restrictions on his responsibilities and routines. Reassure him that the restrictions are temporary.
- Keep the patient on a low-sodium diet; consult with the dietitian to ensure that the patient receives as many favorite foods as possible during the restriction.
- Monitor the patient for left-sided heart failure, pulmonary edema, and adverse reactions to drug therapy. Provide oxygen to prevent tissue hypoxia as needed.
- If the patient has surgery, monitor him postoperatively for hypotension, arrhythmias, and thrombus formation.

• Monitor the patient's vital signs, arterial blood gas levels, intake and output, daily weight, blood chemistry results, chest X-rays, and pulmonary artery catheter readings.
• Teach the patient about diet restrictions, medications, signs and symptoms that should be reported, and the importance of consistent follow-up care.
• Explain all tests and treatments.
• Make sure the patient and his family understand the need to comply with prolonged antibiotic therapy and follow-up care.
• Tell the parents or patient to stop the drug and call the practitioner immediately if the patient develops a rash, fever, chills, or other signs or symptoms of allergy at any time during penicillin therapy.
• Instruct the patient and his family to watch for and report early signs and symptoms of heart failure, such as dyspnea and a hacking, nonproductive cough.

Mitral stenosis

In patients with mitral stenosis, valve leaflets become diffusely thickened by fibrosis and calcification. The mitral commissures fuse, the chordae tendineae fuse and shorten, the valvular cusps become rigid, and the apex of the valve becomes narrowed, obstructing blood flow from the left atrium to the left ventricle. (See *Types of valvular heart disease*, page 8.)

CAUSES AND INCIDENCE

Mitral stenosis most commonly results from rheumatic fever. It also may be related to congenital anomalies.

As a result of obstructive changes, left atrial volume and pressure increase and the atrial chamber dilates. The increased resistance to blood flow causes pulmonary hypertension, right ventricular hypertrophy and, eventually, right-sided heart failure. Pulmonary hypertension increases transudation of fluid from pulmonary capillaries, which can cause fibrosis in the alveoli and pulmonary capillaries. This action reduces vital capacity, total lung capacity, maximal breathing capacity, and oxygen uptake per unit of ventilation. Also, inadequate filling of the left ventricle reduces cardiac output.

Mitral stenosis occurs twice as often in women as in men.

SIGNS AND SYMPTOMS

Patients with mild mitral stenosis may have no symptoms. Those with moderate to severe mitral stenosis may have a history of exertional dyspnea, paroxysmal nocturnal dyspnea, orthopnea, weakness, fatigue, and palpitations. A dry cough and dysphagia may occur because of an enlarged left atrium or bronchus. The presence of hemoptysis suggests rupture of pulmonary-bronchial venous connections.

Inspection may reveal peripheral and facial cyanosis, particularly in severe cases. The patient's face may appear pinched and blue, and she may have a malar rash. Jugular vein distention and ascites may be present in a patient with severe pulmonary hypertension or tricuspid stenosis. Palpation may reveal peripheral edema, hepatomegaly, and a diastolic thrill at the cardiac apex. Auscultation may reveal a loud S_1 or opening snap and a diastolic murmur at the apex, along the left sternal border, or at the base of the heart. (See *Identifying the murmur of mitral stenosis*.) In a patient with pulmonary hypertension, S_2 is commonly accentuated, and the two components of S_2 are closely split. A pulmonary systolic ejection click may be heard in a patient with severe pulmonary hypertension. Crackles may be heard when the lungs are auscultated.

COMPLICATIONS

- Pulmonary hypertension
- Pulmonary hemorrhage
- Pulmonary fibrosis
- Thrombi
- Infarction of the brain, kidneys, spleen, or limbs (most common in patients with arrhythmias)

DIAGNOSIS

- Echocardiography is the preferred diagnostic test for mitral stenosis.
- Transthoracic echocardiography is useful in establishing the diagnosis, determining the shape of the valve leaflets, and assessing the hemodynamic response to exercise.
- Transesophageal echocardiography will identify thrombus in the left atrium, a potential source of embolic stroke.
- Cardiac catheterization shows a diastolic pressure gradient across the valve. It also shows elevated pulmonary artery wedge pressure (greater than 15 mm Hg) and pulmonary artery pressure in the left atrium with severe pulmonary hypertension. It detects elevated right ventricular pressure, decreased

IDENTIFYING THE MURMUR OF MITRAL STENOSIS

Mitral stenosis produces a low, rumbling crescendo-decrescendo murmur in the mitral valve area, as diagrammed here.

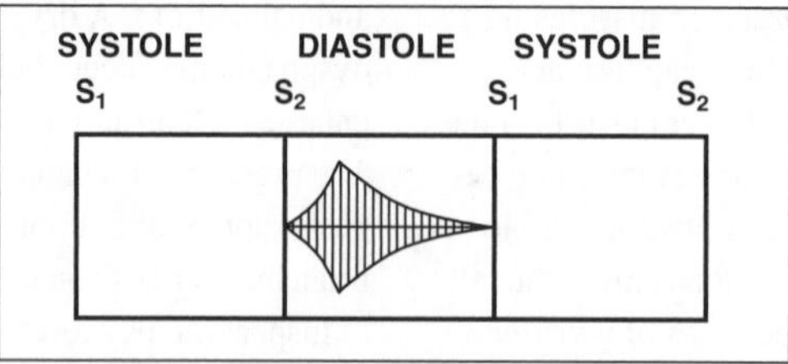

cardiac output, and abnormal contraction of the left ventricle.

- Cardiac catheterization can resolve discrepancies between the clinical presentation of a patient's symptoms and the results of a noninvasive transthoracic echocardiogram. If coronary artery disease is suspected, the need for coronary artery bypass graft surgery can be determined.
- Chest X-rays show left atrial and ventricular enlargement (in patients with severe mitral stenosis), straightening of the left border of the cardiac silhouette, enlarged pulmonary arteries, dilation of the upper lobe pulmonary veins, and mitral valve calcification.
- Electrocardiography reveals left atrial enlargement, right ventricular hypertrophy, right axis deviation and, in 40% to 50% of cases, atrial fibrillation.

TREATMENT

Treatment for the patient with valvular heart disease depends on the nature and severity of associated symptoms. In a young patient with asymptomatic mitral stenosis, endocarditis prophylaxis is important.

If the patient is symptomatic, treatment varies. Heart failure requires bed rest, medication, a sodium-restricted diet and, for acute cases, oxygen.

If hemoptysis develops, the patient requires bed rest, a sodium-restricted diet, and a diuretic to decrease pulmonary venous pressure. Embolization mandates an anticoagulant along with symptomatic treatments.

A patient with severe, medically uncontrollable symptoms may need open-heart surgery with cardiopulmonary bypass for valve replacement or repair. Percutaneous balloon valvuloplasty may be used in a young patient who has no calcification or subvalvular deformity, in the symptomatic pregnant woman, and in an elderly patient with end-stage disease who can't withstand general anesthesia. This procedure is performed in the cardiac catheterization laboratory.

Drugs

- Beta-adrenergic blockers or calcium channel blockers to control heart rate
- Anticoagulants to prevent thrombus formation around diseased, repaired, or replaced valves
- Digoxin (Lanoxin), diuretics, and vasodilators to treat heart failure

SPECIAL CONSIDERATIONS

- Before giving penicillin, ask the patient if she has ever had a hypersensitivity reaction to it. Even if she hasn't, warn her that such a reaction is possible.
- If the patient needs bed rest, stress its importance. Assist with bathing as needed. Provide a bedside commode because using a commode puts less stress on the heart than using a bedpan. Offer the patient diversionary, physically undemanding activities.
- To reduce anxiety, let the patient express concerns about her inability to meet her responsibilities because of activity restrictions. Reassure her

that activity limitations are temporary.

- Watch closely for signs of heart failure, pulmonary edema, and adverse reactions to drug therapy.
- Place the patient in an upright position to relieve dyspnea if needed. Give oxygen to prevent tissue hypoxia as needed.
- If the patient has had surgery, watch for hypotension, arrhythmias, and thrombus formation. Monitor her vital signs, arterial blood gas levels, intake and output, daily weight, blood chemistry results, chest X-rays, and pulmonary artery catheter readings.
- Keep the patient on a low-sodium diet; provide as many favorite foods as possible.
- Explain all tests and treatments.
- Advise the patient to plan for periodic rest in her daily routine to prevent undue fatigue.
- Teach the patient about diet restrictions, medications, symptoms that should be reported, and the importance of consistent follow-up care.
- Make sure the patient and her family understand the need to comply with prolonged antibiotic therapy and follow-up care and the possible need for additional antibiotics during dental or other surgical procedures.

Mitral valve prolapse

Mitral valve prolapse is also called *systolic click-murmur syndrome* and *floppy mitral valve syndrome.* The mitral valve, which separates the left atrium and left ventricle, is prolapsed into the left atrium and it doesn't open and close properly. (See *Valve position in mitral valve prolapse* and *Types of valvular heart disease,* page 8.)

CAUSES AND INCIDENCE

The cause of mitral valve prolapse is unknown. It has been linked to inherited connective tissue disorders, such as Marfan syndrome, Ehlers-Danlos syndrome, and osteogenesis imperfecta.

In this disorder, the cusps of the mitral valve are enlarged, thickened, and scalloped, possibly from collagen abnormalities. The chordae tendineae may be longer than usual, allowing the cusps to stretch upward. Mitral regurgitation occurs when the valve permits blood to leak into the atrium.

Mitral valve prolapse occurs in 3% to 8% of adults and is more common in women than in men.

SIGNS AND SYMPTOMS

Mitral valve prolapse typically produces no symptoms. When they do occur, the patient may complain of chest pain, palpitations, headache, fatigue, exercise intolerance, dyspnea, light-headedness, syncope, mood swings, anxiety, or panic attacks. Auscultation typically reveals a mobile, midsystolic click, with or without a mid-to-late systolic murmur.

COMPLICATIONS

- Ruptured chordae tendineae
- Ventricular failure
- Emboli

VALVE POSITION IN MITRAL VALVE PROLAPSE

This cross section of the left ventricle shows the positions of a normal and a prolapsed mitral valve.

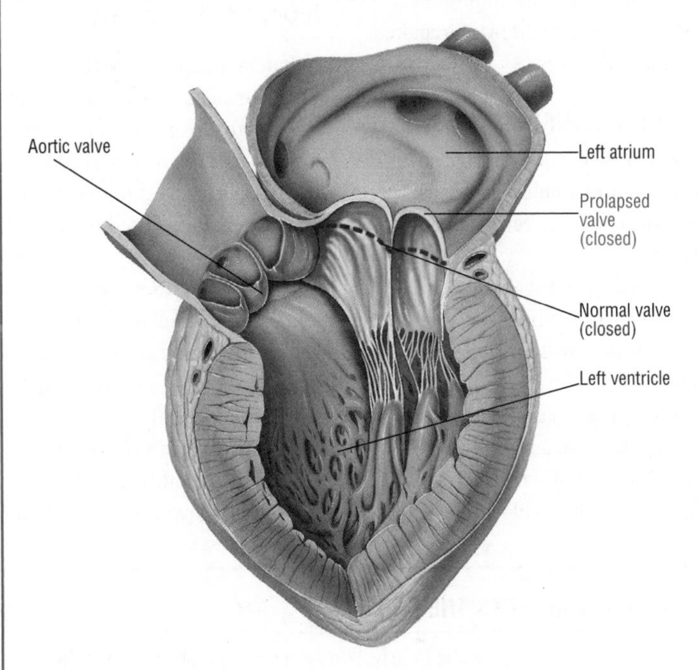

- Bacterial endocarditis
- Sudden death

DIAGNOSIS

- Two-dimensional echocardiography reveals prolapse of the mitral valve leaflets into the left atrium.
- Color-flow Doppler studies show mitral insufficiency.
- Resting electrocardiogram (ECG) demonstrates ST-segment changes and biphasic or inverted T-waves in leads II, III, or AV_F.
- Exercise ECG evaluates chest pain and arrhythmias.

TREATMENT

Treatment corresponds to the degree of mitral insufficiency. Activity restriction may be necessary as well as measures to avoid hypovolemia. Severe disease may necessitate valve repair or replacement.

Drugs

- Antibiotics to treat infective endocarditis
- Angiotensin-converting enzyme inhibitors or beta-adrenergic blockers to treat heart failure

• Digoxin (Lanoxin), calcium channel blockers, or beta-adrenergic blockers to treat arrhythmias
• Anticoagulants (warfarin [Coumadin]) to prevent thrombus formation around diseased, repaired, or replaced valves

SPECIAL CONSIDERATIONS

• Watch closely for evidence of heart failure or pulmonary edema and for adverse effects of drug therapy.
• Teach the patient about diet restrictions, medications, and the importance of consistent follow-up care.
• If the patient has surgery, watch for hypotension, arrhythmias, and thrombus formation. Monitor her vital signs, arterial blood gas values, intake, output, daily weight, blood chemistries, chest X-rays, and pulmonary artery catheter readings.

Myocardial infarction

Myocardial infarction (MI), commonly known as a *heart attack* and part of a broader category of disease known as *acute coronary syndromes* (ACS), results from prolonged myocardial ischemia caused by reduced blood flow through one of the coronary arteries. (See *How ACS affects the body*.) In cardiovascular disease, the leading cause of death in the United States and Western Europe, death usually results from cardiac damage or from complications of MI. Mortality is high when treatment is delayed, and almost half

HOW ACS AFFECTS THE BODY

An acute coronary syndrome (ACS) can have far-reaching physiological effects and requires a multidisciplinary approach to care. Here's what happens in ACS:

Cardiovascular system

- When the heart muscle is damaged by lack of oxygen, the integrity of the cell membrane is impaired.
- Intracellular contents, including cardiac enzymes (such as creatine kinase, lactate dehydrogenase, and aspartate aminotransferase) and proteins (such as troponin T, troponin I, and myoglobin) are released.
- An area of viable ischemic tissue surrounds a zone of injury, which may in turn surround a zone of dead myocardial tissue.
- Within 24 hours, the infarcted area becomes edematous and cyanotic.
- During the next several days, leukocytes infiltrate the necrotic area and begin to remove necrotic cells, thinning the ventricular wall.
- Scar formation begins by the 3rd week after a myocardial infarction (MI); by the 6th week, scar tissue is well established.
- Scar tissue that forms on the necrotic area inhibits contractility.
- Compensatory mechanisms (vascular constriction, increased heart rate, and renal retention of sodium and water) try to maintain cardiac output.

HOW ACS AFFECTS THE BODY *(continued)*

- Ventricular dilation also may occur in a process called remodeling.
- Functionally, an MI may cause reduced contractility with abnormal wall motion, altered left ventricular compliance, reduced stroke volume, reduced ejection fraction, and elevated left ventricular end-diastolic pressure.
- Cardiogenic shock is caused by failure of the heart to perform as an effective pump and can result in low cardiac output, diminished peripheral perfusion, pulmonary congestion, and elevated systemic vascular resistance and pulmonary vascular pressures.
- Ineffective contractility of the heart leads to the accumulation of blood in the venous circulation upstream to the failing ventricle.
- Arrhythmias may occur in a patient with an acute MI as a result of autonomic nervous system imbalance, electrolyte disturbances, ischemia, and slowed conduction in zones of ischemic myocardium.

Neurologic system

- Hypoperfusion of the brain results in altered mental status, involving changes in levels of consciousness, restlessness, irritability, confusion, or disorientation.
- Stupor or coma may result if the decrease in cerebral perfusion continues.

Renal system

- Shock and hypoperfusion from an MI cause the kidneys to respond by conserving salt and water.
- Poor perfusion results in diminished renal blood flow, increased afferent arteriolar resistance, and a decreased glomerular filtration rate.
- Increased amounts of antidiuretic hormone and aldosterone are released to help maintain perfusion. However, urine formation is reduced.
- Depletion of renal adenosine triphosphate stores results from prolonged renal hypoperfusion, causing impaired renal function.

Respiratory system

- Cardiogenic shock with left-sided heart failure results in increased fluid in the lungs. This process can overwhelm the capacity of the pulmonary lymphatics, resulting in interstitial and alveolar edema.
- Lung edema occurs when pulmonary capillary pressure exceeds 18 mm Hg.
- Pulmonary alveolar edema develops when pressures exceed 24 mm Hg, impairing oxygen diffusion.
- Increased interstitial and intra-alveolar fluid causes progressive reduction in lung compliance, increasing the work of ventilation and increasing perfusion of poorly ventilated alveoli.

Collaborative management

A cardiologist will provide an initial assessment and treatment, and a cardiothoracic surgeon may be needed if the patient's condition warrants invasive therapy. After initial therapy and treatment, other specialists may be needed, such as a physical therapist for cardiac rehabilitation and a nutritionist for dietary and lifestyle changes.

of sudden deaths from MI occur before hospitalization, within 1 hour after symptoms begin. The prognosis improves if vigorous treatment begins immediately.

CAUSES AND INCIDENCE

Predisposing risk factors include:
- diabetes mellitus
- drug use, especially cocaine
- elevated serum triglyceride, total cholesterol, and low-density lipoprotein levels
- hypertension
- obesity or excessive intake of saturated fats, carbohydrates, or salt
- family history
- sedentary lifestyle
- smoking
- stress or a type A personality.

Rupture or erosion of plaque—an unstable and lipid-rich substance—launches all coronary syndromes. The rupture results in platelet adhesions, fibrin clot formation, and activation of thrombin. When a thrombus progresses and occludes blood flow, MI results. (See *What happens during a myocardial infarction,* page 132.) The degree of blockage and the time that the affected vessel remains occluded determine the type of infarct that occurs. The underlying effect is an imbalance in myocardial oxygen supply and demand. (See *Stages of myocardial ischemia, injury, and infarct,* page 134.)

For patients with unstable angina, a thrombus full of platelets partially occludes a coronary vessel. The partially occluded vessel may have distal microthrombi that cause necrosis in some myocytes. The smaller vessels infarct, thus placing the patient at higher risk for a non–ST-segment elevation MI (NSTEMI).

If a thrombus fully occludes the vessel for a prolonged time, it's classified as an ST-segment elevation MI (STEMI). This type of MI involves a greater concentration of thrombin and fibrin.

The site of MI depends on the vessels involved.
- Occlusion of the circumflex branch of the left coronary artery causes a lateral wall infarction.
- Occlusion of the anterior descending branch of the left coronary artery causes an anterior wall infarction.
- True posterior or inferior wall MIs typically result from occlusion of the right coronary artery or one of its branches. Right ventricular infarctions can also result from right coronary artery occlusion, can accompany inferior infarctions, and may cause right-sided heart failure.

In a Q-wave (transmural) MI, tissue damage extends through all myocardial layers. In a non–Q-wave (subendocardial) MI, it affects only the innermost and possibly the middle layers.

Incidence is high: About 1 million patients visit the hospital each year with an MI and another 200,000 to 300,000 people die from MI-related complications without seeking medical care. Men and postmenopausal women are more susceptible to MI than premenopausal women, although incidence is rising among women, especially those who smoke and take hormonal contraceptives.

SIGNS AND SYMPTOMS

The cardinal symptom of MI—particularly for men—is persistent, crushing substernal pain that may radiate to the left arm, jaw, neck, or shoulder blades. Such pain is usually described as heavy, squeezing, or crushing and may persist for 12 hours or more. However, in some MI patients—particularly elderly people or those with diabetes—pain may not occur at all; in others, it may be mild and confused with indigestion. In patients with coronary artery disease (CAD), angina of increasing frequency, severity, or duration (especially if not provoked by exertion, a heavy meal, or cold and wind) may signal impending infarction.

Other clinical effects include a feeling of impending doom, fatigue, nausea, vomiting, and shortness of breath. The patient may have no symptoms. He may develop catecholamine responses, such as coolness in the limbs, perspiration, anxiety, and restlessness. Fever is unusual at the onset of an MI, but a low-grade temperature elevation may develop during the next few days. Blood pressure varies; hypotension or hypertension may be present. Auscultation may reveal diminished heart sounds, gallops and, in papillary dysfunction, the apical systolic murmur of mitral insufficiency over the mitral valve area.

COMPLICATIONS

The most common post-MI complications include recurrent or persistent chest pain, arrhythmias, left-sided heart failure (resulting in heart failure or acute pulmonary edema), and cardiogenic shock. Unusual but potentially lethal complications that may develop soon after infarction include thromboembolism; papillary muscle dysfunction or rupture, causing mitral insufficiency; rupture of the ventricular septum, causing ventricular septal defect; rupture of the myocardium; and ventricular aneurysm. Up to several months after infarction, Dressler's syndrome may develop.

Arrhythmias

Electrocardiogram (ECG) shows premature ventricular contractions, ventricular tachycardia, or ventricular fibrillation. In an inferior wall MI, the patient may have bradycardia and junctional rhythms or atrioventricular block. In an anterior wall MI, he may have tachycardia or heart block. Treatment includes antiarrhythmics, atropine, a pacemaker, and cardioversion for tachycardia.

Heart failure

In left-sided heart failure, chest X-rays show venous congestion, cardiomegaly, and Kerley's B lines. Catheterization shows increased pulmonary artery pressure (PAP) and central venous pressure. Treatment includes diuretics, angiotensin-converting enzyme (ACE) inhibitors, vasodilators, inotropic

(*Text continues on page 135.*)

WHAT HAPPENS DURING A MYOCARDIAL INFARCTION

When blood supply to the myocardium is interrupted, the following events occur:

1. Injury to the endothelial lining of the coronary arteries causes platelets, white blood cells, fibrin, and lipids to converge at the injured site. Foam cells, or resident macrophages, congregate under the damaged lining and absorb oxidized cholesterol, forming a fatty streak that narrows the arterial lumen.

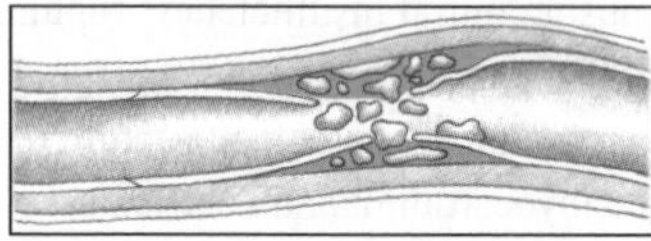

2. Because the arterial lumen narrows gradually, collateral circulation develops and helps maintain myocardial perfusion distal to the obstruction. During this stage, the patient may have angina when myocardial oxygen demand increases.

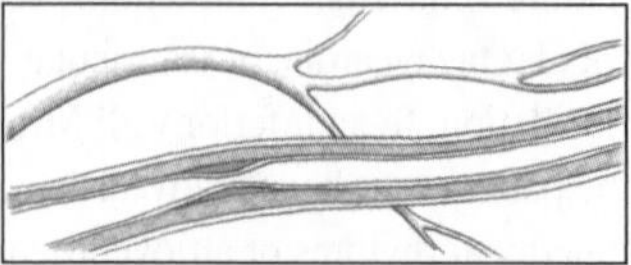

3. When myocardial demand for oxygen is more than the collateral circulation can supply, myocardial metabolism shifts from aerobic to anaerobic, producing lactic acid (A), which stimulates pain nerve endings. The patient develops worsening angina that needs rest and medication for relief.

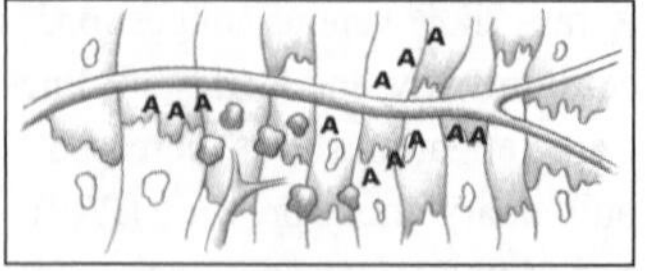

4. If they continue to lack oxygen, the myocardial cells die. This decreases contractility, stroke volume, and blood pressure. The patient develops tachycardia, hypotension, diminished heart sounds, cyanosis, tachypnea, and poor perfusion to vital organs.

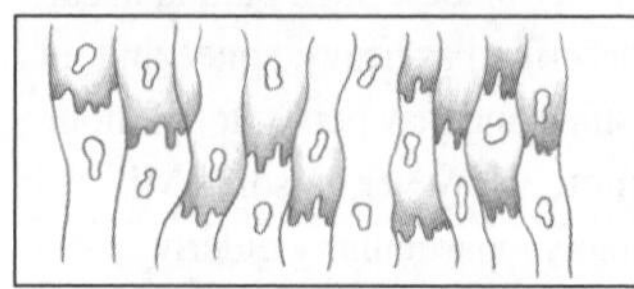

5. Hypoperfusion stimulates baroreceptors, which in turn stimulate the adrenal glands to release epinephrine and norepinephrine. These catecholamines (C) increase the heart rate and cause peripheral vasoconstriction, further increasing myocardial oxygen demand. The patient may have tachyarrhythmias, changes in pulse rates, a decreased level of consciousness, and cold, clammy skin.

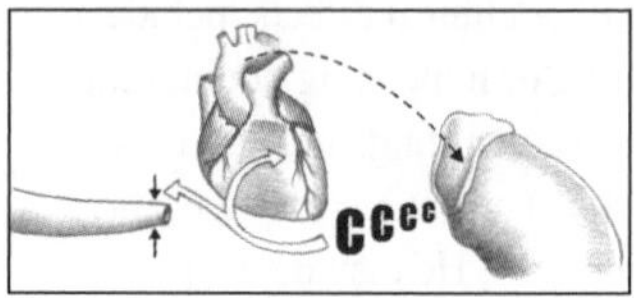

6. Damaged cell membranes in the infarcted area allow intracellular contents to enter the vascular circulation. Ventricular arrhythmias then develop with elevated serum levels of potassium (■), creatine kinase (CK) and CK-MB (▲), troponin (•), and lactate dehydrogenase (○).

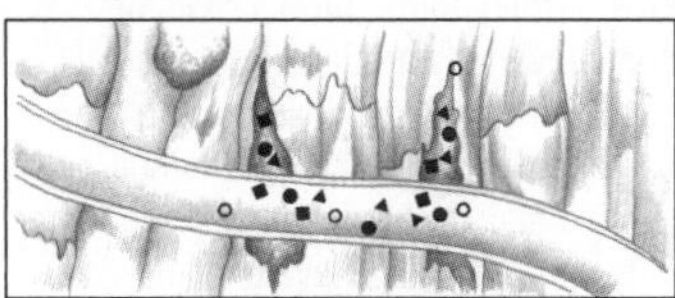

7. All myocardial cells are capable of spontaneous depolarization and repolarization, so the electrical conduction system may be affected by ischemia, injury, and infarct. The patient may have fever, leukocytosis, tachycardia, and electrocardiogram signs of tissue ischemia (altered T waves), injured tissue (altered ST segments), and infarcted tissue (deep Q waves).

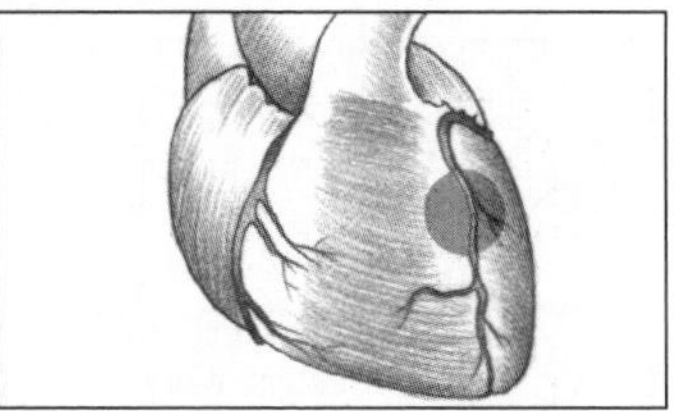

8. Extensive damage to the left ventricle may impair its ability to pump, allowing blood to back up into the left atrium and, eventually, into the pulmonary veins and capillaries. When this occurs, the patient may be dyspneic, orthopneic, tachypneic, and cyanotic. Crackles may be heard in the lungs on auscultation. Pulmonary artery and pulmonary artery wedge pressures are increased.

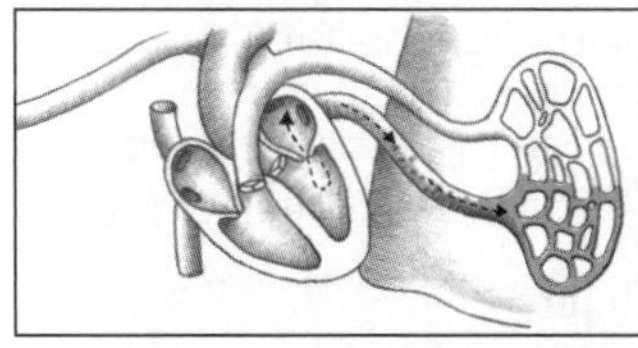

9. As back pressure increases, fluid crosses the alveolar-capillary membrane, impeding diffusion of oxygen (O_2) and carbon dioxide (CO_2). The patient has increasing respiratory distress, and arterial blood gas results may show decreased partial pressure of oxygen and arterial pH and increased partial pressure of carbon dioxide.

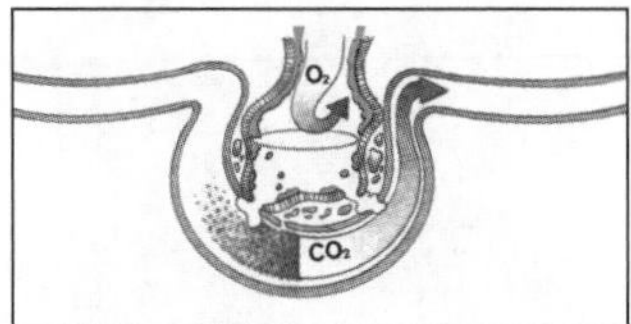

STAGES OF MYOCARDIAL ISCHEMIA, INJURY, AND INFARCT

Occlusion of a coronary artery can cause three stages of myocardial tissue damage: ischemia, injury, and infarction.

Ischemia

Ischemia is the first stage and develops when blood flow is insufficient to meet the heart muscle's oxygen demand. Ischemia can be reversed by improving blood flow or by reducing the oxygen needs of cardiac muscle supplied by the affected artery. During ischemia, an electrocardiogram (ECG) may show ST-segment depression or T-wave changes, as shown below.

Injury

The second stage, injury, occurs when the ischemia lasts long enough to damage the affected area of heart muscle. An ECG usually shows ST-segment elevation (usually in two or more leads).

Infarction

In infarction, the third stage, myocardial cells die from lack of oxygen. Scar tissue eventually replaces the dead area, and damage to the heart muscle is permanent.

Early in a myocardial infarction (MI), hyperacute (very tall and narrow) T waves may appear on the ECG. Within hours, the T waves become inverted and the ST-segment becomes elevated in leads facing the damaged area. Finally, a pathologic Q wave may develop, which is the only permanent ECG evidence of myocardial necrosis.

Q waves are pathologic when they're 0.04 second wide or wider and when their height is more than 25% of the R wave height in that lead. They develop in more than 90% of patients with ST-segment elevation MI and about 25% of patients with a non-ST-segment elevation MI. (The remainder have what's called a non-Q wave MI.)

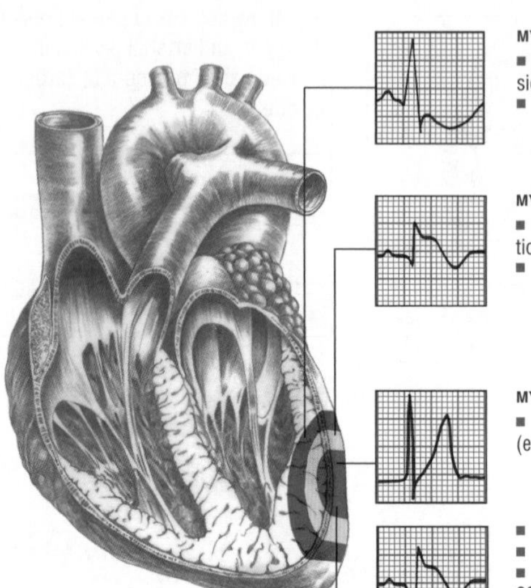

MYOCARDIAL ISCHEMIA
- ST-segment depression
- T-wave inversion

MYOCARDIAL INJURY
- ST-segment elevation
- T-wave inversion

MYOCARDIAL INFARCTION
- Hyperacute T waves (earliest stage)

- ST-segment elevation
- T-wave inversion
- Pathologic Q waves in 90% of ST-segment elevation MIs and 25% of non-ST-segment elevation MIs

agents, cardiac glycosides, and beta-adrenergic blockers.

Cardiogenic shock

In cardiogenic shock, catheterization shows decreased cardiac output and increased PAP and pulmonary artery wedge pressure (PAWP). Signs include hypertension, tachycardia, S_3, S_4, decreased level of consciousness, decreased urine output, jugular vein distension, and cool, pale skin. Treatment includes I.V. fluids, vasodilators, diuretics, cardiac glycosides, an intra-aortic balloon pump (IABP), a ventricular assist device (VAD), and beta-adrenergic agonists.

Thromboembolism

A patient with thromboembolism has severe dyspnea and chest pain or neurologic changes. A nuclear scan shows a ventilation-perfusion mismatch, and angiography shows arterial blockage. Treatment includes oxygen and heparin.

Rupture of left ventricular papillary muscle

A ruptured left papillary muscle causes hypotension and pulmonary edema. Auscultation reveals an apical holosystolic murmur. Inspection of jugular vein pulse or hemodynamic monitoring shows increased *v* waves. Dyspnea is prominent. Color-flow and Doppler echocardiogram show mitral insufficiency. Pulmonary artery catheterization shows increased PAP and PAWP. Treatment includes nitroprusside (Nitropress), an IABP, a VAD, and surgical replacement of the mitral valve with possible myocardial revascularization (in patients with significant CAD).

Ventricular septal rupture

In a left-to-right shunt, auscultation reveals a holosystolic murmur and thrill. Catheterization shows increased PAP and PAWP. Confirmation is by increased oxygen saturation of the right ventricle and pulmonary artery. Treatment includes surgical correction, an IABP, nitroglycerin, nitroprusside, low-dose inotropic agents, or a pacemaker.

Ventricular aneurysm

In a ventricular aneurysm, a chest X-ray may show cardiomegaly. An ECG may show arrhythmias and persistent ST-segment elevation. Left ventriculography shows altered or paradoxical left ventricular motion. Treatment includes cardioversion, defibrillation, antiarrhythmics, vasodilators, anticoagulants, cardiac glycosides, and diuretics. If conservative treatment fails, surgical resection is needed.

Pericarditis or Dressler's syndrome

Dressler's syndrome causes pericarditis, a pericardial friction rub, chest pain, fever, leukocytosis, and possibly pleurisy or pneumonitis. Chest pain is relieved by sitting up. A 12-lead ECG shows diffuse ST-segment changes. Treatment includes aspirin and nonsteroidal anti-inflammatory drugs (NSAIDs).

DIAGNOSIS

- In a serial 12-lead ECG, abnormalities may be absent or inconclusive during the first few hours after an MI. When present, characteristic abnormalities include serial ST-segment depression in non–Q-wave (subendocardial) MI and ST-segment elevation in Q-wave (transmural) MI. (See *ECG characteristics in acute coronary syndromes*.)

ECG CHARACTERISTICS IN ACUTE CORONARY SYNDROMES

The initial step in assessing a patient complaining of chest pain is to obtain an electrocardiogram (ECG). This should be done within 10 minutes of being seen by the practitioner. It's crucial in determining the presence of myocardial ischemia, and the findings direct the treatment plan.

Angina

Most patients with angina show ischemic changes on an ECG only during the attack. Because these changes may be fleeting, always obtain an order for and perform a 12-lead ECG as soon as the patient reports chest pain.

MI

According to the American Heart Association, patients should be classified as having ST-segment elevation or new left bundle-branch block (LBBB), ST-segment depression or dynamic T-wave inversion, or nondiagnostic or normal ECG.

ST-segment elevation or new LBBB

- Patients with an ST-segment elevation of 1 mm or more in two or more contiguous leads or with new LBBB need to be treated for an acute myocardial infarction (MI).
- More than 90% of patients with this presentation will develop new Q waves and have positive serum cardiac markers.
- Repeating the ECG may be helpful for patients who present with hyperacute T waves.

ST-segment depression or dynamic T-wave inversion

- Patients with ST-segment depression, indicating a posterior MI, benefit most when an acute MI is diagnosed.
- Ischemia should be suspected with findings of ST-segment depression of 0.5 mm or more, marked symmetrical T-wave inversion in multiple precordial leads, and dynamic ST-T changes with pain.
- Patients with persistent symptoms and recurrent ischemia, diffuse or widespread ECG abnormalities, heart failure, and positive serum markers are considered high risk.

Nondiagnostic or normal ECG

- A normal ECG won't show ST-segment changes or arrhythmias.
- If the ECG is nondiagnostic, it may show ST-segment depression of less than 0.5 mm or T-wave inversion or flattening in leads with dominant R waves.
- Continue assessing myocardial changes with serial ECGs, ST-segment monitoring, and serum cardiac markers.
- If further assessment is warranted, perform perfusion radionuclide imaging and stress echocardiography.

• In serial serum enzyme levels, creatine kinase (CK) levels are elevated, specifically the CK-MB isoenzyme.
• Troponin T or troponin I is also used in the diagnosis because both are specific to cardiac necrosis, and levels rise 6 to 8 hours after the onset of ischemia.
• Echocardiography may show abnormalities of ventricular wall motion in patients with a Q-wave (transmural) MI.
• Nuclear ventriculography scans (multiple gated acquisition or radionuclide ventriculography) using an I.V. radioactive substance can identify acutely damaged muscle by picking up radioactive nucleotides, producing a "hot spot" on the film that's useful in localizing a recent MI.

TREATMENT

The goals of treatment are to relieve chest pain, stabilize heart rhythm, reduce cardiac workload, revascularize the coronary arteries, and preserve myocardial tissue. (See *Treating an MI,* pages 138.) Arrhythmias, the main problem during the first 48 hours after MI, may require antiarrhythmics, possibly a pacemaker and, rarely, cardioversion. Arrhythmias are best detected using a 12-lead ECG.

The preferred method of reperfusing myocardial tissue during STEMI is percutaneous intervention (PCI) as long as the procedure can start within 12 hours of symptom onset and if the balloon can be inflated within 90 minutes of arrival to the hospital. If PCI isn't available at the presenting hospital, rapid transport to another hospital results in a better outcome than fibrinolysis as long as door-to-balloon time (including transport) is less than 90 minutes. If total door-to-balloon time is expected to exceed 90 minutes, then a fibrinolytic is given, followed by emergency transfer to a center capable of performing a PCI within 6 hours, even if reperfusion is successful. Door-to-needle time for fibrinolytics should be less than 30 minutes.

The PCI should be performed by an experienced operator who performs more than 75 PCIs per year and in a center that performs more than 200 PCIs annually. All patients undergoing PCI should be premedicated with aspirin and clopidogrel (Plavix). Preferred thrombolytics include streptokinase (Streptose), alteplase (Activase), tenecteplase (TNKase), and reteplase (Retavase). (See *Comparing thrombolytics,* page 140.)

NSTEMI is treated with cardiac catheterization, PCI, or both within 48 hours of symptom onset. In contrast to STEMI, patients with NSTEMI shouldn't receive thrombolytic therapy.

Other treatments may include:
• pulmonary artery catheterization, an IABP, or a VAD for cardiogenic shock or left- or right-sided heart failure
• transcutaneous pacing, a transvenous pacemaker, or defibrillation if

(*Text continues on page 141.*)

TREATING AN MI

This flowchart shows treatments that may be provided for various stages of myocardial infarction (MI).

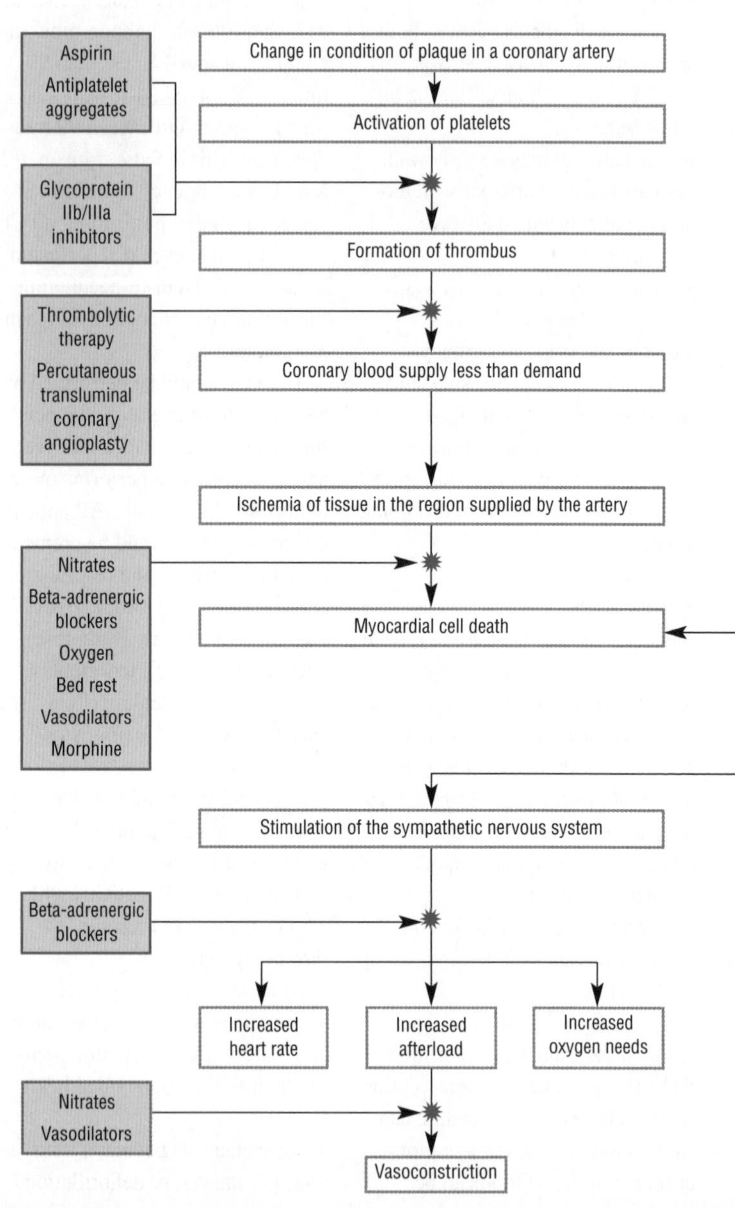

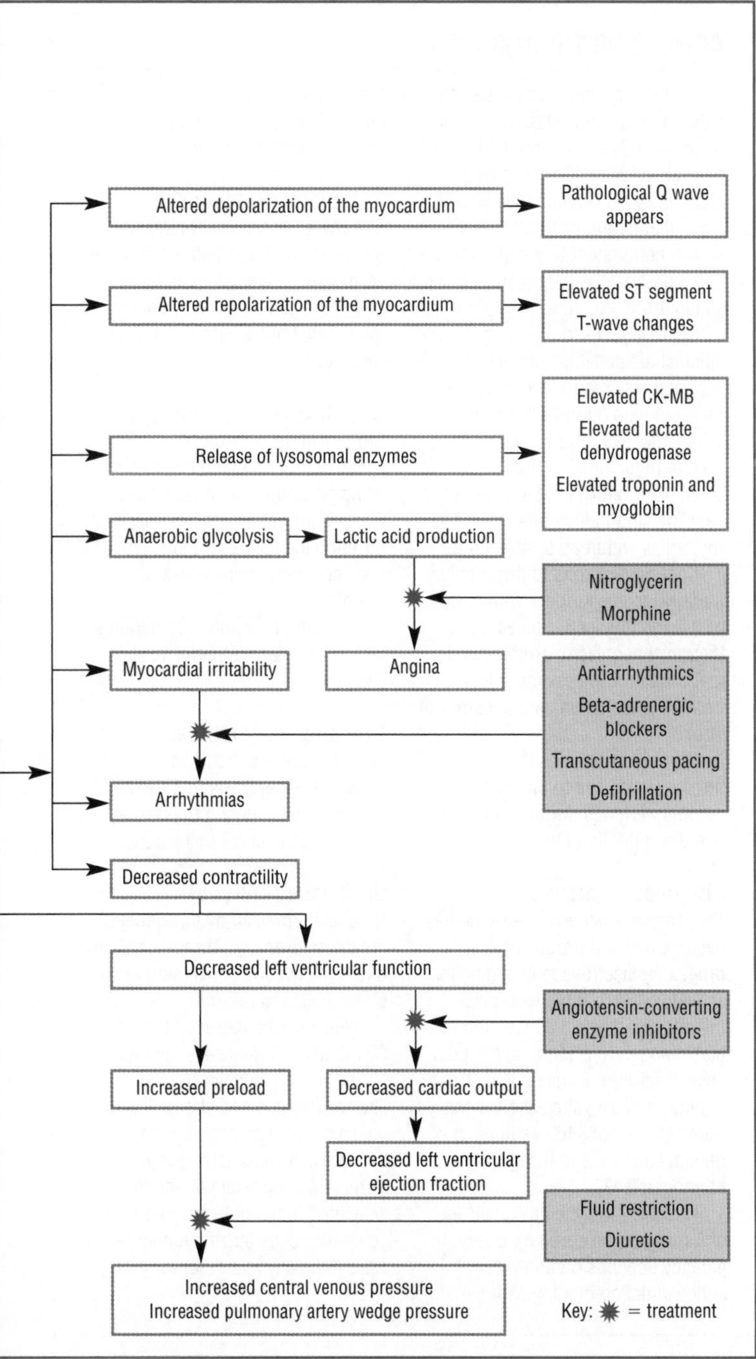

Altered depolarization of the myocardium
Pathological Q wave appears
Altered repolarization of the myocardium
Elevated ST segment
T-wave changes
Release of lysosomal enzymes
Elevated CK-MB
Elevated lactate dehydrogenase
Elevated troponin and myoglobin
Anaerobic glycolysis
Lactic acid production
Nitroglycerin
Morphine
Myocardial irritability
Angina
Antiarrhythmics
Beta-adrenergic blockers
Transcutaneous pacing
Defibrillation
Arrhythmias
Decreased contractility
Decreased left ventricular function
Angiotensin-converting enzyme inhibitors
Increased preload
Decreased cardiac output
Decreased left ventricular ejection fraction
Fluid restriction
Diuretics
Increased central venous pressure
Increased pulmonary artery wedge pressure
Key: = treatment

COMPARING THROMBOLYTICS

Thrombolytic drugs are tissue activators that convert plasminogen to plasmin, thus enhancing the body's natural ability to dissolve blood clots. Plasmin is a nonspecific protease that degrades fibrin (the essential component of a clot), fibrinogen, and procoagulant factors (such as factors V, VII, and XII).

Candidates for thrombolytic therapy include patients with acute ST-segment elevation and chest pain of no more than 6 hours' duration. When effective, thrombolytics can restore myocardial perfusion, relieve chest pain, return the ST segment to baseline, and induce reperfusion arrhythmias within 30 to 45 minutes.

Contraindications to thrombolytic therapy include surgery within the past 2 months, active bleeding, intracranial neoplasm, arteriovenous malformation, aneurysm, uncontrolled hypertension, and a history of stroke.

Here's a review of selected thrombolytics use to open occluded coronary arteries during acute myocardial infarction (MI).

Alteplase (Activase)

This naturally occurring enzyme has been cloned and produced as a drug, alteplase (tissue plasminogen activator [tPA]). It binds to plasminogen, catalyzing conversion of plasminogen to plasmin in the presence of fibrin. Because it has strong affinity for fibrin, alteplase concentrates at the clot site, resulting in a minimal decrease in the systemic fibrinogen level.

This thrombolytic has a half-life of 5 minutes, so coronary artery patency depends on continued anticoagulation therapy with heparin. Alteplase doesn't induce antigenic responses, and doses may be repeated at any time.

Reteplase (Retavase)

Reteplase, recombinant plasminogen activator, has a half-life of 13 to 16 minutes. Because of its longer half-life, it can be given in bolus form. Two boluses are needed for treatment.

Streptokinase (Streptase)

Streptokinase, a thrombolytic, is a bacterial protein that binds to circulating plasminogen and catalyzes plasmin formation. Its low specificity for fibrin induces a systemic lytic state and increases the risk of bleeding.

The half-life is about 20 minutes. Like anistreplase, streptokinase is antigenic.

Tenecteplase (TNKase)

Tenecteplase is a modified form of human tPA that binds to fibrin and converts plasminogen to plasmin. It's given as a single bolus dose.

Urokinase (Kinlytic)

Naturally produced by the kidneys, urokinase promotes thrombolysis by directly activating conversion of plasminogen to plasmin.

With a serum half-life of 10 to 20 minutes, urokinase is rapidly cleared by the kidneys and liver. Unlike anistreplase and streptokinase, it doesn't induce an antigenic response. Urokinase isn't given through a peripheral I.V. line to treat an acute MI, but patients who undergo cardiac catheterization may receive it directly in a coronary artery.

the patient has ventricular fibrillation or pulseless ventricular tachycardia
- percutaneous transluminal coronary angioplasty or coronary artery bypass graft surgery for obstructive lesions.

Drugs

- Oxygen administration (a lower concentration if the patient has chronic obstructive pulmonary disease)
- Thrombolytics for STEMI when PCI will be delayed by 90 minutes
- Heparin and glycoprotein IIb/IIIa inhibitors to minimize platelet aggregation
- Nitrates to reduce myocardial oxygen demand while possibly increasing supply (sublingual, I.V., and then oral or topical)
- Beta-adrenergic blockers to reduce myocardial work (I.V. and then oral)
- Statins to stabilize atherosclerotic plaque and lower serum lipids (oral)
- ACE inhibitors to reduce myocardial work (oral) or angiotensin II receptor blockers (oral) if the patient can't tolerate ACE inhibitors
- Calcium channel blockers (oral) when beta-adrenergic blockers are contraindicated and the patient doesn't have left ventricular dysfunction or heart failure (immediate-release nifedipine [Procardia] is contraindicated)
- Anticoagulation (I.V. and then oral) for patients at high risk for thromboembolism (such as those with atrial fibrillation, a left ventricular thrombus or aneurysm, a left ventricular ejection fraction (LVEF) less than 30%, or a history of thromboembolism)
- Antiarrhythmics (I.V. and then oral) for patients with atrial or ventricular arrhythmias
- Aldosterone antagonists to reduce myocardial work for patients with a low LVEF or diabetes (oral)
- Atropine I.V. or a temporary pacemaker for heart block or bradycardia
- Low-dose unfractionated or low–molecular-weight heparin for deep vein thrombosis prophylaxis for immobile patients
- Morphine (I.V.) for pain and preload reduction after the MI has been diagnosed
- Positive inotropes, diuretics, vasoactive medications, left ventricular support (with IABP, left ventricular assist device, percutaneous bypass), PCI, or open-heart surgery to treat cardiogenic shock

SPECIAL CONSIDERATIONS

- Care for a patient with an MI is directed toward detecting complications, preventing further myocardial damage, and promoting comfort, rest, and emotional well-being. The patient usually receives treatment in the intensive care unit (ICU), where he's under constant observation for complications.
- On admission to the ICU, monitor and record the patient's ECG, blood pressure, intake and output, oxygen saturation, temperature, and heart and breath sounds. To decrease

cardiac workload, maintain bed rest and provide a bedside commode.

- Assess and record the severity and duration of pain, and give analgesics. Avoid I.M. injections; absorption from the muscle is unpredictable, and bleeding is likely if the patient receives thrombolytic therapy.
- Check the patient's blood pressure after giving nitroglycerin, especially the first dose.
- Monitor telemetry to detect rate changes or arrhythmias. Place rhythm strips in the patient's chart periodically for evaluation.
- Daily, during episodes of chest pain, and before and after nitroglycerin therapy, obtain a 12-lead ECG, blood pressure, and pulmonary artery catheter measurements. Monitor them for changes.
- Watch for signs and symptoms of fluid retention (crackles, cough, tachypnea, decreased oxygenation, increased filling pressures, jugular vein distention, and edema), which may indicate impending heart failure. Carefully monitor daily weight, intake and output, respirations, serum enzyme levels, and blood pressure. Auscultate for adventitious breath sounds periodically (patients on bed rest commonly have atelectatic crackles that disappear after coughing), for S_3 or S_4 gallops, and for new-onset heart murmurs.
- If the patient receives an ACE inhibitor, an aldosterone antagonist, or both, watch for increased potassium levels.
- Don't give beta-adrenergic blockers to patients with cardiogenic shock, bradycardia, heart block, or reactive airway disease.
- Nitrates are contraindicated in patients who have taken a phosphodiesterase inhibitor within the previous 24 hours, and they should be used cautiously or avoided in patients with severe aortic stenosis or right ventricular infarction.
- Keep the serum potassium level above 4 mEq/L and the magnesium level above 2 mEq/L to reduce arrhythmias.
- NSAIDs (except aspirin) should be discontinued.
- Organize patient care and activities to maximize periods of uninterrupted rest.
- Start a cardiac rehabilitation program. This usually includes education about heart disease, exercise, and emotional support for the patient and his family.
- Ask the dietary department to provide a clear liquid diet until nausea subsides. A low-carbohydrate, low-cholesterol, low-sodium, low-fat, high-fiber diet may be prescribed.
- Provide a stool softener to prevent straining during defecation, which causes vagal stimulation and may slow the heart rate. Allow the use of a bedside commode, and provide as much privacy as possible.
- Assist with range-of-motion exercises. If the patient is completely immobilized by a severe MI, turn him often. Antiembolism stockings

help prevent venostasis and thrombophlebitis.

- Provide emotional support, and help reduce stress and anxiety; give tranquilizers as needed. Explain procedures and answer questions. Explaining the ICU environment and routine can ease the patient's anxiety. Involve the patient's family in his care as much as possible.

Preparing for discharge

- Thoroughly explain dosages and therapy to promote compliance with the prescribed medication regimen and other treatment measures. Warn about adverse drug effects, and advise the patient to watch for and report evidence of toxicity (anorexia, nausea, vomiting, and yellow vision, for example, if the patient is receiving digoxin [Lanoxin]).
- Review diet restrictions with the patient. If he must follow a special diet, provide a list of foods that he should avoid. Ask the dietitian to speak to the patient and his family.
- Counsel the patient about when to resume sexual activity, and instruct him to do so progressively.
- Advise the patient to report typical or atypical chest pain. Postinfarction syndrome may develop, producing chest pain that must be differentiated from recurrent MI, pulmonary infarct, or heart failure.
- If the patient has a Holter monitor in place, explain its purpose and use.
- Provide information about smoking cessation, if needed.
- Encourage participation in a cardiac rehabilitation program.
- Review follow-up procedures, such as office visits and treadmill testing, with the patient.
- Instruct the patient to practice heart-healthy living, with a heart-healthy diet, regular exercise, stress reduction, preventive care, weight control, smoking cessation, and abstinence from alcohol and illegal drugs, especially cocaine.
- Suggest a daily aspirin regimen for patients with CAD.

Myocarditis

Myocarditis is a focal or diffuse inflammation of the cardiac muscle (myocardium). It may be acute or chronic and may occur at any age. In many cases, myocarditis produces no specific cardiovascular symptoms or electrocardiogram (ECG) abnormalities, and recovery is spontaneous and without residual defects. Occasionally, myocarditis is complicated by heart failure; in rare cases, it leads to cardiomyopathy.

CAUSES AND INCIDENCE

Myocarditis may result from:

- bacterial infections, such as diphtheria, tuberculosis, typhoid fever, tetanus, and staphylococcal, pneumococcal, and gonococcal infections
- chemical poisons such as chronic alcoholism
- helminthic infections such as trichinosis
- hypersensitive immune reactions, such as acute rheumatic fever and postcardiotomy syndrome

- parasitic infections, such as toxoplasmosis and especially South American trypanosomiasis (Chagas' disease) in infants and immunosuppressed adults
- radiation therapy, particularly large doses of radiation to the chest in treating lung or breast cancer
- viral infections (most common cause in the United States and western Europe), such as coxsackievirus A and B strains and possibly poliomyelitis, influenza, rubeola, rubella, and adenoviruses and echoviruses.

Damage to the myocardium occurs when an infectious organism triggers an autoimmune, cellular, and humoral reaction. The resulting inflammation may lead to hypertrophy, fibrosis, and inflammatory changes of the myocardium and conduction system. The heart muscle weakens, and contractility is reduced. The heart muscle becomes flabby and dilated, and pinpoint hemorrhages may develop.

Myocarditis occurs in 1 to 10 of every 100,000 people in the United States. It causes up to 20% of all cases of sudden death in young adults. The median age for this disorder is 42, and incidence is equal in men and women. Children, especially neonates, and people who are immunocompromised or pregnant (especially pregnant black women) are at higher risk for this disorder.

SIGNS AND SYMPTOMS

Myocarditis usually causes nonspecific symptoms—such as fatigue, dyspnea, palpitations, and fever—that reflect the accompanying systemic infection. Signs and symptoms may relate to either the actual inflammation of the myocardium or the weakness of the heart muscle due to the inflammation. Occasionally, it may produce mild, continuous pressure or soreness in the chest (unlike the recurring, stress-related pain of angina pectoris). Physical examination shows supraventricular and ventricular arrhythmias, S_3 and S_4 gallops, a faint S_1, possibly a murmur of mitral insufficiency (from papillary muscle dysfunction) and, if pericarditis is present, a pericardial friction rub.

Although myocarditis usually is self-limiting, it may induce myofibril degeneration that results in right- and left-sided heart failure, with cardiomegaly, jugular vein distention, dyspnea, persistent fever with resting or exertional tachycardia disproportionate to the degree of fever, and supraventricular and ventricular arrhythmias. Sometimes myocarditis recurs or produces chronic valvulitis (when it results from rheumatic fever), cardiomyopathy, arrhythmias, and thromboembolism.

COMPLICATIONS

- Arrhythmias
- Thromboembolism
- Pericarditis
- Chronic valvulitis (when disease results from rheumatic fever)
- Recurrence of disease

• Left-sided heart failure (occasional)
• Cardiomyopathy (rare)

DIAGNOSIS

History reveals recent febrile upper respiratory tract infection. These tests help confirm the diagnosis of myocarditis:

• Laboratory testing may reveal elevated levels of creatine kinase (CK), CK-MB, troponin I, troponin T, aspartate aminotransferase, and lactate dehydrogenase. Also, inflammation and infection can cause an elevated white blood cell count and erythrocyte sedimentation rate.
• Antibody titers, such as antistreptolysin-O titer in rheumatic fever, may be elevated.
• ECG may reveal diffuse ST-segment and T-wave abnormalities, conduction defects (prolonged PR interval, bundle-branch block, or complete heart block), supraventricular arrhythmias, and ventricular extrasystoles.
• Chest X-rays may show an enlarged heart and pulmonary vascular congestion.
• Echocardiography may show some degree of left ventricular dysfunction.
• Radionuclide scanning may identify inflammatory and necrotic changes characteristic of myocarditis.
• Laboratory cultures of stool, throat, and other body fluids may identify bacterial or viral causes of infection.
• Endomyocardial biopsy may confirm the diagnosis. A negative biopsy doesn't exclude the diagnosis.

TREATMENT

Treatment includes drugs, modified bed rest to decrease the workload on the heart, and careful management of complications. Heart failure requires restriction of activity to minimize myocardial oxygen consumption, supplemental oxygen therapy, sodium restriction, diuretics, and cardiac glycosides. Surgical treatment may include left ventricular assistive devices and extracorporeal membrane oxygenation for support of cardiogenic shock. Heart transplantation has been beneficial for giant cell myocarditis.

Drugs

• Antibiotics to treat bacterial infection
• Antipyretics to reduce fever and decrease stress on the heart
• Diuretics to decrease fluid retention
• Angiotensin-converting enzyme inhibitors and digoxin (Lanoxin) to increase myocardial contractility for patients with heart failure. (Give digoxin cautiously because some patients may have a paradoxical sensitivity even to small doses.)
• Antiarrhythmics, such as quinidine or procainamide, to treat arrhythmias. (Use antiarrhythmics cautiously because they may depress myocardial contractility. A temporary pacemaker may be inserted if

complete atrioventricular block occurs.)
- Anticoagulation to prevent thromboembolism
- Corticosteroids and immunosuppressants (controversial) to combat life-threatening complications such as intractable heart failure

SPECIAL CONSIDERATIONS

ALERT

Keep in mind that nonsteroidal anti-inflammatory drugs are contraindicated during the acute phase (first 2 weeks) of myocardial infarction because they increase myocardial damage.

- Assess the patient's cardiovascular status often, watching for signs of heart failure, such as dyspnea, hypotension, and tachycardia. Check for changes in cardiac rhythm or conduction.
- Observe for signs of digoxin (Lanoxin) toxicity (anorexia, nausea, vomiting, blurred vision, and cardiac arrhythmias) and for complicating factors that may potentiate toxicity, such as electrolyte imbalance or hypoxia.
- Stress the need for bed rest. Assist with bathing as needed. Provide a bedside commode because it stresses the heart less than using a bedpan. Reassure the patient that activity limitations are temporary. Offer diversional activities that are physically undemanding.
- During recovery, recommend that the patient resume normal activities slowly and avoid competitive sports.
- Urge the patient to obtain prompt treatment of causative disorders.
- Instruct the patient to practice good hygiene, including thorough hand washing.
- Tell the patient to thoroughly wash and cook his food.
- Educate the patient about the importance of vaccinations and how they reduce the risk of myocarditis from measles, rubella, mumps, polio, and influenza.

Patent ductus arteriosus

The ductus arteriosus is a fetal blood vessel connecting the pulmonary artery to the descending aorta, just distal to the left subclavian artery. During fetal development, the ductus directs blood from the right ventricle away from the fetus's fluid-filled lungs. Normally, the ductus closes within days after birth.

In patent ductus arteriosus (PDA), the lumen of the ductus remains open after birth. (See *Understanding patent ductus arteriosus,* page 148). This creates a left-to-right shunt of blood from the aorta to the pulmonary artery and results in recirculation of arterial blood through the lungs. Initially, PDA may produce no clinical effects. In time, however, it can cause pulmonary vascular disease, causing symptoms to appear by age 40. The prognosis is good if the shunt is small or surgical repair is effective. Otherwise, PDA may advance to intractable heart failure, which may be fatal.

CAUSES AND INCIDENCE

Normally, the ductus closes within days to weeks after birth. Failure to close is most prevalent in premature neonates, probably as a result of abnormalities in oxygenation or the relaxant action of prostaglandin E, which prevents the ductal spasm and contracture needed for closure. PDA commonly accompanies rubella syndrome and may be linked to other congenital defects, such as coarctation of the aorta, ventricular septal defect, and pulmonary and aortic stenoses.

The ductus arteriosus normally closes as prostaglandin levels from the placenta fall and oxygen levels rise. This process typically begins as soon as the neonate takes its first breath but may take as long as 3 months in some children.

In PDA, relative resistances in pulmonary and systemic vasculature and the size of the ductus determine the amount of left-to-right shunting. Because of increased aortic pressure, oxygenated blood is shunted from the aorta through the ductus arteriosus to the pulmonary artery. The blood returns to the left side of the heart and is pumped out to the aorta once more.

The left atrium and left ventricle must accommodate the increased pulmonary venous return, which increases filling pressure and workload on the left side of the heart, possibly causing heart failure. In the final stages of untreated PDA, the left-to-right shunt leads to chronic

UNDERSTANDING PATENT DUCTUS ARTERIOSUS

This anomaly occurs when the ductus arteriosus—a tubular connection that shunts blood away from the fetal pulmonary circulation—fails to close after birth. Blood then shunts from the aorta to the pulmonary artery.

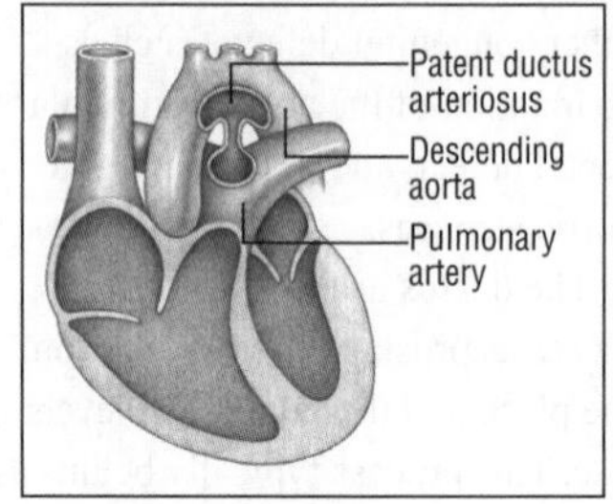

pulmonary artery hypertension that becomes fixed and unreactive. This causes the shunt to reverse; unoxygenated blood thus enters systemic circulation, causing cyanosis.

PDA is found in 1 of every 2,500 to 5,000 infants and is the most common congenital heart defect in adults. It affects twice as many females as males.

SIGNS AND SYMPTOMS

In neonates, especially those who are premature, a large PDA usually produces respiratory distress and signs of heart failure from the tremendous volume of blood shunted to the lungs through a patent ductus and the increased workload on the left side of the heart. Other characteristic features may include heightened susceptibility to respiratory tract infections, slow motor development, and failure to thrive.

Most children with PDA have no symptoms except cardiac ones. Others may show signs of heart disease, such as physical underdevelopment, fatigability, and frequent respiratory tract infections. Adults with undetected PDA may develop pulmonary vascular disease and, by age 40, may have fatigability and dyspnea on exertion. About 10% of them develop infective endocarditis.

Auscultation reveals the classic machinery murmur (Gibson murmur) in 85% of children with PDA. This is a continuous murmur (during systole and diastole) best heard at the heart's base, at the second left intercostal space under the left clavicle. The murmur may obscure S_2. (See *Auscultating for patent ductus arteriosus*.) However, with a right-to-left shunt, such a murmur may be absent.

Palpation may reveal a thrill at the left sternal border and a prominent left ventricular impulse. Peripheral arterial pulses are bounding (Corrigan's pulse); pulse pressure will be widened because of a drop in diastolic blood pressure and, secondarily, a rise in systolic pressure.

COMPLICATIONS

- Left-sided heart failure
- Pulmonary artery hypertension
- Respiratory distress (children)
- Infective endocarditis
- Recurrent pneumonia

AUSCULTATING FOR PATENT DUCTUS ARTERIOSUS

To detect patent ductus arteriosus (PDA), auscultate the base of the heart at the second left intercostal space under the left clavicle. You'll hear systolic clicks (C) and a continuous murmur during systole and diastole, possibly not through the entire cycle but through S_2 in a crescendo-decrescendo manner, as shown below.

NORMAL

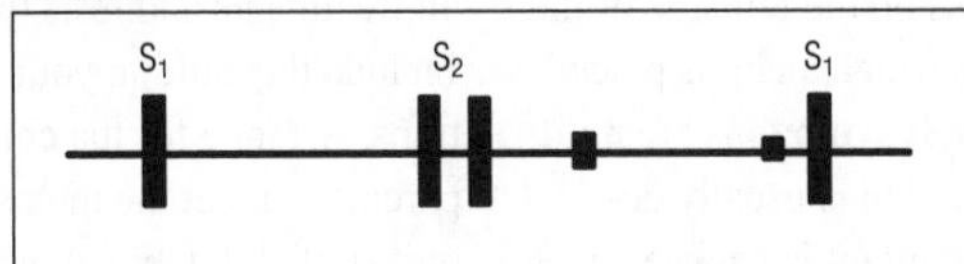

PDA

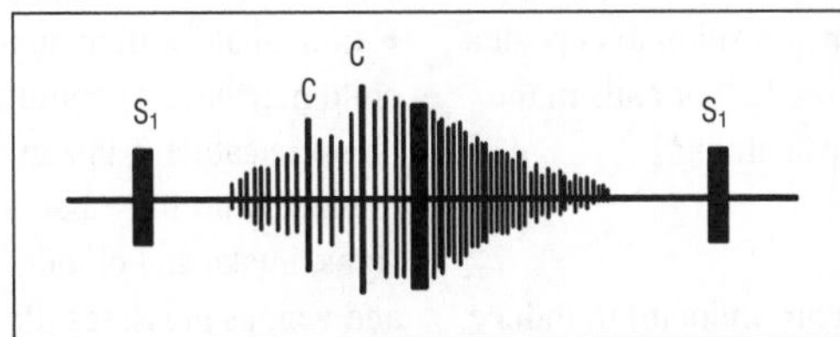

DIAGNOSIS

- Chest X-ray may show increased pulmonary vascular markings, prominent pulmonary arteries, and left ventricle and aorta enlargement.
- Electrocardiograph (ECG) may be normal or may indicate left atrial or ventricular hypertrophy and, in pulmonary vascular disease, biventricular hypertrophy.
- Echocardiography detects and helps estimate the size of a PDA. It also reveals an enlarged left atrium and left ventricle or right ventricular hypertrophy from pulmonary vascular disease.
- Cardiac catheterization shows pulmonary arterial oxygen content higher than right ventricular content because of the influx of aortic blood. Increased pulmonary artery pressure indicates a large shunt or, if it exceeds systemic arterial pressure, severe pulmonary vascular disease. Catheterization allows calculation of blood volume crossing the ductus and can rule out associated cardiac defects. Dye injection definitively demonstrates PDA.

TREATMENT

Asymptomatic infants with PDA need no immediate treatment. Those with heart failure need fluid restriction, diuretics, and cardiac glycosides to minimize or control symptoms. If these measures can't control heart failure, surgery is needed to ligate the ductus. Surgery can be performed via a left thoracotomy or visual assisted thoracoscopic surgery (VATS). VATS may be done at the bedside or in a procedure room. This technique involves three small incisions on the left side of the chest through which a clip is placed on the ductus. If symptoms are mild, surgical correction is usually delayed until the infant is between ages 6 months and 3 years, unless problems develop. Other options include a cardiac catheterization to deposit a plug (or "umbrella") or coils in the ductus to stop shunting.

Drugs

- Indomethacin (Indocin) to induce ductus spasm and closure in premature infants
- A prophylactic antibiotic to protect against infective endocarditis
- Diuretic and digoxin (Lanoxin) to treat heart failure

SPECIAL CONSIDERATIONS

- PDA requires careful monitoring, patient and family teaching, and emotional support.
- Watch carefully for signs of PDA in all premature neonates.
- Be alert for respiratory distress symptoms resulting from heart failure, which may develop rapidly in a premature neonate. Assess vital signs, ECG, electrolyte levels, and intake and output. Record the patient's response to diuretics and other therapy. Watch for evidence of digoxin toxicity, such as poor feeding and vomiting.
- If the infant receives indomethacin for ductus closure, watch for possible adverse effects, such as diarrhea, jaundice, bleeding, and renal dysfunction.
- Before surgery, carefully explain all treatments and tests to parents. Include the child in your explanations. Arrange for the child and her parents to meet the intensive care unit staff. Tell them about expected I.V. lines, monitoring equipment, and postoperative procedures.
- Immediately after surgery, the child may have a central venous pressure catheter and an arterial line in place. Carefully assess vital signs, intake and output, and arterial and venous pressures. Provide pain relief as needed.
- Before discharge, review instructions to the parents about activity restrictions based on the child's tolerance and energy levels. Advise parents not to become overprotective as their child's tolerance for physical activity increases.
- Stress the need for regular follow-up examinations. Advise parents to inform any practitioner who treats their child about her history of surgery for PDA—even if the child is being treated for an unrelated medical problem.

Pericarditis

Pericarditis is an inflammation of the pericardium, which is the fibroserous sac that envelops, supports, and protects the heart. The disorder may be acute or chronic. Acute pericarditis can be fibrinous or effusive, with purulent serous or hemorrhagic exudates. Chronic constrictive pericarditis is characterized by dense fibrous pericardial thickening. The prognosis depends on the underlying cause and usually is good in acute pericarditis, unless constriction occurs.

CAUSES AND INCIDENCE

Common causes of this disease include bacterial, fungal, or viral infection (infectious pericarditis); neoplasms (primary or metastatic from lungs, breasts, or other organs); high-dose radiation to the chest; uremia; hypersensitivity or autoimmune disease, such as acute rheumatic fever (most common cause in children), systemic lupus erythematosus, and rheumatoid arthritis; postcardiac injury such as myocardial infarction (MI), which later causes an autoimmune reaction (Dressler's syndrome) in the pericardium; trauma or surgery that leaves the pericardium intact but causes blood to leak into the pericardial cavity; drugs, such as hydralazine (Apresazide), procainamide, isoniazid (Nydrazid), cyclosporine (Gengraf), or tetracyclines; and idiopathic factors (most common in acute pericarditis).

Less common causes include aortic aneurysm with pericardial leakage and myxedema with cholesterol deposits in the pericardium.

Pericardial tissue damaged by bacteria or other substances results in the release of chemical mediators of inflammation (prostaglandins, histamines, bradykinins, and serotonin) into the surrounding tissue, thereby initiating the inflammatory process. Friction occurs as the inflamed pericardial layers rub against each other. Histamines and other chemical mediators dilate vessels and increase vessel permeability. Vessel walls then leak fluids and protein (including fibrinogen) into tissues causing extracellular edema. Macrophages already present in the tissue begin to phagocytize the invading bacteria and are joined by neutrophils and monocytes. After several days, the area fills with an exudate composed of necrotic tissue and dead and dying bacteria, neutrophils, and macrophages. Eventually the contents of the cavity autolyze and are gradually reabsorbed into healthy tissue. (See *Understanding pericarditis,* page 152).

A pericardial effusion develops if fluid accumulates in the pericardial cavity. Cardiac tamponade results when fluid accumulates rapidly in the pericardial space, compressing the heart, preventing it from filling during diastole, and reducing cardiac output.

Chronic constrictive pericarditis develops if the pericardium becomes thick and stiff from chronic or recurrent pericarditis, encasing the heart in a stiff shell and preventing it from properly filling during diastole. This causes an increase in

UNDERSTANDING PERICARDITIS

Pericarditis occurs when a pathogen or other substance attacks the pericardium, leading to the following events.

Inflammation

Pericardial tissue damaged by bacteria or other substances releases chemical mediators of inflammation (such as prostaglandins, histamines, bradykinins, and serotonins) into the surrounding tissue, starting the inflammatory process. The inflamed pericardial layers rub against each other, creating friction.

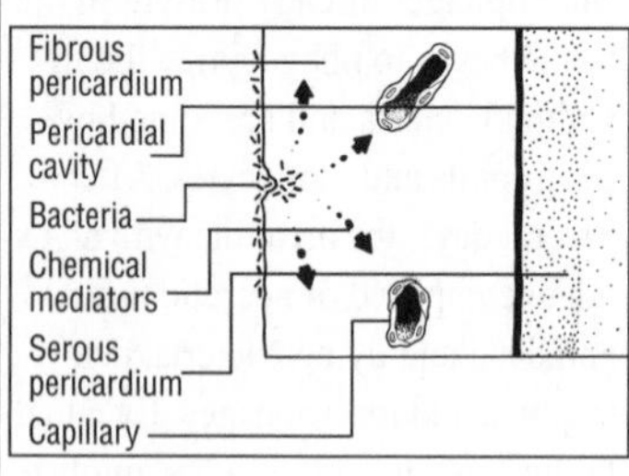

Vasodilation and clotting

Histamines and other chemical mediators cause vasodilation and increased vessel permeability. Local blood flow (hyperemia) increases. Vessel walls leak fluids and proteins (including fibrinogen) into tissues, causing extracellular edema. Clots of fibrinogen and tissue fluid form a wall, blocking tissue spaces and lymph vessels in the injured area. This wall prevents the spread of bacteria and toxins to adjoining healthy tissues.

Initial phagocytosis

Macrophages already present in the tissues begin to phagocytize the invading bacteria but usually fail to stop the infection.

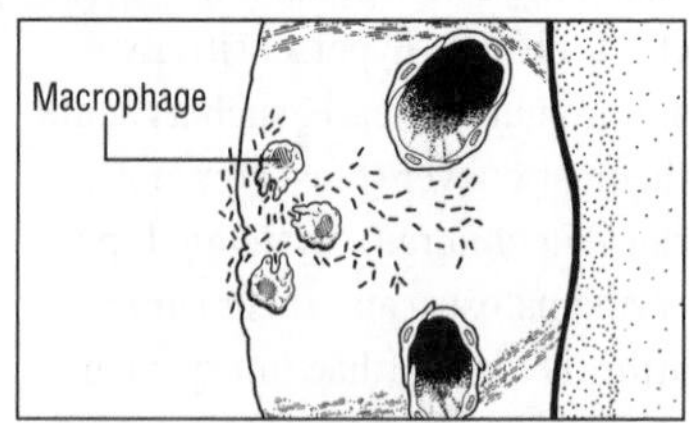

left- and right-sided filling pressures, leading to a drop in stroke volume and cardiac output.

Pericarditis most commonly affects men ages 20 to 50, but it can also occur in children following infection with an adenovirus or coxsackievirus.

SIGNS AND SYMPTOMS

Acute pericarditis usually produces a sharp, sudden pain that starts over the sternum and radiates to the neck, shoulders, back, and arms. However, unlike the pain of MI, pericardial pain often is pleuritic, increasing with deep inspiration and decreasing when the patient sits up and leans forward, pulling the heart away from the diaphragmatic pleurae of the lungs.

Pericardial friction rub, a classic sign, is a grating sound heard as the heart moves. Usually, it can best be auscultated during forced expiration, while the patient leans forward or is on his hands and knees in bed. It may have up to three components,

Enhanced phagocytosis
Substances released by the injured tissue stimulate neutrophil production in the bone marrow. Neutrophils then travel to the injury site through the bloodstream and join macrophages in destroying pathogens. Meanwhile, additional macrophages and monocytes migrate to the injured area and continue phagocytosis.

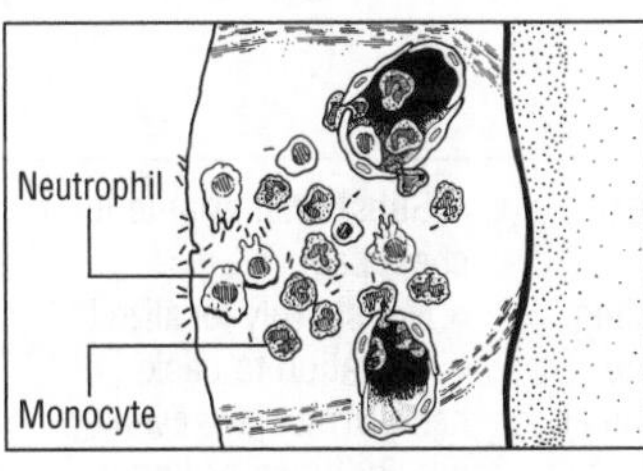

Exudation
After several days, the infected area fills with an exudate composed of necrotic tissue and dead and dying bacteria, neutrophils, and macrophages. This exudate, which is thinner than pus, forms until all infection ceases, creating a cavity that remains until tissue destruction stops. The contents of the cavity autolyze and are gradually reabsorbed into healthy tissue.

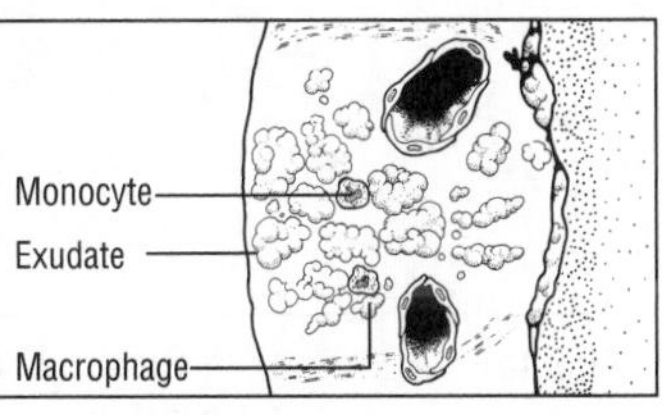

Fibrosis and scarring
As the end products of the infection slowly disappear, fibrosis and scar tissue may form. Scarring, which can be extensive, can ultimately cause heart failure if it restricts movement.

corresponding to the timing of atrial systole, ventricular systole, and the rapid-filling phase of ventricular diastole. Occasionally, this friction rub is heard only briefly or not at all.

Pericardial effusion, the major complication of acute pericarditis, may produce effects of heart failure (such as dyspnea, orthopnea, and tachycardia), ill-defined substernal chest pain, and a feeling of fullness in the chest. (See *Patterns of cardiac pain,* page 154.) If acute pericarditis has caused very large pericardial effusions, physical examination reveals increased cardiac dullness and diminished or absent apical impulse and distant heart sounds.

Chronic constrictive pericarditis causes a gradual increase in systemic venous pressure and produces symptoms similar to those of chronic right-sided heart failure (fluid retention, ascites, and hepatomegaly).

PATTERNS OF CARDIAC PAIN

Although everyone feels the effects of cardiac disorders uniquely, the disorders listed here tend to produce certain kinds of pain.

Cause	Onset and duration	Location and radiation
Pericarditis	■ Sudden onset ■ Continuous pain lasting days ■ Residual soreness	■ Substernal pain to left of midline ■ Radiation to back or subclavicular area
Angina	■ Gradual or sudden onset ■ Pain usually lasting less than 15 and no more than 30 minutes (average, 3 minutes)	■ Substernal or anterior chest pain ■ Not sharply localized ■ Radiation to back, neck, arms, jaw, even upper abdomen or fingers
Myocardial infarction	■ Sudden onset ■ Pain lasting 30 minutes to 2 hours ■ Waxes and wanes ■ Residual soreness for 1 to 3 days	■ Substernal, midline, or anterior chest pain ■ Radiation to jaw, neck, back, shoulders, or one or both arms

COMPLICATIONS

- Pericardial effusion
- Constrictive pericarditis
- Cardiac tamponade
- Shock
- Cardiovascular collapse
- Death

DIAGNOSIS

- Diagnosis includes typical clinical features and elimination of other possible causes.
- Chest X-ray, echocardiogram, magnetic resonance imaging of the chest and heart, computed tomography scan of the heart, and radionuclide scanning can detect fluid that

Quality and intensity	Signs and symptoms	Precipitating factors
▪ Mild ache to severe pain ▪ Deep or superficial ▪ May be described as stabbing or knifelike	▪ Precordial friction rub ▪ Increased pain with movement, inspiration, laughing, coughing ▪ Decreased pain with sitting or leaning forward (which pulls heart away from diaphragm)	▪ Myocardial infarction ▪ Upper respiratory tract infection ▪ Invasive cardiac trauma
▪ Mild to moderate pressure ▪ Deep sensation ▪ Varied pattern of attacks ▪ May be described as tightness, squeezing, crushing, pressure	▪ Dyspnea ▪ Diaphoresis ▪ Nausea ▪ Desire to void ▪ Belching ▪ Apprehension	▪ Exertion ▪ Stress ▪ Eating ▪ Cold weather ▪ Hot, humid weather
▪ Persistent, severe pressure ▪ Deep sensation ▪ May be described as crushing, squeezing, heavy, oppressive	▪ Nausea, vomiting ▪ Apprehension ▪ Feeling of impending doom ▪ Dyspnea ▪ Diaphoresis ▪ Increased or decreased blood pressure ▪ Gallop heart sound	▪ Physical exertion ▪ Emotional stress ▪ May occur at rest

has accumulated in the pericardial sac. They may also show enlargement of the heart and signs of inflammation or scarring, depending on the cause of pericarditis. In pericardial effusion, echocardiography is diagnostic when it shows an echo-free space between the ventricular wall and the pericardium.

• Laboratory results reflect inflammation and may identify its cause. They may include a normal or elevated white blood cell count, especially in infectious pericarditis, an elevated erythrocyte sedimentation rate, and slightly elevated cardiac enzyme levels with associated myocarditis. Culture of pericardial fluid obtained by open surgical drainage or cardiocentesis sometimes identifies a causative organism in bacterial or fungal pericarditis.

- Electrocardiography shows the following changes in acute pericarditis: elevation of ST segments in the standard limb leads and most precordial leads without the significant changes in QRS morphology that occur with MI, atrial ectopic rhythms such as atrial fibrillation and, in pericardial effusion, diminished QRS voltage.
- Blood urea nitrogen levels are used to check for uremia.
- Antistreptolysin-O titers reveal rheumatic fever.
- A purified protein derivative skin test may be used to check for tuberculosis.

TREATMENT

The goal of treatment is to relieve symptoms and manage the underlying systemic disease. In acute idiopathic pericarditis and postthoracotomy pericarditis, treatment includes nonsteroidal anti-inflammatory drugs (NSAIDs) and bed rest as long as fever and pain persist. If NSAIDs fail to relieve symptoms, corticosteroids may be used. Post-MI patients should avoid NSAIDs and steroids because they may interfere with myocardial scar formation.

Infectious pericarditis that results from disease of the left pleural space, mediastinal abscesses, or septicemia requires antibiotics (possibly by direct pericardial injection), surgical drainage, or both. Pericardiocentesis, guided by echocardiography, is the technique used to drain the effusion.

Recurrent pericarditis may require partial pericardectomy to create a window through which fluid can drain into the pleural space. In constrictive pericarditis, the patient may need total pericardectomy to permit adequate filling and contraction of the heart. Treatment also must include management of rheumatic fever, uremia, tuberculosis, and other underlying disorders.

Drugs

- An NSAID, such as aspirin or indomethacin (Indocin), to relieve pain and reduce inflammation
- A corticosteroid if the NSAID is ineffective and no infection exists (Corticosteroids must be administered cautiously because episodes may recur when therapy is discontinued.)
- Antibacterial, antifungal, or antiviral therapy if an infectious cause is suspected

SPECIAL CONSIDERATIONS

- A patient with pericarditis needs complete bed rest.
- Assess pain in relation to respiration and body position to distinguish pericardial pain from myocardial ischemic pain.
- Place the patient in an upright position to relieve dyspnea and chest pain, provide analgesics and oxygen, and reassure the patient with acute pericarditis that his condition is temporary and treatable.

• Watch for signs of cardiac compression or cardiac tamponade, possible complications of pericardial effusion. Signs include decreased blood pressure, increased central venous pressure, and pulsus paradoxus. Because cardiac tamponade requires immediate treatment, keep a pericardiocentesis set handy whenever pericardial effusion is suspected.
• Explain tests and treatments to the patient. If surgery is needed, teach deep-breathing and coughing exercises beforehand. Postoperative care is similar to that given after cardiothoracic surgery.

Peripheral artery disease

Peripheral artery disease (PAD), also known as *arterial occlusive disease,* is the obstruction or narrowing of the lumen of the aorta and its major branches, causing an interruption of blood flow, usually to the legs and feet. PAD may affect the carotid, vertebral, innominate, subclavian, mesenteric, and celiac arteries. (See *Possible sites of major artery occlusion,* page 158.) Occlusions may be acute or chronic and commonly cause severe ischemia, skin ulceration, and gangrene.

The prognosis depends on the occlusion's location, the development of collateral circulation to counteract reduced blood flow and, in acute disease, the time elapsed between occlusion and its removal.

CAUSES AND INCIDENCE

PAD is a common complication of atherosclerosis. The occlusive mechanism may be endogenous or exogenous. (See *What causes acute arterial occlusion?* page 159.) Predisposing factors include smoking; aging; such conditions as hypertension, hyperlipidemia, and diabetes; and a family history of vascular disorders, myocardial infarction, or stroke.

In this disease, fibrous plaques narrow the lumens of blood vessels. This occlusion can occur acutely or progressively over 20 to 40 years, with areas of vessel branching, or bifurcation, being the most common sites. The narrowing of the lumens reduces the blood volume that can flow through them, causing arterial insufficiency to the affected area. Ischemia usually occurs after the vessel lumens have narrowed by at least 50%, reducing blood flow to a level at which it no longer meets the needs of tissue and nerves.

PAD has no racial predilection. Aging causes sclerotic changes in blood vessels, which leads to decreased elasticity and lumen narrowing, further contributing to the development of the disease. In people older than age 70, the prevalence of the disease is about 10% to 18%. Men older than age 50 are at increased risk for intermittent claudication, a common sign of PAD.

SIGNS AND SYMPTOMS

The signs and symptoms of PAD depend on the site of the occlusion.

POSSIBLE SITES OF MAJOR ARTERY OCCLUSION

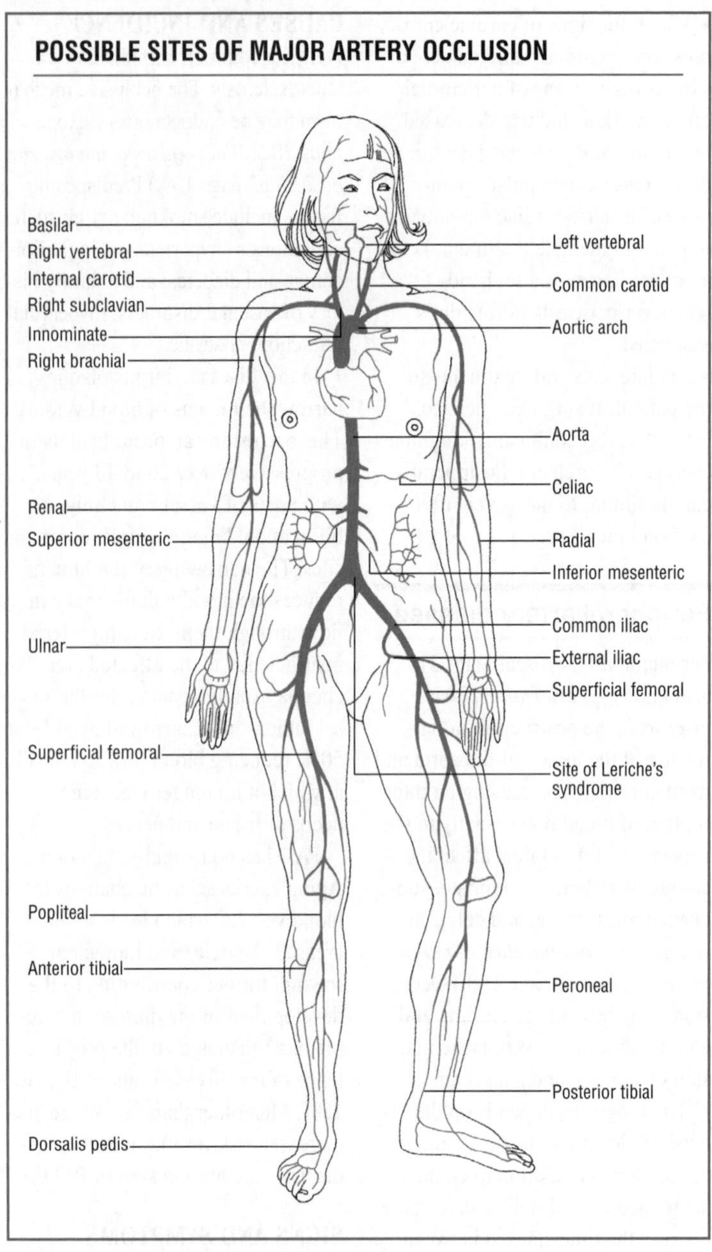

WHAT CAUSES ACUTE ARTERIAL OCCLUSION?

The most common cause of acute arterial occlusion is obstruction of a major artery by a clot. The occlusion may result from an endogenous mechanism, such as embolism, thrombosis, or plaque, or it may have an exogenous cause.

Embolism

Often, arterial occlusion results from an embolus originating in the heart. Emboli typically lodge in the arms and legs, where blood vessels narrow or branch. In the arms, they usually lodge in the brachial artery, although they may occlude the subclavian or axillary arteries. Common sites in the legs include the iliac, femoral, and popliteal arteries. Emboli originating in the heart can cause neurologic damage if they enter the cerebral circulation.

Thrombosis

In a patient with atherosclerosis and marked arterial narrowing, thrombosis may cause acute intrinsic arterial occlusion. This complication typically arises in areas with severely stenotic vessels, especially in a patient who also has heart failure, hypovolemia, polycythemia, or traumatic injury.

Plaque

Atheromatous debris (plaque) from proximal arterial lesions may intermittently obstruct small vessels, usually in the hands or feet. These plaques also may develop in the brachiocephalic vessels and travel to the cerebral circulation, where they may lead to transient cerebral ischemia or infarction.

Exogenous causes

Acute arterial occlusion may stem from insertion of an indwelling arterial catheter or intra-arterial drug abuse. In addition, extrinsic arterial occlusion can result from direct blunt or penetrating trauma to the artery.

(See *Types of peripheral artery disease*, page 160.)

COMPLICATIONS

- Severe ischemia and necrosis
- Skin ulceration
- Gangrene, which can lead to limb amputation
- Impaired nail and hair growth
- Stroke or transient ischemic attack
- Peripheral or systemic embolism

DIAGNOSIS

- Diagnosis includes a patient history and physical examination.
- Ankle-brachial index (ABI) (the ratio of systolic blood pressure at the ankle to that at the arm) decreases with worsening arterial occlusive disease. An ABI less than 0.9 indicates some degree of arterial occlusive disease.
- Arteriography demonstrates the type (thrombus or embolus), location,

TYPES OF PERIPHERAL ARTERY DISEASE

Site of occlusion	Signs and symptoms
Carotid arterial system ▪ Internal carotids ▪ External carotids	▪ Absent or decreased pulsation with an auscultatory bruit over the affected vessels ▪ Neurologic dysfunction (recurrent features that usually last 5 to 10 minutes but may persist up to 24 hours and may herald a stroke: transient ischemic attack (TIA) from reduced cerebral circulation producing unilateral sensory or motor dysfunction (transient monocular blindness and hemiparesis); possible aphasia or dysarthria, confusion, decreased mentation, and headache
Vertebrobasilar system ▪ Vertebral arteries ▪ Basilar arteries	▪ Neurologic dysfunction: TIA of the brain stem and cerebellum producing binocular vision disturbances, vertigo, dysarthria, and "drop attacks" (falling down without loss of consciousness); less common than carotid TIA
Innominate ▪ Brachiocephalic artery	▪ Indications of ischemia (claudication) of the right arm ▪ Neurologic dysfunction: signs and symptoms of vertebrobasilar occlusion ▪ Possible bruit over the right side of the neck
Subclavian artery	▪ Clinical effects of vertebrobasilar occlusion and exercise-induced arm claudication ▪ Subclavian steal syndrome (characterized by backflow of blood from the brain through the vertebral artery on the same side as the occlusion into the subclavian artery distal to the occlusion) ▪ Possibly gangrene (usually limited to the digits)
Mesenteric artery ▪ Superior (most commonly affected) ▪ Celiac axis ▪ Inferior	▪ Bowel ischemia, infarct necrosis, and gangrene ▪ Diarrhea ▪ Leukocytosis ▪ Nausea and vomiting ▪ Shock from massive intraluminal fluid and plasma loss ▪ Sudden, acute abdominal pain

TYPES OF PERIPHERAL ARTERY DISEASE *(continued)*

Site of occlusion	Signs and symptoms
Aortic bifurcation ▪ Saddle block occlusion, a medical emergency associated with cardiac embolization	▪ Sensory and motor deficits (muscle weakness, numbness, paresthesias, and paralysis) in both legs ▪ Signs of ischemia (sudden pain and cold, pale legs with decreased or absent peripheral pulses) in both legs
Iliac artery ▪ Leriche's syndrome	▪ Absent or reduced femoral or distal pulses ▪ Impotence ▪ Intermittent claudication of the lower back, buttocks, and thighs, relieved by rest ▪ Possible bruit over femoral arteries
Femoral and popliteal artery ▪ Associated with aneurysm formation	▪ Gangrene ▪ Intermittent claudication of the calves on exertion ▪ Ischemic pain in the feet ▪ Leg pallor and coolness, with blanching of the feet on elevation ▪ No palpable pulses in the ankles and feet ▪ Pretrophic pain (heralds necrosis and ulceration)

and degree of obstruction and the collateral circulation. It's particularly useful in chronic disease or for evaluating candidates for reconstructive surgery.

• Doppler ultrasonography and plethysmography are noninvasive tests that show decreased blood flow distal to the occlusion in acute disease.

• Ophthalmodynamometry helps determine the degree of obstruction in the internal carotid artery by comparing ophthalmic artery pressure to brachial artery pressure on the affected side. More than a 20% difference between pressures suggests insufficiency.

• EEG and computed tomography scan may be necessary to rule out brain lesions.

TREATMENT

Treatment depends on the obstruction's cause, location, and size. For mild chronic disease, supportive measures include smoking cessation, hypertension control, hyperlipidemia control, and mild exercise such as walking. Acute PAD usually requires surgery to restore circulation to the affected area. It may include the following:

• atherectomy, which involves excision of plaque using a drill or slicing mechanism

- balloon angioplasty, in which the obstruction is compressed using balloon inflation
- bypass graft, in which blood flow is diverted through an anastomosed autogenous or Dacron graft past the thrombosed segment
- combined therapy, which combines any of the treatments described above
- embolectomy (used mainly for mesenteric, femoral, or popliteal artery occlusion), in which a balloon-tipped Fogarty catheter is used to remove thrombotic material from the artery
- laser angioplasty, which uses excision and hot-tip lasers to vaporize the obstruction
- lumbar sympathectomy, which may be used as an adjunct to surgery, depending on the sympathetic nervous system's condition
- patch grafting, which involves removal of the thrombosed arterial segment and replacement with an autogenous vein or Dacron graft
- stent placement, which may follow laser angioplasty or atherectomy and involves insertion of wire mesh that stretches and molds to the arterial wall to prevent reocclusion
- thromboendarterectomy (usually performed after angiography and commonly used with autogenous vein or Dacron femoral-popliteal or aortofemoral bypass surgery), which involves opening the occluded artery and direct removal of the obstructing thrombus and the medial layer of the arterial wall
- amputation, if arterial reconstructive surgery fails or if the patient develops gangrene, persistent infection, or intractable pain.

Other therapy includes bowel resection after restoration of blood flow (for mesenteric artery occlusion).

Drugs

- Life-long aspirin therapy for carotid artery occlusion
- Aspirin (first-line agent), clopidogrel (Plavix), or ticlopidine (Ticlid) for chronic occlusive disease
- Cilostazol (Pletal) for patients with disabling intermittent claudication who are poor candidates for surgery
- Heparin to prevent emboli (for embolic occlusion)
- Thrombolytics (urokinase [Kinlytic], streptokinase [Streptase], or alteplase [Activase]) to cause lysis of the clot around or in the plaque

SPECIAL CONSIDERATIONS

- Provide comprehensive patient teaching, including proper foot care. Explain diagnostic tests and procedures. Advise the patient to stop smoking and to follow the prescribed medical regimen.

Responding to an acute episode

- Assess the patient's circulatory status by checking for the most distal pulses and by inspecting his skin color and temperature.
- Provide pain relief as needed.

• Give heparin by continuous I.V. drip, as ordered. Use an infusion monitor or pump to ensure the proper flow rate.
• Wrap the patient's affected foot in soft cotton batting and reposition it often to prevent pressure on any one area. Don't elevate or apply heat to the affected leg.
• Watch for signs of fluid and electrolyte imbalance, and monitor intake and output for evidence of renal failure (urine output less than 30 ml/hour).
• If the patient has carotid, innominate, vertebral, or subclavian artery occlusion, watch for evidence of stroke, such as numbness in an arm or leg and intermittent blindness.

Postoperative care

• Monitor the patient's vital signs. Continuously assess his circulatory function by inspecting skin color and temperature and by checking for distal pulses. In charting, compare earlier assessments and observations. Watch closely for signs of hemorrhage (tachycardia and hypotension) and check dressings for excessive bleeding.
• In carotid, innominate, vertebral, or subclavian artery occlusion, assess neurologic status often for changes in level of consciousness or muscle strength and pupil size.
• In mesenteric artery occlusion, set the nasogastric tube to low intermittent suction. Monitor intake and output. (Low urine output may indicate damage to renal arteries during surgery.) Check bowel sounds for return of peristalsis. Increasing abdominal distention and tenderness may indicate extension of bowel ischemia with resulting gangrene, necessitating further excision, or it may indicate peritonitis.
• In saddle block occlusion, check distal pulses for adequate circulation. Watch for signs of renal failure and mesenteric artery occlusion (severe abdominal pain), and for cardiac arrhythmias, which may precipitate embolus formation.
• In iliac artery occlusion, monitor urine output for signs of renal failure from decreased perfusion to the kidneys as a result of surgery. Provide meticulous catheter care.
• In both femoral and popliteal artery occlusions, assist with early ambulation, but discourage prolonged sitting.
• After amputation, check the patient's stump carefully for drainage and record its color and amount, and the time. Elevate the stump as ordered, and administer adequate analgesic medication. Because phantom limb pain is common, explain this phenomenon to the patient.
• When preparing the patient for discharge, instruct him to watch for signs of recurrence (pain, pallor, numbness, paralysis, and absence of pulse) that can result from graft occlusion or occlusion at another site. Warn him against wearing constrictive clothing.

Pulmonary edema

Pulmonary edema is the accumulation of fluid in the extravascular spaces of the lung. In cardiogenic pulmonary edema, fluid accumulation results from elevations in pulmonary venous and capillary hydrostatic pressures. A common complication of cardiac disorders, pulmonary edema can occur as a chronic condition or it can develop quickly and cause death.

CAUSES AND INCIDENCE

Pulmonary edema usually results from left-sided heart failure caused by arteriosclerotic, hypertensive, cardiomyopathic, or valvular cardiac disease. In such disorders, the compromised left ventricle is unable to maintain adequate cardiac output, and increased pressures are transmitted to the left atrium, pulmonary veins, and pulmonary capillary bed. This increased pulmonary capillary hydrostatic force promotes transudation of intravascular fluids into the pulmonary interstitium, decreasing lung compliance and interfering with gas exchange.

Other factors that may predispose a patient to pulmonary edema include:

- excessive infusion of I.V. fluids
- decreased serum colloid osmotic pressure as a result of nephrosis, protein-losing enteropathy, extensive burns, hepatic disease, or nutritional deficiency
- impaired lung lymphatic drainage from Hodgkin's lymphoma or obliterative lymphangitis after radiation
- mitral stenosis, which impairs left atrial emptying, and pulmonary veno-occlusive disease
- lung damage from a severe infection or exposure to poisonous gas
- kidney failure.

SIGNS AND SYMPTOMS

The early symptoms of pulmonary edema reflect interstitial fluid accumulation and diminished lung compliance: dyspnea on exertion, paroxysmal nocturnal dyspnea, orthopnea, and coughing. Clinical features include tachycardia, tachypnea, dependent crackles, jugular venous distention, and a diastolic (S_3) gallop. With severe pulmonary edema, the alveoli and bronchioles may fill with fluid and intensify the early symptoms. Respiration becomes labored and rapid, with more diffuse crackles and coughing that produces frothy, bloody sputum. Tachycardia increases, and arrhythmias may occur. Skin becomes cold, clammy, diaphoretic, and cyanotic. Blood pressure falls, and the pulse becomes thready as cardiac output falls.

Symptoms of severe heart failure with pulmonary edema also may include signs and symptoms of hypoxemia, such as anxiety, restlessness, and changes in the patient's level of consciousness.

COMPLICATIONS

- Respiratory failure
- Respiratory acidosis
- Cardiac arrest

DIAGNOSIS

- Arterial blood gas (ABG) analysis usually shows hypoxia; the partial pressure of arterial carbon dioxide is variable. Profound respiratory alkalosis and acidosis may occur.
- Chest X-ray shows diffuse haziness of the lung fields and, commonly, cardiomegaly and pleural effusions.
- Ultrasound (echocardiogram) may show weak heart muscle, leaking or narrow heart valves, and fluid surrounding the heart.
- Pulmonary artery catheterization helps identify left-sided heart failure by showing elevated pulmonary wedge pressures. This helps to rule out acute respiratory distress syndrome—in which pulmonary wedge pressure is usually normal.

TREATMENT

Treatment measures for pulmonary edema are designed to reduce extravascular fluid, improve gas exchange and myocardial function and, if possible, correct any underlying pathologic conditions.

Administration of high concentrations of oxygen by a cannula, a face mask and, if the patient fails to maintain an acceptable partial pressure of arterial oxygen level, assisted ventilation improves oxygen delivery to the tissues and usually improves acid base disturbances.

Drugs

- Diuretics—furosemide (Lasix) and bumetanide (Bumex), for example—to promote diuresis, which reduces extravascular fluid
- Angiotensin-converting enzyme inhibitors, diuretics, inotropic drugs (such as digoxin [Lanoxin]), antiarrhythmic agents, beta-adrenergic blockers, and human B-type natriuretic peptide to treat heart failure
- Morphine to reduce anxiety and dyspnea, as well as dilate the systemic venous bed, promoting blood flow from the pulmonary circulation to the periphery

SPECIAL CONSIDERATIONS

- Carefully monitor the vulnerable patient for early signs of pulmonary edema, especially tachypnea, tachycardia, and abnormal breath sounds. Report any abnormalities. Assess for peripheral edema and weight gain, which may indicate that fluid is accumulating in tissue.
- Administer oxygen, as ordered.
- Monitor the patient's vital signs every 15 to 30 minutes while giving nitroprusside (Nitropress) in dextrose 5% in water by I.V. drip. Protect the nitroprusside solution from light by wrapping the bottle or bag with aluminum foil, and discard unused solution after 4 hours. Watch for arrhythmias in a patient receiving cardiac glycosides and for marked respiratory depression in a patient receiving morphine.
- Assess the patient's condition often, and record the response to treatment. Monitor ABG levels, oral and IV. fluid intake, urine output and, in the patient with a pulmonary artery catheter, pulmonary end diastolic and wedge pressures. Check the

cardiac monitor often. Report changes immediately.

- Carefully record the time and amount of morphine given.
- Reassure the patient who is anxious due to hypoxia and respiratory distress. Explain all procedures. Provide emotional support to his family as well.

Pulmonary embolism

The most common pulmonary complication in hospitalized patients, pulmonary embolism is an obstruction of the pulmonary arterial bed by a dislodged thrombus, heart valve vegetation, or foreign substance. Although pulmonary infarction that results from embolism may be so mild as to be asymptomatic, massive embolism (more than 50% obstruction of pulmonary arterial circulation) and the accompanying infarction can be rapidly fatal.

CAUSES AND INCIDENCE

Pulmonary embolism typically results from dislodged thrombi originating in the leg veins. More than half of such thrombi arise in the deep veins of the legs. Other less common sources of thrombi are the pelvic veins, renal veins, hepatic vein, right side of the heart, and arms.

Such thrombus formation results directly from vascular wall damage, venostasis, or hypercoagulability of the blood. Trauma, clot dissolution, sudden muscle spasm, intravascular pressure changes, or a change in peripheral blood flow can cause the thrombus to loosen or fragment. Then the thrombus—now called an embolus—floats to the heart's right side and enters the lung through the pulmonary artery. There, the embolus may dissolve, continue to fragment, or grow.

By occluding the pulmonary artery, the embolus prevents alveoli from producing enough surfactant to maintain alveolar integrity. As a result, alveoli collapse and atelectasis develops. If the embolus enlarges, it may clog most or all of the pulmonary vessels and cause death. Rarely, emboli contain air, fat, bacteria, amniotic fluid, talc (from drugs intended for oral administration that are injected intravenously by addicts), or tumor cells.

Predisposing factors for pulmonary embolism include long-term immobility, chronic pulmonary disease, heart failure or atrial fibrillation, thrombophlebitis, polycythemia vera, thrombocytosis, autoimmune hemolytic anemia, sickle cell disease, varicose veins, recent surgery, advanced age, pregnancy, leg fractures or surgery, burns, obesity, vascular injury, cancer, I.V. drug abuse, or hormonal contraceptives.

SIGNS AND SYMPTOMS

Total occlusion of the main pulmonary artery is rapidly fatal; smaller or fragmented emboli produce symptoms that vary with the size, number, and location of the emboli. Usually, the first symptom of pulmonary embolism is dyspnea, which may be accompanied by angina or pleuritic chest pain. Other clinical features include tachycardia, productive cough (sputum may be blood-tinged), low-grade fever, and pleural effusion. Less common signs include massive hemoptysis, chest splinting, leg edema and, with a large embolus, cyanosis, syncope, and distended jugular veins.

In addition, pulmonary embolism may cause pleural friction rub and signs of circulatory collapse (weak, rapid pulse and hypotension) and hypoxia (restlessness and anxiety).

COMPLICATIONS

- Pulmonary infarction
- Death

DIAGNOSIS

- The patient history typically reveals predisposing conditions for pulmonary embolism. A triad of deep vein thrombosis (DVT) formation is stasis, endothelial injury, and hypercoagulability. Risk factors include long car or plane trips, cancer, pregnancy, hypercoagulability, prior DVT, and pulmonary emboli.
- Chest X-ray helps to rule out other pulmonary diseases; areas of atelectasis, an elevated diaphragm and pleural effusion, a prominent pulmonary artery and, occasionally, the characteristic wedge-shaped infiltrate suggestive of pulmonary infarction, or focal oligemia of blood vessels, are apparent.
- Lung scan shows perfusion defects in areas beyond occluded vessels; however, it doesn't rule out microemboli.
- Pulmonary angiography is the most definitive test but requires a skilled angiographer and radiologic equipment; it also poses some risk to the patient. Its use depends on the uncertainty of the diagnosis and the need to avoid unnecessary anticoagulant therapy in a high-risk patient.
- Electrocardiography may show right axis deviation; right bundle-branch block; tall, peaked P waves; depression of ST segments and T-wave inversions (indicative of right-sided heart strain); and supraventricular tachyarrhythmias in extensive pulmonary embolism. A pattern sometimes observed is S_1, Q_3, and T_3 (S wave in lead I, Q wave in lead III, and inverted T wave in lead III).
- Auscultation occasionally reveals a right ventricular S_3 gallop and an increased intensity of a pulmonic component of S_2. Also, crackles and a pleural rub may be heard at the embolism site.
- Arterial blood gas (ABG) analysis showing a decreased partial pressure of arterial oxygen and partial pressure of arterial carbon dioxide are characteristic but don't always occur.
- If pleural effusion is present, thoracentesis may rule out empyema, which indicates pneumonia.

TREATMENT

Treatment is designed to maintain adequate cardiovascular and pulmonary function during resolution of the obstruction and to prevent recurrence of embolic episodes. Because most emboli resolve within 10 to 14 days, treatment consists of oxygen therapy as needed and anticoagulation with heparin to inhibit new thrombus formation, followed by oral warfarin (Coumadin). Heparin therapy is monitored by daily coagulation studies (partial thromboplastin time [PTT]).

Surgery is performed on patients who can't take anticoagulants, who have recurrent emboli during anticoagulant therapy, or who have been treated with thrombolytic agents or pulmonary thromboendarterectomy. This procedure (which shouldn't be performed without angiographic evidence of pulmonary embolism) consists of vena caval ligation, plication, or insertion of an inferior vena cava device to filter blood returning to the heart and lungs.

Drugs

- Heparin, then warfarin, to prevent new thrombus formation
- Patients with massive pulmonary embolism and shock may need fibrinolytic therapy with thrombolytic therapy (streptokinase [Streptase], urokinase [Kinlytic], or tissue plasminogen activator) to enhance fibrinolysis of the pulmonary emboli and remaining thrombi
- Vasopressors to treat hypotension
- Antibiotics to treat septic emboli

SPECIAL CONSIDERATIONS

- Give oxygen by nasal cannula or mask. Check ABG levels if the patient develops fresh emboli or worsening dyspnea. Be prepared to provide endotracheal intubation with assisted ventilation if breathing is severely compromised.
- Give heparin, as ordered, through I.V. push or continuous drip. Monitor coagulation studies daily. Effective heparin therapy raises the PTT to more than 1½ times normal. Watch closely for nosebleeds, petechiae, and other signs of abnormal bleeding; check stools for occult blood. Protect patients from trauma and injury, avoid I.M. injections, and maintain pressure over venipuncture sites for 5 minutes, or until bleeding stops, to reduce hematoma.
- After the patient is stable, urge him to move about often, and help with isometric and range-of-motion exercises. Check pedal pulses, temperature, and the color of his feet to detect venostasis. Never massage the patient's legs. Offer diversional activities to promote rest and relieve restlessness.
- Help the patient walk as soon as possible after surgery to prevent venostasis.
- Maintain adequate nutrition and fluid balance to promote healing.
- Report frequent pleuritic chest pain, so that analgesics can be prescribed. Also, incentive spirometry can assist in deep breathing. Provide tissues and a bag for easy disposal of sputum.
- Warn the patient not to cross his legs; this promotes thrombus formation.
- To relieve anxiety, explain procedures and treatments. Encourage the

patient's family to participate in his care.

- Most patients need treatment with an oral anticoagulant (warfarin) for 3 to 6 months after a pulmonary embolism. Advise these patients to watch for signs of bleeding (bloody stools, blood in urine, and large ecchymoses), to take the prescribed medication exactly as ordered, not to change the dosage without consulting the practitioner, and to avoid taking additional medication (including aspirin and vitamins). Stress the need for follow-up laboratory tests (International Normalized Ratio) to monitor anticoagulant therapy.

Pulmonary hypertension

Pulmonary hypertension occurs when pulmonary artery pressure (PAP) rises above normal for reasons other than aging or altitude. No definitive set of values is used to diagnose pulmonary hypertension, but the National Institutes of Health requires a mean PAP of 25 mm Hg or more. The prognosis depends on the cause of the underlying disorder, but the long-term prognosis is poor. Within 5 years of diagnosis, only 25% of patients are still alive.

CAUSES AND INCIDENCE

Primary (or idiopathic) pulmonary hypertension is rare, occurring most commonly—and with no known cause—in women between ages 20 and 40. Secondary pulmonary hypertension results from existing cardiac, pulmonary, thromboembolic, or collagen vascular diseases or from the use of certain drugs.

In primary pulmonary hypertension, the smooth muscle in the pulmonary artery wall hypertrophies for no detectable reason, narrowing the small pulmonary artery (arterioles) or obliterating it completely. Fibrous lesions also form around the vessels, impairing distensibility and increasing vascular resistance. Pressures in the left ventricle, which receives blood from the lungs, remain normal. However, the increased pressures generated in the lungs are transmitted to the right ventricle, which supplies the pulmonary artery. Eventually, the right ventricle fails (cor pulmonale). Although oxygenation isn't severely affected initially, hypoxia and cyanosis eventually occur. Death results from cor pulmonale.

Alveolar hypoventilation can result from diseases caused by alveolar destruction, such chronic obstructive pulmonary disease (most common cause in the United States), sarcoidosis, diffuse interstitial disease, pulmonary metastasis, and certain diseases such as scleroderma. Other disorders that cause alveolar hypoventilation without lung tissue damage include obesity, kyphoscoliosis, and obstructive sleep apnea. In any of these disorders, pulmonary vascular resistance increases secondary to hypoxemia and destruction of the alveolocapillary bed. The resulting hypoxemia also causes vasoconstriction, further increasing vascular resistance and leading to pulmonary hypertension.

Vascular obstruction from pulmonary embolism, vasculitis, and disorders that cause obstruction of small or large pulmonary veins, such as left atrial myxoma, idiopathic veno-occlusive disease, fibrosing mediastinitis, and mediastinal neoplasm, also cause pulmonary hypertension. This is because blood isn't allowed to flow appropriately through the vessels.

Primary cardiac diseases may be congenital or acquired. Congenital defects that cause left-to-right shunting of blood—such as patent ductus arteriosus or atrial or ventricular septal defect—increase blood flow into the lungs and, consequently, raise pulmonary vascular pressure. Acquired cardiac diseases, such as rheumatic valvular disease and mitral stenosis, increase pulmonary venous pressure by restricting blood flow returning to the heart.

Secondary pulmonary hypertension can be reversed if the disorder is resolved. If hypertension persists, hypertrophy occurs in the medial smooth muscle layer of the arterioles. The larger arteries stiffen, and hypertension progresses. Pulmonary pressures begin to equal systemic blood pressure, causing right ventricular hypertrophy and, eventually, cor pulmonale.

SIGNS AND SYMPTOMS

Most patients complain of increasing dyspnea on exertion, weakness, syncope, and fatigability. Many also show signs of right-sided heart failure, including peripheral edema, ascites, jugular vein distention, and hepatomegaly. Other clinical effects vary with the underlying disorder.

COMPLICATIONS

- Cor pulmonale
- Cardiac failure
- Cardiac arrest

DIAGNOSIS

- Arterial blood gas (ABG) analysis indicates hypoxemia (decreased partial pressure of arterial oxygen).
- Electrocardiography shows right axis deviation and tall or peaked P waves in inferior leads in a patient with right ventricular hypertrophy.
- Cardiac catheterization reveals pulmonary systolic pressure above 30 mm Hg as well as increased pulmonary artery wedge pressure (PAWP) if the underlying cause is left atrial myxoma, mitral stenosis, or left-sided heart failure (otherwise normal).
- Pulmonary angiography detects filling defects in pulmonary vasculature such as those that develop in patients with pulmonary emboli.
- Pulmonary function tests may show decreased flow rates and increased residual volume in underlying obstructive disease and decreased total lung capacity in underlying restrictive disease.
- Radionuclide imaging detects abnormalities in right and left ventricular functioning.
- Open lung biopsy may determine the type of disorder.

• Echocardiography allows the assessment of ventricular wall motion and possible valvular dysfunction. It can also demonstrate right ventricular enlargement, abnormal septal configuration consistent with right ventricular pressure overload, and reduction in left ventricular cavity size.
• Perfusion lung scanning may produce normal or abnormal results, with multiple patchy and diffuse filling defects that don't suggest pulmonary embolism.

TREATMENT

Treatment usually includes oxygen therapy to decrease hypoxemia and pulmonary vascular resistance. Fluid restriction is implemented to decrease the heart's workload in right-sided heart failure. In severe cases, heart-lung transplantation is needed.

Drugs

• Digoxin (Lanoxin) to increase cardiac output
• Diuretic to decrease intravascular volume and extravascular fluid accumulation
• Vasodilator to reduce myocardial workload and oxygen consumption
• Calcium channel blocker to reduce myocardial workload and oxygen consumption
• Bronchodilator to relax smooth muscles and increase airway patency
• Beta-adrenergic blocker to improve oxygenation

SPECIAL CONSIDERATIONS

• Pulmonary hypertension requires keen observation and careful monitoring as well as skilled supportive care.
• Administer oxygen therapy as ordered, and observe the patient's response. Report signs of increasing dyspnea so treatment can be adjusted accordingly.
• Monitor ABG levels for acidosis and hypoxemia. Report any change in the patient's level of consciousness at once.
• When caring for a patient with right-sided heart failure, especially one receiving diuretics, record his weight daily, carefully measure intake and output, and explain all medications and diet restrictions. Check for worsening jugular vein distention, which may indicate fluid overload.
• Monitor the patient's vital signs, especially blood pressure and heart rate. Watch for hypotension and tachycardia. If he has a pulmonary artery catheter, check PAP and PAWP, as indicated. Report any changes.
• Before discharge, help the patient adjust to the limitations imposed by this disorder. Advise against overexertion, and suggest frequent rest periods between activities. Refer the patient to the social services department if he'll need special equipment, such as oxygen equipment, for home use. Make sure that he understands the prescribed medications and diet and the need to weigh himself daily.

Pulmonic insufficiency

In patients with pulmonic insufficiency, blood ejected into the pulmonary artery during systole flows back into the right ventricle during diastole. (See *Types of valvular heart disease,* page 8.)

CAUSES

Pulmonic insufficiency may be congenital or may result from pulmonary hypertension. The most common acquired cause is dilation of the pulmonic valve ring from severe pulmonary hypertension. Rarely, pulmonic insufficiency may result from prolonged use of a pressure monitoring catheter in the pulmonary artery.

The backflow of blood into the right ventricle leads to fluid overload in the ventricle, ventricular hypertrophy, and eventual right-sided heart failure.

SIGNS AND SYMPTOMS

The patient may complain of exertional dyspnea, fatigue, chest pain, and syncope. Peripheral edema may cause discomfort. A patient with severe insufficiency that progresses to right-sided heart failure may appear malnourished and jaundiced with severe peripheral edema and ascites. Auscultation may reveal a high-pitched, decrescendo, diastolic blowing murmur along the left sternal border (Graham Steell's murmur). This murmur may be difficult to distinguish from the murmur of aortic insufficiency. (See *Identifying the murmur of pulmonic insufficiency.*) Palpation may reveal hepatomegaly if the patient has right-sided heart failure.

IDENTIFYING THE MURMUR OF PULMONIC INSUFFICIENCY

In a patient with pulmonic insufficiency, you'll hear a high-pitched, blowing decrescendo murmur at Erb's point, as depicted here.

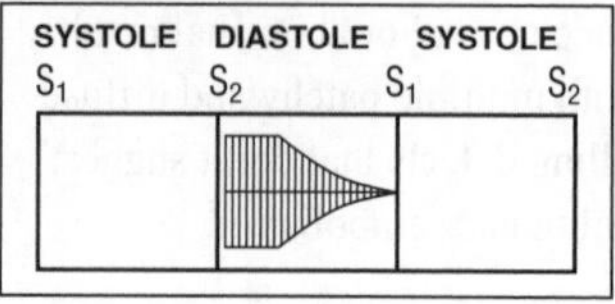

COMPLICATIONS

- Right-sided heart failure

DIAGNOSIS

- Cardiac catheterization shows pulmonic insufficiency, increased right ventricular pressure, and associated cardiac defects.
- Chest X-rays show right ventricular and pulmonary arterial enlargement.
- Echocardiography can be used to visualize the pulmonic valve abnormality.
- Electrocardiography findings may be normal in mild cases or reveal right ventricular hypertrophy.

TREATMENT

Treatment for pulmonic insufficiency is based on the patient's symptoms and typically includes a low-sodium diet to reduce hepatic congestion before surgery. Valvulotomy or valve replacement may be required in severe cases.

Drugs

- Diuretic to reduce hepatic congestion prior to surgery

SPECIAL CONSIDERATIONS

- Alternate periods of activity and rest to prevent extreme fatigue and dyspnea.
- Keep the patient's legs elevated while he sits in a chair to improve venous return to the heart.
- Elevate the head of the bed to improve ventilation.
- Keep the patient on a low-sodium diet. Consult with a dietitian to make sure the patient receives foods that he likes while adhering to diet restrictions.
- Monitor the patient for signs and symptoms of heart failure, pulmonary edema, and adverse reactions to drug therapy.
- To reduce anxiety, allow the patient to express his concerns about the effects of activity restrictions on his responsibilities and routines. Reassure him that the restrictions are temporary.
- If the patient has surgery, watch for hypotension, arrhythmias, and thrombus formation. Monitor his vital signs, arterial blood gas levels, intake and output, daily weights, blood chemistry results, chest X-rays, and pulmonary artery catheter readings.
- Teach the patient about diet restrictions, medications, symptoms that should be reported, and the importance of consistent follow-up care.
- Tell the patient to elevate his legs whenever he sits.

Pulmonic stenosis

In patients with pulmonic stenosis, obstructed right ventricular outflow causes right ventricular hypertrophy as the right ventricle attempts to overcome resistance to the narrow valvular opening. Eventually, right-sided heart failure results.

CAUSES AND INCIDENCE

A congenital defect, pulmonic stenosis is associated with other congenital heart defects such as tetralogy of Fallot. It's rare among elderly patients. (See *Types of valvular heart disease,* page 8.)

SIGNS AND SYMPTOMS

Depending on the severity of the obstruction, a patient with mild stenosis may be asymptomatic. A patient with moderate to severe stenosis may complain of exertional dyspnea, fatigue, chest pain, peripheral edema, and syncope.

Inspection may reveal a prominent *a* wave in the jugular venous pulse. If severe stenosis has progressed to right-sided heart failure, the patient may appear malnourished and jaundiced with severe peripheral edema and ascites. Auscultation may reveal a fourth heart sound, a thrill at the upper left sternal border, a harsh systolic ejection murmur, and a holosystolic decrescendo murmur of tricuspid insufficiency, particularly if the patient has heart failure. (See *Identifying the murmur of pulmonic stenosis*.) Palpation may detect hepatomegaly if the patient has right-sided heart failure, presystolic pulsations of the liver, and a right parasternal lift.

COMPLICATIONS

- Right-sided heart failure

DIAGNOSIS

- Chest X-ray usually shows a normal heart size and normal lung vascularity, although the pulmonary arteries may be evident. With severe obstruction and right-sided heart failure, the right atrium and ventricle typically appear enlarged.
- Echocardiography can be used to visualize the pulmonic valve abnormality.
- Cardiac catheterization may be recommended if the stenosis is more pronounced, in order to evaluate the need for balloon dilatation.
- Electrocardiography results may be normal in mild cases, or they may show right-axis deviation and right ventricular hypertrophy. High-amplitude P waves in leads II and V_1 indicate right atrial enlargement.

> **IDENTIFYING THE MURMUR OF PULMONIC STENOSIS**
>
> In a patient with pulmonic stenosis, you'll hear a medium-pitched, harsh, crescendo-decrescendo murmur in the area of the pulmonic valve, as depicted here.
>
> 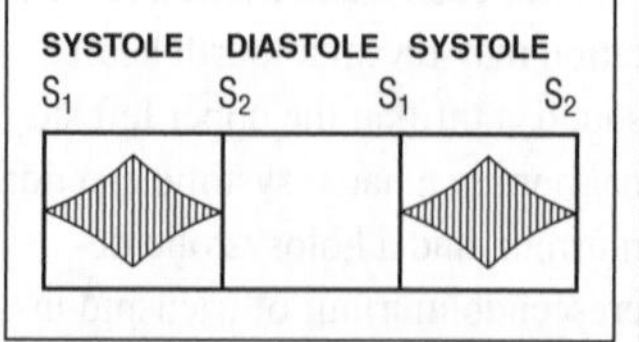
>

TREATMENT

A low-sodium diet helps reduce hepatic congestion before surgery. Additionally, cardiac catheter balloon valvuloplasty is usually effective, even with moderate to severe obstruction.

Drugs

- Diuretic to reduce hepatic congestion before surgery

SPECIAL CONSIDERATIONS

- Alternate periods of activity with periods of rest to prevent extreme fatigue and dyspnea.
- Keep the patient's legs elevated while he sits in a chair to improve venous return to the heart.
- Elevate the head of the bed to improve ventilation.
- Keep the patient on a low-sodium diet. Consult with a dietitian to make sure the patient receives foods that he likes while adhering to the diet restrictions.
- Monitor the patient for signs and symptoms of heart failure, pulmonary edema, and adverse reactions to drug therapy.
- To reduce anxiety, allow the patient to express his concerns about

the effects of activity restrictions on his responsibilities and routines. Reassure him that the restrictions are temporary.

- After cardiac catheterization, apply firm pressure to the catheter insertion site, usually in the groin. Monitor the site for signs of bleeding every 15 minutes for at least 6 hours. If the site bleeds, remove the pressure dressing and manually apply firm pressure to the site.
- Notify the practitioner of changes in peripheral pulses distal to the insertion site, changes in cardiac rhythm and vital signs, and complaints of chest pain.
- Teach the patient about diet restrictions, medications, signs and symptoms that should be reported, and the importance of consistent follow-up care.
- Teach the patient to elevate his legs when sitting.

R

Raynaud's disease

Raynaud's disease is one of several primary arteriospastic disorders characterized by episodic vasospasm in the small peripheral arteries and arterioles. It's triggered by exposure to cold or stress. This condition occurs bilaterally and usually affects the hands or, less often, the feet. Raynaud's disease is most prevalent in women, particularly those between puberty and age 40. It's a benign condition requiring no specific treatment and causing no serious sequelae.

Raynaud's phenomenon, in contrast, is commonly linked to a connective tissue disorder—such as scleroderma, systemic lupus erythematosus (SLE), or polymyositis—and has a progressive course, leading to ischemia, gangrene, and amputation. Distinguishing between the two disorders is difficult because some patients who experience mild symptoms of Raynaud's disease for several years may later develop overt connective tissue disease, especially scleroderma. (See *Causes of Raynaud's phenomenon.*)

CAUSES AND INCIDENCE

Although the cause is unknown, several theories account for the reduced digital blood flow: intrinsic vascular wall hyperactivity to cold, increased vasomotor tone due to sympathetic stimulation, and antigen-antibody immune response (the most likely theory because abnormal immunologic test results accompany Raynaud's phenomenon). Risk factors include associated diseases (Buerger's disease, atherosclerosis, rheumatoid arthritis, scleroderma, and SLE) and smoking.

This disorder affects women more often than men.

SIGNS AND SYMPTOMS

After exposure to cold or stress, the skin on the fingers typically blanches and then becomes cyanotic before changing to red and before changing from cold to normal temperature. Numbness and tingling may also occur. These symptoms are relieved by warmth. In longstanding disease, trophic changes, such as sclerodactyly, ulcerations, or chronic paronychia, may result. Although it's extremely uncommon, minimal cutaneous gangrene necessitates amputation of one or more phalanges.

COMPLICATIONS

- Ischemia
- Gangrene
- Amputation

CAUSES OF RAYNAUD'S PHENOMENON

Patients with primary or idiopathic Raynaud's have Raynaud's disease. Raynaud's phenomenon, on the other hand, may result from the disorders and other factors listed here.

Collagen vascular disease
- Dermatomyositis
- Polymyositis
- Rheumatoid arthritis
- Scleroderma
- Systemic lupus erythematosus

Arterial occlusive disease
- Acute arterial occlusion
- Atherosclerosis of the extremities
- Thoracic outlet syndrome
- Thromboangiitis obliterans

Neurologic disorders
- Carpal tunnel syndrome
- Invertebral disk disease
- Poliomyelitis
- Spinal cord tumors
- Stroke
- Syringomyelia

Blood dyscrasias
- Cold agglutinins
- Cryofibrinogenemia
- Myeloproliferative disorders
- Waldenström's disease

Trauma
- Cold injury
- Electric shock
- Hammering
- Keyboarding
- Piano playing
- Vibration injury

Drugs
- Beta-adrenergic blockers
- Bleomycin (Blenoxane)
- Cisplatin (Platinol)
- Ergot derivatives such as ergotamine (Ergomar)
- Methysergide
- Vinblastine

Other
- Pulmonary hypertension

DIAGNOSIS

- Clinical criteria that establish Raynaud's disease include skin color changes induced by cold or stress; bilateral involvement; absence of gangrene or, if present, minimal cutaneous gangrene; normal arterial pulses; and a history of clinical symptoms of longer than 2 years' duration.
- Diagnosis must also rule out secondary disease processes, such as chronic arterial occlusive or connective tissue disease.
- Antinuclear antibody (ANA) titer is used to identify autoimmune disease as an underlying cause of Raynaud's phenomenon. Further testing must be performed if ANA titer is positive.
- Arteriography rules out arterial occlusive disease.
- Doppler ultrasonography may show reduced blood flow if symptoms result from arterial occlusive disease.
- A cold-stimulation test measures the temperature of each finger after

they are placed in an ice-water bath. Raynaud's phenomenon may be diagnosed if the finger temperature takes greater than 20 minutes to return to pre-bath temperature.

- Nailfold capillaroscopy is useful to determine the presence of a connective tissue disorder.

TREATMENT

Initially, treatment includes avoidance of cold, mechanical, or chemical injury; cessation of smoking; and reassurance that symptoms are benign. Because adverse drug effects, especially from vasodilators, may be more bothersome than the disease itself, drug therapy is reserved for unusually severe symptoms. Sympathectomy may be helpful when conservative treatment fails to prevent ischemic ulcers; it becomes necessary in less than 25% of patients.

Drugs

- Calcium channel blocker, such as nifedipine (Procardia), diltiazem (Cardizem), or nicardipine (Cardene), to produce vasodilation and prevent vasospasm
- Alpha blocker, such as prazosin (Minipress) or doxazosin (Cardura), which may improve blood flow
- Vasodilator, such as topical nitroglycerin, to relax blood vessels and help heal skin ulcers

SPECIAL CONSIDERATIONS

- Warn the patient to avoid exposure to the cold. Tell him to wear mittens or gloves in cold weather or when handling cold items or defrosting the freezer.
- Advise the patient to avoid stressful situations and to stop smoking.
- Instruct the patient to inspect the skin often and to seek immediate care for signs of skin breakdown or infection.
- Teach the patient about drugs, their use, and their adverse effects.
- Provide psychological support and reassurance to allay the patient's fear of amputation and disfigurement.

Renovascular hypertension

Renovascular hypertension is a rise in systemic blood pressure resulting from stenosis of the major renal arteries or their branches or from intrarenal atherosclerosis. This narrowing or sclerosis may be partial or complete, and the resulting blood pressure elevation may be benign or malignant. Renovascular hypertension is the most common type of secondary hypertension. (See *What happens in renovascular hypertension,* page 180.)

CAUSES AND INCIDENCE

Stenosis or occlusion of the renal artery stimulates the affected kidney to release the enzyme renin, which converts angiotensinogen—a plasma protein—to angiotensin I. As angiotensin I circulates through the lungs and liver, it converts to angiotensin II, which causes peripheral vasoconstriction, increased arterial pressure and aldosterone secretion and, eventually, hypertension.

Atherosclerosis (especially in older men) and fibromuscular diseases of the renal artery wall layers—such as medial fibroplasia and, less commonly, intimal and subadventitial fibroplasias—are the primary causes in 95% of patients with renovascular hypertension. Other causes include arteritis, anomalies of the renal arteries, embolism, trauma, tumor, and dissecting aneurysm. Less than 5% of patients with high blood pressure have renovascular hypertension; it's most common in those younger than age 30 or older than age 50.

SIGNS AND SYMPTOMS

In addition to elevated systemic blood pressure, renovascular hypertension usually produces symptoms common to hypertensive states, such as headache, palpitations, tachycardia, anxiety, light-headedness, decreased tolerance of temperature extremes, retinopathy, and mental sluggishness. An altered level of consciousness and pitting edema may occur if renal failure ensues.

COMPLICATIONS

- Heart failure
- Myocardial infarction
- Stroke
- Renal failure (occasionally)

DIAGNOSIS

- Arterial digital subtraction angiography with assays of venous renin is the definitive diagnostic procedure. When stenosis is significant, transluminal angioplasty can be done during the same procedure.
- Gadolinium enhanced magnetic resonance angiography can identify turbulent blood flow indicative of renal stenosis.
- Duplex Doppler ultrasonography scans the renal artery and will reveal stenosis but results vary.
- Oral captopril (Capoten) renography is the simplest noninvasive test for detection of renovascular hypertension but has a relatively high false-positive rate.

TREATMENT

Surgery, the treatment of choice, is performed to restore circulation and to control severe hypertension or severely impaired renal function. It involves renal artery bypass, endarterectomy, arterioplasty or, as a last resort, nephrectomy. Balloon catheter renal artery dilatation is used in certain cases to correct renal artery stenosis without the risks and morbidity of surgery. Symptomatic measures include antihypertensives, diuretics, and a sodium-restricted diet. Response to medications is highly individual, and the dosage or specific drug used may need frequent adjustment.

Lifestyle changes may be needed, including weight loss, exercise, dietary adjustments, smoking cessation, and avoidance of alcohol. These habits add to the effects of hypertension in causing complications.

WHAT HAPPENS IN RENOVASCULAR HYPERTENSION

The kidneys normally play a key role in maintaining blood pressure and volume through vasoconstriction and regulation of sodium and fluid levels. In renovascular hypertension, these regulatory mechanisms fail.

Certain conditions, such as renal artery stenosis and tumors, reduce blood flow to the kidneys. This causes juxtaglomerular cells to continuously secrete renin.

In this stage, be alert for flank pain, systolic bruit in the epigastric vein over the upper abdomen, reduced urine output, and an elevated renin level.

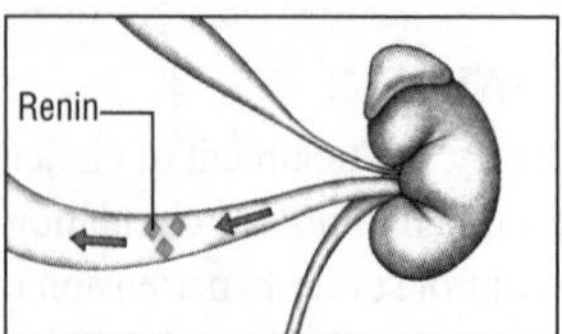

In the liver, renin and angiotensinogen combine to form angiotensin I, which converts to angiotensin II in the lungs. This potent vasoconstrictor heightens peripheral resistance and blood pressure.

Check for headache, nausea, anorexia, an elevated renin level, and hypertension.

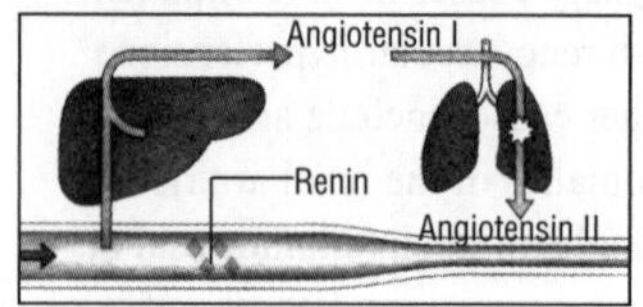

Angiotensin II acts directly on the kidneys, causing them to reabsorb sodium and water.

Assess the patient for hypertension, decreased urine output, albuminuria, hypokalemia, and hypernatremia.

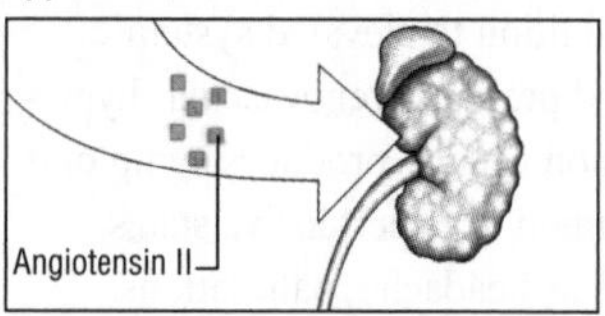

Drugs

- Diuretics, beta-adrenergic blockers, calcium channel blockers, angiotensin-converting enzyme inhibitors, angiotensin receptor blockers, and alpha adrenergic blockers to control blood pressure
- Diazoxide (Proglycem) or nitroprusside (Nitropress) while hospitalized, if symptoms are acute

SPECIAL CONSIDERATIONS

- The care plan must emphasize helping the patient and his family understand renovascular hypertension and the importance of following the prescribed treatment.
- Accurately monitor intake and output and daily weight. Check blood pressure in both arms regularly with the patient lying down and standing. A drop of 20 mm Hg or more on arising may necessitate an adjustment in antihypertensive medications. Assess renal function daily.
- Maintain fluid and sodium restrictions. Explain the purpose of a low-sodium diet.
- Explain the diagnostic tests, and prepare the patient appropriately; for

Angiotensin II stimulates the adrenal cortex to secrete aldosterone. This also causes the kidneys to retain sodium and water, elevating blood volume and pressure.

Expect worsening symptoms.

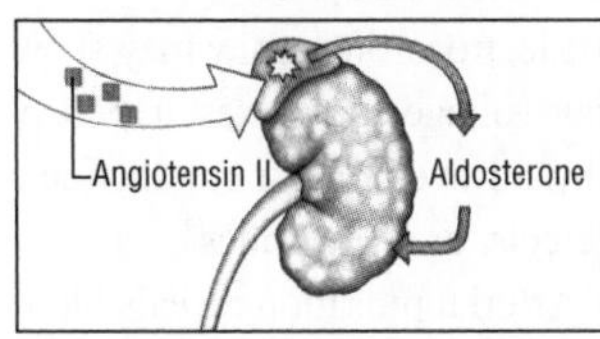

Intermittent pressure diuresis causes excretion of sodium and water, reduced blood volume, and decreasing cardiac output.

Check for blood pressure that increases slowly, drops (but not as low as before), and then increases again. Headache, high urine specific gravity, hyponatremia, fatigue, and heart failure also occur.

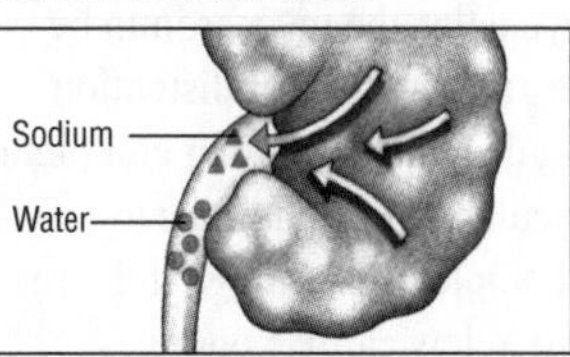

A high aldosterone level causes further sodium retention, but it can't curtail renin secretion. Excessive aldosterone and angiotensin II can damage renal tissue, leading to renal failure. Expect to find hypertension, pitting edema, anemia, decreased level of consciousness, and increased blood urea nitrogen and serum creatinine levels.

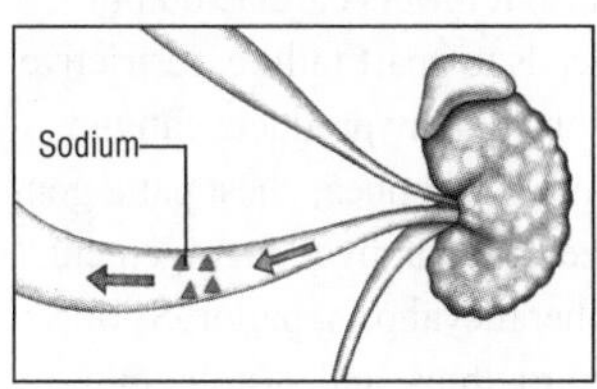

example, adequately hydrate the patient before tests that use contrast media. Make sure the patient isn't allergic to the dye used in diagnostic tests. After excretory urography or arteriography, watch for complications.

- If a nephrectomy is needed, reassure the patient that the remaining kidney is adequate for renal function.

Restrictive cardiomyopathy

Restrictive cardiomyopathy, a disorder of the myocardial musculature, is characterized by restricted ventricular filling (the result of left ventricular hypertrophy) and endocardial fibrosis and thickening. If severe, it's irreversible. (See *Comparing cardiomyopathies,* page 68.)

CAUSES AND INCIDENCE

Primary restrictive cardiomyopathy is an extremely rare disorder of unknown cause. Restrictive cardiomyopathy syndrome, in contrast, is a manifestation of amyloidosis and results from infiltration of amyloid into the intracellular spaces in the myocardium, endocardium, and subendocardium.

In both forms of restrictive cardiomyopathy, the myocardium becomes rigid, with poor distention during diastole, inhibiting complete ventricular filling, and fails to contract completely during systole, resulting in low cardiac output.

Restrictive cardiomyopathy is rare. It occurs most often in children and young adults. There's no racial predilection, but people living in Africa, South America, and India are at increased risk.

SIGNS AND SYMPTOMS

Because it lowers cardiac output and leads to heart failure, restrictive cardiomyopathy produces fatigue, dyspnea, orthopnea, chest pain, generalized edema, liver engorgement, peripheral cyanosis, pallor, S_3 or S_4 gallop rhythms, and systolic murmurs of mitral and tricuspid insufficiency.

COMPLICATIONS

- Heart failure
- Arrhythmias
- Systemic or pulmonary embolization
- Sudden death

DIAGNOSIS

- In advanced stages of this disease, chest X-ray shows massive cardiomegaly affecting all four chambers of the heart, pericardial effusion, and pulmonary congestion.
- Echocardiography, computed tomography scan, or magnetic resonance imaging rules out constrictive pericarditis as the cause of restricted filling by detecting increased left ventricular muscle mass and differences in end-diastolic pressures between the ventricles.
- Electrocardiography may show low-voltage complexes, hypertrophy, atrioventricular conduction defects, or arrhythmias.
- Arterial pulsation reveals blunt carotid upstroke with small volume.
- Cardiac catheterization shows increased left ventricular end-diastolic pressure and rules out constrictive pericarditis as the cause of restricted filling.
- Restrictive cardiomyopathy may be difficult to differentiate from constrictive pericarditis. A biopsy of heart muscle may be used to confirm the diagnosis. A cardiac catheterization procedure can also help differentiate the type of cardiomyopathy through simultaneous left- and right-heart catheterization. In some cases, surgical exploration and biopsies are the only means to distinguish the type of cardiomyopathy or to differentiate it from pericarditis. (See *Comparing diagnostic tests in cardiomyopathy,* page 72.)

TREATMENT

Although no therapy exists for restricted ventricular filling, certain medications and a low-sodium diet can ease symptoms of heart failure. A heart transplant may be considered in those with poor myocardial function.

Drugs

- Cardiac glycoside and diuretic to treat heart failure
- Oral vasodilator—such as isosorbide dinitrate (Isordil), prazosin [Minipress], or hydralazine (Apresazide)—which may control intractable heart failure
- Anticoagulant therapy to prevent thrombophlebitis in a patient on prolonged bed rest
- Treatment of the underlying cause, such as deferoxamine (Desferal) to bind iron in restrictive cardiomyopathy resulting from hemochromatosis

SPECIAL CONSIDERATIONS

- In the acute phase, monitor heart rate and rhythm, blood pressure, urine output, and pulmonary artery pressure readings to help guide treatment.
- Give psychological support. Provide appropriate diversionary activities for a patient restricted to prolonged bed rest. Because a poor prognosis may cause profound anxiety and depression, be especially supportive and understanding, and encourage the patient to express his fears. Refer him for psychosocial counseling, as needed, for assistance in coping with his restricted lifestyle. Be flexible with visiting hours whenever possible.
- Before discharge, teach the patient to watch for and report signs and symptoms of digoxin toxicity (anorexia, nausea, vomiting, yellow vision); to record and report weight gain; and, if sodium restriction is ordered, to avoid canned foods, pickles, smoked meats, and use of table salt.

Rheumatic fever and rheumatic heart disease

Acute rheumatic fever is a systemic inflammatory disease of childhood, commonly recurrent, that follows a group A beta-hemolytic streptococcal infection. Rheumatic heart disease refers to the cardiac manifestations of rheumatic fever and includes pancarditis (myocarditis, pericarditis, endocarditis) during the early acute phase and chronic valvular disease later.

Long-term antibiotic therapy can minimize the recurrence of rheumatic fever, reducing the risk of permanent cardiac damage and eventual valvular deformity. However, severe pancarditis occasionally produces fatal heart failure during the acute phase. Of the patients who survive this complication, about 20% die within 10 years.

CAUSES AND INCIDENCE

Rheumatic fever appears to be a hypersensitivity reaction to a group A beta-hemolytic streptococcal infection, in which antibodies produced to combat streptococci react and produce characteristic lesions at specific tissue sites, especially in the heart and joints. Because few people (3%) with streptococcal infections contract rheumatic fever, altered host resistance must be involved in its development or recurrence. The antigens of group A streptococci bind to receptors in the heart, muscle, brain, and synovial joints, causing an autoimmune response. Because of a similarity between the antigens of the body's own cells, antibodies may attack healthy body cells by mistake.

Although rheumatic fever tends to be familial, this may merely reflect contributing environmental factors. For example, in lower socioeconomic groups, incidence is highest in children between ages 5 and 15, probably as a result of malnutrition and crowded living conditions. This disease strikes generally during cool, damp weather in the winter and early spring. In the United States, it's most common in the northern states.

SIGNS AND SYMPTOMS

In 95% of patients, rheumatic fever characteristically follows a streptococcal infection that appeared a few days to 6 weeks earlier. A temperature of at least 100.4° F (38° C) occurs, and most patients complain of migratory joint pain or polyarthritis. Swelling, redness, and signs of effusion usually accompany such pain, which most commonly affects the knees, ankles, elbows, or hips. In 5% of patients (usually those with carditis), rheumatic fever causes skin lesions such as erythema marginatum, a nonpruritic, macular, transient rash that gives rise to red lesions with blanched centers. Rheumatic fever also may produce firm, movable, nontender, subcutaneous nodules about 3 mm to 2 cm in diameter, usually near tendons or bony prominences of joints (especially the elbows, knuckles, wrists, and knees) and less often on the scalp and backs of the hands. These nodules persist for a few days to several weeks and, like erythema marginatum, often accompany carditis.

Later, rheumatic fever may cause transient chorea, which develops up to 6 months after the original streptococcal infection. Mild chorea may produce hyperirritability, deterioration in handwriting, or an inability to concentrate. Severe chorea (Sydenham's chorea) causes purposeless, nonrepetitive, involuntary muscle spasms; poor muscle coordination; and weakness. Chorea resolves without residual neurologic damage.

The most destructive effect of rheumatic fever is carditis, which develops in up to 50% of patients and may affect the endocardium, myocardium, pericardium, or the heart valves. Pericarditis causes a pericardial friction rub and, occasionally, pain and effusion. Myocarditis produces characteristic lesions called *Aschoff bodies* (in the acute stages) and cellular swelling and fragmentation of interstitial collagen, leading to formation of a progressively fibrotic nodule and interstitial scars. Endocarditis causes valve leaflet swelling, erosion along the lines of leaflet closure, and blood, platelet, and fibrin deposits, which form beadlike vegetations. Endocarditis affects the mitral valve most often in females; the aortic, most often in males. In both females and males, endocarditis affects the tricuspid valves occasionally and the pulmonic valve only rarely.

Severe rheumatic carditis may cause heart failure with dyspnea; right upper quadrant pain; tachycardia; tachypnea; a hacking, nonproductive cough; edema; and significant mitral and aortic murmurs. The most common of such murmurs include:

- a systolic murmur of mitral insufficiency (high-pitched, blowing, holosystolic, loudest at apex, possibly radiating to the anterior axillary line)
- a midsystolic murmur from stiffening and swelling of the mitral leaflet
- occasionally, a diastolic murmur of aortic insufficiency (low-pitched, rumbling, almost inaudible).

Valvular disease may eventually result in chronic valvular stenosis and insufficiency, including mitral stenosis and insufficiency, and aortic insufficiency. In children, mitral insufficiency remains the major sequela of rheumatic heart disease.

COMPLICATIONS

- Destruction of mitral and aortic valves
- Severe pancarditis
- Pericardial effusion
- Fatal heart failure

DIAGNOSIS

- Diagnosis depends on recognition of one or more of the classic symptoms (carditis, rheumatic fever without carditis, polyarthritis, chorea, erythema marginatum, or subcutaneous nodules) and a detailed patient history.
- White blood cell count and erythrocyte sedimentation rate may be elevated (during the acute phase); blood studies show slight anemia due to suppressed erythropoiesis during inflammation.
- C-reactive protein is positive (especially during acute phase).
- Cardiac enzyme levels may be increased in severe carditis.
- Antistreptolysin-O titer is elevated in 95% of patients within 2 months of onset.
- Electrocardiogram changes aren't diagnostic, but the PR interval is prolonged in 20% of patients.
- Chest X-rays show normal heart size (except with myocarditis, heart failure, or pericardial effusion).
- Echocardiography helps evaluate valvular damage, chamber size, and ventricular function.
- Cardiac catheterization evaluates valvular damage and left ventricular function in severe cardiac dysfunction.

TREATMENT

Effective management eradicates the streptococcal infection, relieves symptoms, and prevents recurrence, reducing the chance of permanent cardiac damage. Supportive treatment requires strict bed rest for about 5 weeks during the acute phase with active carditis, followed by a progressive increase in physical activity, depending on clinical and laboratory findings and the response to treatment.

Heart failure demands continued bed rest and diuretics. Severe mitral or aortic valve dysfunction that causes persistent heart failure requires corrective valvular surgery, including commissurotomy (separation of the adherent, thickened leaflets of the mitral valve), valvuloplasty (inflation of a balloon within a valve), or valve replacement (with prosthetic valve). Such surgery is seldom necessary before late adolescence.

Drugs

- Penicillin, sulfadiazine, or erythromycin (E-mycin) during the acute phase
- Salicylates, such as aspirin, to relieve fever and minimize joint swelling and pain
- Corticosteroids if carditis is present or salicylates fail to relieve pain and inflammation
- Low-dose antibiotics after the acute phase subsides to prevent recurrence (usually continues for 5 years or until age 21, whichever is longer)

SPECIAL CONSIDERATIONS

- Because rheumatic fever and rheumatic heart disease require prolonged treatment, the care plan should include comprehensive patient teaching to promote compliance with the prescribed therapy.
- Before giving penicillin, ask the patient or his parents if he has ever had a hypersensitive reaction to it. If he hasn't, warn that such a reaction is possible. Tell them to stop the drug and call the practitioner immediately if he develops a rash, fever, chills, or other signs of allergy at any time during penicillin therapy.
- Instruct the patient and his family to watch for and report early signs of heart failure, such as dyspnea and a hacking, nonproductive cough.
- Stress the need for bed rest during the acute phase, and suggest appropriate, physically undemanding diversions. After the acute phase, encourage family and friends to spend as much time as possible with the patient to minimize boredom. Advise parents to secure tutoring services to help a child keep up with schoolwork during the long convalescence.
- Help parents overcome guilty feelings they may have about their child's illness. Tell them that failure to seek treatment for streptococcal infection is common because this illness often seems no worse than a cold. Urge the child and his parents to vent their frustrations during the long, tedious recovery. If the child has severe carditis, help them prepare for permanent changes in his lifestyle.
- Teach the patient and family about the disease and its treatment. Warn parents to watch for and immediately report signs and

symptoms of recurrent streptococcal infection—sudden sore throat, diffuse throat redness and oropharyngeal exudate, swollen and tender cervical lymph glands, pain on swallowing, temperature of 101° to 104° F (38.3° to 40° C), headache, and nausea. Urge them to keep the child away from people with respiratory tract infections.

- Promote good dental hygiene to prevent gingival infection. Make sure the patient and his family understand the need to comply with prolonged antibiotic therapy and follow-up care and the need for additional antibiotics during dental surgery or procedures. Arrange for a home health nurse to oversee home care if necessary.
- Teach the patient to follow current recommendations of the American Heart Association for prevention of bacterial endocarditis. Antibiotic regimens used to prevent recurrence of acute rheumatic fever are inadequate for preventing bacterial endocarditis.

Septic shock

Second only to cardiogenic shock as the leading cause of shock-related death, septic shock involves inadequate tissue perfusion, abnormalities of oxygen supply and demand, metabolic changes, and circulatory collapse. It typically occurs among hospitalized patients, usually as a result of bacterial infection. About 25% of patients who develop gram-negative bacteremia go into shock. Unless vigorous treatment begins promptly, preferably before symptoms fully develop, septic shock rapidly progresses to death (in many cases within a few hours) in up to 80% of these patients. Septic shock is the most common cause of death in acute care units in the United States.

CAUSES AND INCIDENCE

In two-thirds of patients, septic shock results from infection with the gram-negative bacteria *Escherichia coli, Klebsiella, Enterobacter, Proteus, Pseudomonas,* or *Bacteroides;* in a minority of patients, it results from the gram-positive bacteria *Streptococcus pneumoniae, Streptococcus pyogenes, Staphylococcus aureus,* or *Actinomyces.* Infections with viruses, rickettsiae, chlamydiae, and protozoa may be complicated by shock.

These organisms produce septicemia in people whose resistance is already compromised by an existing condition; infection also results from translocation of bacteria from other areas of the body through surgery, I.V. therapy, and catheters. Septic shock commonly occurs in patients hospitalized for primary infection of the genitourinary, biliary, GI, or gynecologic tract. Other predisposing factors include immunodeficiency, advanced age, trauma, burns, diabetes mellitus, cirrhosis, and disseminated cancer.

SIGNS AND SYMPTOMS

Signs and symptoms of septic shock vary according to the stage of shock, the organism causing it, and the patient's immune response and age. In the early stage, they include oliguria, sudden fever (over 101° F [38.3° C]), chills, tachypnea, tachycardia, full bounding pulse, hyperglycemia, nausea, vomiting, diarrhea, and prostration. In the late stage, they include restlessness, apprehension, irritability, thirst from decreased cerebral tissue perfusion, hypoglycemia, hypothermia, and anuria. Hypotension, an altered level of consciousness, and hyperventilation may be the only signs among infants and the elderly.

COMPLICATIONS

- Disseminated intravascular coagulation
- Renal failure
- Heart failure
- GI ulcers
- Hepatic dysfunction

DIAGNOSIS

- One or more typical symptoms (fever, confusion, nausea, vomiting, and hyperventilation) in a patient suspected of having an infection suggests septic shock and requires immediate treatment.
- In early stages, arterial blood gas (ABG) levels indicate respiratory alkalosis (low partial pressure of carbon dioxide [$Paco_2$], low or normal bicarbonate [HCO_3^-], and high pH). As shock progresses, metabolic acidosis develops with hypoxemia, indicated by decreasing $Paco_2$ (may increase as respiratory failure ensues); partial pressure of oxygen; HCO_3^-, and pH.
- Blood cultures isolate the organism.
- Laboratory tests show a decreased platelet count and leukocytosis (15,000 to 30,000/mm^3) increased blood urea nitrogen and creatinine levels, decreased creatinine clearance, and abnormal prothrombin consumption and partial thromboplastin time.
- Simultaneous measurement of urine and plasma osmolalities for renal failure shows urine osmolality below 400 mOsm, with a ratio of urine to plasma below 1.5.
- The patient will have decreased central venous pressure (CVP), pulmonary artery pressure, and pulmonary artery wedge pressure (PAWP); decreased cardiac output (in early septic shock, cardiac output increases); and low systemic vascular resistance.
- An electrocardiogram shows ST-segment depression, inverted T waves, and arrhythmias resembling myocardial infarction.

TREATMENT

The first goal of treatment is to monitor for and then reverse shock through volume expansion with I.V. fluids and insertion of a pulmonary artery catheter to check PAWP. Administration of whole blood or plasma can then raise PAWP to a high normal to slightly elevated level of 14 to 18 mm Hg. A ventilator may be needed to overcome hypoxia. Urinary catheterization allows accurate measurement of hourly urine output.

Treatment also requires immediate administration of I.V. antibiotics to control the infection. Other measures to combat infection include surgery to drain and excise abscesses and débridement.

Drugs

- Depending on the organism, an antibiotic combination that usually includes an aminoglycoside (such as amikacin [Amikin], gentamicin, or tobramycin) for gram-negative bacteria combined with a penicillin

(such as ticarcillin [Timentin] or piperacillin [Zosyn])
- Sometimes a cephalosporin or vancomycin (Vancocin) for suspected staphylococcal infection
- Possibly chloramphenicol for nonsporulating anaerobes (*Bacteroides*), which may cause bone marrow depression, and clindamycin (Cleocin), which may produce pseudomembranous enterocolitis
- Metronidazole (Flagyl) for anaerobic infection
- Appropriate antibiotics for other causes of septic shock, depending on the suspected organism
- Vasopressors, such as dopamine, to maintain adequate blood perfusion in the brain, liver, GI tract, kidneys, and skin
- Drotrecogin alfa (Xigris) to interrupt the sepsis cascade
- I.V. bicarbonate to correct acidosis
- Corticosteroids (especially in patients with gram-negative septic shock)
- Opioid antagonists, prostaglandin inhibitors, and calcium channel blockers to block the rapid inflammatory process

SPECIAL CONSIDERATIONS

- Determine which of your patients are at high risk for septic shock. Know the signs of impending septic shock, but don't rely solely on technical aids to judge the patient's status. Consider any change in mental status and urine output as significant as a change in CVP. Report such changes promptly.
- Carefully maintain the pulmonary artery catheter. Check ABG levels for adequate oxygenation or gas exchange, and report any changes immediately.
- Record intake and output and daily weight. Maintain adequate urine output (0.5 to 1 ml/kg/hour) and systolic pressure. Avoid fluid overload.
- Monitor serum antibiotic level, and administer drugs as ordered.

Tetralogy of Fallot

Tetralogy of Fallot is a combination of four cardiac defects: ventricular septal defect (VSD), right ventricular outflow tract obstruction (pulmonic stenosis), right ventricular hypertrophy, and dextroposition of the aorta, with overriding of the VSD. (See *Defects in tetralogy of Fallot,* page 192.)

Blood shunts right to left through the VSD, permitting unoxygenated blood to mix with oxygenated blood, resulting in cyanosis. Tetralogy of Fallot sometimes coexists with other congenital heart defects, such as patent ductus arteriosus or atrial septal defect.

CAUSES AND INCIDENCE

The cause of tetralogy of Fallot is unknown, but it results from embryologic hypoplasia of the outflow tract of the right ventricle. Multiple factors, such as Down syndrome, have been linked to it. Prenatal risk factors include maternal rubella or other viral illnesses, poor prenatal nutrition, maternal alcoholism, mother older than age 40, and diabetes.

In tetralogy of Fallot, unoxygenated venous blood returning to the right side of the heart may pass through the VSD to the left ventricle, bypassing the lungs, or it may enter the pulmonary artery, depending on the extent of the pulmonic stenosis. Rather than originating from the left ventricle, the aorta overrides both ventricles.

The VSD usually lies in the outflow tract of the right ventricle and is generally large enough to permit equalization of right and left ventricular pressures. However, the ration of systemic vascular resistance to pulmonic stenosis affects the direction and magnitude of shunt flow across the VSD. Severe obstruction of right ventricular outflow produces a right-to-left shunt, causing decreased systemic arterial oxygen saturation, cyanosis, reduced pulmonary blood flow, and hypoplasia of the entire pulmonary vasculature. Right ventricular hypertrophy develops in response to the extra force needed to push blood into the stenotic pulmonary artery. Milder forms of pulmonic stenosis result in a left-to-right shunt or no shunt at all.

Tetralogy of Fallot occurs in about 5 of every 10,000 infants and accounts for about 10% of all congenital heart diseases. It occurs equally in boys and girls. Before surgical advances made correction possible, about one-third of these children died in infancy.

SIGNS AND SYMPTOMS

The degree of pulmonary stenosis, interacting with the VSD's size and location, determines the clinical and hemodynamic effects of this complex defect. Generally, the hallmark of the disorder is cyanosis, which usually becomes evident within several months after birth but may be present at birth if the neonate has severe pulmonary stenosis. Between ages 2 months and 2 years, children with tetralogy of Fallot may experience cyanotic or "blue" spells. Such spells result from increased right-to-left shunting, possibly caused by spasm of the right ventricular outflow tract, increased systemic venous return, or decreased systemic arterial resistance.

Exercise, crying, straining, infection, or fever can precipitate blue spells. They're characterized by dyspnea; deep, sighing respirations; bradycardia; fainting; seizures; and loss of consciousness. Older children may develop additional signs of poor oxygenation, such as clubbing, diminished exercise tolerance, increasing dyspnea on exertion, growth retardation, and eating difficulties. These children habitually squat when they feel short of breath; this is thought to decrease venous return of unoxygenated blood from the legs and increase systemic arterial resistance.

Auscultation reveals a loud systolic heart murmur (best heard along the left sternal border), which may diminish or obscure the pulmonic component of S_2. In a patient with a large patent ductus, the continuous murmur of the ductus obscures the systolic murmur. Palpation may reveal a cardiac thrill at the left sternal border and an obvious right ventricular impulse. The inferior sternum appears prominent.

Children with tetralogy of Fallot also risk developing cerebral abscesses, pulmonary thrombosis, venous thrombosis or cerebral embolism, and infective endocarditis.

In females with tetralogy of Fallot who live to childbearing age, incidence of spontaneous abortion,

DEFECTS IN TETRALOGY OF FALLOT

This four-part complex includes a ventricular septal defect, an overriding aorta, right ventricular outflow obstruction (pulmonic stenosis), and right ventricular hypertrophy. The severity of these defects influences hemodynamic changes. Milder defects may produce a left-to-right shunt. More severe defects produce a right-to-left shunt, through which unoxygenated blood enters the aorta directly.

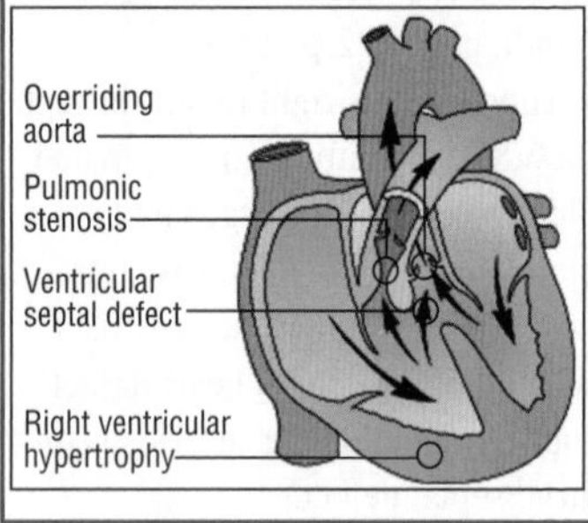

premature births, and low birth weight rises.

COMPLICATIONS

- Cerebral abscess
- Pulmonary thrombosis
- Venous thrombosis
- Cerebral embolism
- Infective endocarditis

DIAGNOSIS

- Chest X-ray may demonstrate decreased pulmonary vascular marking, depending on the pulmonary obstruction's severity, and a boot-shaped cardiac silhouette.
- Electrocardiography shows right ventricular hypertrophy, right axis deviation and, possibly, right atrial hypertrophy.
- Echocardiography identifies septal overriding of the aorta, the VSD, and pulmonary stenosis and detects the hypertrophied walls of the right ventricle.
- Laboratory findings reveal diminished arterial oxygen saturation and polycythemia (hematocrit may be more than 60%) if the cyanosis is severe and long-standing, predisposing the patient to thrombosis.
- Cardiac catheterization confirms the diagnosis by visualizing pulmonary stenosis, the VSD, and the overriding aorta and ruling out other cyanotic heart defects. This test also measures the degree of oxygen saturation in aortic blood.

TREATMENT

Effective management of tetralogy of Fallot requires prevention and treatment of complications, measures to relieve cyanosis, and palliative or corrective surgery. During cyanotic spells, the knee-chest position and administration of oxygen and morphine improve oxygenation.

Palliative surgery is performed on infants with potentially fatal hypoxic spells. The goal of surgery is to enhance blood flow to the lungs to reduce hypoxia; this is often accomplished by joining the subclavian artery to the pulmonary artery (Blalock-Taussig procedure). Management may also include phlebotomy in children with polycythemia.

Complete corrective surgery to relieve pulmonary stenosis and close the VSD, directing left ventricular outflow to the aorta, requires cardiopulmonary bypass with hypothermia to decrease oxygen utilization during surgery, especially in young children. An infant may have this corrective surgery without prior palliative surgery. It's usually done when progressive hypoxia and polycythemia impair the quality of his life, rather than at a specific age. However, most children require surgery before they reach school age.

Drugs

- Propranolol (Inderal)—a beta-adrenergic blocker—which may prevent blue spells
- Prophylactic antibiotics to prevent infective endocarditis or cerebral abscess administered before, during, and after bowel, bladder, or any other surgery or dental treatments

SPECIAL CONSIDERATIONS

- Explain tetralogy of Fallot to parents. Explain that their child will set his own exercise limits and will know when to rest. Make sure they understand that their child can engage in physical activity, and advise them not to be overprotective.
- Teach parents to recognize serious hypoxic spells, which can dramatically increase cyanosis; deep, sighing respirations; and loss of consciousness. Tell them to place their child in the knee-chest position and to report such spells immediately. Emergency treatment may be necessary.
- Instruct parents on ways to prevent overexerting their child, such as feeding him slowly and providing smaller and more frequent meals. Tell them that remaining calm may decrease his anxiety and that anticipating his needs may minimize crying. Urge parents to recruit other family members in the child's care to help prevent their own exhaustion.
- To prevent infective endocarditis and other infections, warn parents to keep their child away from people with infections. Urge them to maintain the child's dental hygiene, and tell them to watch for ear, nose, and throat infections and dental caries, all of which require immediate treatment. When dental care, infections, or surgery requires prophylactic antibiotics, tell the parents to make sure the child completes the prescribed regimen.
- If the child needs medical attention for an unrelated problem, advise parents to immediately inform the practitioner of the child's history of tetralogy of Fallot because any treatment must take this serious heart defect into consideration.
- During hospitalization, alert the staff to the child's condition. Because of the right-to-left shunt through the VSD, treat I.V. lines like arterial lines. A clot dislodged from a catheter tip in a vein can cross the VSD and cause cerebral embolism. The same thing can happen if air enters the venous lines.

After palliative surgery

- Monitor oxygenation and arterial blood gas (ABG) values closely in the intensive care unit.
- If the child has had the Blalock-Taussig procedure, don't use the arm on the operative side for checking blood pressure, inserting I.V. lines, or drawing blood samples because blood perfusion on this side diminishes greatly until collateral circulation develops. Note this on the child's chart and at his bedside.

After corrective surgery

- Watch for right bundle-branch block or more serious disturbances of atrioventricular conduction and for ventricular ectopic beats.
- Be alert for other postoperative complications, such as bleeding, right-sided heart failure, and respiratory failure. After surgery, transient heart failure is common and may require treatment with digoxin (Lanoxin) and diuretics.
- Monitor left atrial pressure directly. A pulmonary artery catheter may

also be used to check central venous and pulmonary artery pressures.

- Frequently check color and vital signs. Obtain ABG measurements regularly to assess oxygenation. Suction to prevent atelectasis and pneumonia, as needed. Monitor mechanical ventilation.
- Monitor and record intake and output accurately.
- If atrioventricular block develops with a low heart rate, a temporary external pacemaker may be necessary.
- If blood pressure or cardiac output is inadequate, catecholamines may be ordered by continuous I.V. infusion. To decrease left ventricular workload, give nitroprusside (Nitropress), if ordered, and provide analgesics as needed.
- Keep parents informed about their child's progress. After discharge, the child may need digoxin, diuretics, and other drugs. Stress the importance of complying with the prescribed regimen and make sure the parents know how and when to administer these medications. Teach parents to watch for signs and symptoms of digoxin toxicity (anorexia, nausea, vomiting). Prophylactic antibiotics to prevent infective endocarditis will still be needed. Advise parents to avoid becoming overprotective as the child's tolerance of physical activity rises.

Thoracic aortic aneurysm

Thoracic aortic aneurysm is an abnormal widening of the ascending, transverse, or descending part of the aorta. Aneurysm of the ascending aorta is the most common type and has the highest mortality. Aneurysms may be dissecting, saccular, or fusiform. (See *Types of aortic aneurysms,* page 196.) Some aneurysms progress to serious or, eventually, lethal complications, such as rupture of an untreated thoracic dissecting aneurysm into the pericardium with resulting tamponade.

CAUSES AND INCIDENCE

Thoracic aortic aneurysms commonly result from atherosclerosis, which weakens the aortic wall and gradually distends the lumen. An intimal tear in the ascending aorta initiates dissecting aneurysm in about 60% of affected patients. Regardless of the cause, these aneurysms affect 6 of every 100,000 people.

Ascending aortic aneurysms, the most common type, usually occur in hypertensive men younger than age 60. Descending aortic aneurysms, usually found just below the origin of the subclavian artery, are most common in elderly hypertensive men.

Descending aortic aneurysms are also seen in younger patients with a history of traumatic chest injury, less often in those with infection. Transverse aortic aneurysms are the least common type.

Other causes include:

- fungal infection (mycotic aneurysms) of the aortic arch and descending segments

TYPES OF AORTIC ANEURYSMS

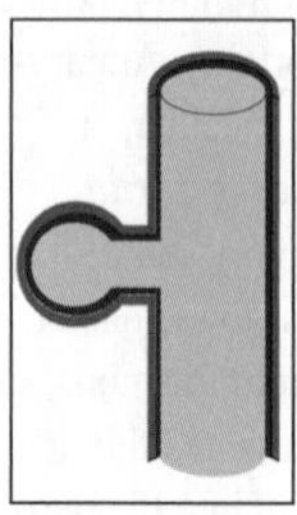

Saccular
A unilateral pouch-like bulge with a narrow neck

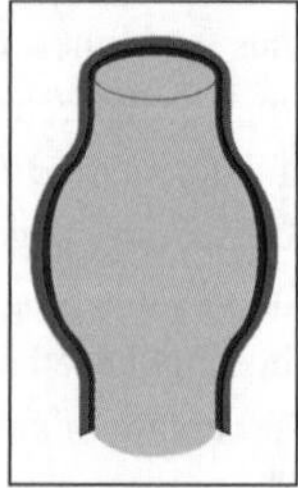

Fusiform
A spindle-shaped bulge encompassing the vessel's entire diameter

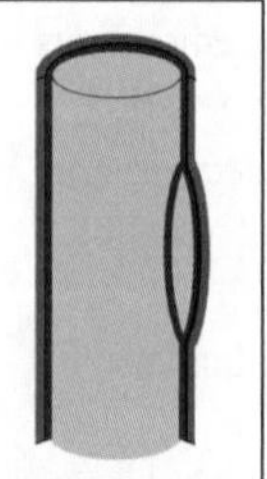

Dissecting
A hemorrhagic separation of the medial layer of the vessel wall, which creates a false lumen

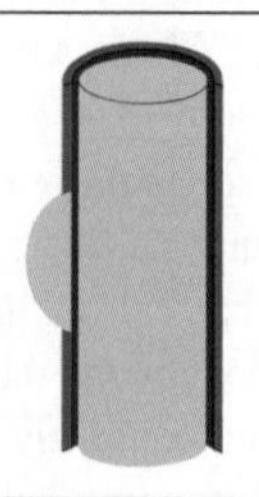

False aneurysm
A pulsating hematoma resulting from trauma and usually seen in the femoral artery after catheterization

- congenital disorders, such as coarctation of the aorta and Marfan syndrome
- trauma, usually of the descending thoracic aorta, from an accident that shears the aorta transversely (acceleration-deceleration injuries)
- syphilis, usually of the ascending aorta (uncommon because of antibiotics)
- hypertension (in dissecting aneurysm).

SIGNS AND SYMPTOMS

The most common symptom of thoracic aortic aneurysm is pain. With ascending aneurysm, the pain is described as severe, boring, and ripping and extends to the neck, shoulders, lower back, or abdomen but seldom radiates to the jaw and arms. Pain is more severe on the right side.

Other signs of ascending aneurysm may include bradycardia, aortic insufficiency, pericardial friction rub caused by a hemopericardium, unequal intensities of the right carotid and left radial pulses, and a difference in blood pressure between the right and left arms. These signs are absent in descending aneurysm. If dissection involves the carotids, an abrupt onset of neurologic deficits may occur.

With descending aneurysm, pain usually starts suddenly between the shoulder blades and may radiate to the chest; it's described as sharp and tearing. Transverse aneurysm

CLASSIFYING AORTIC DISSECTION

These drawings illustrate the DeBakey classification of aortic dissections (shaded areas) according to location. Dissections also can be classified by their location in relation to the aortic valve. Thus, types I and II are proximal and type III is distal.

Type I

In type I dissection, which is the most common and lethal type, intimal tearing occurs in the ascending aorta, and the dissection extends into the descending aorta.

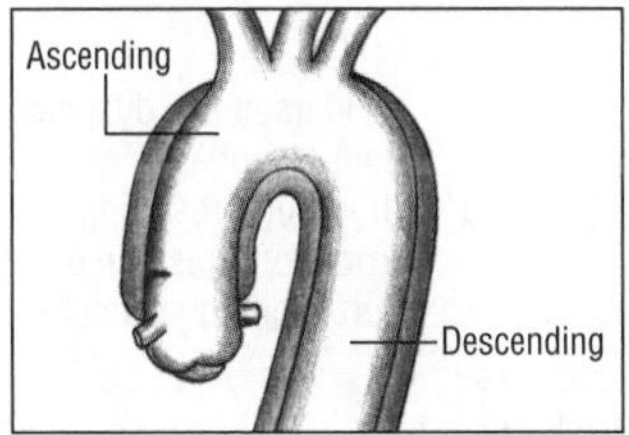

Type II

In type II, which appears most commonly in Marfan syndrome, dissection is limited to the ascending aorta.

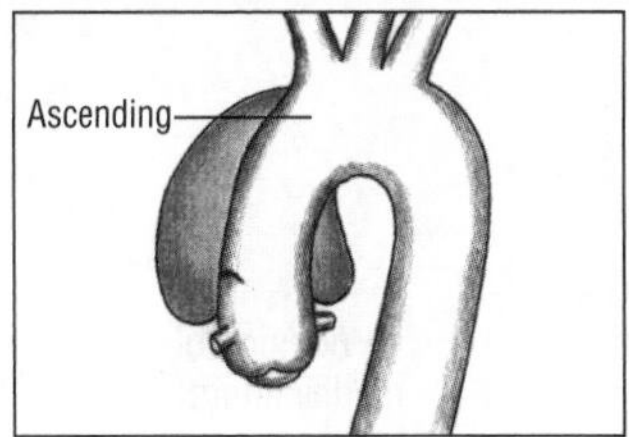

Type III

Type III dissection includes two formations. In type IIIa, the intimal tear is located in the descending aorta with distal propagation of the dissection that's confined to the thorax. Type IIIb has the same origin site but may extend beyond the diaphragm.

Type IIIa

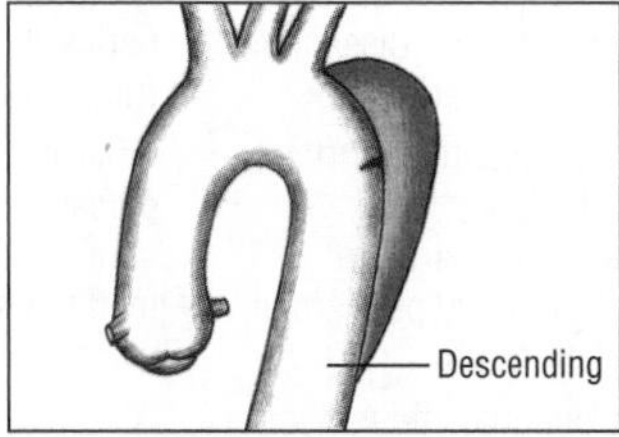

TYPE IIIb

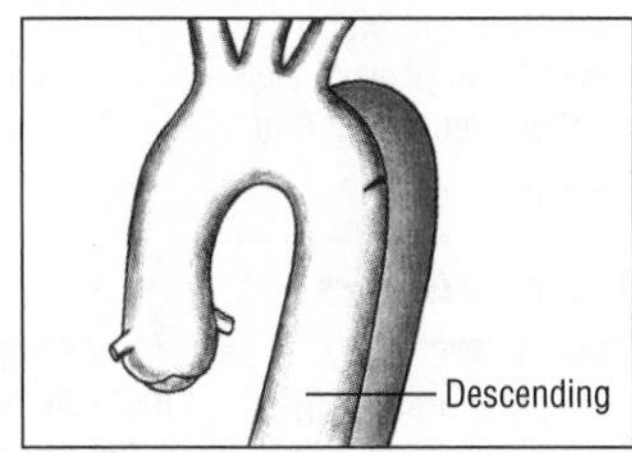

causes a sudden, sharp, tearing pain radiating to the shoulders. It also may cause hoarseness, dyspnea, dysphagia, and a dry cough because of compression of surrounding structures in this area. (See *Classifying aortic dissection* and *Clinical characteristics of thoracic dissection,* page 198.)

COMPLICATIONS

- Rupture and hemorrhage
- Cardiac tamponade
- Superior vena cava obstruction (ascending)

CLINICAL CHARACTERISTICS OF THORACIC DISSECTION

Ascending aorta	Descending aorta	Transverse aorta
Character of pain		
▪ Severe, boring, ripping ▪ Extending to neck, shoulders, lower back, or abdomen (rarely to jaw and arms) ▪ More severe on right side	▪ Sudden onset ▪ Sharp, tearing, usually between the shoulder blades ▪ May radiate to the chest ▪ Most diagnostic feature	▪ Sudden onset ▪ Sharp, boring, tearing ▪ Radiates to shoulders
Other symptoms and effects		
▪ Abrupt onset of neurologic deficits (usually intermittent) if dissection involves carotids ▪ Bradycardia, aortic insufficiency, and hemopericardium detected by pericardial friction rub ▪ Unequal intensity of right and left carotid pulses and radial pulses ▪ Difference in blood pressure, especially systolic, between right and left arms	▪ Aortic insufficiency without murmur, hemopericardium, or pleural friction rub ▪ Carotid and radial pulses and blood pressure in both arms that tend to stay equal	▪ Hoarseness, dyspnea, pain, dysphagia, and dry cough resulting from compression of surrounding structures
Diagnostic features		
Chest X-ray ▪ Best diagnostic tool ▪ Widening of mediastinum ▪ Enlargement of ascending aorta	▪ Widening of mediastinum ▪ Descending aorta larger than ascending	▪ Widening of mediastinum ▪ Descending aorta larger than ascending ▪ Widened transverse arch
Aortography ▪ False lumen ▪ Narrowing of lumen of aorta in ascending section	▪ False lumen ▪ Narrowing of lumen of aorta in descending section	▪ False lumen ▪ Narrowing of lumen of aorta in transverse arch

CLINICAL CHARACTERISTICS OF THORACIC DISSECTION *(continued)*

Ascending aorta	Descending aorta	Transverse aorta
Treatment		
▪ This is a medical emergency requiring immediate, aggressive treatment to reduce blood pressure (usually with nitroprusside [Nitropress] or trimethaphan). ▪ Surgical repair is also required.	▪ Surgical repair is required but is less urgent than for the ascending dissection. ▪ Nitroprusside and propranolol (Inderal) may be used to control hypertension if bradycardia and heart failure are absent.	▪ Immediate surgical repair (mortality as high as 50%) and control of hypertension are required.

- Aortic insufficiency (ascending)
- Laryngeal nerve damage (aortic arch)
- Tracheal or bronchial compression (descending)
- Spinal cord compression or thrombosis of spinal arteries (descending)

DIAGNOSIS

- Diagnosis relies on patient history, clinical features, and appropriate tests.
- In an asymptomatic patient, diagnosis often occurs accidentally when chest X-rays show widening of the aorta.
- Aortography, the most definitive test, shows the lumen of the aneurysm, its size and location, and the false lumen in dissecting aneurysm.
- Electrocardiograph (ECG) helps distinguish thoracic aneurysm from myocardial infarction.
- Echocardiography may help identify dissecting aneurysm of the aortic root.
- Hemoglobin levels may be normal or low, due to blood loss from a leaking aneurysm.
- Computed tomography scan can confirm and locate the aneurysm and may be used to monitor its progression.
- Magnetic resonance imaging may aid diagnosis.
- Transesophageal echocardiography is used to diagnose and size an aneurysm in either the ascending or the descending aorta.

TREATMENT

Dissecting aortic aneurysm is an emergency that requires prompt surgery and stabilizing measures, including antihypertensives such as nitroprusside (Nitropress); negative inotropic drugs that decrease contractility force, such as propranolol (Inderal); oxygen for respiratory distress; opioids for pain; I.V. fluids; and, possibly, whole blood transfusions.

Surgery involves resecting the aneurysm, restoring normal blood flow through a Dacron or Teflon graft replacement and, with aortic valve insufficiency, replacing the aortic valve. Groin catheter placement may be used for aortic stenting. This procedure, which may be used for aneurysms of the descending aorta, eliminates the need for a chest incision.

Postoperative measures include careful monitoring and continuous assessment in the intensive care unit, antibiotics, endotracheal (ET) and chest tubes, ECG monitoring, and pulmonary artery catheterization.

Long-term management includes treatment of underlying conditions, such as heart disease and diabetes.

Drugs

- Antihypertensives to control hypertension
- Negative inotropes to control cardiac output
- Opioids to treat pain

SPECIAL CONSIDERATIONS

- Monitor blood pressure, pulmonary artery wedge pressure (PAWP), and central venous pressure (CVP). Assess pain, breathing, and carotid, radial, and femoral pulses.
- Make sure laboratory tests include complete blood count, differential, electrolyte levels, type and crossmatching for whole blood, arterial blood gas studies, and urinalysis.
- Insert an indwelling urinary catheter. Administer dextrose 5% in water or lactated Ringer's solution and antibiotics, as ordered. Carefully monitor nitroprusside I.V.; use a separate I.V. line for infusion. Adjust the dose by slowly increasing the infusion rate. Meanwhile, check blood pressure every 5 minutes until it stabilizes. With suspected bleeding from aneurysm, give whole blood transfusion.
- Explain diagnostic tests. If surgery is scheduled, explain the procedure and expected postoperative care (I.V. lines, ET and drainage tubes, cardiac monitoring, and ventilation).

After repair of thoracic aneurysm

- Assess level of consciousness. Monitor vital signs; pulmonary artery pressure, PAWP, and CVP; pulse rate; urine output; and pain.
- Check respiratory function. Carefully observe and record type and amount of chest-tube drainage, and frequently assess heart and breath sounds.
- Assess for spinal cord ischemia. Manage and monitor cerebrospinal fluid pressure and drainage as indicated.
- Monitor I.V. therapy.
- Give medications as appropriate.
- Watch for signs of infection (especially fever) and excessive wound drainage.
- Assist with range-of-motion exercises for the legs to prevent thromboembolism from venostasis during prolonged bed rest.

• After stabilization of vital signs and respiration, encourage and assist the patient in turning, coughing, and deep breathing. If needed, provide intermittent positive-pressure breathing to promote lung expansion. Help the patient walk as soon as he's able.
• Before discharge, ensure compliance with antihypertensive therapy by explaining the need for such drugs and the expected adverse effects. Teach the patient how to monitor his blood pressure. Refer him to community agencies for continued support and assistance, as needed.
• Throughout hospitalization, offer the patient and his family psychological support. Answer all of their questions honestly and provide reassurance.

Thrombophlebitis

An acute condition characterized by inflammation and thrombus formation, thrombophlebitis may occur in deep (intermuscular or intramuscular) or superficial (subcutaneous) veins. Deep vein thrombosis (DVT) or thrombophlebitis affects small veins, such as the soleal venous sinuses, or large veins, such as the vena cava and the femoral, iliac, and subclavian veins, causing venous insufficiency. (See *Chronic venous insufficiency*.) This disorder typically is progressive, leading to pulmonary embolism, a potentially lethal complication. Superficial thrombophlebitis usually is self-limiting and seldom leads to pulmonary embolism. Thrombophlebitis often begins with localized inflammation

CHRONIC VENOUS INSUFFICIENCY

Chronic venous insufficiency occurs when valves are destroyed in deep vein thrombophlebitis, usually in the iliac and femoral veins, and occasionally the saphenous veins. Often, changes include incompetence of the communicating veins at the ankle, causing increased venous pressure and fluid migration into the interstitial tissue. Clinical effects include chronic edema and swelling of the affected leg, leading to tissue fibrosis and induration, skin discoloration from extravasation of blood in subcutaneous tissue, and stasis ulcers around the ankle.

Treatment of small ulcers includes bed rest, elevation of the legs, warm soaks, and antimicrobial therapy for infection. Treatment to counteract increased venous pressure (the result of reflux from the deep venous system to surface veins) may include compression dressings, such as a sponge rubber pressure dressing or a zinc gelatin boot (Unna's boot). This therapy begins after massive swelling subsides with leg elevation and bed rest.

Large stasis ulcers unresponsive to conservative treatment may require excision and skin grafting. Patient care includes daily inspection to assess healing. Other care measures are the same as for varicose veins.

alone (phlebitis), but such inflammation rapidly provokes thrombus formation. Rarely, venous thrombosis develops without associated inflammation of the vein (phlebothrombosis).

CAUSES AND INCIDENCE

A thrombus occurs when alteration in the epithelial lining causes platelet aggregation and consequent fibrin entrapment of red and white blood cells and additional platelets. Thrombus formation is more rapid in areas where blood flow is slower, due to greater contact between platelet and thrombin accumulation. The rapidly expanding thrombus initiates a chemical inflammatory process in the vessel epithelium, which leads to fibrosis. The enlarging clot may occlude the vessel lumen partially or totally, or it may detach and embolize to lodge elsewhere in the systemic circulation. (See *Patient-teaching aid: DVT*.)

DVT may be idiopathic, but it usually results from endothelial damage, accelerated blood clotting, and reduced blood flow known as *Virchow's triad*. Predisposing factors are prolonged bed rest, trauma, surgery, childbirth, and use of hormonal contraceptives such as estrogen. It occurs in about 80 of every 100,000 people; 1 of every 20 people is affected at some point during his lifetime. Men are at slightly greater risk than women. People older than age 40 are also at increased risk.

Causes of superficial thrombophlebitis include trauma, infection, I.V. drug abuse, and chemical irritation due to extensive use of the I.V. route for medications and diagnostic tests.

SIGNS AND SYMPTOMS

Some patients may have signs of inflammation and, possibly, a positive Homans' sign (pain on dorsiflexion of the foot) during physical examination; others are asymptomatic. Physical findings are usually nonspecific and not reliable for making a DVT diagnosis.

In both types of thrombophlebitis, clinical features vary with the site and length of the affected vein. Although DVT may produce no symptoms, it also may produce severe pain, fever, chills, malaise, and possible swelling and cyanosis of the affected arm or leg. Superficial thrombophlebitis produces visible and palpable signs, such as heat, pain, swelling, rubor, tenderness, and induration along the length of the affected vein. Varicose veins also may be present. Extensive vein involvement may cause lymphadenitis.

COMPLICATIONS

- Pulmonary embolism
- Chronic venous insufficiency

DIAGNOSIS

- Duplex Doppler ultrasonography and impedance plethysmography make it possible to noninvasively examine the major veins (but not calf veins).

PATIENT-TEACHING AID: DVT

Dear Patient:

Your physician has determined that you have deep vein thrombosis (DVT). This handout will help you understand how DVT can affect your body.

- DVT is a type of thrombophlebitis that affects the deep veins of the lower leg and thigh.
- Thrombophlebitis is an inflammation of a vein with thrombus (blood clot) formation. Thrombophlebitis can occur in any leg vein, but it usually occurs at valve sites.
- Inflammation of the vein causes a blood clot, or thrombus, to form. The clot is formed of elements in blood, such as platelets, red blood cells, white blood cells, and fibrin.
- The thrombus can rapidly expand as inflammation worsens and can block blood from flowing through the vessel, causing swelling and pain below it and reducing blood flow above it (see illustration 1 below).
- If a piece of clot breaks off, it's called an embolus (see illustration 2 below). An embolus can travel through the blood vessels and may lodge elsewhere, blocking blood flow to any tissue or organ supplied by that blood vessel. If the embolus travels to the lungs, it's called a pulmonary embolus, a life-threatening condition.

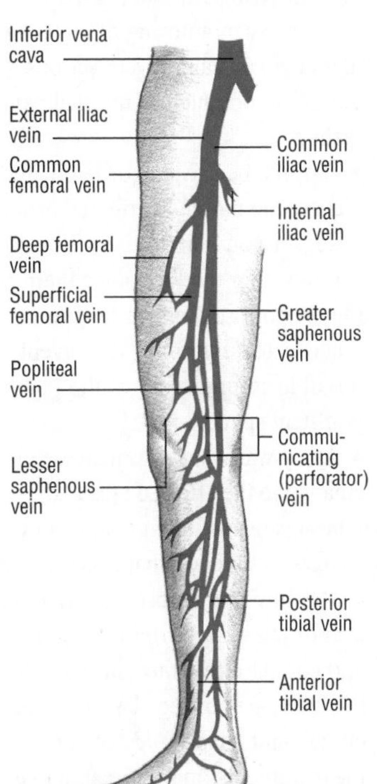

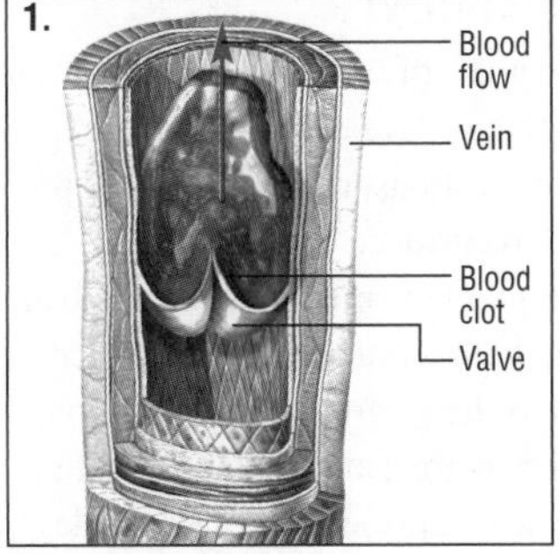

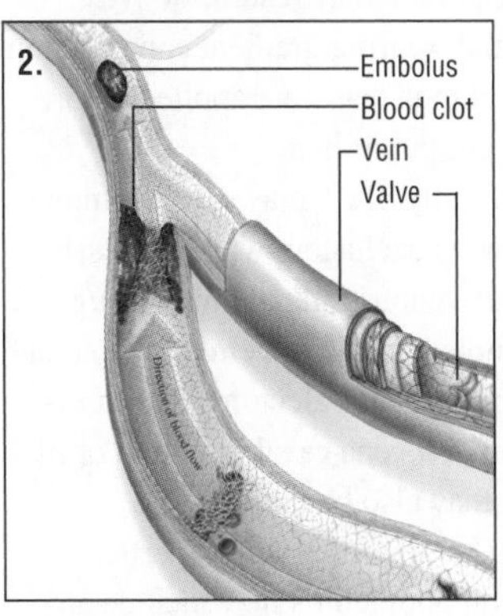

- Plethysmography shows decreased circulation distal to the affected area; this test is more sensitive than ultrasound in detecting DVT.
- Magnetic resonance venography, or phlebography, which shows filling defects and diverted blood flow, usually confirms the diagnosis.
- Diagnosis must also rule out peripheral artery disease, lymphangitis, cellulitis, and myositis.
- Diagnosis of superficial thrombophlebitis is based on physical examination (redness and warmth over the affected area, palpable vein, and pain during palpation or compression).

TREATMENT

The goals of treatment are to control thrombus development, prevent complications, relieve pain, and prevent recurrence of the disorder. Symptomatic measures include bed rest, with elevation of the affected arm or leg; warm, moist soaks to the affected area; and analgesics. After the acute episode of DVT subsides, the patient may resume activity while wearing gradient compression stockings that were applied before he got out of bed.

Rarely, DVT may cause complete venous occlusion, which necessitates venous interruption through simple ligation to vein plication, or clipping. Embolectomy and insertion of a vena caval umbrella or filter may also be done.

Therapy for severe superficial thrombophlebitis may include an anti-inflammatory drug, compression stockings, warm soaks, and elevation of the leg.

Drugs

- Anticoagulants (initially, heparin; later, warfarin [Coumadin]) to prolong clotting time
- Streptokinase (Streptase) for lysis of acute, extensive DVT
- An anti-inflammatory drug, such as indomethacin (Indocin), for severe superficial thrombophlebitis
- Analgesics to relieve pain

SPECIAL CONSIDERATIONS

- Patient teaching, identification of high-risk patients, and measures to prevent venostasis can prevent DVT; close monitoring of anticoagulant therapy can prevent serious complications such as internal hemorrhage.
- Enforce bed rest as ordered, and elevate the patient's affected arm or leg. If you plan to use pillows for elevating the leg, place them so they support the entire length of the affected extremity to prevent possible compression of the popliteal space.
- Apply warm soaks to increase circulation to the affected area and to relieve pain and inflammation. Give analgesics to relieve pain, as ordered.
- Measure and record the affected arm or leg's circumference daily and compare this measurement to the other arm or leg. To ensure accuracy and consistency of serial measurements, mark the skin over the area and measure at the same spot daily.

• Administer heparin I.V., as ordered, with an infusion monitor or pump to control the flow rate.
• Low-molecular-weight (LMW) heparin is effective in treating DVT. Although LMW heparin is more expensive, it requires no monitoring of anticoagulant effect. Full anticoagulant doses must be discontinued during any operative period because of the risk of hemorrhage. After some types of surgery, especially major abdominal or pelvic operations, prophylactic doses of anticoagulants may reduce the risk of DVT and pulmonary embolism.
• Measure partial thromboplastin time regularly for a patient on heparin therapy. Check prothrombin time and International Normalized Ratio (INR) for a patient on warfarin. (For prothrombin time, therapeutic anticoagulation values are 1½ to 2 times control values; for INR, therapeutic values are 2 to 3.) Watch for signs and symptoms of bleeding, such as dark, tarry stools; coffee-ground vomitus; and ecchymoses. Urge the patient to use an electric razor and to avoid products that contain aspirin.

Preparing for discharge

• Emphasize the need for follow-up blood studies to monitor anticoagulant therapy.
• If the patient is being discharged on heparin therapy, teach him or his family how to give subcutaneous injections. If he needs further assistance, arrange for a home health nurse.

PREVENTION

PREVENTING THROMBOPHLEBITIS

To prevent thrombophlebitis in a high-risk patient, do the following:
■ Perform range-of-motion exercises while the patient is on bed rest.
■ Use intermittent pneumatic calf massage during lengthy surgical or diagnostic procedures.
■ Apply gradient compression stockings postoperatively.
■ Encourage early ambulation.

After some types of surgery, especially major abdominal or pelvic operations, prophylactic anticoagulation may reduce the risk of deep vein thrombosis and pulmonary embolism.

• Tell the patient to avoid prolonged sitting or standing to help prevent recurrence.
• Teach the patient how to properly apply and use compression stockings. Tell him to report any complications such as cold, blue toes. (See *Preventing thrombophlebitis*.)

Transposition of the great arteries

In this congenital heart defect, the great arteries are reversed: the aorta arises from the right ventricle and the pulmonary artery from the left ventricle, producing two noncommunicating circulatory systems (pulmonary and systemic). (See *Understanding transposition of the great arteries*, page 206.)

UNDERSTANDING TRANSPOSITION OF THE GREAT ARTERIES

In this anomaly, the aorta arises from the right ventricle and the pulmonary artery from the left ventricle, preventing the pulmonary and systemic circulations from mixing. Without associated defects that allow these circulatory systems to mix—such as patent ductus arteriosus or a septal defect—the neonate will die.

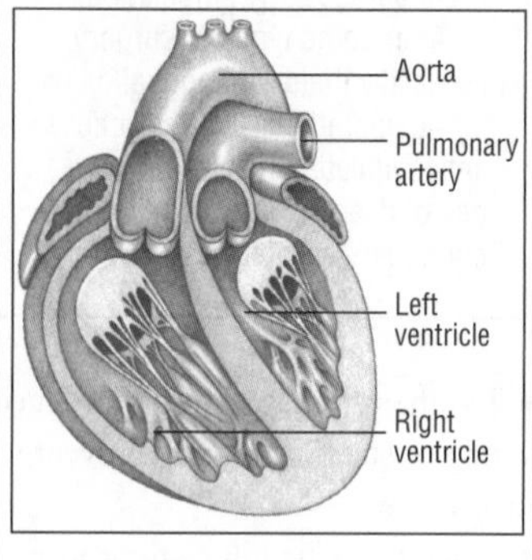

Transposition accounts for about 5% of all congenital heart defects and often coexists with other congenital heart defects, such as ventricular septal defect (VSD), VSD with pulmonary stenosis (PS), atrial septal defect (ASD), and patent ductus arteriosus (PDA). It affects two to three times more male than female infants.

CAUSES AND INCIDENCE

Transposition of the great arteries results from faulty embryonic development, but the cause of such development is unknown. In transposition, oxygenated blood returning to the left side of the heart is carried back to the lungs by a transposed pulmonary artery; unoxygenated blood returning to the right side of the heart is carried to the systemic circulation by a transposed aorta.

Communication between the pulmonary and systemic circulations is necessary for survival. In infants with isolated transposition, blood mixes only at the patent foramen ovale and at the PDA, resulting in slight mixing of unoxygenated systemic blood and oxygenated pulmonary blood. In infants with concurrent cardiac defects, greater mixing of blood occurs.

Transposition of the great arteries occurs in about 40 of every 100,000 infants.

SIGNS AND SYMPTOMS

Within the first few hours after birth, neonates with transposition of the great arteries and no other heart defects typically show cyanosis and tachypnea that worsen with crying. After several days or weeks, such neonates usually develop signs of heart failure (gallop rhythm, tachycardia, dyspnea, hepatomegaly, and cardiomegaly). S_2 is louder than normal because the anteriorly transposed aorta is directly behind the sternum. In many cases, however, no murmur can be heard during the first few days of life. Associated defects (ASD, VSD, or PDA) cause their typical murmurs and may minimize cyanosis but also may cause other complications (especially severe heart failure). VSD with PS produces a characteristic murmur and severe cyanosis.

As infants with this defect grow older, cyanosis is their most prominent abnormality. However, they also develop diminished exercise tolerance, fatigability, coughing, clubbing, and more pronounced murmurs if ASD, VSD, PDA, or PS is present.

COMPLICATIONS

- Chronic heart failure
- Infective endocarditis
- Poor oxygenation
- Arrhythmias
- Right-sided heart failure

DIAGNOSIS

- Chest X-rays are normal in the first days of life. Within days to weeks, right atrial and right ventricular enlargement characteristically cause the heart to appear oblong. X-rays also show increased pulmonary vascular markings, except when pulmonary stenosis coexists.
- Electrocardiography typically reveals right axis deviation and right ventricular hypertrophy but may be normal in a neonate.
- Echocardiography shows the reversed position of the aorta and pulmonary artery and records echoes from both semilunar valves simultaneously due to aortic valve displacement. It also detects other cardiac defects.
- Cardiac catheterization reveals decreased oxygen saturation in left ventricular blood and aortic blood; increased right atrial, right ventricular, and pulmonary artery oxygen saturation; and right ventricular systolic pressure equal to systemic pressure. Dye injection reveals the transposed vessels and the presence of any other cardiac defects.
- Arterial blood gas (ABG) measurements indicate hypoxia and secondary metabolic acidosis.

TREATMENT

An infant with transposition may undergo atrial balloon septostomy (Rashkind procedure) during cardiac catheterization. This procedure enlarges the patent foramen ovale, which improves oxygenation by allowing more mixing of the pulmonary and systemic circulations. Atrial balloon septostomy requires passage of a balloon-tipped catheter through the foramen ovale and subsequent inflation and withdrawal across the atrial septum. This procedure alleviates hypoxia to a certain degree. Afterward, digoxin (Lanoxin) and diuretics can lessen heart failure until the infant is ready to withstand corrective surgery (usually between birth and age 1).

One of three surgical procedures can correct transposition, depending on the defect's physiology. The Mustard procedure replaces the atrial septum with a Dacron or pericardial partition that allows systemic venous blood to be channeled to the pulmonary artery—which carries the blood to the lungs for oxygenation—and oxygenated blood returning to the heart to be channeled from the pulmonary veins into the aorta. (See *Mustard procedure*.)

The Senning procedure accomplishes the same result, using the atrial septum to create partitions to redirect blood flow. In the arterial switch, or Jatene procedure, transposed arteries are surgically anastomosed to the correct ventricle. For this procedure to be successful, the left ventricle must be used to pump at systemic pressure, as it does in neonates or in children with a left ventricular outflow obstruction or a large VSD. Surgery also corrects other heart defects.

Drugs

- Digoxin and diuretics to treat heart failure
- Prostaglandin infusion to keep the ductus arteriosus open until surgical correction

SPECIAL CONSIDERATIONS

- Explain cardiac catheterization and all needed procedures to the parents. Offer emotional support.
- Monitor vital signs, ABG values, urine output, and central venous pressure, watching for signs of heart failure. Give digoxin and I.V. fluids, being careful to avoid fluid overload.
- Teach the parents to recognize signs of heart failure and digoxin toxicity (poor feeding and vomiting). Stress the importance of regular checkups to monitor cardiovascular status.

MUSTARD PROCEDURE

In the Mustard procedure, a Dacron patch (1) is sutured in the excised atrial septum (2) to divert pulmonary venous return to the tricuspid valve and systemic venous return to the mitral valve (3).

1

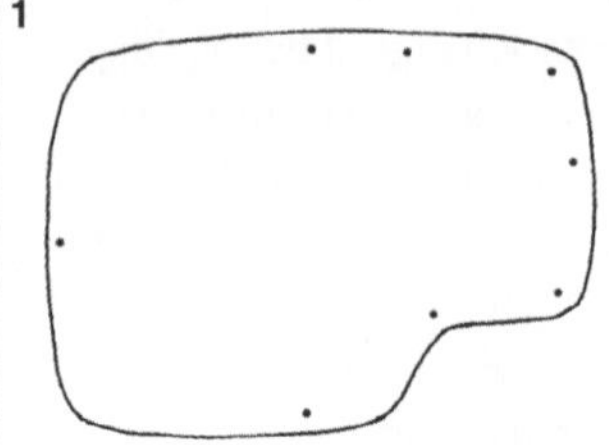

2

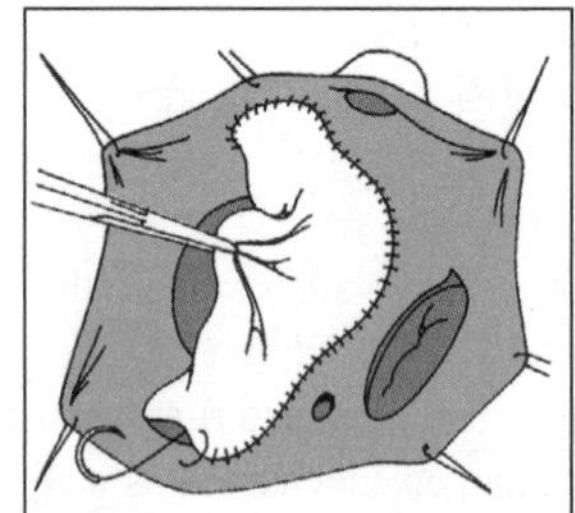

3

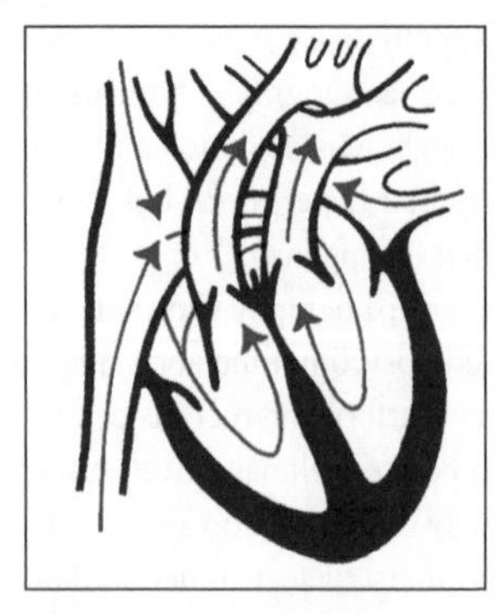

- Teach parents to protect their infant from infection and to give antibiotics.
- Tell parents to let their child develop normally. They need not restrict activities; he'll set his own limits.
- If the patient is scheduled for surgery, explain the procedure to parents and child, if old enough. Teach them about the intensive care unit and introduce them to the staff. Also explain postoperative care.
- Preoperatively, monitor ABG values, acid-base balance, intake and output, and vital signs.

After corrective surgery

- Monitor cardiac output by checking blood pressure, skin color, heart rate, urine output, central venous and left atrial pressures, and level of consciousness. Report abnormalities or changes.
- Carefully monitor ABG levels and report changes in trends.
- To detect supraventricular conduction blocks and arrhythmias, monitor the patient closely. Watch for signs of atrioventricular block, atrial arrhythmias, and faulty sinoatrial function.
- After Mustard or Senning procedures, watch for signs of baffle obstruction such as marked facial edema.
- Encourage parents to help their child assume new activity levels and independence. Teach them about postoperative antibiotic prophylaxis for endocarditis.

Tricuspid insufficiency

In patients with tricuspid insufficiency (also known as *tricuspid regurgitation*), an incompetent tricuspid valve allows blood to flow back into the right atrium from the right ventricle. (See *Types of valvular heart disease,* page 8.)

CAUSES AND INCIDENCE

Tricuspid insufficiency results from marked dilation of the right ventricle and tricuspid valve ring. It most commonly occurs in the late stages of heart failure because of rheumatic or congenital heart disease. Mitral stenosis, pulmonic valve stenosis, and pulmonary hypertension can elevate pressure in the right ventricle during contraction, which can lead to tricuspid insufficiency.

Less commonly, it results from congenitally deformed tricuspid valves, atrioventricular canal defects, or Ebstein's malformation of the tricuspid valve. Other causes include infarction of the right ventricular papillary muscles, tricuspid valve prolapse, carcinoid heart disease, endomyocardial fibrosis, infective endocarditis, and trauma.

In patients with tricuspid insufficiency, blood flows back into the right atrium during systole, decreasing blood flow to the lungs and left side of the heart. Cardiac output also decreases. Cardiac output also lessens. Fluid overload in the right side of the heart can eventually lead to right-sided heart failure.

SIGNS AND SYMPTOMS

The patient may complain of dyspnea, fatigue, weakness, syncope, and pain due to peripheral edema. Inspection may reveal jugular vein distention with prominent *v* waves in a patient with normal sinus rhythm. A patient with severe tricuspid insufficiency that has progressed to right-sided heart failure may appear jaundiced, with severe peripheral edema and ascites.

Auscultation may disclose a blowing holosystolic murmur at the lower left sternal border that increases with inspiration and decreases with expiration and Valsalva's maneuver. (See *Identifying the murmur of tricuspid insufficiency*.) Palpation may reveal hepatomegaly when the patient has right-sided heart failure, systolic pulsations of the liver, and a positive hepatojugular reflex. A prominent right ventricular pulsation along the left parasternal region may also be palpable.

IDENTIFYING THE MURMUR OF TRICUSPID INSUFFICIENCY

In a patient with tricuspid insufficiency, you'll hear a high-pitched, blowing holosystolic murmur in the tricuspid area, as depicted below.

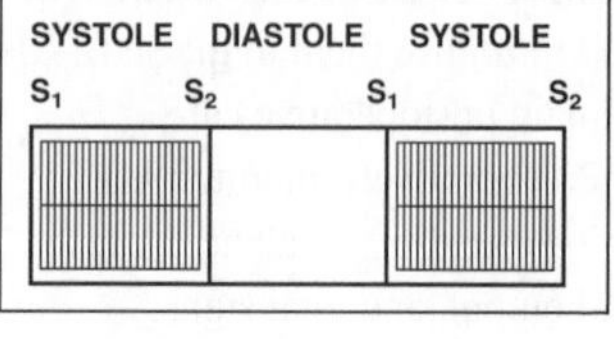

COMPLICATIONS

- Right-sided heart failure

DIAGNOSIS

- Cardiac catheterization shows markedly decreased cardiac output. The right atrial pressure pulse may show no x descent during early systole, but instead a prominent c-v wave with a rapid y descent. The mean right atrial and right ventricular end-diastolic pressures typically are elevated.
- Chest X-rays reveal right atrial and right ventricular enlargement.
- Echocardiography reveals the specific tricuspid valve leaflet structure and degree of prolapse or flail. It may also show other cardiac abnormalities such as right ventricular dilation.
- Electrocardiography discloses right atrial hypertrophy, right or left ventricular hypertrophy, atrial fibrillation, and incomplete right bundle-branch block.

TREATMENT

The cause of the tricuspid insufficiency determines the need for medical versus surgical treatment. For example, if the tricuspid insufficiency is caused by mitral stenosis, repair or replacement of the mitral valve may be indicated. A sodium-restricted diet and a diuretic help reduce hepatic congestion before surgery. When rheumatic fever has deformed the tricuspid valve, resulting in severe insufficiency, the patient usually needs open-heart surgery for tricuspid annuloplasty or tricuspid valve replacement.

Drugs

- Diuretics to treat heart failure and reduce hepatic congestion preoperatively

SPECIAL CONSIDERATIONS

- Alternate periods of activity with periods of rest to prevent extreme fatigue and dyspnea.
- Keep the patient's legs elevated while he's sitting to improve venous return to his heart.
- Elevate the head of the bed to improve ventilation.
- Maintain a low-sodium diet. Consult with a dietitian to make sure the patient receives foods that he likes while adhering to the diet restrictions.
- Monitor the patient for signs of heart failure, pulmonary edema, and adverse reactions to drug therapy.
- To reduce anxiety, allow the patient to express his concerns about the effects of activity restrictions on his responsibilities and routines. Reassure him that the restrictions are temporary.
- If the patient has surgery, watch for hypotension, arrhythmias, and thrombus formation. Monitor his vital signs, arterial blood gas levels, intake and output, daily weights, blood chemistry results, chest X-rays, and pulmonary artery catheter readings.
- Teach the patient about diet restrictions, medications, signs and symptoms that should be reported, and the importance of consistent follow-up care.
- Tell the patient to elevate his legs whenever he's sitting.

Tricuspid stenosis

Tricuspid stenosis is a relatively uncommon disorder in which blood flow from the right atrium to the right ventricle is obstructed. (See *Types of valvular heart disease,* page 8.)

CAUSES AND INCIDENCE

Although tricuspid stenosis usually is caused by rheumatic fever, it also may be congenital or a result of infective endocarditis. Rheumatic disease may produce both forms of tricuspid valve disease: insufficiency and stenosis.

Tricuspid stenosis seldom occurs alone and is usually associated with mitral stenosis. It's most common in women.

In patients with tricuspid stenosis, the right atrium dilates and becomes hypertrophied. Eventually, this leads to right-sided heart failure and increases pressure in the vena cava.

SIGNS AND SYMPTOMS

A patient with tricuspid stenosis may report dyspnea, fatigue, weakness, syncope, and discomfort associated with peripheral edema. Inspection may reveal jugular vein distention with giant *a* waves in a patient who has normal sinus rhythm. A patient with severe tricuspid stenosis that has progressed to right-sided heart failure may appear malnourished and jaundiced with severe peripheral edema and ascites.

Auscultation may reveal a diastolic murmur at the lower left sternal border and over the xiphoid process. It's most prominent during presystole in sinus rhythm. The murmur increases with inspiration and decreases with expiration and during Valsalva's maneuver. (See *Identifying the murmur of tricuspid stenosis.*) Palpation may reveal hepatomegaly in a patient with right-sided heart failure.

COMPLICATIONS

- Right-sided heart failure

DIAGNOSIS

- Cardiac catheterization shows an increased pressure gradient across the valve, increased right atrial pressure, and decreased cardiac output.
- Chest X-rays demonstrate right atrial and superior vena cava enlargement.
- Echocardiography reveals the specific tricuspid valve leaflet structure and degree of stenotic obstruction. It can also show the severity of right atrial enlargement.
- Electrocardiography reveals right atrial hypertrophy, right or left ventricular hypertrophy, and atrial fibrillation. Tall, peaked P waves appear in lead II and prominent, upright P waves appear in lead V_1.

IDENTIFYING THE MURMUR OF TRICUSPID STENOSIS

In tricuspid stenosis, you'll hear a low, rumbling, crescendo-decrescendo murmur in the tricuspid area, as depicted here.

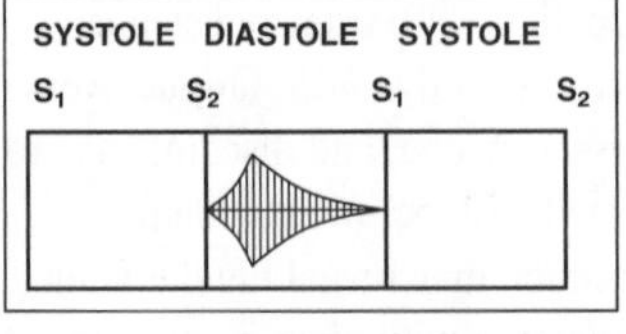

TREATMENT

Treatment for tricuspid stenosis is based on the patient's symptoms. A sodium-restricted diet and a diuretic can help to reduce hepatic congestion before surgery. A patient with moderate to severe stenosis probably requires open-heart surgery for valvulotomy or valve replacement. Valvuloplasty may be performed on elderly patients with end-stage disease in the cardiac catheterization laboratory.

Drugs

- Diuretic to treat heart failure and reduce hepatic congestion preoperatively

SPECIAL CONSIDERATIONS

- Alternate periods of activity and rest to prevent extreme fatigue and dyspnea.

- When the patient sits in a chair, elevate her legs to improve venous return to the heart.
- Elevate the head of the bed to improve ventilation.
- Keep the patient on a low-sodium diet. Consult with a dietitian to make sure the patient receives foods that she likes while adhering to the diet restrictions.
- Monitor the patient for signs of heart failure, pulmonary edema, and adverse reactions to the drug therapy.
- Allow the patient to express her fears and concerns about the disorder, its impact on her life, and upcoming surgery. Provide reassurance as needed.
- If the patient has surgery, watch for hypotension, arrhythmias, and thrombus formation. Monitor vital signs, arterial blood gas levels, intake and output, daily weight, blood chemistry results, chest X-rays, and pulmonary artery catheter readings.
- Teach the patient about diet restrictions, medications, signs and symptoms that should be reported, and the importance of consistent follow-up care.
- Urge the patient to elevate her legs whenever she sits.

V-Z

Varicose veins

Varicose veins are dilated, tortuous veins that are engorged with blood. They result from improper venous valve function, and they may be primary, originating in the superficial veins, or secondary, occurring in the deep veins. Without treatment, varicose veins continue to enlarge. Although there's no cure, certain measures, such as walking and using compression stockings, can reduce the symptoms. Surgery may remove varicose veins, but the condition can occur in other veins.

CAUSES AND INCIDENCE

Primary varicose veins can arise from conditions that produce prolonged venous stasis or increased intra-abdominal pressure, such as pregnancy, obesity, constipation, or wearing tight clothes. They also may occur because of a congenital weakness of the valves or venous wall. Occupations that require standing for an extended period are another influential factor.

Secondary varicose veins may be caused by arteriovenous fistulas, deep vein thrombosis, occlusion, trauma to the venous system, or venous malformation.

To understand the pathophysiology of varicose veins, remember that veins are thin-walled, distensible vessels with valves that keep blood flowing in one direction. Any condition that weakens, destroys, or distends these valves allows blood to flow backward to the previous valve. If a valve can't hold the pooling blood, it can become incompetent, allowing even more blood to flow backward. As the volume of venous blood builds, pressure in the vein increases and the vein becomes distended. As the veins stretch, their walls weaken and lose elasticity, becoming enlarged, lumpy, and tortuous. As hydrostatic pressure increases, plasma is forced out of the veins and into the surrounding tissues, resulting in edema. (See *Vascular changes in varicose veins*.)

People who stand for long periods may develop venous pooling because muscle contractions in the legs are inadequate to force blood back up to the heart. If valves in the veins are too weak to hold the pooling blood, they begin to leak, allowing blood to flow backward.

Primary varicose veins tend to be familial and to affect both legs; they're twice as common in women as in men. They account for about 90% of varicose veins; 10% to 20% of Americans have primary varicose veins. Usually, secondary varicose veins occur in one leg. Both types are more common in middle adulthood.

VASCULAR CHANGES IN VARICOSE VEINS

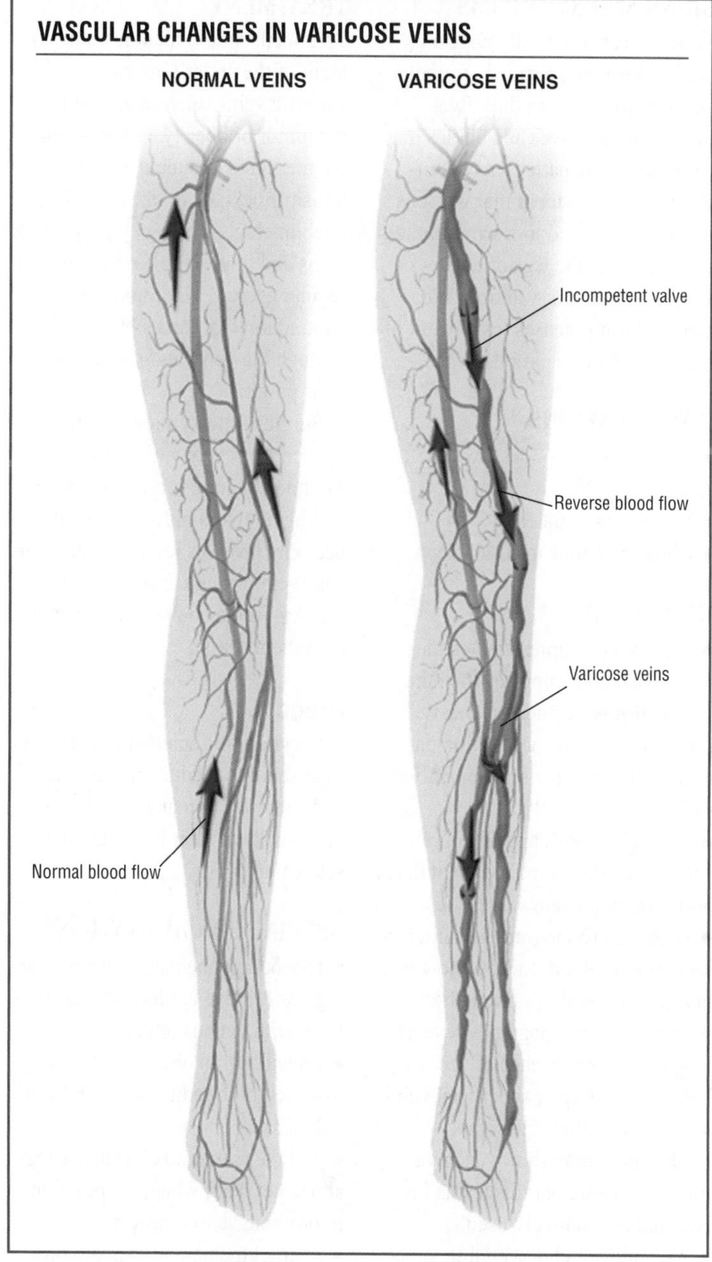

SIGNS AND SYMPTOMS

Varicose veins typically appear as dilated, tortuous, purplish, ropelike veins, particularly in the calves. Edema of the calves and ankles may be present. The patient may complain of leg heaviness that worsens in the evening and in warm weather, dull aching in the legs after prolonged standing or walking, and aching during menses (as a result of increased fluid retention).

COMPLICATIONS

- Blood clots secondary to venous stasis
- Venous stasis ulcers
- Chronic venous insufficiency

DIAGNOSIS

- A manual compression test detects a palpable impulse when the vein is firmly occluded at least 8″ (20 cm) above the point of palpation, indicating incompetent valves in the vein.
- Trendelenburg's test (retrograde filling test) shows incompetent deep and superficial vein valves.
- Photoplethysmography characterizes venous blood flow by showing changes in the skin's circulation.
- Doppler ultrasonography reveals the presence or absence of venous backflow in deep or superficial veins.
- Venous outflow and reflux plethysmography shows deep venous occlusion, but this test is invasive and not routinely used.
- Ascending and descending venography demonstrates venous occlusion and patterns of collateral flow.

TREATMENT

Treatment should include management of the underlying cause of varicose veins, such as an abdominal tumor or obesity. Other supportive measures include use of antiembolism stockings or elastic bandages to counteract swelling by supporting veins and improving circulation and regular exercise to promote muscle contraction that forces blood through the veins and reduces venous pooling.

Surgical intervention may be needed for severe varicose veins. Methods include surgical stripping and ligation and phlebectomy. Phlebectomy involves removing the varicose vein through small incisions in the skin; it may be performed in an outpatient setting.

Drugs

- Injection of a sclerosing agent to treat small to medium varicosities
- Analgesics to manage pain postoperatively or after injection of a sclerosing agent

SPECIAL CONSIDERATIONS

- Discourage the patient from wearing constrictive clothing that interferes with venous return.
- Encourage an obese patient to lose weight to reduce intra-abdominal pressure.
- Tell the patient to elevate her legs above her heart whenever possible to promote venous return.
- Instruct the patient to avoid prolonged standing or sitting because

these actions enhance venous pooling.

- After surgery, check circulation often in the toes (color and temperature) and observe elastic bandages for bleeding. As ordered, rewrap bandages at least once per shift, wrapping from toe to thigh with the leg elevated.

Vasculitis

Vasculitis includes a broad spectrum of disorders characterized by inflammation and necrosis of blood vessels. Its clinical effects, which reflect tissue ischemia caused by obstructed blood flow, and confirming laboratory procedures depend on the vessels involved. The prognosis is variable. For example, hypersensitivity vasculitis usually is a benign disorder limited to the skin; more extensive polyarteritis nodosa can be rapidly fatal.

Vasculitis may occur at any age, except for mucocutaneous lymph node syndrome, which occurs only during childhood. Vasculitis may be a primary disorder or occur secondary to other disorders, such as rheumatoid arthritis or systemic lupus erythematosus.

CAUSES AND INCIDENCE

How vascular damage develops in vasculitis isn't well understood. It has been linked to a history of serious infectious disease, such as hepatitis B or bacterial endocarditis, and high-dose antibiotic therapy. It may result from excessive circulating antigen that triggers formation of soluble antigen-antibody complexes. These complexes can't be cleared effectively by the reticuloendothelial system, so they're deposited in blood vessel walls (type III hypersensitivity). Increased vascular permeability from release of vasoactive amines by platelets and basophils enhances such deposition. The deposited complexes activate the complement cascade, resulting in chemotaxis of neutrophils, which release lysosomal enzymes. In turn, these enzymes cause vessel damage and necrosis, which may trigger thrombosis, occlusion, hemorrhage, and ischemia.

Another mechanism that may contribute to vascular damage is the cell-mediated (T-cell) immune response, in which circulating antigen triggers release of soluble mediators by sensitized lymphocytes, which attracts macrophages. The macrophages release intracellular enzymes, which cause vascular damage. They can also transform into the epithelioid and multinucleated giant cells that typify the granulomatous vasculitides. Phagocytosis of immune complexes by macrophages enhances granuloma formation.

SIGNS AND SYMPTOMS

The clinical effects of vasculitis vary according to the blood vessels involved. (See *Types of vasculitis*, page 218.)

(*Text continues on page 221.*)

TYPES OF VASCULITIS

Vasculitis occurs in various forms; diagnosis depends on the presenting signs and symptoms.

Type of vasculitis and vessels involved	Signs and symptoms	Diagnosis
Polyarteritis nodosa (Kussmaul disease, Kussmaul-Meier disease) Small to medium arteries throughout the body (Lesions tend to be segmental, occur at bifurcations and branchings of arteries, and spread distally to arterioles. In severe cases, lesions circumferentially involve adjacent veins.)	▪ Hypertension ▪ Abdominal pain ▪ Myalgias ▪ Headache ▪ Joint pain ▪ Weakness	▪ History of symptoms ▪ Elevated erythrocyte sedimentation rate (ESR) and blood urea nitrogen and creatinine levels ▪ Leukocytosis ▪ Anemia ▪ Thrombocytosis ▪ Depressed C3 complement ▪ Rheumatoid factor more than 1:60 ▪ Circulating immune complexes ▪ Tissue biopsy showing necrotizing vasculitis
Allergic angiitis and granulomatosis (Churg-Strauss syndrome) Small to medium arteries (including arterioles, capillaries, and venules), mainly of lungs and kidneys but also other organs	▪ Resembles polyarteritis nodosa with hallmark of severe pulmonary involvement	▪ History of asthma ▪ Eosinophilia ▪ Increased immunoglobulin (Ig) E level ▪ Tissue biopsy showing granulomatous inflammation with eosinophilic infiltration
Polyangiitis overlap syndrome (microscopic polyangiitis) Small to medium arteries (including arterioles, capillaries, and venules) of the lungs and other organs	▪ Combines symptoms of polyarteritis nodosa, allergic angiitis, and granulomatosis	▪ Possible history of allergy ▪ Eosinophilia ▪ Tissue biopsy showing granulomatous inflammation with eosinophilic infiltration

TYPES OF VASCULITIS *(continued)*

Type of vasculitis and vessels involved	Signs and symptoms	Diagnosis
Wegener's granulomatosis Medium to large; vessels of the respiratory tract and kidney; may also involve small arteries and veins	▪ Fever ▪ Pulmonary congestion ▪ Cough ▪ Malaise ▪ Anorexia ▪ Weight loss ▪ Mild to severe hematuria	▪ Tissue biopsy showing necrotizing vasculitis with granulomatous inflammation ▪ Leukocytosis ▪ Elevated ESR and IgA and IgG levels ▪ Low rheumatoid factor titer ▪ Circulating immune complexes ▪ Antineutrophil cytoplasmic antibody in more than 90% of patients
Temporal arteritis (Giant cell arteritis) Medium to large arteries, most commonly branches of the carotid artery	▪ Fever, myalgia, jaw claudication, visual changes, and headache (associated with polymyalgia rheumatica syndrome)	▪ Decreased hemoglobin (Hb) level ▪ Elevated ESR ▪ Tissue biopsy showing panarteritis with infiltration of mononuclear cells, giant cells within vessel wall, fragmentation of internal elastic lamina, and proliferation of intima
Takayasu's arteritis (aortic arch syndrome) Medium to large arteries, particularly the aortic arch, its branches and, possibly, the pulmonary artery	▪ Malaise ▪ Pallor ▪ Nausea ▪ Night sweats ▪ Arthralgias ▪ Anorexia ▪ Weight loss ▪ Pain or paresthesia distal to affected area ▪ Bruits ▪ Loss of distal pulses ▪ Syncope	▪ Decreased Hb level ▪ Leukocytosis ▪ Positive lupus erythematosus cell preparation and elevated ESR ▪ Arteriography showing calcification and obstruction of affected vessels

(continued)

TYPES OF VASCULITIS *(continued)*

Type of vasculitis and vessels involved	Signs and symptoms	Diagnosis
Takayasu's arteritis (aortic arch syndrome) *(continued)*	▪ If a carotid artery is involved, diplopia and transient blindness ▪ May progress to heart failure or stroke	▪ Tissue biopsy showing inflammation of adventitia and intima of vessels and thickening of vessel walls
Hypersensitivity vasculitis Small vessels, especially of the skin	▪ Palpable purpura ▪ Papules ▪ Nodules ▪ Vesicles ▪ Bullae, ulcers, or chronic or recurrent urticaria	▪ History of exposure to antigen, such as a microorganism or drug ▪ Tissue biopsy showing leukocytoclastic angiitis, usually in postcapillary venules, with infiltration of polymorphonuclear leukocytes, fibrinoid necrosis, and extravasation of erythrocytes
Mucocutaneous lymph node syndrome (Kawasaki disease) Small to medium vessels, primarily of the lymph nodes; may progress to involve coronary arteries	▪ Fever ▪ Nonsuppurative cervical adenitis ▪ Edema ▪ Congested conjunctivae ▪ Erythema of oral cavity, lips, and palms ▪ Desquamation of fingertips ▪ May progress to arthritis, myocarditis, pericarditis, myocardial infarction, and cardiomegaly	▪ History of symptoms ▪ Elevated ESR ▪ Tissue biopsy showing intimal proliferation and infiltration of vessel walls with mononuclear cells ▪ Echocardiography needed
Behçet's disease Small vessels, primarily of the mouth and genitalia, but also of the eyes, skin, joints, GI tract, and central nervous system	▪ Recurrent oral ulcers, eye lesions, genital lesions, and cutaneous lesions	▪ History of symptoms

TYPES OF VASCULITIS *(continued)*

Type of vasculitis and vessels involved	Signs and symptoms	Diagnosis
Henoch-Schönlein purpura Any blood vessel in the skin	■ Red to purple papule skin lesions ■ Pain ■ Infarction ■ Joint pain ■ Numbness ■ Weakness ■ Fever ■ Fatigue ■ Dysmenorrhea ■ Pyrosis ■ Dysphonia ■ Dysphagia	■ History of symptoms ■ Muscle biopsy ■ Chest X-ray ■ Sedimentation rate

COMPLICATIONS

- Renal failure
- Renal hypertension
- Glomerulitis
- Fibrous scarring of lung tissue
- Stroke
- GI bleeding
- Necrotizing vasculitis
- Spontaneous hemorrhage
- Intestinal obstruction
- Myocardial infarction
- Pericarditis
- Rupture or mesenteric aneurysms

DIAGNOSIS

Laboratory tests performed to confirm a diagnosis of vasculitis depend on the blood vessels involved.

TREATMENT

Treatment of vasculitis aims to minimize irreversible tissue damage from ischemia. In primary vasculitis, treatment may involve removal of an offending antigen or use of anti-inflammatory or immunosuppressant drugs. For example, antigenic drugs, food, and other environmental substances should be identified and eliminated, if possible.

In secondary vasculitis, treatment focuses on the underlying disorder.

Drugs

- In primary vasculitis, low-dose cyclophosphamide (2 mg/kg daily) with daily corticosteroids
- In rapidly fulminant vasculitis, increased cyclophosphamide dosage (4 mg/kg daily) for the first 2 to 3 days, followed by the regular dose
- Prednisone (1 mg/kg daily) in divided doses for 7 to 10 days, to a single morning dose by 2 to 3 weeks (when vasculitis appears to be in remission or when prescribed cytotoxic drugs take full effect), and then to an alternate-day schedule for 3 to 6 months before slow discontinuation

SPECIAL CONSIDERATIONS

- Assess patients with Wegener's granulomatosis for dry nasal mucosa. Instill nose drops to lubricate the mucosa and help diminish crusting, or irrigate the nasal passages with warm normal saline solution.
- Monitor vital signs. Use a Doppler ultrasonic flowmeter, if available, to auscultate blood pressure in patients with Takayasu's arteritis, whose peripheral pulses are generally difficult to palpate.
- Monitor intake and output. Check daily for edema. Keep the patient well hydrated (3 L daily) to reduce the risk of hemorrhagic cystitis from cyclophosphamide therapy.
- Provide emotional support to help the patient and his family cope with an altered body image—the result of the disorder or its therapy. (For example, Wegener's granulomatosis may be associated with saddle nose, steroids may cause weight gain, and cyclophosphamide may cause alopecia.)
- Teach the patient how to recognize drug adverse effects. Monitor the patient's white blood cell count during cyclophosphamide therapy to prevent severe leukopenia.

Ventricular aneurysm

A ventricular aneurysm is an outpouching, almost always of the left ventricle, that produces ventricular wall dysfunction in about 20% of patients after myocardial infarction (MI). It may develop within weeks after MI. Untreated ventricular aneurysm can lead to arrhythmias, systemic embolization, or heart failure, and it may cause sudden death. Resection improves the prognosis in patients with heart failure or refractory patients who have developed ventricular arrhythmias.

CAUSES AND INCIDENCE

When MI destroys a large muscular section of the left ventricle, necrosis reduces the ventricular wall to a thin sheath of fibrous tissue. Under intracardiac pressure, this thin layer stretches and forms a separate noncontractile sac (aneurysm). Abnormal muscular wall movement accompanies ventricular aneurysm and includes akinesia (lack of movement), dyskinesia (paradoxical movement), asynergia (decreased and inadequate movement), and asynchrony (uncoordinated movement).

During systolic ejection, the abnormal muscular wall movements associated with the aneurysm cause the remaining normally functioning myocardial fibers to increase the force of contraction in order to maintain stroke volume and cardiac output. At the same time, a portion of the stroke volume is lost to passive distention of the noncontractile sac. (See *Understanding ventricular aneurysm*.)

SIGNS AND SYMPTOMS

Ventricular aneurysm may cause arrhythmias—such as premature ventricular contractions or ventricular tachycardia—palpitations, signs of

UNDERSTANDING VENTRICULAR ANEURYSM

When myocardial infarction destroys a large, muscular section of the left ventricle, necrosis reduces the ventricular wall to a thin layer of fibrous tissue. The thin wall stretches under intracardiac pressure and forms a ventricular aneurysm. Ventricular aneurysms usually occur on the anterior or apical surface of the heart.

Ventricular aneurysms balloon outward with each systole (dyskinesia). Blood is diverted to the distended muscle wall of the aneurysm, which doesn't contract (akinesia). Mural thrombus is present about 50% of the time; thromboembolism rarely is. Calcification of the thrombus is common.

To maintain stroke volume and cardiac output, the remaining normally functioning myocardial fibers increase contractile force. If they can't, overall ventricular function is impaired and complications, such as heart failure and ventricular arrhythmias, may develop.

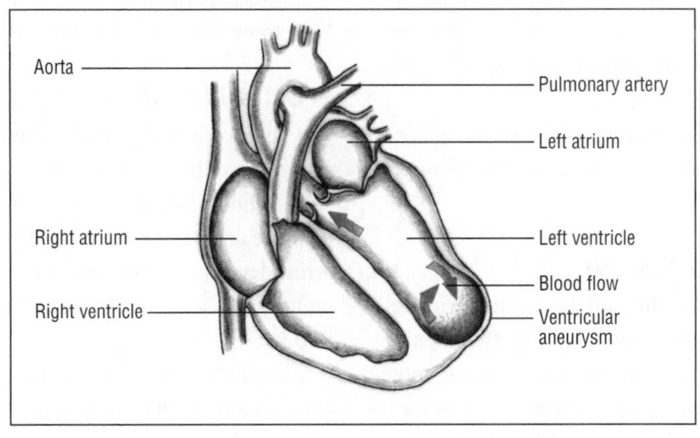

cardiac dysfunction (weakness on exertion, fatigue, and angina) and, occasionally, a visible or palpable systolic precordial bulge. This condition also may lead to left ventricular dysfunction with chronic heart failure (dyspnea, fatigue, edema, crackles, gallop rhythm, and jugular vein distention); pulmonary edema; systemic embolization; and, with left-sided heart failure, pulsus alternans. Ventricular aneurysms enlarge but seldom rupture.

COMPLICATIONS

- Ventricular arrhythmias
- Cerebral embolism
- Heart failure
- Death

DIAGNOSIS

- Persistent ventricular arrhythmias, onset of heart failure, or systemic embolization in a patient with left-sided heart failure and a history of MI strongly suggests ventricular aneurysm.

• Left ventriculography reveals left ventricular enlargement, with an area of akinesia or dyskinesia (during cineangiography) and diminished cardiac function.
• Electrocardiography may show persistent ST-T wave elevations after infarction.
• Chest X-ray may demonstrate an abnormal bulge distorting the heart's contour if the aneurysm is large; the X-ray may be normal if the aneurysm is small.
• Noninvasive nuclear cardiology scan may indicate the site of infarction and suggest the area of aneurysm.
• Echocardiography shows abnormal motion in the left ventricular wall.

TREATMENT

Depending on the aneurysm's size and the complications, treatment varies from routine follow-up monitoring to aggressive measures for intractable ventricular arrhythmias, heart failure, and emboli.

Refractory ventricular tachycardia, heart failure, recurrent arterial embolization, and persistent angina with coronary artery occlusion may necessitate surgery, of which the most effective procedure is aneurysmectomy with myocardial revascularization.

Drugs

• Antiarrhythmics I.V. or cardioversion for emergency treatment of ventricular arrhythmia
• Oral antiarrhythmics, such as procainamide, quinidine, or disopyramide (Norpace), for continued preventive treatment
• Oxygen, cardiac glycosides I.V., furosemide (Lasix) I.V., morphine I.V. and, possibly nitroprusside (Nitropress) I.V. and intubation as emergency treatment for heart failure with pulmonary edema
• Nitrates, prazosin (Minipress), and oral hydralazine (Apresazide) as maintenance treatment
• Anticoagulation therapy or embolectomy in systemic embolization

SPECIAL CONSIDERATIONS

• If ventricular tachycardia occurs, give a prescribed antiarrhythmic such as lidocaine. Monitor blood pressure and heart rate. If cardiac arrest develops, start cardiopulmonary resuscitation (CPR) and call a code.
• In a patient with heart failure, closely monitor vital signs, heart sounds, intake and output, fluid and electrolyte balance, and blood urea nitrogen and creatinine levels. Because of the threat of systemic embolization, check peripheral pulses and limb color and temperature often. Be alert for sudden changes in sensorium that indicate cerebral embolization and for any signs that suggest renal failure or progressive MI.
• If arrhythmias warrant cardioversion, use enough conducting jelly to prevent chest burns. If the patient is conscious, give diazepam (Valium) or methohexital (Brevital). I.V., as ordered, before cardioversion.

Explain that cardioversion is a lifesaving method using brief electroshock to the heart. If the patient is receiving antiarrhythmics, check appropriate laboratory tests. For instance, if the patient takes procainamide, check antinuclear antibodies because this drug may induce symptoms that mimic lupus erythematosus.

- If the patient will have a resection, explain expected postoperative care in the intensive care unit (including use of such things as endotracheal tube, ventilator, hemodynamic monitoring, chest tubes, and drainage bottle).
- After resection, monitor vital signs, intake and output, heart sounds, and pulmonary artery catheter. Watch for signs of infection, such as fever and drainage.

Preparing for discharge

- Teach him how to check for pulse irregularity and rate changes. Encourage him to follow his prescribed medication regimen—even during the night—and to watch for adverse effects.
- Because arrhythmias can cause sudden death, refer the family to a community-based CPR training program.
- Provide psychological support for the patient and his family.

Ventricular septal defect

In ventricular septal defect (VSD), the most common congenital heart disorder, an opening in the septum between the ventricles allows blood to shunt between the left and right ventricles. This disease accounts for up to 30% of all congenital heart defects. The prognosis is good for defects that close spontaneously or are correctable surgically but poor for untreated defects, which are sometimes fatal by age 1, usually from secondary complications.

CAUSES AND INCIDENCE

In neonates with VSD, the ventricular septum fails to close completely by the eighth week of gestation, as it would normally. VSD occurs in some neonates with fetal alcohol syndrome, but a causal relationship hasn't been established. Although most children with congenital heart defects are otherwise normal, in some, VSD coexists with additional birth defects, especially Down syndrome and other autosomal trisomies, renal anomalies, and such cardiac defects as patent ductus arteriosus and coarctation of the aorta.

VSDs are located in the membranous or muscular portion of the ventricular septum and vary in size. Some defects close spontaneously; in other defects, the entire septum is absent, creating a single ventricle. (See *Types of ventricular septal defects,* page 226.)

VSD isn't readily apparent at birth because right and left ventricular pressures are about equal, so blood doesn't shunt through the defect. As the pulmonary vasculature gradually relaxes, 4 to 8 weeks after birth, right ventricular pressure

TYPES OF VENTRICULAR SEPTAL DEFECTS

The names for ventricular septal defects correspond to their anatomic locations, as shown. Defects of different types may appear together or converge.

Subpulmonary defects

Subpulmonic defects are located in the right ventricular outflow. Viewed from the left ventricle, they appear just below the aortic valve.

Membranous or perimembranous defects

When viewed from either ventricle, membranous or perimembranous defects involve the subaortic region of the membranous septum. Some experts use the term *perimembranous* because this type of defect may not be confined to the membranous septum.

Atrioventricular canal defects

Atrioventricular canal defects appear in the inflow of the right ventricle.

Muscular defects

Defects in the lower trabecular septum are known as *muscular* defects and, more specifically, as *apical, midmuscular, anterior,* and *posterior defects.* A large apical muscular defect may look like a single hole when viewed from the left ventricle but have a "swiss cheese" appearance when viewed from the right ventricle. Right ventricular trabeculations cause this defect by partially covering the defect.

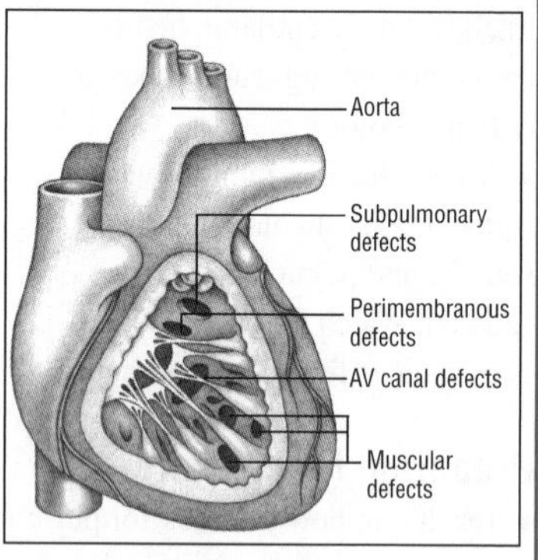

decreases, allowing blood to shunt from the left to the right ventricle.

Less than 1% of neonates are born with VSD. In 80% to 90% of neonates who are born with this disorder, the hole is small and will usually close spontaneously. In the remaining 10% to 20% of neonates, surgery is needed to close the hole.

SIGNS AND SYMPTOMS

Clinical features of VSD vary with the defect's size, the shunting's effect on the pulmonary vasculature, and the infant's age. In a small VSD, shunting is minimal, and pulmonary artery pressure and heart size remain normal. Such defects may eventually close spontaneously without ever causing symptoms.

Initially, large VSD shunts cause left atrial and left ventricular hypertrophy. Later, an uncorrected VSD will cause right ventricular hypertrophy due to increasing pulmonary vascular resistance. Eventually, biventricular heart failure and cyanosis (from reversal of shunt direction) occur. Resulting cardiac hypertrophy may make the anterior chest wall prominent. A large VSD increases the risk of pneumonia.

Infants with large VSDs are thin and small and gain weight slowly. They may develop heart failure with dusky skin; liver, heart, and spleen enlargement because of systemic venous congestion; diaphoresis; feeding difficulties; rapid, grunting respirations; and increased heart rate. They may also develop severe pulmonary hypertension. Fixed pulmonary hypertension may occur much later in life with right-to-left shunt (Eisenmenger's syndrome), causing cyanosis and clubbing of the nail beds.

The typical murmur of a VSD is blowing or rumbling and varies in frequency. In the neonate, a moderately loud early systolic murmur may be heard along the lower left sternal border. About the second or third day after birth, the murmur may become louder and longer. In infants, the murmur may be loudest near the heart's base and may suggest pulmonary stenosis. A small VSD may produce a functional murmur or a characteristic loud, harsh systolic murmur. Larger VSDs produce audible murmurs (at least a grade 3 pansystolic), loudest at the fourth intercostal space, usually with a thrill; however, a large VSD with minimal pressure gradient may have no audible murmur. In addition, the pulmonic component of S_2 sounds loud and is widely split. Palpation reveals displacement of the point of maximal impulse to the left. When fixed pulmonary hypertension is present, a diastolic murmur may be audible on auscultation, the systolic murmur becomes quieter, and S_2 is greatly accentuated.

COMPLICATIONS

- Right arterial and ventricular hypertrophy
- Heart failure
- Pulmonary hypertension

DIAGNOSIS

- Chest X-ray is normal in small defects; in large VSDs, it shows cardiomegaly, left atrial and left ventricular enlargement, and prominent pulmonary vascular markings.
- Electrocardiograph (ECG) is normal in children with small VSDs; in large VSDs, it shows left and right ventricular hypertrophy, suggesting pulmonary hypertension.
- Echocardiography may detect a large VSD and its location in the septum, estimate the size of a left-to-right shunt, suggest pulmonary hypertension, and identify associated lesions and complications.
- Cardiac catheterization determines the VSD's size and exact location, calculates the degree of shunting by comparing the blood oxygen saturation in each ventricle, determines the extent of pulmonary hypertension, and detects associated defects.

TREATMENT

In mild cases, no treatment is needed, although the infant should be closely followed to make sure the hole closes properly as he grows. Large defects usually require early surgical correction before heart failure and irreversible pulmonary vascular disease develop. For small defects, surgery consists of simple suture closure. Moderate to large defects require insertion of a patch graft using cardiopulmonary bypass. In patients who develop increased pulmonary resistance and irreversible pulmonary vascular changes that produce a reversible right-to-left shunt (Eisenmenger's syndrome), a heart-lung transplant may be required.

If the child has other defects and will benefit from delaying surgery, pulmonary artery banding normalizes pressures and flow distal to the band and prevents pulmonary vascular disease, allowing postponement of surgery. (Pulmonary artery banding is done only when the child has other complications.) A rare complication of VSD repair is complete heart block from interference with the bundle of His during surgery. (Heart block may require temporary or permanent pacemaker implantation.)

Before surgery, treatment consists of:

- digoxin (Lanoxin), sodium restriction, and diuretics to prevent heart failure
- careful monitoring by physical examination, X-ray, and ECG to detect increased pulmonary hypertension, which indicates a need for early surgery
- measures to prevent infection (prophylactic antibiotics, for example, to prevent infective endocarditis).

Typically, postoperative treatment includes a brief period of mechanical ventilation. The patient will need analgesics and may also require diuretics to increase urine output, continuous infusions of nitroprusside (Nitropress) or adrenergic agents to regulate blood pressure and cardiac output and, in rare cases, a temporary pacemaker.

Drugs

- Digoxin and diuretics to control symptoms in patients with heart failure
- Prophylactic antibiotics to prevent infective endocarditis
- Analgesics to treat postoperative pain
- Nitroprusside or adrenergic agents to regulate blood pressure and cardiac output postoperatively

SPECIAL CONSIDERATIONS

- Although the parents of an infant with VSD often suspect something is wrong with their child before diagnosis, they need psychological support to help them accept the reality of a serious cardiac disorder. Because surgery may take place months after diagnosis, parent teaching is vital to prevent complications until the child is scheduled for surgery or the defect closes. Thorough explanations of all tests are also essential.

- Instruct parents to watch for signs of heart failure, such as poor feeding, sweating, and heavy breathing.
- If the child is receiving digoxin or another medication, tell parents how to give it and how to recognize adverse effects. Caution them to keep medications out of the reach of all children.
- Teach parents to recognize and report early signs of infection and to avoid exposing the child to people with obvious infections.
- Encourage parents to let the child engage in normal activities.
- Tell parents to follow up with their pediatrician. Also tell them that child life therapy may be appropriate if their child has delayed growth and development or failure to thrive.
- Stress the importance of prophylactic antibiotics before and after surgery.

After surgery

- Monitor vital signs and intake and output. Maintain the infant's body temperature with an overbed warmer. Give catecholamines, nitroprusside, and diuretics, as ordered; analgesics as needed.
- Monitor central venous pressure, intra-arterial blood pressure, and left atrial or pulmonary artery pressure readings. Assess heart rate and rhythm for signs of conduction block.
- Check oxygenation, particularly in a child who needs mechanical ventilation. Suction to maintain a patent airway and to prevent atelectasis and pneumonia, as needed.
- Monitor pacemaker effectiveness if needed. Watch for signs of failure, such as bradycardia and hypotension.
- Reassure parents and allow them to participate in their child's care.

Part 2

Drugs

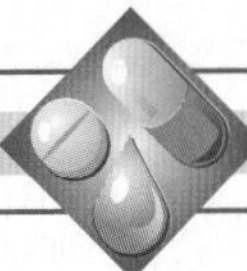

abciximab
ab-SIX-ah-mab

ReoPro

Pharmacologic class: antiplatelet aggregator
Pregnancy risk category C

AVAILABLE FORMS
Injection: 2 mg/ml

INDICATIONS & DOSAGES
➤ **Adjunct to percutaneous coronary intervention (PCI) to prevent acute cardiac ischemic complications**
Adults: 0.25 mg/kg as an I.V. bolus given 10 to 60 minutes before start of PCI; then, a continuous I.V. infusion of 0.125 mcg/kg/minute to maximum 10 mcg/minute for 12 hours.
➤ **Unstable angina not responding to conventional medical therapy in patients scheduled for PCI within 24 hours**
Adults: 0.25 mg/kg as an I.V. bolus; then an 18- to 24-hour infusion of 10 mcg/minute concluding 1 hour after PCI.

ADMINISTRATION
I.V.
- Give drug in a separate I.V. line. Don't add other drugs to infusion solution.
- Inspect solution for particulate matter before administration. If opaque particles are visible, discard solution and obtain new vial.
- For bolus, withdraw needed amount of drug through a low–protein-binding 0.2- or 5-micron syringe filter.
- Give bolus 10 to 60 minutes before procedure.
- For continuous infusion, filter drug either by withdrawing needed amount of drug through a low–protein-binding 0.2- or 5-micron syringe filter into a syringe or by infusing with a continuous infusion set equipped with a low–protein-binding 0.2- or 0.22-micron in-line filter. Use normal saline solution or D_5W.
- Infuse at 0.125 mcg/kg/minute (maximum, 10 mcg/minute) for 12 hours via a continuous infusion pump.
- Discard unused portion after 12-hour infusion.
- **Incompatibilities:** None reported.

ACTION
Binds to the glycoprotein IIb/IIIa (GPIIb/IIIa) receptor of human platelets and inhibits platelet aggregation.

Route	Onset	Peak	Duration
I.V.	Immediate	Immediate	48 hr

Half-life: 10 to 30 minutes.

ADVERSE REACTIONS
CNS: confusion, headache, hyperesthesia, hypoesthesia, pain.
CV: *hypotension, **bradycardia,*** peripheral edema.
EENT: abnormal vision.
GI: *nausea,* abdominal pain, vomiting.
Hematologic: ***bleeding, thrombocytopenia,*** anemia, leukocytosis.
Respiratory: pleural effusion, pleurisy, pneumonia.

INTERACTIONS
Drug-drug. *Antiplatelet drugs, dipyridamole, heparin, NSAIDs, other anticoagulants, thrombolytics, ticlopidine:* May increase risk of bleeding. Monitor patient closely.

EFFECTS ON LAB TEST RESULTS
- May decrease hemoglobin level.
- May increase WBC count. May decrease platelet count.

CONTRAINDICATIONS & CAUTIONS
• Contraindicated in patients hypersensitive to drug, its ingredients, or murine proteins.
• Contraindicated in those with active internal bleeding, significant GI or GU bleeding within 6 weeks, stroke within past 2 years, or significant residual neurologic deficit, bleeding diathesis, thrombocytopenia (platelet count lower than 100,000/mm^3), major surgery or trauma within 6 weeks, intracranial neoplasm, intracranial arteriovenous malformation, intracranial aneurysm, severe uncontrolled hypertension, or history of vasculitis.
• Contraindicated when oral anticoagulants have been given within past 7 days unless PT is 1.2 times control or less, or when I.V. dextran is used before or during PCI.
• Use with caution in patients at increased risk for bleeding, including those who weigh less than 75 kg (165 lb) or who are older than age 65, those who have a history of GI disease, and those who are receiving thrombolytics. Conditions that increase patient's risk of bleeding include PCI within 12 hours of onset of symptoms for acute MI, prolonged PCI (lasting longer than 70 minutes), or failed PCI. Heparin use may also increase the risk of bleeding.

NURSING CONSIDERATIONS
• The risk of bleeding is reduced by using low-dose, weight-adjusted heparin, early sheath removal, and careful maintenance of access site immobility.
• Drug is intended for use with aspirin and heparin; review and monitor other drugs patient is taking.
• ***Alert:*** Keep epinephrine, dopamine, theophylline, antihistamines, and corticosteroids readily available in case of anaphylaxis.
• Monitor patient closely for bleeding at the arterial access site used for cardiac catheterization and internal bleeding involving the GI or GU tract or retroperitoneal sites.
• Institute bleeding precautions. Keep patient on bed rest for 6 to 8 hours after sheath removal or end of drug infusion, whichever is later. Minimize arterial and venous punctures, I.M. injections, urinary catheters, nasogastric tubes, automatic blood pressure cuffs, and nasotracheal intubation; avoid, if possible.
• During infusion, remove sheath only after heparin has been stopped and its effects largely reversed.
• Before treatment, obtain platelet count, PT, ACT, and activated PTT.
• Monitor platelet count closely. Obtain levels 2 to 4 hours after bolus dose, and 24 hours after bolus dose or before discharge, whichever is first.
• Anticipate stopping drug and giving platelets for severe bleeding or thrombocytopenia.
• ***Look alike–sound alike:*** Don't confuse abciximab with infliximab.

PATIENT TEACHING
• Explain use and administration of drug to patient and family.
• Instruct patient to report adverse reactions immediately.

acetazolamide
ah-set-a-ZOLE-ah-mide

Acetazolam†, Diamox Sequels

acetazolamide sodium

Pharmacologic class: carbonic anhydrase inhibitor
Pregnancy risk category C

AVAILABLE FORMS
acetazolamide
Capsules (extended-release): 500 mg
Tablets: 125 mg, 250 mg
acetazolamide sodium
Powder for injection: 500-mg vial

INDICATIONS & DOSAGES
➤ **Secondary glaucoma; preoperative treatment of acute angle-closure glaucoma**
Adults: 250 mg P.O. every 4 hours or 250 mg P.O. b.i.d. for short-term therapy. In acute cases, 500 mg P.O.; then 125 to 250 mg P.O. every 4 hours. To rapidly lower intraocular pressure (IOP), initially, 500 mg I.V.; may repeat in 2 to 4 hours, if

needed, followed by 125 to 250 mg P.O. every 4 to 6 hours.
Children: 10 to 15 mg/kg P.O. daily in divided doses every 6 to 8 hours. For acute angle-closure glaucoma, 5 to 10 mg/kg I.V. every 6 hours.

➤ **Chronic open-angle glaucoma**
Adults: 250 mg to 1 g P.O. daily in divided doses q.i.d., or 500 mg extended-release P.O. b.i.d.

➤ **To prevent or treat acute mountain sickness (high-altitude sickness)**
Adults: 500 mg to 1 g (regular or extended-release) P.O. daily in divided doses every 12 hours. Start 24 to 48 hours before ascent and continue for 48 hours while at high altitude. When rapid ascent is required, start with 1,000 mg P.O. daily.

➤ **Adjunct for epilepsy and myoclonic, refractory, generalized tonic-clonic, absence, or mixed seizures**
Adults and children: 8 to 30 mg/kg P.O. daily in divided doses. For adults, 375 mg to 1 g daily is ideal. If given with other anticonvulsants, start at 250 mg P.O. once daily, and increase to 375 mg to 1 g daily.

➤ **Edema caused by heart failure; drug-induced edema**
Adults: 250 mg to 375 mg (5 mg/kg) P.O. daily in the morning. For best results, use every other day or 2 days on followed by 1 to 2 days off.
Children: 5 mg/kg or 150 mg/m^2 P.O. or I.V. daily in the morning.

ADMINISTRATION

P.O.

- Give drug with food to minimize GI upset.
- Don't crush or open extended-release capsules.
- If patient can't swallow oral form, pharmacist may make a suspension using crushed tablets in a highly flavored syrup, such as cherry, raspberry, or chocolate to mask the bitter flavor. Although concentrations up to 500 mg/5 ml are possible, concentrations of 250 mg/5 ml are more palatable.
- Refrigeration improves palatability but doesn't improve stability. Suspensions are stable for 1 week.

I.V.

- Reconstitute drug in 500-mg vial with at least 5 ml of sterile water for injection. Use within 12 hours of reconstitution.
- Inject 100 to 500 mg/minute into a large vein using a 21G or 23G needle.
- Direct I.V. injection is the preferred route.
- Intermittent and continuous infusions aren't recommended.
- **Incompatibilities:** Multivitamins.

ACTION

Promotes renal excretion of sodium, potassium, bicarbonate, and water. As anticonvulsant, drug normalizes neuronal discharge. In mountain sickness, drug stimulates ventilation and increases cerebral blood flow. In glaucoma, drug reduces IOP.

Route	Onset	Peak	Duration
P.O.	60–90 min	1–4 hr	8–12 hr
P.O. (extended-release)	2 hr	3–6 hr	18–24 hr
I.V.	2 min	15 min	4–5 hr

Half-life: 10 to 15 hours.

ADVERSE REACTIONS

CNS: ***seizures,*** drowsiness, paresthesia, confusion, depression, weakness, ataxia.
EENT: transient myopia, hearing dysfunction, tinnitus.
GI: nausea, vomiting, anorexia, metallic taste, diarrhea, black tarry stools, constipation.
GU: polyuria, hematuria, crystalluria, glycosuria, phosphaturia, renal calculus.
Hematologic: ***aplastic anemia, leukopenia, thrombocytopenia,*** hemolytic anemia.
Metabolic: hypokalemia, asymptomatic hyperuricemia, hyperchloremic acidosis.
Skin: *pain at injection site,* ***Stevens-Johnson syndrome,*** rash, urticaria.
Other: sterile abscesses.

INTERACTIONS

Drug-drug. *Amphetamines, anticholinergics, mecamylamine, procainamide, quinidine:* May decrease renal clearance of these drugs, increasing toxicity. Monitor patient for toxicity.

Cyclosporine: May increase cyclosporine level, causing nephrotoxicity and neurotoxicity. Monitor patient for toxicity.
Diflunisal: May increase acetazolamide adverse effects; may significantly decrease IOP. Use together cautiously.
Lithium: May increase lithium excretion, decreasing its effect. Monitor lithium level.
Methenamine: May reduce methenamine effect. Avoid using together.
Primidone: May decrease serum and urine primidone levels. Monitor patient closely.
Salicylates: May cause accumulation and toxicity of acetazolamide, including CNS depression and metabolic acidosis. Monitor patient for toxicity.
Drug-lifestyle. *Sun exposure:* May increase risk of photosensitivity reactions. Advise patient to avoid excessive sunlight exposure.

EFFECTS ON LAB TEST RESULTS

- May increase uric acid level. May decrease potassium and hemoglobin levels and hematocrit.
- May decrease WBC and platelet counts.
- May decrease iodine uptake by the thyroid in hyperthyroid and euthyroid patients. May cause false-positive urine protein test result.

CONTRAINDICATIONS & CAUTIONS

- Contraindicated in patients hypersensitive to drug and in those with hyponatremia or hypokalemia, renal or hepatic disease or dysfunction, renal calculi, adrenal gland failure, hyperchloremic acidosis, or severe pulmonary obstruction.
- Contraindicated in those receiving long-term treatment for chronic noncongestive angle-closure glaucoma.
- Use cautiously in patients receiving other diuretics and in those with respiratory acidosis or COPD.

NURSING CONSIDERATIONS

- Cross-sensitivity between antibacterial sulfonamides and sulfonamide-derivative diuretics such as acetazolamide has been reported.
- Monitor fluid intake and output, glucose, and electrolytes, especially potassium, bicarbonate, and chloride. When drug is used in diuretic therapy, consult prescriber and dietitian about providing a high-potassium diet.
- Monitor elderly patients closely because they are especially susceptible to excessive diuresis.
- Weigh patient daily. Rapid or excessive fluid loss may cause weight loss and hypotension.
- Diuretic effect decreases when acidosis occurs but can be reestablished by using intermittent administration schedules.
- Monitor patient for signs of hemolytic anemia (pallor, weakness, and palpitations).
- Drug may increase glucose level and cause glycosuria.
- ***Look alike–sound alike:*** Don't confuse acetazolamide with acetaminophen or acyclovir.

PATIENT TEACHING

- Tell patient to take oral form with food to minimize GI upset.
- Tell patient not to crush, chew, or open capsules.
- Caution patient not to perform hazardous activities if adverse CNS reactions occur.
- Instruct patient to avoid prolonged exposure to sunlight because drug may cause phototoxicity.
- Instruct patient to notify prescriber of any unusual bleeding, bruising, tingling, or tremors.

adenosine

a-DEN-oh-seen

Adenocard

Pharmacologic class: nucleoside
Pregnancy risk category C

AVAILABLE FORMS

Injection: 3 mg/ml in 2-ml, 4-ml, and 5-ml vials and syringes

INDICATIONS & DOSAGES

➤ **To convert paroxysmal supraventricular tachycardia (PSVT) to sinus rhythm**
Adults and children who weigh 50 kg (110 lb) or more: 6 mg I.V. by rapid bolus injection over 1 to 2 seconds. If PSVT isn't

eliminated in 1 to 2 minutes, give 12 mg by rapid I.V. push and repeat, if needed.
Children who weigh less than 50 kg: Initially, 0.05 to 0.1 mg/kg I.V. by rapid bolus injection followed by a saline flush. If PSVT isn't eliminated in 1 to 2 minutes, give additional bolus injections, increasing the amount given by 0.05- to 0.1-mg/kg increments, followed by a saline flush. Continue, as needed, until conversion or a maximum single dose of 0.3 mg/kg is given.

ADMINISTRATION

I.V.

- Don't give single doses exceeding 12 mg.
- In adults, avoid giving drug through a central line because more prolonged asystole may occur.
- Give by rapid I.V. injection to ensure drug action.
- Give directly into a vein, if possible. When giving through an I.V. line, use the port closest to the patient.
- Flush immediately and rapidly with normal saline solution to ensure that drug quickly reaches the systemic circulation.
- **Incompatibilities:** Other I.V. drugs.

ACTION

Naturally occurring nucleoside that acts on the AV node to slow conduction and inhibit reentry pathways. Drug is also useful in treating PSVTs, including those with accessory bypass tracts (Wolff-Parkinson-White syndrome).

Route	Onset	Peak	Duration
I.V.	Immediate	Immediate	Unknown

Half-life: Less than 10 seconds.

ADVERSE REACTIONS

CNS: dizziness, light-headedness, numbness, tingling in arms, headache.
CV: chest pressure, *facial flushing.*
GI: nausea.
Respiratory: *dyspnea, shortness of breath.*

INTERACTIONS

Drug-drug. *Carbamazepine:* May cause high-level heart block. Use together cautiously.
Digoxin, verapamil: May cause ventricular fibrillation. Monitor ECG closely.
Dipyridamole: May increase adenosine's effects. Adenosine dose may need to be reduced. Use together cautiously.
Methylxanthines (caffeine, theophylline): May decrease adenosine's effects. Adenosine dose may need to be increased or patients may not respond to adenosine therapy.
Drug-herb. *Guarana:* May decrease patient's response to drug. Monitor patient.

EFFECTS ON LAB TEST RESULTS

None reported.

CONTRAINDICATIONS & CAUTIONS

- Contraindicated in patients hypersensitive to drug.
- Contraindicated in those with second- or third-degree heart block or sinus node disease (such as sick sinus syndrome and symptomatic bradycardia), except those with a pacemaker.
- Use cautiously in patients with asthma, emphysema, or bronchitis because bronchoconstriction may occur.

NURSING CONSIDERATIONS

- ***Alert:*** By decreasing conduction through the AV node, drug may produce first-, second-, or third-degree heart block. Patients who develop high-level heart block after a single dose shouldn't receive additional doses.
- ***Alert:*** New arrhythmias, including heart block and transient asystole, may develop; monitor cardiac rhythm and treat as indicated.
- If solution is cold, crystals may form; gently warm solution to room temperature. Don't use solutions that aren't clear.
- Drug lacks preservatives. Discard unused portion.
- ***Alert:*** Don't confuse adenosine with adenosine phosphate.

PATIENT TEACHING

- Instruct patient to report adverse reactions promptly.

• Tell patient to report discomfort at I.V. site.
• Inform patient that he may experience flushing or chest pain lasting 1 to 2 minutes.

✳ NEW DRUG

aliskiren
a-LIS-ke-ren

Tecturna

Pharmacologic class: renin inhibitor
Pregnancy risk category C for 1st trimester; D for 2nd and 3rd trimesters

AVAILABLE FORMS
Tablets: 150 mg, 300 mg

INDICATIONS & DOSAGES
➤ **Hypertension, alone or with other antihypertensives**
Adults: 150 mg P.O. daily; may increase to 300 mg P.O. daily.

ADMINISTRATION
P.O.
• Don't give drug with high-fat meal because this may decrease the drug's effectiveness.

ACTION
Inhibits conversion of angiotensin I to angiotensin II, decreasing vasoconstriction and lowering blood pressure.

Route	Onset	Peak	Duration
P.O.	Unknown	1–3 hr	Unknown

Half-life: Unknown.

ADVERSE REACTIONS
CNS: *headache,* dizziness, fatigue, ***seizures.***
CV: *hypotension.*
EENT: nasopharyngitis.
GI: abdominal pain, diarrhea, dyspepsia, gastroesophageal reflux.
Metabolic: hyperuricemia, ***hyperkalemia.***
Musculoskeletal: back pain.
Respiratory: cough, upper respiratory tract infection.
Skin: rash.
Other: ***angioedema.***

INTERACTIONS
Drug-drug. *Atorvastatin:* May increase aliskiren levels. Use cautiously together.
Ketoconazole: May significantly increase aliskiren levels. Use cautiously together.
Irbesartan: May decrease aliskiren levels. Monitor patient for effectiveness.
Furosemide: May reduce furosemide peak levels. Monitor patient for effectiveness.
Drug-food. *High fat meals:* May substantially decrease plasma levels of drug. Monitor patient for effectiveness.

EFFECTS ON LAB TEST RESULTS
• May increase potassium, creatine kinase, BUN, and serum creatinine levels.

CONTRAINDICATIONS & CAUTIONS
• Contraindicated in patients hypersensitive to drug or its components.
• ***Alert:*** Contraindicated in pregnant women. Because of risk of fetal toxicity, stop drug as soon as possible if patient becomes pregnant.
• Contraindicated in breast-feeding patients.
• Use cautiously in patients with history of angioedema, severe renal dysfunction (creatinine of 1.7 mg/dl in women and 2 mg/dl in men, or GFR $<$ 30 ml/minute), history of dialysis, nephrotic syndrome, or renovascular hypertension.

NURSING CONSIDERATIONS
• Monitor blood pressure for hypotension, especially if used in combination with other antihypertensives.
• Monitor potassium levels, especially in patients also taking ACE inhibitors.
• ***Alert:*** Rarely, angioedema occurs. Supportive measures may include antihistamines, steroids, and epinephrine.
• Monitor renal function. It's unknown how patients with significant renal disorders will respond to the use of this drug.
• Effect of any dose is usually seen within 2 weeks.

PATIENT TEACHING
• Instruct patient not to take drug with a high fat meal because this may decrease the drug's effectiveness.

• Instruct patient to monitor blood pressure daily, if possible, and to report low readings, dizziness, and headaches to prescriber.
• Tell patient to immediately report swelling of the face or neck or difficulty breathing.
• Advise patient of need for regular laboratory tests to monitor for adverse effects.

SAFETY ALERT!

alprostadil

al-PROSS-ta-dil

Prostin VR Pediatric

Pharmacologic class: prostaglandin
Pregnancy risk category NR

AVAILABLE FORMS

Injection: 500 mcg/ml

INDICATIONS & DOSAGES

➤ **Palliative therapy for temporary maintenance of patency of ductus arteriosus until surgery can be performed**
Neonates: 0.05 to 0.1 mcg/kg/minute by I.V. infusion. When therapeutic response is achieved, reduce infusion rate to lowest dose that will maintain response. Maximum dose is 0.4 mcg/kg/minute. Or, give drug through umbilical artery catheter placed at ductal opening.

ADMINISTRATION

I.V.
• Dilute drug before giving. Prepare fresh solution daily; discard solution after 24 hours.
• For infusion, dilute 1 ml of concentrate labeled as containing 500 mcg in normal saline solution or D_5W injection to yield a solution containing 2 to 20 mcg/ml.
• When using a device with a volumetric infusion chamber, add appropriate volume of diluent to the chamber; then add 1 ml of alprostadil concentrate.
• During dilution, avoid direct contact between concentrate and wall of plastic volumetric infusion chamber because solution may become hazy. If this occurs, discard solution.
• Don't use diluents that contain benzyl alcohol. Fatal toxic syndrome may occur.
• Drug isn't recommended for direct injection or intermittent infusion. Give by continuous infusion using an infusion pump. Infuse through a large peripheral or central vein or through an umbilical artery catheter placed at the level of the ductus arteriosus. If flushing from peripheral vasodilation occurs, reposition catheter.
• Reduce infusion rate if patient develops fever or significant hypotension.
• **Incompatibilities:** None reported.

ACTION

Relaxes smooth muscle of ductus arteriosus.

Route	Onset	Peak	Duration
I.V.	20 min	1–2 hr	Length of infusion

Half-life: About 5 to 10 minutes.

ADVERSE REACTIONS

CNS: *fever, **seizures.***
CV: *flushing, **bradycardia, cardiac arrest,*** edema, hypotension, tachycardia.
GI: diarrhea.
Hematologic: ***DIC.***
Metabolic: hypokalemia.
Respiratory: **APNEA.**
Other: ***sepsis.***

INTERACTIONS

None significant.

EFFECTS ON LAB TEST RESULTS

• May decrease potassium level.

CONTRAINDICATIONS & CAUTIONS

• Contraindicated in neonates before making differential diagnosis between respiratory distress syndrome and cyanotic heart disease and in those with respiratory distress syndrome.
• Use cautiously in neonates with bleeding tendencies because drug inhibits platelet aggregation.

NURSING CONSIDERATIONS

• Keep respiratory support available.
• In infants with restricted pulmonary blood flow, measure drug's effectiveness by monitoring blood oxygenation. In

infants with restricted systemic blood flow, measure drug's effectiveness by monitoring systemic blood pressure and blood pH.
• Monitor arterial pressure by umbilical artery catheter, auscultation, or Doppler transducer. If arterial pressure falls significantly, slow infusion rate.
• Carefully monitor neonates receiving drug at recommended doses for longer than 120 hours for gastric outlet obstruction and antral hyperplasia.
• ***Alert:*** Apnea is most often seen in neonates weighing less than 2 kg (4.5 lb) at birth and usually appears during the 1st hour of drug infusion. CV and CNS adverse reactions occur more often in infants weighing less than 2 kg and in those receiving infusions for longer than 48 hours.
• ***Alert:*** Apnea and bradycardia may reflect drug overdose; if either occurs, stop infusion immediately.
• ***Look alike–sound alike:*** Don't confuse alprostadil with alprazolam.

PATIENT TEACHING

• Tell parents why this drug is needed, and explain its use.
• Encourage parents to ask questions and express concerns.

SAFETY ALERT!

alteplase (tissue plasminogen activator, recombinant; t-PA)

al-ti-PLAZE

Activase, Cathflo Activase

Pharmacologic class: enzyme
Pregnancy risk category C

AVAILABLE FORMS

Cathflo Activase injection: 2-mg single-patient vials
Injection: 50-mg (29 million international units), 100-mg (58 million international units) vials

INDICATIONS & DOSAGES

➤ Lysis of thrombi obstructing coronary arteries in acute MI

3-hour infusion
Adults who weigh 65 kg (143 lb) or more: 100 mg by I.V. infusion over 3 hours, as follows: 60 mg in first hour, 6 to 10 mg of which is given as a bolus over first 1 to 2 minutes. Then 20 mg/hour infused for 2 hours.
Adults who weigh less than 65 kg: Give 1.25 mg/kg in a similar fashion (60% in first hour, 10% of which is given as a bolus; then 20% of total dose per hour for 2 hours. Don't exceed total dose of 100 mg.
Accelerated infusion
Adults who weigh more than 67 kg (147 lb): 100 mg maximum total dose. Give 15 mg I.V. bolus over 1 to 2 minutes, followed by 50 mg infused over the next 30 minutes; then 35 mg infused over the next hour.
Adults who weigh 67 kg or less: 15 mg I.V. bolus over 1 to 2 minutes, followed by 0.75 mg/kg (not to exceed 50 mg) infused over the next 30 minutes; then 0.5 mg/kg (not to exceed 35 mg) infused over the next hour. Don't exceed total dose of 100 mg.

➤ To manage acute massive pulmonary embolism

Adults: 100 mg by I.V. infusion over 2 hours. Begin heparin at end of infusion when PTT or thrombin time returns to twice normal or less. Don't exceed 100-mg dose. Higher doses may increase risk of intracranial bleeding.

➤ Acute ischemic stroke

Adults: 0.9 mg/kg by I.V. infusion over 1 hour with 10% of total dose given as an initial I.V. bolus over 1 minute. Maximum total dose is 90 mg.

➤ To restore function to central venous access devices

Cathflo Activase
Adults and children older than age 2: For patients who weigh more than 30 kg (66 lb), instill 2 mg in 2 ml sterile water into catheter. For patients who weigh 10 kg (22 lb) to 30 kg, instill 110% of the internal lumen volume of the catheter, not to exceed 2 mg in 2 ml sterile water. After 30 minutes of dwell time, assess catheter function by aspirating blood. If function is restored, aspirate 4 to 5 ml of blood to remove drug and residual clot, and gently irrigate the catheter with normal saline

solution. If catheter function isn't restored after 120 minutes, instill a second dose.

➤ **Lysis of arterial occlusion in a peripheral vessel or bypass graft ♦**
Adults: 0.05 to 0.1 mg/kg/hour infused intra-arterially for 1 to 8 hours.

ADMINISTRATION

I.V.

- Immediately before use, reconstitute solution with unpreserved sterile water for injection. Check manufacturer's labeling for specific information.
- Don't use 50-mg vial if vacuum isn't present; 100-mg vials don't have a vacuum.
- Using an 18G needle, direct stream of sterile water at lyophilized cake. Don't shake.
- Slight foaming is common. Let it settle before giving drug. Solution should be colorless or pale yellow.
- Drug may be given reconstituted (at 1 mg/ml) or diluted with an equal volume of normal saline solution or D_5W to yield 0.5 mg/ml.
- Give drug using a controlled infusion device.
- Discard any unused drug after 8 hours.

Cathflo Activase

- Assess the cause of catheter dysfunction before using drug. Possible causes of occlusion include catheter malposition, mechanical failure, constriction by a suture, and lipid deposits or drug precipitates in the catheter lumen. Don't try to suction the catheter because you risk damaging the vessel wall or collapsing a soft-walled catheter.
- Reconstitute Cathflo Activase with 2.2 ml sterile water to yield 1 mg/ml. Dissolve completely to produce a colorless to pale yellow solution.
- Don't use excessive pressure while instilling drug into catheter; doing so could rupture the catheter or expel a clot into circulation.
- Solution is stable up to 8 hours at room temperature.
- **Incompatibilities:** None reported, but don't mix with other drugs.

ACTION

Converts plasminogen to plasmin by directly cleaving peptide bonds at two sites, causing fibrinolysis.

Route	Onset	Peak	Duration
I.V.	Unknown	Unknown	Unknown

Half-life: Less than 10 minutes.

ADVERSE REACTIONS

CNS: ***cerebral hemorrhage,*** fever.
CV: ***arrhythmias,*** hypotension, edema, ***cholesterol embolization, venous thrombosis.***
GI: ***bleeding (Cathflo Activase),*** nausea, vomiting.
GU: ***bleeding.***
Hematologic: ***spontaneous bleeding.***
Skin: ecchymosis.
Other: ***anaphylaxis, sepsis (Cathflo Activase),*** bleeding at puncture sites, hypersensitivity reactions.

INTERACTIONS

Drug-drug. *Aspirin,* ***clopidogrel,*** *dipyridamole, drugs affecting platelet activity (abciximab), heparin, warfarin anticoagulants:* May increase risk of bleeding. Monitor patient carefully.
Nitroglycerin: May decrease alteplase antigen level. Avoid using together. If use together is unavoidable, use the lowest effective dose of nitroglycerin.

EFFECTS ON LAB TEST RESULTS

- May alter coagulation and fibrinolytic test results.

CONTRAINDICATIONS & CAUTIONS

- Contraindicated in patients with active internal bleeding, intracranial neoplasm, arteriovenous malformation, aneurysm, severe uncontrolled hypertension, or history or current evidence of intracranial hemorrhage, suspicion of subarachnoid hemorrhage, or seizure at onset of stroke when used for acute ischemic stroke.
- Contraindicated in patients with history of stroke, intraspinal or intracranial trauma or surgery within 2 months, or known bleeding diathesis.

• Use cautiously in patients having major surgery within 10 days (when bleeding is difficult to control because of its location); organ biopsy; trauma (including cardiopulmonary resuscitation); GI or GU bleeding; cerebrovascular disease; systolic pressure of 180 mm Hg or higher or diastolic pressure of 110 mm Hg or higher; mitral stenosis, atrial fibrillation, or other conditions that may lead to left heart thrombus; acute pericarditis or subacute bacterial endocarditis; hemostatic defects caused by hepatic or renal impairment; septic thrombophlebitis; or diabetic hemorrhagic retinopathy.
• Use cautiously in patients receiving anticoagulants, in patients age 75 and older, and during pregnancy and the first 10 days postpartum.

NURSING CONSIDERATIONS

• *Alert:* When used for acute ischemic stroke, give drug within 3 hours after symptoms occur and only when intracranial bleeding has been ruled out.
• Drug may be given to menstruating women.
• To recanalize occluded coronary arteries and to improve heart function, begin treatment as soon as possible after symptoms start.
• Anticoagulant and antiplatelet therapy is commonly started during or after treatment, to decrease risk of another thrombosis.
• Monitor vital signs and neurologic status carefully. Keep patient on strict bed rest.
• Coronary thrombolysis is linked with arrhythmias caused by reperfusion of ischemic myocardium. Such arrhythmias don't differ from those commonly linked with MI. Have antiarrhythmics readily available, and carefully monitor ECG.
• Avoid invasive procedures during thrombolytic therapy. Closely monitor patient for signs of internal bleeding, and frequently check all puncture sites. Bleeding is the most common adverse effect and may occur internally and at external puncture sites.
• If uncontrollable bleeding occurs, stop infusion (and heparin) and notify prescriber.
• Avoid I.M. injections.

PATIENT TEACHING

• Explain use and administration of drug to patient and family.
• Tell patient to report adverse reactions promptly.

SAFETY ALERT!

✱ *NEW DRUG*

ambrisentan

am-bree-SEN-tan

Pharmacologic class: endothelin-receptor antagonist
Pregnancy risk category X

AVAILABLE FORMS

Tablets: 5 mg, 10 mg

INDICATIONS & DOSAGES

➤ **Pulmonary arterial hypertension (PAH) in patients with World Health Organization class II (with significant exertion) or III (with mild exertion) symptoms to improve exercise tolerance and decrease rate of clinical worsening**
Adults: 5 mg P.O. once daily; may increase to 10 mg P.O. once daily if tolerated.
Adjust-a-dose: Don't start therapy in patients with elevated aminotransferase levels (ALT and AST) of more than three times the upper limit of normal (ULN) at baseline. If ALT elevations during therapy are between three and five times the ULN, remeasure. If confirmed level is in the same range, reduce dose or stop therapy and remeasure every 2 weeks until levels are less than three times the ULN. If ALT and AST are between five and eight times the ULN, stop therapy and monitor until levels are less than three times the ULN. Restart therapy with more frequent monitoring. If ALT and AST exceed eight times the ULN, stop therapy and don't restart.

ADMINISTRATION

P.O.
• Give drug without regard for food.
• Give drug whole; don't crush or split tablets.

ACTION

Blocks endothelin-1 receptors on vascular endothelin and smooth muscle. Stimulation of these receptors in smooth muscle cells is associated with vasoconstriction and PAH.

Route	Onset	Peak	Duration
P.O.	Rapid	2 hr	Unknown

Half-life: 9 hours.

ADVERSE REACTIONS

CNS: *headache.*
CV: *peripheral edema,* flushing, palpitations.
EENT: nasal congestion, sinusitis, nasopharyngitis.
GI: abdominal pain, constipation.
Hematologic: anemia.
Hepatic: hepatic impairment.
Respiratory: dyspnea.

INTERACTIONS

Drug-drug. *CYP enzyme inducers, such as carbamazepine, phenobarbital, phenytoin, and rifampin:* May decrease effects of ambrisentan. Use together cautiously.
CYP enzyme inhibitors, such as atanazavir, clarithromycin, fluvoxamine, fluconazole, indinavir, itraconazole, ketoconazole, nefazodone, nelfinavir, omeprazole, ritonavir, saquinavir, telithromycin, and ticlopidine: May increase the effects of ambrisentan. Use together cautiously.
Cyclosporine: May increase ambrisentan levels. Use together cautiously and monitor patient for increased adverse effects.

EFFECTS ON LAB TEST RESULTS

- May increase AST, ALT, and bilirubin levels. May decrease hemoglobin level and hematocrit.

CONTRAINDICATIONS & CAUTIONS

- Contraindicated in patients hypersensitive to drug or its components.
- Contraindicated in pregnant women because it may harm the fetus.
- Contraindicated in those with moderate to severe hepatic impairment; don't begin therapy in those with elevated baseline ALT and AST levels of more than three times the ULN.
- Use cautiously in those with mild hepatic impairment.
- Use cautiously in those with renal impairment; drug hasn't been studied in those with severe renal impairment.

PATIENT TEACHING

- Inform female patient that she'll need to have a pregnancy test done monthly and to report suspected pregnancy to her prescriber immediately.
- ***Alert:*** Teach woman of childbearing age to use two reliable birth control methods unless she has had tubal sterilization or has a Copper T 380A intrauterine device (IUD) or an LNg 20 IUD inserted.
- Tell patient that monthly blood tests will be done to monitor for adverse effects.
- Advise patient to take the pill whole and not to split, crush, or chew the tablet.
- ***Alert:*** Teach patient to notify prescriber immediately of signs or symptoms of liver injury, including anorexia, nausea, vomiting, fever, malaise, fatigue, right upper quadrant abdominal discomfort, itching, and jaundice.
- Tell the patient to report edema and weight gain.

amikacin sulfate

am-i-KAY-sin

Amikin

Pharmacologic class: aminoglycoside
Pregnancy risk category D

AVAILABLE FORMS

Injection: 50 mg/ml (pediatric) vial, 250 mg/ml vial, 250 mg/ml disposable syringe

INDICATIONS & DOSAGES

➤ **Serious infections caused by sensitive strains of *Pseudomonas aeruginosa, Escherichia coli, Proteus, Klebsiella,* or *Staphylococcus***
Adults and children: 15 mg/kg/day I.M. or I.V. infusion, in divided doses every 8 to 12 hours for 7 to 10 days.

Neonates: Initially, loading dose of 10 mg/kg I.V.; then 7.5 mg/kg every 12 hours for 7 to 10 days.

➤ **Uncomplicated UTI caused by organisms not susceptible to less toxic drugs**

Adults: 250 mg I.M. or I.V. b.i.d.

➤ **Active tuberculosis, with other antituberculotics ♦**

Adults and children age 15 and older: 15 mg/kg (up to 1 g) I.M. or I.V. once daily five to seven times per week for 2 to 4 months or until culture conversion. Then reduce dose to 15 mg/kg daily given two or three times weekly depending on other drugs in regimen. Patients older than age 59 may receive a reduced dose of 10 mg/kg (up to 750 mg) daily.

Children younger than age 15: Give 15 to 30 mg/kg (up to 1 g) I.M. or I.V. once daily or twice weekly.

➤ ***Mycobacterium avium* complex infection ♦**

Adults: 15 mg/kg/day I.V. in divided doses every 8 to 12 hours as part of a multiple-drug regimen.

Adjust-a-dose: For adults with impaired renal function, initially, 7.5 mg/kg I.M. or I.V. Subsequent doses and frequency determined by amikacin levels and renal function studies. For adults receiving hemodialysis, give supplemental doses of 50% to 75% of initial loading dose at end of each dialysis session. Monitor drug levels and adjust dosage accordingly.

ADMINISTRATION

I.V.

- Obtain specimen for culture and sensitivity tests before giving first dose. Begin therapy while awaiting results.
- For adults, dilute I.V. drug in 100 to 200 ml of D_5W or normal saline solution. For children, the amount of fluid will depend on the ordered dose.
- In adults and children, infuse over 30 to 60 minutes. In infants, infuse over 1 to 2 hours.
- After infusion, flush line with normal saline solution or D_5W.
- **Incompatibilities:** Allopurinol, aminophylline, amphotericin B, ampicillin, azithromycin, bacitracin, cefazolin, ceftazidime, chlorothiazide sodium, cisplatin, heparin sodium, hetastarch in 0.9% sodium chloride, oxacillin, phenytoin, propofol, thiopental, vancomycin, vitamin B complex with C.

I.M.

- Obtain specimen for culture and sensitivity tests before giving first dose. Begin therapy while awaiting results.
- Obtain blood for peak level 1 hour after I.M. injection and 30 minutes to 1 hour after I.V. infusion ends; for trough levels, draw blood just before next dose. Don't collect blood in a heparinized tube; heparin is incompatible with aminoglycosides.

ACTION

Inhibits protein synthesis by binding directly to the 30S ribosomal subunit; bactericidal.

Route	Onset	Peak	Duration
I.V.	Immediate	30 min	8–12 hr
I.M.	Unknown	1 hr	8–12 hr

Half-life: Adults, 2 to 3 hours. Patients with severe renal damage, 30 to 86 hours.

ADVERSE REACTIONS

CNS: ***neuromuscular blockade.***
EENT: *ototoxicity.*
GU: *azotemia,* ***nephrotoxicity,*** increase in urinary excretion of casts.
Musculoskeletal: arthralgia.
Respiratory: ***apnea.***

INTERACTIONS

Drug-drug. *Acyclovir, amphotericin B, bacitracin, cephalosporins, cidofovir, cisplatin, methoxyflurane, vancomycin, other aminoglycosides:* May increase nephrotoxicity. Use together cautiously, and monitor renal function test results.

Atracurium, pancuronium, rocuronium, vecuronium: May increase effects of nondepolarizing muscle relaxants, including prolonged respiratory depression. Use together only when necessary, and expect to reduce dosage of nondepolarizing muscle relaxant.

Dimenhydrinate: May mask ototoxicity symptoms. Monitor patient's hearing.

General anesthetics: May increase neuromuscular blockade. Monitor patient for increased effects.

Indomethacin: May increase trough and peak amikacin levels. Monitor amikacin level.
I.V. loop diuretics such as furosemide: May increase ototoxicity. Use together cautiously, and monitor patient's hearing.
Parenteral penicillins: May inactivate amikacin in vitro. Don't mix.

EFFECTS ON LAB TEST RESULTS
- May increase BUN, creatinine, nonprotein nitrogen, and urine urea levels.

CONTRAINDICATIONS & CAUTIONS
- Contraindicated in patients hypersensitive to drug or other aminoglycosides.
- Use cautiously in patients with impaired renal function or neuromuscular disorders, in neonates and infants, and in elderly patients.

NURSING CONSIDERATIONS
- ***Alert:*** Evaluate patient's hearing before and during therapy if he'll be receiving the drug for longer than 2 weeks. Notify prescriber if patient has tinnitus, vertigo, or hearing loss.
- Weigh patient and review renal function studies before therapy begins.
- Correct dehydration before therapy because of increased risk of toxicity.
- Peak drug levels more than 35 mcg/ml and trough levels more than 10 mcg/ml may be linked to a higher risk of toxicity.
- ***Alert:*** Monitor renal function: urine output, specific gravity, urinalysis, BUN and creatinine levels, and creatinine clearance. Report to prescriber evidence of declining renal function.
- Watch for signs and symptoms of superinfection (especially of upper respiratory tract), such as continued fever, chills, and increased pulse rate.
- ***Alert:*** Neuromuscular blockage and respiratory paralysis have been reported after aminoglycoside administration. Monitor patient closely.
- Therapy usually continues for 7 to 10 days. If no response occurs after 3 to 5 days, stop therapy and obtain new specimens for culture and sensitivity testing.
- ***Look alike–sound alike:*** Don't confuse Amikin with Amicar. Don't confuse amikacin with anakinra.

PATIENT TEACHING
- Instruct patient to promptly report adverse reactions to prescriber.
- Encourage patient to maintain adequate fluid intake.

SAFETY ALERT!

amiodarone hydrochloride
am-ee-OH-dah-rohn

Cordarone, Pacerone

Pharmacologic class: benzofuran derivative
Pregnancy risk category D

AVAILABLE FORMS
Injection: 50 mg/ml in 3-ml ampules, vials
Tablets: 100 mg, 200 mg, 400 mg

INDICATIONS & DOSAGES
➤ **Life-threatening recurrent ventricular fibrillation or recurrent hemodynamically unstable ventricular tachycardia unresponsive to adequate doses of other antiarrhythmics or when alternative drugs can't be tolerated**
Adults: Give loading dose of 800 to 1,600 mg P.O. daily divided b.i.d. for 1 to 3 weeks until first therapeutic response occurs; then 600 to 800 mg P.O. daily for 1 month, followed by maintenance dose 200 to 600 mg P.O. daily.

Or, give loading dose of 150 mg I.V. over 10 minutes (15 mg/minute); then 360 mg I.V. over next 6 hours (1 mg/minute), followed by 540 mg I.V. over next 18 hours (0.5 mg/minute). After first 24 hours, continue with maintenance I.V. infusion of 720 mg/24 hours (0.5 mg/minute).

ADMINISTRATION
P.O.
- Divide oral loading dose into two or three equal doses and give with meals to decrease GI intolerance. Give maintenance

dose once daily or divide into two doses, with meals to decrease GI intolerance.

I.V.

- Give drug I.V. only if continuous ECG and electrophysiologic monitoring are available.
- Mix first dose of 150 mg in 100 ml of D_5W solution.
- If infusion will last 2 hours or longer, mix solution in glass or polyolefin bottles.
- If concentration is 2 mg/ml or more, give drug through a central line. If possible, use a dedicated line.
- Use an in-line filter.
- Continuously monitor patient's cardiac status. If hypotension occurs, reduce infusion rate.
- Cordarone I.V. leaches out plasticizers from I.V. tubing and adsorbs to polyvinyl chloride (PVC) tubing, which can adversely affect male reproductive tract development in fetuses, infants, and toddlers when used at concentrations or flow rates outside of recommendations.
- **Incompatibilities:** Aminophylline, ampicillin sodium and sulbactam sodium, bivalirudin, cefazolin sodium, ceftazidime, digoxin, furosemide, heparin sodium, imipenem and cilastatin sodium, magnesium sulfate, normal saline solution, piperacillin sodium, piperacillin and tazobactam sodium, quinidine gluconate, sodium bicarbonate, sodium nitroprusside, sodium phosphates.

ACTION

Effects result from blockade of potassium chloride leading to a prolongation of action potential duration.

Route	Onset	Peak	Duration
P.O.	Variable	3–7 hr	Variable
I.V.	Unknown	Unknown	Variable

Half-life: 25 to 110 days (usually 40 to 50 days).

ADVERSE REACTIONS

CNS: *fatigue, malaise, tremor,* peripheral neuropathy, ataxia, paresthesia, insomnia, sleep disturbances, headache.
CV: *hypotension,* ***bradycardia, arrhythmias, heart failure, heart block, sinus arrest,*** edema.
EENT: *asymptomatic corneal microdeposits, visual disturbances,* optic neuropathy or neuritis resulting in visual impairment, abnormal smell.
GI: *nausea, vomiting,* abnormal taste, anorexia, constipation, abdominal pain.
Hematologic: ***coagulation abnormalities.***
Hepatic: ***hepatic failure,*** hepatic dysfunction.
Metabolic: *hypothyroidism,* hyperthyroidism.
Respiratory: ***acute respiratory distress syndrome,*** **SEVERE PULMONARY TOXICITY.**
Skin: *photosensitivity,* solar dermatitis, blue-gray skin.

INTERACTIONS

Drug-drug. *Antiarrhythmics:* May reduce hepatic or renal clearance of certain antiarrhythmics, especially flecainide, procainamide, and quinidine. Use of amiodarone with other antiarrhythmics, especially mexiletine, propafenone, disopyramide, and procainamide, may induce torsades de pointes. Avoid using together.
Azole antifungals, disopyramide, pimozide: May increase the risk of arrhythmias, including torsades de pointes. Avoid using together.
Beta blockers, calcium channel blockers: May potentiate bradycardia, sinus arrest, and AV block; may increase hypotensive effect. Use together cautiously.
Cimetidine: May increase amiodarone level. Use together cautiously.
Cyclosporine: May increase cyclosporine level, resulting in an increase in the serum creatinine level and renal toxicity. Monitor cyclosporine levels and renal function tests.
Digoxin: May increase digoxin level 70% to 100%. Monitor digoxin level closely and reduce digoxin dosage by half or stop drug completely when starting amiodarone therapy.
Fentanyl: May cause hypotension, bradycardia, and decreased cardiac output. Monitor patient closely.
Fluoroquinolones: May increase risk of arrhythmias, including torsades de pointes. Avoid using together.

Macrolide antibiotics (azithromycin, clarithromycin, erythromycin, telithromycin): May cause additive or prolongation of the QT interval. Use with caution. Avoid use with telithromycin.
Methotrexate: May impair methotrexate metabolism, causing toxicity. Use together cautiously.
Phenytoin: May decrease phenytoin metabolism and amiodarone level. Monitor phenytoin level and adjust dosages of drugs if needed.
Protease inhibitors (amprenavir, atazanavir, indinavir, lopinavir and ritonavir, nelfinavir, ritonavir, and saquinavir): May increase the risk of amiodarone toxicity. Use of ritonavir or nelfinavir with amiodarone is contraindicated. Use other protease inhibitors cautiously.
Quinidine: May increase quinidine level, causing life-threatening cardiac arrhythmias. Avoid using together, or monitor quinidine level closely if use together can't be avoided. Adjust quinidine dosage as needed.
Rifamycins: May decrease amiodarone level. Monitor patient closely.
Theophylline: May increase theophylline level and cause toxicity. Monitor theophylline level.
Warfarin: May increase anticoagulant response with the potential for serious or fatal bleeding. Decrease warfarin dosage 33% to 50% when starting amiodarone. Monitor patient closely.
Drug-herb. *Pennyroyal:* May change rate of formation of toxic metabolites of pennyroyal. Discourage use together.
St. John's wort: May decrease amiodarone levels. Discourage use together.
Drug-food. *Grapefruit juice:* May inhibit CYP3A4 metabolism of drug in the intestinal mucosa, causing increased levels and risk of toxicity. Discourage use together.
Drug-lifestyle. *Sun exposure:* May cause photosensitivity reaction. Advise patient to avoid excessive sunlight exposure and to take precautions while in the sun.

EFFECTS ON LAB TEST RESULTS

- May increase alkaline phosphatase, ALT, AST, GGT, reverse T_3, and T_4 levels. May decrease T_3 level.
- May increase PT and INR.

CONTRAINDICATIONS & CAUTIONS

- Contraindicated in patients hypersensitive to drug or to iodine.
- Contraindicated in those with cardiogenic shock, second- or third-degree AV block, severe SA node disease resulting in bradycardia unless an artificial pacemaker is present, and in those for whom bradycardia has caused syncope.
- Use cautiously in patients receiving other antiarrhythmics.
- Use cautiously in patients with pulmonary, hepatic, or thyroid disease.

NURSING CONSIDERATIONS

- Be aware of the high risk of adverse reactions.
- Obtain baseline pulmonary, liver, and thyroid function test results and baseline chest X-ray.
- Give loading doses in a hospital setting and with continuous ECG monitoring because of the slow onset of antiarrhythmic effect and the risk of life-threatening arrhythmias.
- ***Alert:*** Drug may pose life-threatening management problems in patients at risk for sudden death. Use only in patients with life-threatening, recurrent ventricular arrhythmias unresponsive to or intolerant of other antiarrhythmics or alternative drugs. Amiodarone can cause fatal toxicities, including hepatic and pulmonary toxicity.
- ***Alert:*** Drug is highly toxic. Watch carefully for pulmonary toxicity. Risk increases in patients receiving doses over 400 mg/day.
- Watch for evidence of pneumonitis, exertional dyspnea, nonproductive cough, and pleuritic chest pain. Monitor pulmonary function tests and chest X-ray.
- Monitor liver and thyroid function test results and electrolyte, particularly potassium and magnesium, levels.
- Monitor PT and INR if patient takes warfarin and digoxin level if he takes digoxin.
- Instill methylcellulose ophthalmic solution during amiodarone therapy to minimize corneal microdeposits. About 1 to 4 months after starting amiodarone, most patients develop corneal microdeposits, although 10% or less have vision

disturbances. Regular ophthalmic examinations are advised.
- Monitor blood pressure and heart rate and rhythm frequently. Perform continuous ECG monitoring when starting or changing dosage. Notify prescriber of significant change in assessment results.
- Life-threatening gasping syndrome may occur in neonates given I.V. solutions containing benzyl alcohol.
- During or after treatment with I.V. form, patient may be transferred to oral therapy.
- ***Look alike–sound alike:*** Don't confuse amiodarone with amiloride.

PATIENT TEACHING
- Advise patient to wear sunscreen or protective clothing to prevent sensitivity reaction to the sun. Monitor patient for skin burning or tingling, followed by redness and blistering. Exposed skin may turn blue-gray.
- Tell patient to take oral drug with food if GI reactions occur.
- Inform patient that adverse effects of drug are more common at high doses and become more frequent with treatment lasting longer than 6 months, but are generally reversible when drug is stopped. Resolution of adverse reactions may take up to 4 months.
- Tell patient not to stop taking this medication without consulting with his prescriber.

amlodipine besylate
am-LOE-di-peen

Norvasc

Pharmacologic class: calcium channel blocker
Pregnancy risk category C

AVAILABLE FORMS
Tablets: 2.5 mg, 5 mg, 10 mg

INDICATIONS & DOSAGES
➤ Chronic stable angina, vasospastic angina (Prinzmetal's or variant angina)
Adults: Initially, 5 to 10 mg P.O. daily. Most patients need 10 mg daily.
Elderly patients: Initially, 5 mg P.O. daily.
Adjust-a-dose: For patients who are small or frail or have hepatic insufficiency, initially, 5 mg P.O. daily.
➤ Hypertension
Adults: Initially, 2.5 to 5 mg P.O. daily. Dosage adjusted according to patient response and tolerance. Maximum daily dose is 10 mg.
Elderly patients: Initially, 2.5 mg P.O. daily.
Adjust-a-dose: For patients who are small or frail, are taking other antihypertensives, or have hepatic insufficiency, initially, 2.5 mg P.O. daily.

ADMINISTRATION
P.O.
- Give drug without regard for food.

ACTION
Inhibits calcium ion influx across cardiac and smooth-muscle cells, dilates coronary arteries and arterioles, and decreases blood pressure and myocardial oxygen demand.

Route	Onset	Peak	Duration
P.O.	Unknown	6–12 hr	24 hr

Half-life: 30 to 50 hours.

ADVERSE REACTIONS
CNS: headache, somnolence, fatigue, dizziness, light-headedness, paresthesia.
CV: *edema,* flushing, palpitations.
GI: nausea, abdominal pain.
GU: sexual difficulties.
Musculoskeletal: muscle pain.
Respiratory: dyspnea.
Skin: rash, pruritus.

INTERACTIONS
None reported.

EFFECTS ON LAB TEST RESULTS
None reported.

CONTRAINDICATIONS & CAUTIONS
- Contraindicated in patients hypersensitive to drug.
- Use cautiously in patients receiving other peripheral vasodilators, especially those with severe aortic stenosis, and in those with heart failure. Because drug is

metabolized by the liver, use cautiously and in reduced dosage in patients with severe hepatic disease.

NURSING CONSIDERATIONS

- ***Alert:*** Monitor patient carefully. Some patients, especially those with severe obstructive coronary artery disease, have developed increased frequency, duration, or severity of angina or acute MI after initiation of calcium channel blocker therapy or at time of dosage increase.
- Monitor blood pressure frequently during initiation of therapy. Because drug-induced vasodilation has a gradual onset, acute hypotension is rare.
- Notify prescriber if signs of heart failure occur, such as swelling of hands and feet or shortness of breath.
- ***Alert:*** Abrupt withdrawal of drug may increase frequency and duration of chest pain. Taper dose gradually under medical supervision.
- ***Look alike–sound alike:*** Don't confuse amlodipine with amiloride.

PATIENT TEACHING

- Caution patient to continue taking drug, even when he feels better.
- Tell patient S.L. nitroglycerin may be taken as needed when angina symptoms are acute. If patient continues nitrate therapy during adjustment of amlodipine dosage, urge continued compliance.

---

ampicillin
am-pi-SILL-in

Apo-Ampi†, Nu-Ampi†

ampicillin sodium

ampicillin trihydrate
Principen

Pharmacologic class: aminopenicillin
Pregnancy risk category B

AVAILABLE FORMS

Capsules: 250 mg, 500 mg
Injection: 250 mg, 500 mg, 1 g, 2 g
Oral suspension: 125 mg/5 ml, 250 mg/5 ml

INDICATIONS & DOSAGES

➤ Respiratory tract or skin and skin-structure infections
Adults and children who weigh 40 kg (88 lb) or more: 250 to 500 mg P.O. every 6 hours.
Children who weigh less than 40 kg: 25 to 50 mg/kg/day P.O. in equally divided doses every 6 to 8 hours. Pediatric dosages shouldn't exceed recommended adult dosages.

➤ GI infections or UTIs
Adults and children who weigh 40 kg (88 lb) or more: 500 mg P.O. every 6 hours. For severe infections, larger doses may be needed.
Children who weigh less than 40 kg: 50 to 100 mg/kg/day P.O. in equally divided doses every 6 hours.

➤ Bacterial meningitis or septicemia
Adults: 150 to 200 mg/kg/day I.V. in divided doses every 3 to 4 hours. May be given I.M. after 3 days of I.V. therapy. Maximum recommended daily dose is 14 g.
Children: 150 to 200 mg/kg I.V. daily in divided doses every 3 to 4 hours. Give I.V. for 3 days; then give I.M.

➤ Uncomplicated gonorrhea
Adults and children who weigh more than 45 kg (99 lb): 3.5 g P.O. with 1 g probenecid given as a single dose.

➤ To prevent endocarditis in patients having dental, GI, and GU procedures ♦
Adults: 2 g I.M. or I.V. within 30 minutes before procedure. For high-risk patients, also give 1.5 mg/kg gentamicin 30 minutes before the procedure; 6 hours later, give 1 g ampicillin I.M. or I.V. or 1 g amoxicillin P.O.
Children: 50 mg/kg I.M. or I.V. within 30 minutes before procedure. For high-risk patients, also give 1.5 mg/kg gentamicin 30 minutes before the procedure; 6 hours later, give 25 mg/kg ampicillin I.M. or I.V. or 25 mg/kg amoxicillin P.O.
Adjust-a-dose: In patients with creatinine clearance of 10 to 50 ml/minute, use same dose but increase dosing interval to 6 to 12 hours; for those with a clearance less than 10 ml/minute, increase dosing interval to 12 to 24 hours.

ADMINISTRATION

P.O.

- Before giving drug, ask patient about allergic reactions to penicillin. A negative history of penicillin allergy is no guarantee against a future allergic reaction.
- Obtain specimen for culture and sensitivity tests before giving. Begin therapy while awaiting results.
- Give drug 1 to 2 hours before or 2 to 3 hours after meals. When given orally, drug may cause GI disturbances. Food may interfere with absorption.
- Give drug I.M. or I.V. if infection is severe or if patient can't take oral dose.

I.V.

- Before giving drug, ask patient about allergic reactions to penicillin. A negative history of penicillin allergy is no guarantee against a future allergic reaction.
- Obtain specimen for culture and sensitivity tests before giving. Begin therapy while awaiting results.
- Give drug I.M. or I.V. only if infection is severe or if patient can't take oral dose.
- Give drug intermittently to prevent vein irritation. Change site every 48 hours.
- For direct injection, reconstitute with bacteriostatic water for injection. Use 5 ml for 250-mg or 500-mg vials, 7.4 ml for 1-g vials, and 14.8 ml for 2-g vials. Give drug over 10 to 15 minutes to avoid seizures. Don't exceed 100 mg/minute.
- For intermittent infusion, dilute in 50 to 100 ml of normal saline solution for injection. Give drug over 15 to 30 minutes.
- Use first dilution within 1 hour. Follow manufacturer's directions for stability data when drug is further diluted for I.V. infusion.
- **Incompatibilities:** Amikacin, amino acid solutions, chlorpromazine, dextran solutions, dextrose solutions, dopamine, erythromycin lactobionate, 10% fat emulsions, fructose, gentamicin, heparin sodium, hetastarch, hydrocortisone sodium succinate, hydromorphone, kanamycin, lidocaine, lincomycin, polymyxin B, prochlorperazine edisylate, sodium bicarbonate, streptomycin, tobramycin.

I.M.

- Before giving drug, ask patient about allergic reactions to penicillin. A negative history of penicillin allergy is no guarantee against a future allergic reaction.
- Obtain specimen for culture and sensitivity tests before giving. Begin therapy while awaiting results.
- Give drug I.M. or I.V. only if infection is severe or if patient can't take oral dose.

ACTION

Inhibits cell-wall synthesis during bacterial multiplication.

Route	Onset	Peak	Duration
P.O.	Unknown	2 hr	6–8 hr
I.V.	Immediate	Immediate	Unknown
I.M.	Unknown	1 hr	Unknown

Half-life: 1 to 1½ hours (10 to 24 hours in severe renal impairment).

ADVERSE REACTIONS

CNS: ***seizures,*** agitation, anxiety, confusion, depression, dizziness, hallucinations, lethargy, fatigue.
CV: thrombophlebitis, vein irritation.
GI: *diarrhea, nausea,* ***pseudomembranous colitis,*** abdominal pain, black hairy tongue, enterocolitis, gastritis, glossitis, stomatitis, vomiting.
GU: interstitial nephritis, nephropathy, vaginitis.
Hematologic: ***leukopenia, thrombocytopenia, thrombocytopenic purpura,*** anemia, eosinophilia, hemolytic anemia, ***agranulocytosis.***
Skin: pain at injection site.
Other: hypersensitivity reactions, overgrowth of nonsusceptible organisms.

INTERACTIONS

Drug-drug. *Allopurinol:* May increase risk of rash. Monitor patient for rash.
H_2 antagonists, proton pump inhibitors: May decrease ampicillin absorption and level. Separate administration times. Monitor patient for continued antibiotic effectiveness.
Hormonal contraceptives: May decrease hormonal contraceptive effectiveness. Advise use of another form of contraception during therapy.
Oral anticoagulants: May increase risk of bleeding. Monitor PT and INR.

Probenecid: May increase levels of ampicillin and other penicillins. Probenecid may be used for this purpose.

EFFECTS ON LAB TEST RESULTS

- May decrease hemoglobin level.
- May increase eosinophil count. May decrease granulocyte, platelet, and WBC counts.
- May falsely decrease aminoglycoside level. May alter results of urine glucose tests that use cupric sulfate, such as Benedict reagent and Clinitest.

CONTRAINDICATIONS & CAUTIONS

- Contraindicated in patients hypersensitive to drug or other penicillins.
- Use cautiously in patients with other drug allergies (especially to cephalosporins) because of possible cross-sensitivity, and in those with mononucleosis because of high risk of maculopapular rash.

NURSING CONSIDERATIONS

- Monitor sodium level because each gram of ampicillin contains 2.9 mEq of sodium.
- If large doses are given or if therapy is prolonged, bacterial or fungal superinfection may occur, especially in elderly, debilitated, or immunosuppressed patients.
- Watch for signs and symptoms of hypersensitivity, such as erythematous maculopapular rash, urticaria, and anaphylaxis.
- In patients with impaired renal function, decrease dosage.
- In pediatric meningitis, drug may be given with parenteral chloramphenicol for 24 hours, pending cultures.
- To prevent bacterial endocarditis in patients at high risk, give drug with gentamicin.

PATIENT TEACHING

- Tell patient to take entire quantity of drug exactly as prescribed, even after he feels better.
- Instruct patient to take oral form on an empty stomach 1 hour before or 2 hours after meals.
- Inform patient to notify prescriber if rash, fever, or chills develop. A rash is the most common allergic reaction, especially if allopurinol is also being taken.
- Advise patient to report discomfort at I.V. injection site.

SAFETY ALERT!

argatroban

ahr-GAH-troh-ban

Pharmacologic class: direct thrombin inhibitor
Pregnancy risk category B

AVAILABLE FORMS

Injection: 100 mg/ml

INDICATIONS & DOSAGES

➤ To prevent or treat thrombosis in patients with heparin-induced thrombocytopenia

Adults without hepatic impairment: 2 mcg/kg/minute, given as a continuous I.V. infusion; adjust dose until the steady-state activated PTT is $1\frac{1}{2}$ to 3 times the initial baseline value, not to exceed 100 seconds; maximum dose 10 mcg/kg/minute. See current manufacturer's label for recommended doses and infusion rates.

Adjust-a-dose: For patients with moderate hepatic impairment, reduce first dose to 0.5 mcg/kg/minute, given as a continuous infusion. Monitor PTT closely and adjust dosage as needed.

➤ Anticoagulation in patients with or at risk for heparin-induced thrombocytopenia during percutaneous coronary intervention (PCI)

Adults: 350 mcg/kg I.V. bolus over 3 to 5 minutes. Start a continuous I.V. infusion at 25 mcg/kg/minute. Check activated clotting time (ACT) 5 to 10 minutes after the bolus dose is completed.

Adjust-a-dose: Use the following table to adjust the dosage.

Activated clotting time	Additional I.V. bolus	Continuous I.V. infusion
< 300 sec	150 mcg/kg	30 mcg/kg/min*
300–450 sec	None needed	25 mcg/kg/min
> 450 sec	None needed	15 mcg/kg/min*

*Check ACT again after 5 to 10 minutes.

In case of dissection, impending abrupt closure, thrombus formation during the procedure, or inability to achieve or maintain an ACT exceeding 300 seconds, give an additional bolus of 150 mcg/kg and increase infusion rate to 40 mcg/kg/minute. Check ACT again after 5 to 10 minutes.

ADMINISTRATION

I.V.

- Before starting therapy, obtain a complete list of patient's prescription and OTC drugs and supplements, including herbs.
- Stop all parenteral anticoagulants before giving drug. Giving with antiplatelets, thrombolytics, and other anticoagulants may increase risk of bleeding.
- Before starting drug, get results of baseline coagulation tests, platelet count, hemoglobin level, and hematocrit, and report any abnormalities to prescriber.
- Dilute in normal saline solution, D_5W, or lactated Ringer's injection to a final concentration of 1 mg/ml.
- Dilute each 2.5-ml vial 100-fold by mixing it with 250 ml of diluent.
- Mix the solution by repeated inversion of the diluent bag for 10 minutes.
- Don't expose solution to direct sunlight.
- Prepared solutions are stable for up to 24 hours at 77° F (25° C).
- **Incompatibilities:** Other I.V. drugs.

ACTION

Reversibly binds to the thrombin-active site and inhibits thrombin-catalyzed or -induced reactions: fibrin formation; coagulation factor V, VIII, and XIII activation; protein C activation; and platelet aggregation. May inhibit the action of free and clot-associated thrombin.

Route	Onset	Peak	Duration
I.V.	Rapid	1–3 hr	Duration of infusion

Half-life: 39 to 51 minutes.

ADVERSE REACTIONS

CNS: ***cerebrovascular disorder, hemorrhage,*** fever, pain.
CV: ***atrial fibrillation, cardiac arrest,*** hypotension, ***ventricular tachycardia.***
GI: abdominal pain, diarrhea, ***GI bleeding,*** nausea, vomiting.
GU: abnormal renal function, groin bleeding, *hematuria,* UTI.
Respiratory: cough, dyspnea, pneumonia, hemoptysis.
Other: allergic reactions, brachial bleeding, infection, ***sepsis.***

INTERACTIONS

Drug-drug. *Antiplatelet drugs, heparin, thrombolytics:* May increase risk of intracranial bleeding. Avoid using together.
Oral anticoagulants: May prolong PT and INR and may increase risk of bleeding. Monitor patient closely.
Drug-herb. *Angelica (dong quai), boldo, bromelains, capsicum, chamomile, dandelion, danshen, devil's claw, fenugreek, feverfew, garlic, ginger, ginkgo, ginseng, horse chestnut, licorice, meadowsweet, onion, passion flower, red clover, willow:* May increase risk of bleeding. Discourage use together.

EFFECTS ON LAB TEST RESULTS

- May decrease hemoglobin level and hematocrit.

CONTRAINDICATIONS & CAUTIONS

- Contraindicated in patients who have overt major bleeding who are hypersensitive to drug or any of its components.
- Use cautiously in patients with hepatic disease or conditions that increase the risk of hemorrhage, such as severe hypertension.
- Use cautiously in patients who have just had lumbar puncture, spinal anesthesia, or major surgery, especially of the brain, spinal cord, or eye; patients with hematologic conditions causing increased bleeding tendencies, such as congenital or acquired bleeding disorders; and patients with GI ulcers or other lesions.

NURSING CONSIDERATIONS

- Check activated PTT 2 hours after giving drug; dose adjustments may be required to get a targeted activated PTT of 1.5 to 3 times the baseline, no longer than

100 seconds. Steady state is achieved 1 to 3 hours after starting drug.

- Draw blood for additional ACT about every 20 to 30 minutes during prolonged PCI.
- Patients can hemorrhage from any site in the body. Any unexplained decrease in hematocrit or blood pressure or any other unexplained symptoms may signify a hemorrhagic event.
- To convert to oral anticoagulant therapy, give warfarin P.O. with argatroban at up to 2 mcg/kg/minute until the INR exceeds 4 on combined therapy. After argatroban is stopped, repeat the INR in 4 to 6 hours. If the repeat INR is less than the desired therapeutic range, resume the I.V. argatroban infusion. Repeat the procedure daily until the desired therapeutic range on warfarin alone is reached.
- Use cautiously in breast-feeding women; it's unknown if drug appears in breast milk.
- ***Look alike–sound alike:*** Don't confuse argatroban with Aggrastat.

PATIENT TEACHING

- Tell patient that this drug can cause bleeding, and ask him to report any unusual bruising or bleeding (nosebleeds, bleeding gums) or tarry stools to the prescriber immediately.
- Advise patient to avoid activities that carry a risk of injury, and to use a soft toothbrush and an electric razor during therapy.
- Advise patient to consult with prescriber before initiating any herbal therapy; many herbs have anticoagulant, antiplatelet, and fibrinolytic properties.
- Instruct patient to notify prescriber if he has wheezing, trouble breathing, or skin rash.
- Instruct woman who is pregnant, has recently delivered, or is breast-feeding to notify her prescriber.
- Tell patient to notify prescriber if he has GI ulcers or liver disease, or has had recent surgery, radiation treatment, falling episodes, or injury.

aspirin (acetylsalicylic acid, ASA)

ASS-pir-in

Aspergum ◊, Bayer ◊, Ecotrin ◊, Empirin ◊, Halfprin, Heartline ◊, Norwich ◊, Novasen† ◊, St Joseph's ◊, ZORprin ◊

Pharmacologic class: salicylate
Pregnancy risk category D

AVAILABLE FORMS

Chewing gum: 227.5 mg ◊
Suppositories: 120 mg ◊, 200 mg ◊, 300 mg ◊, 600 mg ◊
Tablets: 325 mg ◊, 500 mg ◊
Tablets (chewable): 81 mg ◊
Tablets (controlled-release): 800 mg
Tablets (enteric-coated): 81 mg ◊, 165 mg ◊, 325 mg ◊, 500 mg ◊, 650 mg ◊, 975 mg
Tablets (extended-release): 650 mg ◊

INDICATIONS & DOSAGES

➤ Rheumatoid arthritis, osteoarthritis, or other polyarthritic or inflammatory conditions

Adults: Initially, 2.4 to 3.6 g P.O. daily in divided doses. Maintenance dosage is 3.2 to 6 g P.O. daily in divided doses.

➤ Juvenile rheumatoid arthritis

Children who weigh more than 25 kg (55 lb): 2.4 to 3.6 g P.O. daily in divided doses.
Children who weigh 25 kg or less: 60 to 130 mg/kg daily P.O. in divided doses. Increase by 10 mg/kg daily at no more than weekly intervals. Maintenance dosages usually range from 80 to 100 mg/kg daily; up to 130 mg/kg daily.

➤ Mild pain or fever

Adults and children older than age 11: 325 to 650 mg P.O. or P.R. every 4 hours p.r.n.
Children ages 2 to 11: 10 to 15 mg/kg/dose P.O. or P.R. every 4 hours up to 80 mg/kg daily.

➤ To prevent thrombosis

Adults: 1.3 g P.O. daily, divided b.i.d. to q.i.d.

➤ To reduce risk of MI in patients with previous MI or unstable angina
Adults: 75 to 325 mg P.O. daily.
➤ Kawasaki syndrome (mucocutaneous lymph node syndrome)
Children: 80 to 100 mg/kg P.O. daily, divided q.i.d. with immune globulin I.V. After the fever subsides, reduce dosage to 3 to 5 mg/kg once daily. Aspirin therapy usually continues for 6 to 8 weeks.
➤ Acute rheumatic fever
Adults: 5 to 8 g P.O. daily.
Children: 100 mg/kg daily P.O. for 2 weeks; then 75 mg/kg daily P.O. for 4 to 6 weeks.
➤ To reduce risk of recurrent transient ischemic attacks and stroke or death in patients at risk
Adults: 50 to 325 mg P.O. daily.
➤ Acute ischemic stroke
Adults: 160 to 325 mg P.O. daily, started within 48 hours of stroke onset and continued for up to 2 to 4 weeks.
➤ Acute pericarditis after MI
Adults: 160 to 325 mg P.O. daily. Higher doses (650 mg P.O. every 4 to 6 hours) may be needed.

ADMINISTRATION

P.O.

- For patient with swallowing difficulties, crush non–enteric-coated aspirin and dissolve in soft food or liquid. Give liquid immediately after mixing because drug will break down rapidly.
- Give drug with food, milk, antacid, or large glass of water to reduce GI effects.
- Give sustained-release or enteric-coated forms whole; don't crush or break these tablets.

Rectal

- Refrigerate suppositories.

ACTION

Thought to produce analgesia and exert its anti-inflammatory effect by inhibiting prostaglandin and other substances that sensitize pain receptors. Drug may relieve fever through central action in the hypothalamic heat-regulating center. In low doses, drug also appears to interfere with clotting by keeping a platelet-aggregating substance from forming.

Route	Onset	Peak	Duration
P.O. (buffered)	5–30 min	1–2 hr	1–4 hr
P.O. (enteric-coated)	5–30 min	Variable	1–4 hr
P.O. (extended-release)	5–30 min	1–4 hr	1–4 hr
P.O. (solution)	5–30 min	15–40 min	1–4 hr
P.O. (tablet)	5–30 min	25–40 min	1–4 hr
P.R.	Unknown	3–4 hr	Unknown

Half-life: 15 to 20 minutes.

ADVERSE REACTIONS

EENT: *tinnitus, hearing loss.*
GI: *nausea,* ***GI bleeding,*** dyspepsia, GI distress, occult bleeding.
Hematologic: *prolonged bleeding time,* ***leukopenia, thrombocytopenia.***
Hepatic: ***hepatitis.***
Skin: *rash,* bruising, urticaria.
Other: ***angioedema, Reye syndrome,*** hypersensitivity reactions.

INTERACTIONS

Drug-drug. *ACE inhibitors:* May decrease antihypertensive effects. Monitor blood pressure closely.
Ammonium chloride and other urine acidifiers: May increase levels of aspirin products. Watch for aspirin toxicity.
Antacids in high doses and other urine alkalinizers: May decrease levels of aspirin products. Watch for decreased aspirin effect.
Anticoagulants: May increase risk of bleeding. Use with extreme caution if must be used together.
Beta blockers: May decrease antihypertensive effect. Avoid long-term aspirin use if patient is taking antihypertensives.
Corticosteroids: May enhance salicylate elimination and decrease drug level. Watch for decreased aspirin effect.
Heparin: May increase risk of bleeding. Monitor coagulation studies and patient closely if used together.
Ibuprofen, other NSAIDs: May negate the antiplatelet effect of low-dose aspirin therapy. Patients using immediate-release aspirin (not enteric-coated) should take

ibuprofen at least 30 minutes after or more than 8 hours before aspirin. Occasional use of ibuprofen is unlikely to have a negative effect.
Methotrexate: May increase risk of methotrexate toxicity. Avoid using together.
Nizatidine: May increase risk of salicylate toxicity in patients receiving high doses of aspirin. Monitor patient closely.
Oral antidiabetics: May increase hypoglycemic effect. Monitor patient closely.
Probenecid, sulfinpyrazone: May decrease uricosuric effect. Avoid using together.
Valproic acid: May increase valproic acid level. Avoid using together.
Drug-herb. *Dong quai, feverfew, ginkgo, horse chestnut, kelpware, red clover:* May increase risk of bleeding. Monitor patient closely for increased effects. Discourage use together.
White willow: May increase risk of adverse effects. Discourage use together.
Drug-food. *Caffeine:* May increase drug absorption. Watch for increased effects.
Drug-lifestyle. *Alcohol use:* May increase risk of GI bleeding. Discourage use together.

EFFECTS ON LAB TEST RESULTS

- May increase liver function test values. May decrease platelet and WBC counts.
- May falsely increase protein-bound iodine level. May interfere with urine glucose analysis with Diastix, Chemstrip uG, Clinitest, and Benedict solution; with urinary 5-hydroxyindoleacetic acid and vanillylmandelic acid tests; and with Gerhardt test for urine acetoacetic acid.

CONTRAINDICATIONS & CAUTIONS

- Contraindicated in patients hypersensitive to drug and in those with NSAID-induced sensitivity reactions, G6PD deficiency, or bleeding disorders, such as hemophilia, von Willebrand disease, or telangiectasia.
- Use cautiously in patients with GI lesions, impaired renal function, hypoprothrombinemia, vitamin K deficiency, thrombocytopenia, thrombotic thrombocytopenic purpura, or severe hepatic impairment.
- ***Alert:*** Oral and rectal OTC products containing aspirin and nonaspirin salicylates shouldn't be given to children or teenagers who have or are recovering from chickenpox or flulike symptoms because of the risk of Reye syndrome.

NURSING CONSIDERATIONS

- For inflammatory conditions, rheumatic fever, and thrombosis, give aspirin on a schedule rather than as needed.
- Because enteric-coated and sustained-release tablets are slowly absorbed, they aren't suitable for rapid relief of acute pain, fever, or inflammation. They cause less GI bleeding and may be better suited for long-term therapy, such as for arthritis.
- For patients who can't tolerate oral drugs, ask prescriber about using aspirin rectal suppositories. Watch for rectal mucosal irritation or bleeding.
- Febrile, dehydrated children can develop toxicity rapidly.
- Monitor elderly patients closely because they may be more susceptible to aspirin's toxic effects.
- Monitor salicylate level. Therapeutic salicylate level for arthritis is 150 to 300 mcg/ml. Tinnitus may occur at levels above 200 mcg/ml, but this isn't a reliable indicator of toxicity, especially in very young patients and those older than age 60. With long-term therapy, severe toxic effects may occur with levels exceeding 400 mcg/ml.
- During prolonged therapy, assess hematocrit, hemoglobin level, PT, INR, and renal function periodically.
- Drug irreversibly inhibits platelet aggregation. Stop drug 5 to 7 days before elective surgery to allow time for production and release of new platelets.
- Monitor patient for hypersensitivity reactions, such as anaphylaxis and asthma.
- ***Look alike–sound alike:*** Don't confuse aspirin with Asendin or Afrin.

PATIENT TEACHING

- Tell patient who's allergic to tartrazine to avoid aspirin.
- Advise patient on a low-salt diet that 1 tablet of buffered aspirin contains 553 mg of sodium.

- Advise patient to take drug with food, milk, antacid, or large glass of water to reduce GI reactions.
- Tell patient not to crush or chew sustained-release or enteric-coated forms but to swallow them whole.
- Instruct patient to discard aspirin tablets that have a strong vinegar-like odor.
- Tell patient to consult prescriber if giving drug to children for longer than 5 days or adults for longer than 10 days.
- Advise patient receiving prolonged treatment with large doses of aspirin to watch for small, round, red pinprick spots, bleeding gums, and signs of GI bleeding, and to drink plenty of fluids. Encourage use of a soft-bristled toothbrush.
- Because of the many drug interactions with aspirin, warn patient taking prescription drugs to check with prescriber or pharmacist before taking aspirin or OTC products containing aspirin.
- Ibuprofen can interfere with the antiplatelet effect of low-dose aspirin therapy, negating its effect. Tell patient how to safely use ibuprofen in relation to aspirin therapy.
- Urge pregnant woman to avoid aspirin during last trimester of pregnancy unless specifically directed by prescriber.
- Drug is a leading cause of poisoning in children. Caution parents to keep drug out of reach of children. Encourage use of child-resistant containers.

SAFETY ALERT!

atenolol
a-TEN-o-loll

Tenormin

Pharmacologic class: beta blocker
Pregnancy risk category D

AVAILABLE FORMS
Injection: 5 mg/10 ml
Tablets: 25 mg, 50 mg, 100 mg

INDICATIONS & DOSAGES
➤ Hypertension
Adults: Initially, 50 mg P.O. daily alone or in combination with a diuretic as a single dose, increased to 100 mg once daily after 7 to 14 days. Dosages of more than 100 mg daily are unlikely to produce further benefit.

➤ Angina pectoris
Adults: 50 mg P.O. once daily, increased as needed to 100 mg daily after 7 days for optimal effect. Maximum, 200 mg daily.

➤ Acute MI
Adults: 5 mg I.V. over 5 minutes; then another 5 mg after 10 minutes. After another 10 minutes, if patient tolerates the full 10-mg I.V. dose, give 50 mg P.O.; then give another 50 mg P.O. in 12 hours. Subsequently, give 100 mg P.O. daily (as a single dose or 50 mg b.i.d.) for 6 to 9 days or until discharged.

➤ Migraine prophylaxis ♦
Adults: 100 mg P.O. daily.

➤ Unstable angina ♦, non–ST-segment elevation MI in patients at high risk for ischemic events ♦
Adults: Initially, 5 mg I.V. over 2 to 5 minutes, repeat every 5 minutes to maximum of 10 mg. Start oral therapy 1 to 2 hours after last I.V. dose at 50 to 100 mg P.O. daily. Maintenance dose, 50 to 200 mg daily.

Adjust-a-dose: If creatinine clearance is 15 to 35 ml/minute, maximum dose is 50 mg daily; if clearance is below 15 ml/minute, maximum dose is 25 mg daily. Hemodialysis patients need 25 to 50 mg after each dialysis session.

ADMINISTRATION
P.O.
- Check apical pulse before giving drug; if slower than 60 beats/minute, withhold drug and call prescriber.
- Give drug exactly as prescribed, at the same time each day.

I.V.
- Check apical pulse before giving drug; if slower than 60 beats/minute, withhold drug and call prescriber.
- Drug may be mixed with D_5W, normal saline solution, or dextrose and saline solution.
- Give by slow I.V. injection, not exceeding 1 mg/minute.
- Solution is stable for 48 hours after mixing.
- **Incompatibilities:** Other I.V. drugs.

ACTION

Selectively blocks $beta_1$ beta-adrenergic receptors, decreases cardiac output and cardiac oxygen consumption, and depresses renin secretion.

Route	Onset	Peak	Duration
P.O.	1 hr	2–4 hr	24 hr
I.V.	5 min	5 min	12 hr

Half-life: 6 to 7 hours.

ADVERSE REACTIONS

CNS: *dizziness, fatigue,* lethargy, vertigo, drowsiness, fever.
CV: *hypotension,* ***bradycardia, heart failure,*** intermittent claudication.
GI: nausea, diarrhea.
Musculoskeletal: leg pain.
Respiratory: ***bronchospasm,*** dyspnea.
Skin: rash.

INTERACTIONS

Drug-drug. *Amiodarone:* May increase risk of bradycardia, AV block, and myocardial depression. Monitor ECG and vital signs.
Antihypertensives: May increase hypotensive effect. Use together cautiously.
Calcium channel blockers, hydralazine, methyldopa: May cause additive hypotension and bradycardia. Adjust dosage as needed.
Cardiac glycosides, diltiazem, verapamil: May cause excessive bradycardia and increased depressant effect on myocardium. Use together cautiously.
Clonidine: May exacerbate rebound hypertension if clonidine is withdrawn. Atenolol should be withdrawn before clonidine by several days or added several days after clonidine is stopped.
Dolasetron: May decrease clearance of dolasetron and increase risk of toxicity. Monitor patient for toxicity.
Insulin, oral antidiabetics: May alter dosage requirements in previously stabilized diabetic patient. Observe patient carefully.
I.V. lidocaine: May reduce hepatic metabolism of lidocaine, increasing risk of toxicity. Give bolus doses of lidocaine at a slower rate and monitor lidocaine level closely.
NSAIDs: May decrease antihypertensive effects. Monitor blood pressure.
Prazosin: May increase the risk of orthostatic hypotension in the early phases of use together. Help patient stand slowly until effects are known.
Reserpine: May cause hypotension or marked bradycardia. Use together cautiously.

EFFECTS ON LAB TEST RESULTS

- May increase alkaline phosphatase, BUN, creatinine, glucose, LDH, potassium, transaminase, and uric acid levels. May decrease glucose level.
- May increase platelet count.

CONTRAINDICATIONS & CAUTIONS

- Contraindicated in patients with sinus bradycardia, heart block greater than first degree, overt cardiac failure, untreated pheochromocytoma, or cardiogenic shock.
- Use cautiously in patients at risk for heart failure and in those with bronchospastic disease, diabetes, hyperthyroidism, and impaired renal or hepatic function.

NURSING CONSIDERATIONS

- Monitor patient's blood pressure.
- Monitor hemodialysis patients closely because of hypotension risk.
- Beta blockers may mask tachycardia caused by hyperthyroidism. In patients with suspected thyrotoxicosis, withdraw beta blocker gradually to avoid thyroid storm.
- Drug may mask signs and symptoms of hypoglycemia in diabetic patients.
- Drug may cause changes in exercise tolerance and ECG.
- ***Alert:*** Withdraw drug gradually over 2 weeks to avoid serious adverse reactions.
- ***Look alike–sound alike:*** Don't confuse atenolol with timolol or albuterol.

PATIENT TEACHING

- Instruct patient to take drug exactly as prescribed, at the same time every day.
- Caution patient not to stop drug suddenly, but to notify prescriber if unpleasant adverse reactions occur.

• Teach patient how to take his pulse. Tell him to withhold drug and call prescriber if pulse rate is below 60 beats/minute.
• Tell woman of childbearing age to notify prescriber about planned, suspected, or known pregnancy. Drug will need to be stopped.
• Advise breast-feeding mother to contact prescriber; drug isn't recommended for breast-feeding women.

atorvastatin calcium

ah-TOR-va-stah-tin

Lipitor

Pharmacologic class: HMG-CoA reductase inhibitor
Pregnancy risk category X

AVAILABLE FORMS

Tablets: 10 mg, 20 mg, 40 mg, 80 mg

INDICATIONS & DOSAGES

✳*NEW INDICATION:* **In patients with clinically evident coronary heart disease, to reduce the risk of nonfatal MI, fatal and nonfatal strokes, angina, heart failure, and revascularization procedures**
Adults: Initially, 10 to 20 mg P.O. daily. May increase based on patient response and tolerance; usual dosage, 10 to 80 mg P.O. daily.

➤ **To reduce the risk of MI, stroke, angina, or revascularization procedures in patients with multiple risk factors for CAD but who don't yet have the disease**
Adults: 10 mg P.O. daily.

➤ **Adjunct to diet to reduce LDL, total cholesterol, apolipoprotein B, and triglyceride levels and to increase HDL levels in patients with primary hypercholesterolemia (heterozygous familial and nonfamilial) and mixed dyslipidemia (Fredrickson types IIa and IIb); adjunct to diet to reduce triglyceride level (Fredrickson type IV); primary dysbetalipoproteinemia (Fredrickson type III) in patients who don't respond adequately to diet**
Adults: Initially, 10 or 20 mg P.O. once daily. Patient who requires a reduction of more than 45% in LDL level may be started at 40 mg once daily. Increase dose, as needed, to maximum of 80 mg daily as single dose. Dosage based on lipid levels drawn within 2 to 4 weeks of starting therapy and after dosage adjustment.

➤ **Alone or as an adjunct to lipid-lowering treatments, such as LDL apheresis, to reduce total and LDL cholesterol in patients with homozygous familial hypercholesterolemia**
Adults: 10 to 80 mg P.O. once daily.

➤ **Heterozygous familial hypercholesterolemia**
Children ages 10 to 17 (girls should be 1 year postmenarche): Initially, 10 mg P.O. once daily. Adjustment intervals should be at least 4 weeks. Maximum daily dose is 20 mg.

ADMINISTRATION

P.O.
• Give drug without regard for meals.

ACTION

Inhibits HMG-CoA reductase, an early (and rate-limiting) step in cholesterol biosynthesis.

Route	Onset	Peak	Duration
P.O.	Unknown	1–2 hr	Unknown

Half-life: 14 hours.

ADVERSE REACTIONS

CNS: *headache,* asthenia, insomnia.
CV: peripheral edema.
EENT: pharyngitis, rhinitis, sinusitis.
GI: abdominal pain, constipation, diarrhea, dyspepsia, flatulence, nausea.
GU: UTI.
Musculoskeletal: ***rhabdomyolysis,*** arthritis, arthralgia, myalgia.
Respiratory: bronchitis.
Skin: rash.
Other: allergic reactions, flulike syndrome, infection.

INTERACTIONS

Drug-drug. *Antacids, cholestyramine, colestipol:* May decrease atorvastatin level. Separate administration times.

Cyclosporine, diltiazem, *fibric acid derivatives,* ***macrolides (azithromycin, clarithromycin, erythromycin, telithromycin), nefazodone,*** *niacin, protease inhibitors,* ***verapamil:*** May decrease metabolism of HMG-CoA reductase inhibitors, increasing toxicity. Monitor patient for adverse effects and report unexplained muscle pain.
Digoxin: May increase digoxin level. Monitor digoxin level and patient for evidence of toxicity.
Fluconazole, itraconazole, ketoconazole, voriconazole: May increase atorvastatin level and adverse effects. Avoid using together; or if unavoidable, reduce dose of atorvastatin.
Hormonal contraceptives: May increase norethindrone and ethinyl estradiol levels. Consider increased drug levels when selecting an oral contraceptive.
Drug-herb. *Eucalyptus, jin bu huan, kava:* May increase risk of hepatotoxicity. Discourage use together.
Red yeast rice: May increase risk of adverse reactions because herb contains compounds similar to those in drug. Discourage use together.
Drug-food. *Grapefruit juice:* May increase drug levels, increasing risk of adverse reactions. Discourage use together.

EFFECTS ON LAB TEST RESULTS

- May increase ALT, AST, and CK levels.

CONTRAINDICATIONS & CAUTIONS

- Contraindicated in patients hypersensitive to drug and in those with active liver disease or unexplained persistent elevations of transaminase levels.
- Contraindicated in pregnant and breast-feeding women and in women of childbearing age.
- Use cautiously in patients with history of liver disease or heavy alcohol use.
- Withhold or stop drug in patients at risk for renal failure caused by rhabdomyolysis resulting from trauma; in serious, acute conditions that suggest myopathy; and in major surgery, severe acute infection, hypotension, uncontrolled seizures, or severe metabolic, endocrine, or electrolyte disorders.
- Limit use in children to those older than age 9 with homozygous familial hypercholesterolemia.

NURSING CONSIDERATIONS

- Patient should follow a standard cholesterol-lowering diet before and during therapy.
- Before treatment, assess patient for underlying causes for hypercholesterolemia and obtain a baseline lipid profile. Obtain periodic liver function test results and lipid levels before starting treatment and at 6 and 12 weeks after initiation, or after an increase in dosage and periodically thereafter.
- Watch for signs of myositis.
- ***Look alike–sound alike:*** Don't confuse Lipitor with Levatol.

PATIENT TEACHING

- Teach patient about proper dietary management, weight control, and exercise. Explain their importance in controlling high fat levels.
- Warn patient to avoid alcohol.
- Tell patient to inform prescriber of adverse reactions, such as muscle pain, malaise, and fever.
- Advise patient that drug can be taken at any time of day, without regard for meals.
- ***Alert:*** Tell woman to stop drug and notify prescriber immediately if she is or may be pregnant or if she's breast-feeding.

SAFETY ALERT!

atropine sulfate

AT-troe-peen

AtroPen, Sal-Tropine

Pharmacologic class: anticholinergic, belladonna alkaloid
Pregnancy risk category C

AVAILABLE FORMS

Injection: 0.05 mg/ml, 0.1 mg/ml, 0.3 mg/ml, 0.4 mg/ml, 0.5 mg/ml, 0.8 mg/ml, 1 mg/ml
Prefilled auto-injectors: 0.5 mg, 1 mg, 2 mg
Tablets: 0.4 mg

INDICATIONS & DOSAGES

➤ Symptomatic bradycardia, bradyarrhythmia (junctional or escape rhythm)
Adults: Usually 0.5 to 1 mg I.V. push, repeated every 3 to 5 minutes to maximum of 2 mg p.r.n.
Children and adolescents: 0.02 mg/kg I.V., with minimum dose of 0.1 mg and maximum single dose of 0.5 mg in children or 1 mg in adolescents. May repeat dose at 5-minute intervals to a maximum total dose of 1 mg in children or 2 mg in adolescents.

➤ Antidote for anticholinesterase-insecticide poisoning
Adults: Initially, 1 to 2 mg I.V.; may repeat with 2 mg I.M. or I.V. every 5 to 60 minutes until muscarinic signs and symptoms disappear or signs of atropine toxicity appear. Severe poisoning may require up to 6 mg hourly.
Children: 0.05 mg/kg I.V. or I.M. repeated every 10 to 30 minutes until muscarinic signs and symptoms disappear (may be repeated if they reappear) or until atropine toxicity occurs.

➤ Preoperatively to diminish secretions and block cardiac vagal reflexes
Adults and children who weigh 20 kg (44 lb) or more: 0.4 to 0.6 mg I.V., I.M., or subcutaneously 30 to 60 minutes before anesthesia.
Children who weigh less than 20 kg: 0.01 mg/kg I.V., I.M., or subcutaneously up to maximum dose of 0.4 mg 30 to 60 minutes before anesthesia. May repeat every 4 to 6 hours p.r.n.
Infants who weigh more than 5 kg (11 lb): 0.03 mg/kg every 4 to 6 hours p.r.n.
Infants who weigh 5 kg or less: 0.04 mg/kg every 4 to 6 hours p.r.n.

➤ Adjunct treatment of peptic ulcer disease; functional GI disorders such as irritable bowel syndrome
Adults: 0.4 to 0.6 mg P.O. every 4 to 6 hours.

ADMINISTRATION

P.O.
- Give drug without regard for food.

I.V.
- Give into a large vein or into I.V. tubing over at least 1 minute.
- Slow delivery may cause slowing of the heart rate.
- **Incompatibilities:** Alkalies, bromides, iodides, isoproterenol, methohexital, norepinephrine, pentobarbital sodium, sodium bicarbonate.

I.M.
- Document administration site.

Subcutaneous
- Auto-injection may be given through clothing.
- Firmly jab tip into outer thigh at 90-degree angle.
- Hold auto-injector in place for at least 10 seconds to allow time for complete administration.
- Make sure needle is visible after removing auto-injector. If needle didn't engage, repeat injection, jabbing more firmly.
- Massage injection site for several seconds after removing auto-injector.
- In very thin or young patients, pinch the skin on the thigh together before injection.

ACTION

Inhibits acetylcholine at parasympathetic neuroeffector junction, blocking vagal effects on SA and AV nodes, enhancing conduction through AV node and increasing heart rate.

Route	Onset	Peak	Duration
P.O.	30–120 min	1–2 hr	4 hr
I.V.	Immediate	2–4 min	4 hr
I.M.	5–40 min	20–60 min	4 hr
Subcut.	Unknown	Unknown	Unknown

Half-life: Initial, 2 hours; second phase, 12½ hours.

ADVERSE REACTIONS

CNS: *headache, restlessness, insomnia, dizziness,* ataxia, disorientation, hallucinations, delirium, excitement, agitation, confusion.
CV: ***bradycardia,*** palpitations, tachycardia.
EENT: *blurred vision, mydriasis,* photophobia, cycloplegia, increased intraocular pressure.

GI: *dry mouth, constipation,* thirst, nausea, vomiting.
GU: urine retention, impotence.
Other: ***anaphylaxis.***

INTERACTIONS
Drug-drug. *Antacids:* May decrease absorption of oral anticholinergics. Separate doses by at least 1 hour.
Anticholinergics, drugs with anticholinergic effects (amantadine, antiarrhythmics, antiparkinsonians, glutethimide, meperidine, phenothiazines, tricyclic antidepressants): May increase anticholinergic effects. Use together cautiously.
Ketoconazole, levodopa: May decrease absorption of these drugs. Separate doses by at least 2 hours, and monitor patient for clinical effect.
Potassium chloride wax-matrix tablets: May increase risk of mucosal lesions. Use together cautiously.
Drug-herb. *Jaborandi tree, pill-bearing spurge:* May decrease effectiveness of drug. Discourage use together.
Jimsonweed: May adversely affect CV function. Discourage use together.
Squaw vine: Tannic acid may decrease metabolic breakdown of drug. Monitor patient.

EFFECTS ON LAB TEST RESULTS
None reported.

CONTRAINDICATIONS & CAUTIONS
- Contraindicated in patients hypersensitive to drug.
- Contraindicated in those with acute angle-closure glaucoma, obstructive uropathy, obstructive disease of GI tract, paralytic ileus, toxic megacolon, intestinal atony, unstable CV status in acute hemorrhage, tachycardia, myocardial ischemia, asthma, or myasthenia gravis.
- Use cautiously in patients with Down syndrome because they may be more sensitive to drug.

NURSING CONSIDERATIONS
- In adults, avoid doses less than 0.5 mg because of risk of paradoxical bradycardia.
- ***Alert:*** Watch for tachycardia in cardiac patients because it may lead to ventricular fibrillation.
- Many adverse reactions (such as dry mouth and constipation) vary with dose.
- Monitor fluid intake and urine output. Drug causes urine retention and urinary hesitancy.

PATIENT TEACHING
- Teach patient receiving oral form of drug how to handle distressing anticholinergic effects such as dry mouth.
- Instruct patient to report serious or persistent adverse reactions promptly.
- Tell patient about potential for sensitivity of the eyes to the sun and suggest use of sunglasses.

benazepril hydrochloride
ben-A-za-pril

Lotensin

Pharmacologic class: ACE inhibitor
Pregnancy risk category C; D in 2nd and 3rd trimesters

AVAILABLE FORMS
Tablets: 5 mg, 10 mg, 20 mg, 40 mg

INDICATIONS & DOSAGES
➤ **Hypertension**
Adults: For patients not receiving a diuretic, 10 mg P.O. daily initially. Adjust dosage as needed and tolerated; usually 20 to 40 mg daily in one or two divided doses. For patients receiving a diuretic, 5 mg P.O. daily initially.
Children age 6 and older: 0.2 mg/kg (up to 10 mg) P.O. daily. Adjust as needed up to 0.6 mg/kg (maximum 40 mg) P.O. daily.
Adjust-a-dose: If creatinine clearance is below 30 ml/minute, give 5 mg P.O. daily. Daily dose may be adjusted up to 40 mg.

ADMINISTRATION
P.O.
- Request oral suspension for patients who can't swallow tablets.

ACTION
Inhibits ACE, preventing conversion of angiotensin I to angiotensin II, a potent vasoconstrictor. Less angiotensin II decreases peripheral arterial resistance,

decreasing aldosterone secretion, which reduces sodium and water retention and lowers blood pressure. Drug also acts as antihypertensive in patients with low-renin hypertension.

Route	Onset	Peak	Duration
P.O.	1 hr	2–4 hr	24 hr

Half-life: benazepril, 0.6 hour.

ADVERSE REACTIONS

CNS: headache, dizziness, drowsiness, fatigue, somnolence.
CV: symptomatic hypotension.
GI: nausea.
GU: impotence.
Metabolic: ***hyperkalemia.***
Musculoskeletal: arthralgia, arthritis, myalgia.
Respiratory: dry, persistent, nonproductive cough.
Skin: increased diaphoresis.
Other: hypersensitivity reactions.

INTERACTIONS

Drug-drug. *Azathioprine:* May increase risk of anemia or leukopenia. Monitor hematologic study results if used together.
Diuretics, other antihypertensives: May cause excessive hypotension. Stop diuretic or lower dosage of benazepril, as needed.
Lithium: May increase lithium level and toxicity. Use together cautiously; monitor lithium level.
Nesiritide: May increase risk of hypotension. Monitor blood pressure.
NSAIDs: May decrease antihypertensive effects. Monitor blood pressure.
Potassium-sparing diuretics, potassium supplements: May cause hyperkalemia. Monitor potassium level and renal function.
Drug-herb. *Capsaicin:* May cause cough. Discourage use together.
Ma huang: May decrease antihypertensive effects. Discourage use together.
Drug-food. *Salt substitutes containing potassium:* May cause hyperkalemia. Monitor potassium level and renal function.

EFFECTS ON LAB TEST RESULTS

- May increase BUN, creatinine, and potassium levels.

CONTRAINDICATIONS & CAUTIONS

- Contraindicated in patients hypersensitive to ACE inhibitors.
- Use cautiously in patients with impaired hepatic or renal function.

NURSING CONSIDERATIONS

- Monitor patient for hypotension. Excessive hypotension can occur when drug is given with diuretics. If possible, diuretic therapy should be stopped 2 to 3 days before starting benazepril to decrease potential for excessive hypotensive response. If drug doesn't adequately control blood pressure, diuretic may be cautiously reinstituted.
- Although ACE inhibitors reduce blood pressure in all races, they reduce it less in blacks taking the ACE inhibitor alone. Black patients should take drug with a thiazide diuretic for a more favorable response.
- Drug may increase risk of angioedema in black patients.
- Measure blood pressure when drug level is at peak (2 to 6 hours after administration) and at trough (just before a dose) to verify adequate blood pressure control.
- Assess renal and hepatic function before and periodically during therapy. Monitor potassium level.
- ***Look alike–sound alike:*** Don't confuse benazepril with Benadryl or Lotensin with Loniten or lovastatin.

PATIENT TEACHING

- Instruct patient to avoid salt substitutes because they may contain potassium, which can cause high potassium level in patients taking drug.
- Inform patient that light-headedness can occur, especially during first few days of therapy. Tell him to rise slowly to minimize this effect and to report dizziness to prescriber. If fainting occurs, he should stop drug and call prescriber immediately.
- Warn patient to use caution in hot weather and during exercise. Inadequate fluid intake, vomiting, diarrhea, and excessive perspiration can lead to light-headedness and fainting.
- Advise patient to report signs of infection, such as fever and sore throat. Tell him to call prescriber if he develops easy

bruising or bleeding; swelling of tongue, lips, face, eyes, mucous membranes, or extremities; difficulty swallowing or breathing; or hoarseness.
• Tell woman of childbearing age to notify prescriber if she becomes pregnant. Drug will need to be stopped.

SAFETY ALERT!

bivalirudin
bye-VAL-ih-roo-din

Angiomax

Pharmacologic class: direct thrombin inhibitor
Pregnancy risk category B

AVAILABLE FORMS
Injection: 250-mg vial

INDICATIONS & DOSAGES
➤ Anticoagulation in patients with unstable angina undergoing percutaneous transluminal coronary angioplasty (PTCA); anticoagulation in patients with unstable angina undergoing percutaneous coronary intervention (PCI), with provisional use of a platelet glycoprotein IIb/IIIa inhibitor (GPI)
Adults: Give 0.75 mg/kg I.V. bolus followed by a continuous infusion of 1.75 mg/kg/hour during the procedure. Check activated clotting time 5 minutes after bolus dose is given. May give additional 0.3 mg/kg bolus dose if needed. Infusion may continue for up to 4 hours after procedure. After 4-hour infusion, may give an additional infusion of 0.2 mg/kg/hour for up to 20 hours, if needed. Use with 300 to 325 mg aspirin.
➤ Patients undergoing PCI who have or are at risk for heparin-induced thrombocytopenia (HIT) or heparin-induced thrombocytopenia and thrombosis syndrome (HITTS)
Adults: 0.75 mg/kg I.V. bolus, followed by a continuous infusion of 1.75 mg/kg/hour throughout the procedure. Consult prescriber about continuing the infusion after PCI.
Adjust-a-dose: For patients with creatinine clearance of 30 ml/minute or less, decrease infusion rate to 1 mg/kg/hour. For patients on hemodialysis, reduce infusion rate to 0.25 mg/kg/hour. No reduction of bolus dose is needed.

ADMINISTRATION
I.V.
• Reconstitute each 250-mg vial with 5 ml of sterile water for injection.
• Dilute each reconstituted vial in 50 ml D_5W or normal saline solution to yield a final concentration of 5 mg/ml.
• To prepare low-rate infusion, further dilute each reconstituted vial in 500 ml D_5W or normal saline solution to yield a final concentration of 0.5 mg/ml.
• Solutions with concentrations of 0.5 to 5 mg/ml are stable at room temperature for 24 hours.
• **Incompatibilities:** Alteplase, amiodarone, amphotericin B, chlorpromazine, diazepam, prochlorperazine, reteplase, streptokinase, vancomycin.

ACTION
Binds specifically and rapidly to thrombin to produce an anticoagulant effect.

Route	Onset	Peak	Duration
I.V.	Rapid	Immediate	1–2 hr

Half-life: 25 minutes in patients with normal renal function.

ADVERSE REACTIONS
CNS: anxiety, *headache,* insomnia, nervousness, fever, *pain.*
CV: ***bradycardia,*** hypertension, *hypotension.*
GI: abdominal pain, dyspepsia, *nausea,* vomiting.
GU: urine retention.
Hematologic: ***severe, spontaneous bleeding (cerebral, retroperitoneal, GU, GI).***
Musculoskeletal: *back pain,* pelvic pain.
Skin: pain at injection site.

INTERACTIONS
Drug-drug. *Heparin, warfarin, other oral anticoagulants:* May increase risk of hemorrhage. Use together cautiously.

Drug-herb. *Angelica (dong quai), boldo, bromelains, capsicum, chamomile, dandelion, danshen, devil's claw, fenugreek, feverfew, garlic, ginger, ginkgo, ginseng, horse chestnut, licorice, meadowsweet, onion, passion flower, red clover, willow:* May increase risk of bleeding. Discourage use together.

EFFECTS ON LAB TEST RESULTS
None reported.

CONTRAINDICATIONS & CAUTIONS
- Contraindicated in patients hypersensitive to drug or its components and in those with active major bleeding. Avoid using in patients with unstable angina who aren't undergoing PTCA or PCI or in patients with other acute coronary syndromes.
- Use cautiously in patients with HIT or HITTS and in those with diseases linked to increased risk of bleeding.
- Use cautiously in breast-feeding women; it's unknown if drug appears in breast milk.

NURSING CONSIDERATIONS
- Monitor coagulation test results, hemoglobin level, and hematocrit before starting therapy and periodically thereafter.
- Circumstances for provisional use of a GPI during PCI include decreased thrombolysis-in-MI, flow; slow reflow; dissection with decreased flow; new or suspected thrombus; persistent residual stenosis; distal embolization; unplanned stent; suboptimal stenting; side-branch closure; abrupt closure; instability; and prolonged ischemia.
- Obtain a complete list of patient's prescription and OTC drugs and supplements, including herbs.
- Hemorrhage can occur at any site in the body. If patient has unexplained decrease in hematocrit, decrease in blood pressure, or other unexplained symptoms, suspect hemorrhage.
- Monitor venipuncture sites for bleeding, hematoma, or inflammation.
- Puncture-site hemorrhage and catheterization-site hematoma may occur in patients age 65 and older more often than in younger patients.
- Don't give drug I.M.

PATIENT TEACHING
- Advise patient that drug can cause bleeding and tell him to report unusual bruising or bleeding (nosebleeds, bleeding gums) or tarry stools immediately.
- Counsel patient that drug is given with aspirin and caution him to avoid other aspirin-containing drugs or NSAIDs while receiving this drug.
- Advise patient to consult with prescriber before initiating any herbal therapy; many herbs have anticoagulant, antiplatelet, and fibrinolytic properties.
- Advise patient to avoid activities that carry a risk of injury, and instruct him to use a soft toothbrush and electric razor while on drug.

bosentan
bow-SEN-tan

Tracleer

Pharmacologic class: endothelin-receptor antagonist
Pregnancy risk category X

AVAILABLE FORMS
Tablets: 62.5 mg, 125 mg

INDICATIONS & DOSAGES
➤ **Pulmonary arterial hypertension in patients with World Health Organization class III (with mild exertion) or IV (at rest) symptoms, to improve exercise ability and decrease rate of clinical worsening**
Adults: 62.5 mg P.O. b.i.d. in the morning and evening for 4 weeks. Increase to maintenance dosage of 125 mg P.O. b.i.d. in the morning and evening.
Adjust-a-dose: For patients who develop ALT and AST abnormalities, the dose may need to be decreased or the therapy stopped until ALT and AST levels return to normal. If therapy is resumed, begin with initial dose. Test levels within 3 days; then give using the table at right. If liver function abnormalities are accompanied by symptoms of liver injury or if bilirubin level is at least twice the upper limit of normal (ULN), stop treatment and don't restart. In patients who weigh less than

40 kg (88 lb), the initial and maintenance dosage is 62.5 mg b.i.d.

ALT and AST levels	Treatment and monitoring recommendations
> 3 and < 5 times upper limit of normal (ULN)	Confirm with repeat test; if confirmed, reduce dose or interrupt treatment and retest every 2 wk. Once ALT and AST levels return to pretreatment levels, continue or reintroduce treatment at starting dose.
> 5 and < 8 times ULN	Confirm with repeat test; if confirmed, stop treatment and retest at least every 2 wk. Once levels return to pretreatment levels, consider reintroduction of treatment.
> 8 times ULN	Stop treatment; don't consider restarting drug.

ADMINISTRATION

P.O.

• Give drug in morning and evening without regard for meals.

ACTION

Specific and competitive antagonist for endothelin-1 (ET-1). ET-1 levels are elevated in patients with pulmonary arterial hypertension, suggesting a pathogenic role for ET-1 in this disease.

Route	Onset	Peak	Duration
P.O.	Unknown	3–5 hr	Unknown

Half-life: About 5 hours.

ADVERSE REACTIONS

CNS: *headache,* fatigue.
CV: edema, flushing, hypotension, palpitations.
EENT: *nasopharyngitis.*
GI: dyspepsia.
Hematologic: *anemia.*
Hepatic: **HEPATOTOXICITY.**
Skin: pruritus.
Other: leg edema.

INTERACTIONS

Drug-drug. ***Cyclosporine A:*** May increase bosentan level and decrease cyclosporine level. Use together is contraindicated.
Glyburide: May increase risk of elevated liver function test values and decrease levels of both drugs. Use together is contraindicated.
Hormonal contraceptives: May cause contraceptive failure. Advise use of an additional method of birth control.
Ketoconazole: May increase bosentan effect. Watch for adverse effects.
Simvastatin, other statins: May decrease levels of these drugs. Monitor cholesterol levels to assess need to adjust statin dose.
Tacrolimus: May increase bosentan levels. Use together cautiously.

EFFECTS ON LAB TEST RESULTS

• May increase liver aminotransferase level. May decrease hemoglobin level and hematocrit.

CONTRAINDICATIONS & CAUTIONS

• Contraindicated in patients hypersensitive to drug, in pregnant patients, and in those taking cyclosporine A or glyburide.
• Generally avoid using in patients with moderate to severe liver impairment or in those with elevated aminotransferase levels greater than three times the ULN.
• Use cautiously in patients with mild liver impairment.
• Drug may harm fetus. Be sure woman isn't pregnant before starting treatment.
• Because it's unknown whether drug appears in breast milk, drug isn't recommended for breast-feeding women.
• Safety and efficacy in children haven't been established.

NURSING CONSIDERATIONS

• Use of this drug can cause serious liver injury. AST and ALT level elevations may be dose dependent and reversible, so measure these levels before treatment and monthly thereafter, adjusting dosage accordingly. If elevations are accompanied by symptoms of liver injury (nausea, vomiting, fever, abdominal pain, jaundice, or unusual lethargy or fatigue) or if bilirubin level increases by greater than twice the ULN, notify prescriber immediately.

• Fluid retention and heart failure may occur. Patient may require diuretics, fluid management, or hospitalization for decompensating heart failure.
• Monitor hemoglobin level after 1 and 3 months of therapy; then every 3 months.
• Gradually reduce dose before stopping drug.

PATIENT TEACHING

• Advise patient to take doses in the morning and evening, with or without food.
• Warn patient to avoid becoming pregnant while taking this drug. Hormonal contraceptives, including oral, implantable, and injectable methods, may not be effective when used with this drug. Advise patient to use a backup method of contraception. A monthly pregnancy test must be performed.
• Advise patient to have liver function tests and blood counts performed regularly.

bumetanide

byoo-MET-a-nide

Bumex

Pharmacologic class: loop diuretic
Pregnancy risk category C

AVAILABLE FORMS

Injection: 0.25 mg/ml
Tablets: 0.5 mg, 1 mg, 2 mg

INDICATIONS & DOSAGES

➤ **Edema caused by heart failure or hepatic or renal disease**
Adults: 0.5 to 2 mg P.O. once daily. If diuretic response isn't adequate, a second or third dose may be given at 4- to 5-hour intervals. Maximum dose is 10 mg daily. May be given parenterally if oral route isn't possible. Usual first dose is 0.5 to 1 mg given I.V. or I.M. If response isn't adequate, a second or third dose may be given at 2- to 3-hour intervals. Maximum, 10 mg daily.

ADMINISTRATION

P.O.
• Give drug with food to minimize GI upset.
• To prevent nocturia, give drug in morning. If second dose is needed, give in early afternoon.

I.V.
• For direct injection, give drug over 1 to 2 minutes using a 21G or 23G needle.
• For intermittent infusion, give diluted drug through an intermittent infusion device or piggyback into an I.V. line containing a free-flowing, compatible solution.
• **Incompatibilities:** Dobutamine, fenoldopam, midazolam.

I.M.
• Document injection site.

ACTION

Inhibits sodium and chloride reabsorption in the ascending loop of Henle.

Route	Onset	Peak	Duration
P.O.	30–60 min	1–2 hr	4–6 hr
I.V.	Within min	15–30 min	30–60 min
I.M.	40 min	Unknown	5–6 hr

Half-life: 1 to 1½ hours.

ADVERSE REACTIONS

CNS: *weakness,* dizziness, headache, vertigo.
CV: orthostatic hypotension, ECG changes, chest pain.
EENT: transient deafness.
GI: nausea, vomiting, upset stomach, dry mouth, diarrhea.
GU: premature ejaculation, difficulty maintaining erection, oliguria.
Hematologic: ***thrombocytopenia,*** azotemia.
Metabolic: volume depletion and dehydration, hypokalemia, hypochloremic alkalosis, ***hypomagnesemia,*** asymptomatic hyperuricemia.
Musculoskeletal: arthritic pain, muscle cramps and pain.
Skin: rash, pruritus, diaphoresis.

INTERACTIONS

Drug-drug. *Aminoglycoside antibiotics:* May increase ototoxicity. Avoid using together if possible.
Antidiabetics: May decrease hypoglycemic effects. Monitor glucose level.
Antihypertensives: May increase hypotensive effects. Consider dosage adjustment.

Cardiac glycosides: May increase risk of digoxin toxicity from bumetanide-induced hypokalemia. Monitor potassium and digoxin levels.
Chlorothiazide, chlorthalidone, hydrochlorothiazide, indapamide, metolazone: May cause excessive diuretic response, causing serious electrolyte abnormalities or dehydration. Adjust doses carefully, and monitor patient closely for signs and symptoms of excessive diuretic response.
Cisplatin: May increase risk of ototoxicity. Monitor patient closely.
Lithium: May decrease lithium clearance, increasing risk of lithium toxicity. Monitor lithium level.
Neuromuscular blockers: May prolong neuromuscular blockade. Monitor patient closely.
NSAIDs, probenecid: May inhibit diuretic response. Use together cautiously.
Other potassium-wasting drugs (such as amphotericin B, corticosteroids): May increase risk of hypokalemia. Use together cautiously.
Warfarin: May increase anticoagulant effect. Use together cautiously.
Drug-herb. *Dandelion:* May interfere with drug activity. Discourage use together.
Licorice: May cause unexpected, rapid potassium loss. Discourage use together.

EFFECTS ON LAB TEST RESULTS

- May increase alkaline phosphatase, ALT, AST, bilirubin, cholesterol, creatinine, glucose, LDH, and urine urea levels. May decrease calcium, magnesium, potassium, sodium, and chloride levels.
- May decrease platelet count.

CONTRAINDICATIONS & CAUTIONS

- Contraindicated in patients hypersensitive to drug or sulfonamides (possible cross-sensitivity) and in patients with anuria, hepatic coma, or severe electrolyte depletion.
- Use cautiously in patients with hepatic cirrhosis and ascites, in elderly patients, and in those with decreased renal function.

NURSING CONSIDERATIONS

- Safest and most effective dosage schedule is alternate days or 3 or 4 consecutive days with 1 or 2 days off between cycles.
- Monitor fluid intake and output, weight, and electrolyte, BUN, creatinine, and carbon dioxide levels frequently.
- Watch for evidence of hypokalemia, such as muscle weakness and cramps. Instruct patient to report these symptoms.
- Consult prescriber and dietitian about a high-potassium diet. Foods rich in potassium include citrus fruits, tomatoes, bananas, dates, and apricots.
- Monitor glucose level in diabetic patients.
- Monitor uric acid level, especially in patients with history of gout.
- Monitor blood pressure and pulse rate during rapid diuresis. Profound water and electrolyte depletion may occur.
- If oliguria or azotemia develops or increases, prescriber may stop drug.
- Drug can be safely used in patients allergic to furosemide; 1 mg of bumetanide equals about 40 mg of furosemide.
- ***Look alike–sound alike:*** Don't confuse Bumex with Buprenex.

PATIENT TEACHING

- Instruct patient to take drug with food to minimize GI upset.
- Advise patient to take drug in morning to avoid need to urinate at night; if patient needs second dose, have him take it in early afternoon.
- Advise patient to avoid sudden posture changes and to rise slowly to avoid dizziness upon standing quickly.
- Instruct patient to notify prescriber about extreme thirst, muscle weakness, cramps, nausea, or dizziness.
- Instruct patient to weigh himself daily to monitor fluid status.

candesartan cilexetil

kan-dah-SAR-tan

Atacand

Pharmacologic class: angiotensin II receptor antagonist
Pregnancy risk category C; D in 2nd and 3rd trimesters

AVAILABLE FORMS

Tablets: 4 mg, 8 mg, 16 mg, 32 mg

INDICATIONS & DOSAGES

➤ Hypertension (used alone or with other antihypertensives)
Adults: Initially, 16 mg P.O. once daily when used alone; usual range is 8 to 32 mg P.O. daily as a single dose or divided b.i.d.

➤ Heart failure
Adults: Initially, 4 mg P.O. once daily. Double the dose about every 2 weeks as tolerated to a target dose of 32 mg once daily.
Adjust-a-dose: If patient takes a diuretic, consider a lower starting dose.

ADMINISTRATION

P.O.

- Give drug without regard for food.

ACTION

Inhibits vasoconstrictive action of angiotensin II by blocking angiotensin II receptor on the surface of vascular smooth muscle and other tissue cells.

Route	Onset	Peak	Duration
P.O.	Unknown	3–4 hr	24 hr

Half-life: 9 hours.

ADVERSE REACTIONS

CNS: dizziness, fatigue, headache.
CV: chest pain, peripheral edema.
EENT: pharyngitis, rhinitis, sinusitis.
GI: abdominal pain, diarrhea, nausea, vomiting.
GU: albuminuria.
Musculoskeletal: arthralgia, back pain.
Respiratory: coughing, bronchitis, upper respiratory tract infection.

INTERACTIONS

Drug-drug. *Lithium:* May increase lithium concentration. Monitor lithium levels closely.
Potassium-sparing diuretics, potassium supplements: May cause hyperkalemia. Monitor patient closely.
Drug-herb. *Ma huang:* May decrease antihypertensive effects. Discourage use together.
Drug-food. *Salt substitutes containing potassium:* May cause hyperkalemia. Monitor patient closely.

EFFECTS ON LAB TEST RESULTS

- May increase potassium, BUN, and serum creatinine levels.

CONTRAINDICATIONS & CAUTIONS

- Contraindicated in patients hypersensitive to drug or its components.
- Use cautiously in patients whose renal function depends on the renin-angiotensin-aldosterone system (such as patients with heart failure) because of risk of oliguria and progressive azotemia with acute renal failure or death.
- Contraindicated in pregnant patients, especially in the second and third trimesters.
- Use cautiously in patients who are volume or salt depleted because they could develop symptoms of hypotension. Start therapy with a lower dosage range, and monitor blood pressure carefully.

NURSING CONSIDERATIONS

- *Alert:* Drugs such as candesartan that act directly on the renin-angiotensin system can cause fetal and neonatal illness and death when given to pregnant women. If pregnancy is suspected, notify prescriber immediately.
- If hypotension occurs after a dose of candesartan, place patient in the supine position and, if needed, give an I.V. infusion of normal saline solution.
- Most of drug's antihypertensive effect occurs within 2 weeks. Maximal effect may take 4 to 6 weeks. Diuretic may be added if blood pressure isn't controlled by drug alone.
- Carefully monitor elderly patients and those with renal disease for therapeutic response and adverse reactions.

PATIENT TEACHING

- Inform woman of childbearing age of the consequences of second and third trimester exposure to drug. Prescriber should be notified immediately if pregnancy is suspected.
- Advise breast-feeding woman of the risk of adverse effects on the infant and the need to stop either breast-feeding or drug.
- Instruct patient to store drug at room temperature and to keep container tightly sealed.
- Inform patient to report adverse reactions without delay.
- Tell patient that drug may be taken without regard to meals.

captopril

KAP-toe-pril

Capoten

Pharmacologic class: ACE inhibitor
Pregnancy risk category C; D in 2nd and 3rd trimesters

AVAILABLE FORMS

Tablets: 12.5 mg, 25 mg, 50 mg, 100 mg

INDICATIONS & DOSAGES

➤ **Hypertension**

Adults: Initially, 25 mg P.O. b.i.d. or t.i.d. If dosage doesn't control blood pressure satisfactorily in 1 or 2 weeks, increase it to 50 mg b.i.d. or t.i.d. If that dosage doesn't control blood pressure satisfactorily after another 1 or 2 weeks, expect to add a diuretic. If patient needs further blood pressure reduction, dosage may be raised to 150 mg t.i.d. while continuing diuretic. Maximum daily dose is 450 mg.

➤ **Diabetic nephropathy**

Adults: 25 mg P.O. t.i.d.

➤ **Heart failure**

Adults: Initially, 25 mg P.O. t.i.d. Patients with normal or low blood pressure who have been vigorously treated with diuretics and who may be hyponatremic or hypovolemic may start with 6.25 or 12.5 mg P.O. t.i.d.; starting dosage may be adjusted over several days. Gradually increase dosage to 50 mg P.O. t.i.d.; once patient reaches this dosage, delay further dosage increases for at least 2 weeks. Maximum dosage is 450 mg daily.
Elderly patients: Initially, 6.25 mg P.O. b.i.d. Increase gradually as needed.

➤ **Left ventricular dysfunction after acute MI**

Adults: Start therapy as early as 3 days after MI with 6.25 mg P.O. for one dose, followed by 12.5 mg P.O. t.i.d. Increase over several days to 25 mg P.O. t.i.d.; then increase to 50 mg P.O. t.i.d. over several weeks.

ADMINISTRATION

P.O.

- Give 1 hour before meals to enhance drug absorption.

ACTION

Inhibits ACE, preventing conversion of angiotensin I to angiotensin II, a potent vasoconstrictor. Less angiotensin II decreases peripheral arterial resistance, decreasing aldosterone secretion, which reduces sodium and water retention and lowers blood pressure.

Route	Onset	Peak	Duration
P.O.	15–60 min	60–90 min	6–12 hr

Half-life: Less than 2 hours.

ADVERSE REACTIONS

CNS: dizziness, fainting, headache, malaise, fatigue, fever.
CV: tachycardia, hypotension, angina pectoris.
GI: abdominal pain, anorexia, constipation, diarrhea, dry mouth, dysgeusia, nausea, vomiting.
Hematologic: ***leukopenia, agranulocytosis, thrombocytopenia, pancytopenia,*** anemia.
Metabolic: hyperkalemia.
Respiratory: *dry, persistent, nonproductive cough,* dyspnea.
Skin: *urticarial rash, maculopapular rash,* pruritus, alopecia.
Other: ***angioedema.***

INTERACTIONS

Drug-drug. *Antacids:* May decrease captopril effect. Separate dosage times.

Digoxin: May increase digoxin level by 15% to 30%. Monitor digoxin level, and observe patient for signs of digoxin toxicity.
Diuretics, other antihypertensives: May cause excessive hypotension. May need to stop diuretic or reduce captopril dosage.
Insulin, oral antidiabetics: May cause hypoglycemia when captopril therapy is started. Monitor patient closely.
Lithium: May increase lithium level; symptoms of toxicity possible. Monitor patient closely.
NSAIDs: May reduce antihypertensive effect. Monitor blood pressure.
Potassium-sparing diuretics, potassium supplements: May cause hyperkalemia. Avoid using together unless hypokalemia is confirmed.
Drug-herb. *Black catechu:* May cause additional hypotensive effect. Discourage use together.
Capsaicin: May worsen cough. Discourage use together.
Drug-food. *Salt substitutes containing potassium:* May cause hyperkalemia. Monitor patient closely.

EFFECTS ON LAB TEST RESULTS
- May increase alkaline phosphatase, bilirubin, and potassium levels. May decrease hemoglobin level and hematocrit.
- May decrease granulocyte, platelet, RBC, and WBC counts.
- May cause false-positive urine acetone test results.

CONTRAINDICATIONS & CAUTIONS
- Contraindicated in patients hypersensitive to drug or other ACE inhibitors.
- Use cautiously in patients with impaired renal function or serious autoimmune disease, especially systemic lupus erythematosus, and in those who have been exposed to other drugs that affect WBC counts or immune response.

NURSING CONSIDERATIONS
- Monitor patient's blood pressure and pulse rate frequently.
- ***Alert:*** Elderly patients may be more sensitive to drug's hypotensive effects.
- Assess patient for signs of angioedema.
- Drug causes the most frequent occurrence of cough, compared with other ACE inhibitors.
- In patients with impaired renal function or collagen vascular disease, monitor WBC and differential counts before starting treatment, every 2 weeks for the first 3 months of therapy, and periodically thereafter.
- ***Look alike–sound alike:*** Don't confuse captopril with Capitrol.

PATIENT TEACHING
- Instruct patient to take drug 1 hour before meals; food in the GI tract may reduce absorption.
- Inform patient that light-headedness is possible, especially during first few days of therapy. Tell him to rise slowly to minimize this effect and to report occurrence to prescriber. If fainting occurs, he should stop drug and call prescriber immediately.
- Tell patient to use caution in hot weather and during exercise. Lack of fluids, vomiting, diarrhea, and excessive perspiration can lead to light-headedness and syncope.
- Advise patient to report signs and symptoms of infection, such as fever and sore throat.
- Tell women to notify prescriber if pregnancy occurs. Drug will need to be stopped.
- Urge patient to promptly report swelling of the face, lips, or mouth or difficulty breathing.

carvedilol
kar-VAH-da-lol

Coreg

carvedilol phosphate
Coreg CR

Pharmacologic class: alpha-nonselective beta blocker
Pregnancy risk category C

AVAILABLE FORMS
Capsules (extended-release): 10 mg, 20 mg, 40 mg, 80 mg
Tablets: 3.125 mg, 6.25 mg, 12.5 mg, 25 mg

INDICATIONS & DOSAGES

➤ Hypertension

Adults: Dosage highly individualized. Initially, 6.25 mg P.O. b.i.d. Measure standing blood pressure 1 hour after first dose. If tolerated, continue dosage for 7 to 14 days. May increase to 12.5 mg P.O. b.i.d. for 7 to 14 days, following same blood pressure monitoring protocol as before. Maximum dose is 25 mg P.O. b.i.d. as tolerated. May be switched to extended-release capsule after controlled on immediate-release tablets.

➤ Left ventricular dysfunction after MI

Adults: Dosage individualized. Start therapy after patient is hemodynamically stable and fluid retention has been minimized. Initially, 6.25 mg P.O. b.i.d. Increase after 3 to 10 days to 12.5 mg b.i.d., then again to a target dose of 25 mg b.i.d. Or start with 3.25 mg b.i.d., or adjust dosage slower if indicated. May be switched to extended-release capsule after controlled on immediate-release tablets.

➤ Mild to severe heart failure

Adults: Dosage highly individualized. Initially, 3.125 mg P.O. b.i.d. for 2 weeks; if tolerated, may increase to 6.25 mg P.O. b.i.d. Dosage may be doubled every 2 weeks, as tolerated. Maximum dose for patients who weigh less than 85 kg (187 lb) is 25 mg P.O. b.i.d.; for those weighing more than 85 kg, dose is 50 mg P.O. b.i.d. May be switched to extended-release capsule after controlled on immediate-release tablets.

Adjust-a-dose: In patient with pulse rate below 55 beats/minute, reduce dosage.

➤ Angina pectoris ♦

Adults: 25 to 50 mg P.O. b.i.d. May be switched to extended-release capsule after controlled on immediate-release tablets.

➤ Idiopathic cardiomyopathy ♦

Adults: 6.25 to 25 mg P.O. b.i.d. May be switched to extended-release capsule after controlled on immediate-release tablets.

ADMINISTRATION

P.O.

- Give drug with food.
- Capsules may be opened, mixed in cool applesauce, and taken immediately; don't store.
- Give capsules in the morning.
- Extended-release equivalent of 3.125 mg immediate-release b.i.d. is 10 mg; 6.25 mg immediate-release b.i.d. is 20 mg; 12.5 mg immediate-release b.i.d. is 40 mg; and 25 mg immediate-release b.i.d. is 80 mg. Dosage may be further titrated based on clinical response.

ACTION

Nonselective beta blocker with alpha-blocking activity.

Route	Onset	Peak	Duration
P.O.	Rapid	1–2 hr	7–10 hr
P.O. (extended-release)	30 min	5 hr	Unknown

Half-life: Immediate release: 7 to 10 hours; extended-release: unknown.

ADVERSE REACTIONS

CNS: *asthenia, dizziness, fatigue,* ***stroke,*** pain, headache, malaise, fever, hypesthesia, paresthesia, vertigo, somnolence, depression, insomnia.

CV: *hypotension, postural hypertension,* ***AV block, bradycardia,*** edema, syncope, angina pectoris, peripheral edema, hypovolemia, fluid overload, hypertension, palpitations, peripheral vascular disorder, chest pain.

EENT: sinusitis, abnormal vision, blurred vision, pharyngitis, rhinitis.

GI: *diarrhea,* vomiting, nausea, melena, periodontitis, abdominal pain, dyspepsia.

GU: impotence, abnormal renal function, albuminuria, hematuria, UTI.

Hematologic: ***thrombocytopenia,*** purpura, anemia.

Metabolic: *hyperglycemia, weight gain,* ***hyperkalemia, hypoglycemia,*** weight loss, hypercholesterolemia, hyperuricemia, hyponatremia, glycosuria, hypervolemia, diabetes mellitus, gout, hypertriglyceridemia.

Musculoskeletal: arthralgia, back pain, muscle cramps, hypotonia, arthritis.

Respiratory: *upper respiratory tract infection,* ***lung edema,*** bronchitis, cough, rales, dyspnea.

Other: *hypersensitivity reactions,* infection, flulike syndrome, viral infection, injury.

INTERACTIONS

Drug-drug. *Amiodarone:* May increase risk of bradycardia, AV block, and myocardial depression. Monitor patient's ECG and vital signs.
Catecholamine-depleting drugs such as MAO inhibitors, reserpine: May cause bradycardia or severe hypotension. Monitor patient closely.
Cimetidine: May increase bioavailability of carvedilol. Monitor vital signs closely.
Clonidine: May increase blood pressure- and heart rate-lowering effects. Monitor vital signs closely.
Cyclosporine: May increase cyclosporine level. Monitor cyclosporine level.
Digoxin: May increase digoxin level by about 15% when given together. Monitor digoxin level.
Diltiazem, verapamil: May cause isolated conduction disturbances. Monitor patient's heart rhythm and blood pressure.
Fluoxetine, paroxetine, propafenone, quinidine: May increase level of carvedilol. Monitor patient for hypotension and dizziness.
Insulin, oral antidiabetics: May enhance hypoglycemic properties. Monitor glucose level.
NSAIDs: May decrease antihypertensive effects. Monitor blood pressure.
Rifampin: May reduce carvedilol level by 70%. Monitor vital signs closely.
Drug-herb. *Ma huang:* May decrease antihypertensive effects. Discourage use together.
Drug-food. *Any food:* May delay rate of absorption of carvedilol with no change in bioavailability. Advise patient to take drug with food to minimize orthostatic effects.

EFFECTS ON LAB TEST RESULTS

- May increase alkaline phosphatase, ALT, AST, BUN, cholesterol, creatinine, GGT, nonprotein nitrogen, potassium, triglyceride, sodium, and uric acid levels. May increase or decrease glucose level.
- May decrease PT and platelet count.

CONTRAINDICATIONS & CAUTIONS

- Contraindicated in patients hypersensitive to drug and in those with New York Heart Association class IV decompensated cardiac failure requiring I.V. inotropic therapy.
- Contraindicated in those with bronchial asthma or related bronchospastic conditions, second- or third-degree AV block, sick sinus syndrome (unless a permanent pacemaker is in place), cardiogenic shock, severe bradycardia, or symptomatic hepatic impairment.
- Use cautiously in hypertensive patients with left-sided heart failure, perioperative patients who receive anesthetics that depress myocardial function (such as cyclopropane and trichloroethylene), and diabetic patients receiving insulin or oral antidiabetics, and in those subject to spontaneous hypoglycemia.
- Use cautiously in patients with thyroid disease (may mask hyperthyroidism; withdrawal may precipitate thyroid storm or exacerbation of hyperthyroidism), pheochromocytoma, Prinzmetal's or variant angina, bronchospastic disease (in those who can't tolerate other antihypertensives), or peripheral vascular disease (may precipitate or aggravate symptoms of arterial insufficiency).
- Use cautiously in breast-feeding women.
- Safety and effectiveness in children younger than age 18 haven't been established.

NURSING CONSIDERATIONS

- ***Alert:*** Patients who have a history of severe anaphylactic reaction to several allergens may be more reactive to repeated challenge (accidental, diagnostic, or therapeutic). They may be unresponsive to dosages of epinephrine typically used to treat allergic reactions.
- Mild hepatocellular injury may occur during therapy. At first sign of hepatic dysfunction, perform tests for hepatic injury or jaundice; if present, stop drug.
- If drug must be stopped, do so gradually over 1 to 2 weeks, if possible.
- Patient should be stable on maximum immediate-release dose before switching to extended-release form.
- Monitor patient with heart failure for worsened condition, renal dysfunction, or fluid retention; diuretics may need to be increased.

- Monitor diabetic patient closely; drug may mask signs of hypoglycemia, or hyperglycemia may be worsened.
- Observe patient for dizziness or lightheadedness for 1 hour after giving each new dose.
- Monitor elderly patients carefully; drug levels are about 50% higher in elderly patients than in younger patients.

PATIENT TEACHING

- Tell patient not to interrupt or stop drug without medical approval.
- Inform patient that improvement of heart failure symptoms might take several weeks of drug therapy.
- Advise patient with heart failure to call prescriber if weight gain or shortness of breath occurs.
- Inform patient that he may experience low blood pressure when standing. If dizziness or fainting occurs (rare), advise him to sit or lie down and to notify prescriber if symptoms persist.
- Caution patient against performing hazardous tasks during start of therapy.
- Advise diabetic patient to promptly report changes in glucose level.
- Inform patient who wears contact lenses that his eyes may feel dry.
- Tell patient to take drug with food. Extended-release capsule may be opened and contents mixed with cool applesauce and taken immediately; don't store.
- Advise patient that capsules shouldn't be crushed, chewed, or contents divided.

chloramphenicol sodium succinate

klor-am-FEN-i-kole

Chloromycetin Sodium Succinate, Pentamycetin†

Pharmacologic class: dichloroacetic acid derivative
Pregnancy risk category C

AVAILABLE FORMS

Injection: 1-g vial

INDICATIONS & DOSAGES

➤ ***Haemophilus influenzae*** **meningitis, acute** ***Salmonella typhi*** **infection, and meningitis, bacteremia, or other severe infections caused by sensitive** ***Salmonella*** **species, rickettsia, lymphogranuloma, psittacosis, or various sensitive gram-negative organisms**

Adults: 50 to 100 mg/kg I.V. daily, divided every 6 hours. Maximum dose is 100 mg/kg daily.

Full-term infants older than age 2 weeks with normal metabolic processes: Up to 50 mg/kg I.V. daily, divided every 6 hours. May use up to 100 mg/kg/day in four divided doses for meningitis.

Premature infants, neonates age 2 weeks and younger, and children and infants with immature metabolic processes: 25 mg/kg I.V. once daily.

ADMINISTRATION

I.V.

- Reconstitute 1-g vial of powder for injection with 10 ml of sterile water to yield 100 mg/ml.
- Give slowly over at least 1 minute.
- Check injection site daily for phlebitis and irritation.
- Solution is stable for 30 days at room temperature, but you should refrigerate it.
- Don't use cloudy solution.
- Obtain specimen for culture and sensitivity tests before giving first dose. Begin therapy while awaiting results.
- **Incompatibilities:** Chlorpromazine, fluconazole, glycopyrrolate, hydroxyzine, metoclopramide, polymyxin B sulfate, prochlorperazine, promethazine, vancomycin.

ACTION

Inhibits bacterial protein synthesis by binding to the 50S subunit of the ribosome; bacteriostatic.

Route	Onset	Peak	Duration
I.V.	Unknown	1–3 hr	Unknown

Half-life: 1½ to 4½ hours.

ADVERSE REACTIONS

CNS: confusion, delirium, headache, mild depression, peripheral neuropathy with prolonged therapy.
EENT: decreased visual acuity, optic neuritis in patients with cystic fibrosis.
GI: diarrhea, enterocolitis, glossitis, nausea, vomiting, stomatitis.
Hematologic: ***aplastic anemia, granulocytopenia, hypoplastic anemia, thrombocytopenia.***
Hepatic: jaundice.
Other: ***anaphylaxis, gray syndrome in neonates,*** hypersensitivity reactions.

INTERACTIONS

Drug-drug. *Anticoagulants, barbiturates, hydantoins, iron salts, sulfonylureas:* May increase levels of these drugs. Monitor patient for toxicity.
Penicillins: May have synergistic or antagonistic effects. Monitor patient for change in effectiveness.
Rifampin: May reduce chloramphenicol level. Monitor patient for changes in effectiveness.
Vitamin B_{12}: May decrease response of vitamin B_{12} in patients with pernicious anemia. Monitor patient closely.

EFFECTS ON LAB TEST RESULTS

- May decrease hemoglobin level.
- May decrease granulocyte and platelet counts.
- May falsely elevate urine PABA levels if given during a bentiromide test for pancreatic function. May cause false-positive results in urine glucose tests that use cupric sulfate (Clinitest).

CONTRAINDICATIONS & CAUTIONS

- Contraindicated in patients hypersensitive to drug.
- Use cautiously in patients with impaired hepatic or renal function, acute intermittent porphyria, and G6PD deficiency.
- Use cautiously in those taking other drugs that cause bone marrow suppression or blood disorders.
- *Alert:* Use cautiously in premature infants and neonates because potentially fatal gray syndrome may occur. Symptoms include abdominal distention, gray cyanosis, vasomotor collapse, respiratory distress, and death within a few hours of symptom onset.

NURSING CONSIDERATIONS

- Obtain drug level measurement; maintain peak level of 10 to 20 mcg/ml and trough level of 5 to 10 mcg/ml.
- *Alert:* Drug has been reported to cause aplastic anemia and other serious blood dyscrasias; use for serious infections only.
- Monitor CBC, iron level, and platelet and reticulocyte counts before and every 2 days during therapy. Stop drug and notify prescriber immediately if anemia, reticulocytopenia, leukopenia, or thrombocytopenia develops.
- Monitor patient for signs and symptoms of superinfection.

PATIENT TEACHING

- Instruct patient to notify prescriber if adverse reactions occur, especially nausea, vomiting, diarrhea, fever, confusion, sore throat, or mouth sores.
- Tell patient receiving drug I.V. to report discomfort at I.V. insertion site.
- Instruct patient to report signs and symptoms of superinfection.

cholestyramine

koe-LESS-tir-a-meen

Prevalite, Questran, Questran Light

Pharmacologic class: bile acid sequestrant
Pregnancy risk category C

AVAILABLE FORMS

Powder: 378-g cans, 9-g single-dose packets; each scoop of powder or single-dose packet contains 4 g of cholestyramine resin

INDICATIONS & DOSAGES

➤ **Primary hyperlipidemia or pruritus caused by partial bile obstruction, adjunct for reduction of increased cholesterol level in patients with primary hypercholesterolemia**

Adults: 4 g once or twice daily. Maintenance dose is 8 to 16 g daily divided into two doses. Maximum daily dose is 24 g. *Children:* 240 mg/kg daily in two to three divided doses, not to exceed 8 g/day.

ADMINISTRATION

P.O.

- Mix thoroughly with 60 to 180 ml of water or other noncarbonated beverage.
- Give drug with a meal.
- Give other drugs 1 hour before or at least 4 hours after cholestyramine to avoid impeding absorption.

ACTION

Binds bile acids in the intestinal tract, impeding their absorption and causing their elimination in feces. In response to this bile acid depletion, LDL cholesterol levels decrease as the liver uses LDL cholesterol to replenish reduced bile acid stores.

Route	Onset	Peak	Duration
P.O.	Unknown	Unknown	2–4 wk

Half-life: Unknown.

ADVERSE REACTIONS

CNS: *dizziness, headache, vertigo,* anxiety, fatigue, insomnia, syncope, tinnitus.
GI: *abdominal discomfort, constipation, fecal impaction, nausea,* anorexia, diarrhea, flatulence, GI bleeding, hemorrhoids, steatorrhea, vomiting.
GU: dysuria, hematuria.
Hematologic: anemia, bleeding tendencies, ecchymoses.
Metabolic: hyperchloremic acidosis.
Musculoskeletal: backache, muscle and joint pains, osteoporosis.
Skin: *rash,* irritation of skin, tongue, and perianal area.
Other: *vitamin A, D, E, and K deficiencies from decreased absorption.*

INTERACTIONS

Drug-drug. *Acetaminophen, beta blockers, cardiac glycosides, corticosteroids, estrogens, fat-soluble vitamins (A, D, E, and K), iron preparations, niacin, penicillin G, phenobarbital, progestins, tetracycline, thiazide diuretics, thyroid hormones, warfarin and other coumarin derivatives:* May decrease absorption of these drugs. Give other drugs 1 hour before or 4 to 6 hours after cholestyramine.

EFFECTS ON LAB TEST RESULTS

- May increase alkaline phosphatase level. May decrease hemoglobin level and hematocrit.
- May increase PT.
- May cause abnormal results in cholecystography that uses iopanoic acid because iopanoic acid is also bound by cholestyramine.

CONTRAINDICATIONS & CAUTIONS

- Contraindicated in patients hypersensitive to bile-acid sequestering resins and in those with complete biliary obstruction.
- Use cautiously in patients predisposed to constipation and in those with conditions aggravated by constipation, such as severe, symptomatic coronary artery disease.

NURSING CONSIDERATIONS

- Monitor cholesterol and triglyceride levels regularly during therapy.
- Monitor levels of cardiac glycosides in patients receiving cardiac glycosides and cholestyramine together. If cholestyramine therapy is stopped, adjust dosage of cardiac glycosides, if necessary, to avoid toxicity.
- Monitor bowel habits. Encourage a diet high in fiber and fluids. If severe constipation develops, decrease dosage, add a stool softener, or stop drug.
- Watch for hyperchloremic acidosis with long-term use or very high doses.
- Long-term use may lead to deficiencies of vitamins A, D, E, and K and folic acid.
- For patients with phenylketonuria, light form contains 28.1 mg of phenylalanine per 6.4-g dose.
- ***Look alike–sound alike:*** Don't confuse Questran with Quarzan.

PATIENT TEACHING

- ***Alert:*** Tell patient never to take drug in its dry form because it may irritate the esophagus or cause severe constipation.
- Tell patient to prepare drug in a large glass containing water, milk, or juice (especially pulpy fruit juice). Tell him to sprinkle powder on the surface of the

beverage, let the mixture stand for a few minutes, and then stir thoroughly. Discourage mixing with carbonated beverages because of excessive foaming. After drinking preparation, patient should swirl a small additional amount of liquid in the same glass and then drink again to make sure he has taken the entire dose.
- Tell patient to avoid sipping or holding the suspension in the mouth because drug may damage tooth surfaces. Advise patient to maintain good oral hygiene.
- Advise patient to take at mealtime, if possible.
- Advise patient to take all other drugs at least 1 hour before or 4 to 6 hours after cholestyramine to avoid blocking their absorption.
- Teach patient about proper dietary management of fats. When appropriate, recommend weight control, exercise, and smoking cessation programs.
- Tell patient that drug may deplete body stores of vitamins A, D, E, and K and folic acid. Patient should discuss need for supplements with prescriber.

cilostazol
sill-AHS-tah-zoll

Pletal

Pharmacologic class: quinolone phosphodiesterase inhibitor
Pregnancy risk category C

AVAILABLE FORMS
Tablets: 50 mg, 100 mg

INDICATIONS & DOSAGES
➤ To reduce symptoms of intermittent claudication
Adults: 100 mg P.O. b.i.d., at least 30 minutes before or 2 hours after breakfast and dinner.
Adjust-a-dose: Decrease dose to 50 mg P.O. b.i.d. when giving with drugs that may interact to cause an increase in cilostazol level.

ADMINISTRATION
P.O.
- Give drug at least 30 minutes before or 2 hours after breakfast and dinner.
- Don't give drug with grapefruit juice.

ACTION
Thought to inhibit the enzyme phosphodiesterase III, thus inhibiting platelet aggregation and causing vasodilation.

Route	Onset	Peak	Duration
P.O.	Unknown	2–4 hr	Unknown

Half-life: 11 to 13 hours.

ADVERSE REACTIONS
CNS: *dizziness, headache,* vertigo.
CV: *palpitations,* peripheral edema, tachycardia.
EENT: *pharyngitis, rhinitis.*
GI: *abnormal stools, diarrhea,* abdominal pain, dyspepsia, flatulence, nausea.
Musculoskeletal: back pain, myalgia.
Respiratory: increased cough.
Other: *infection,* bleeding.

INTERACTIONS
Drug-drug. *Diltiazem:* May increase cilostazol level. Reduce cilostazol dosage to 50 mg b.i.d.
Erythromycin, other macrolides: May increase level of cilostazol and its metabolites. Reduce cilostazol dosage to 50 mg b.i.d.
Omeprazole: May increase level of cilostazol metabolite. Reduce cilostazol dosage to 50 mg b.i.d.
Strong inhibitors of CYP3A4 (such as fluconazole, fluoxetine, fluvoxamine, itraconazole, ketoconazole, miconazole, nefazodone, sertraline): May increase level of cilostazol and its metabolites. Reduce cilostazol dosage to 50 mg b.i.d.
Drug-food. *Grapefruit juice:* May increase drug level. Discourage use together.
Drug-lifestyle. *Smoking:* May decrease drug exposure. Discourage smoking.

EFFECTS ON LAB TEST RESULTS
- May reduce triglyceride levels. May increase HDL level.

CONTRAINDICATIONS & CAUTIONS

- Contraindicated in patients hypersensitive to drug or its components and in those with heart failure of any severity.
- Contraindicated in patients with hemostatic disorders or active bleeding, such as bleeding peptic ulcer and intracranial bleeding.
- Use cautiously in patients with severe underlying heart disease; also use cautiously with other drugs having antiplatelet activity.

NURSING CONSIDERATIONS

- Beneficial effects may not be seen for up to 12 weeks after therapy starts.
- ***Alert:*** Cilostazol and similar drugs that inhibit the enzyme phosphodiesterase decrease the likelihood of survival in patients with class III and IV heart failure.
- ***Alert:*** CV risk is unknown in patients who use drug on long-term basis and in those with severe underlying heart disease.
- Dosage can be reduced or stopped without such rebound effects as platelet hyperaggregation.

PATIENT TEACHING

- Instruct patient to take drug on an empty stomach, at least 30 minutes before or 2 hours after breakfast and dinner.
- Tell patient that beneficial effect of drug on cramping pain isn't likely to be noticed for 2 to 4 weeks and that it may take as long as 12 weeks.
- Advise patient to avoid drinking grapefruit juice during drug therapy.
- Inform patient that CV risk is unknown in patients who use drug on a long-term basis and in those with severe underlying heart disease.
- Tell patient that drug may cause dizziness. Caution patient not to drive or perform other activities that require alertness until response to drug is known.

clindamycin hydrochloride

klin-da-MYE-sin

Cleocin, Dalacin C†

clindamycin palmitate hydrochloride

Cleocin Pediatric, Dalacin C Flavored Granules†

clindamycin phosphate

Cleocin Phosphate, Dalacin C Phosphate Sterile Solution†

Pharmacologic class: lincomycin derivative

Pregnancy risk category B

AVAILABLE FORMS

clindamycin hydrochloride

Capsules: 75 mg, 150 mg, 300 mg

clindamycin palmitate hydrochloride

Granules for oral solution: 75 mg/5 ml

clindamycin phosphate

Injectable infusion (in D_5W): 300 mg (50 ml), 600 mg (50 ml), 900 mg (50 ml)

Injection: 150-mg base/ml, 300-mg base/2 ml, 600-mg base/4 ml, 900-mg base/6 ml

INDICATIONS & DOSAGES

➤ **Infections caused by sensitive staphylococci, streptococci, pneumococci, *Bacteroides, Fusobacterium, Clostridium perfringens,* and other sensitive aerobic and anaerobic organisms**

Adults: 150 to 450 mg P.O. every 6 hours; or 300 to 600 mg I.M. or I.V. every 6, 8, or 12 hours.

Children older than age 1 month: 8 to 20 mg/kg P.O. daily, in divided doses every 6 or 8 hours; or 15 to 40 mg/kg I.M. or I.V. daily, in divided doses every 6 or 8 hours.

➤ **Pelvic inflammatory disease**

Adults and adolescents: 900 mg I.V. every 8 hours, with gentamicin. Continue at least 48 hours after symptoms improve; then switch to oral clindamycin 450 mg q.i.d. for total of 10 to 14 days or doxycycline 100 mg P.O. every 12 hours for total of 10 to 14 days.

➤ ***Pneumocystis jiroveci (carinii)* pneumonia** ♦
Adults: 600 mg I.V. every 6 hours or 900 mg I.V. every 8 hours, with primaquine.

➤ **CNS toxoplasmosis in AIDS patients, as alternative to sulfonamides with pyrimethamine** ♦
Adults: 1,200 to 2,400 mg/day in divided doses.

ADMINISTRATION

P.O.
- Obtain specimen for culture and sensitivity tests before giving first dose. Begin therapy while awaiting results.
- Give capsule form with a full glass of water to prevent esophageal irritation.
- Don't refrigerate reconstituted oral solution because it will thicken. Drug is stable for 2 weeks at room temperature.

I.V.
- Obtain specimen for culture and sensitivity tests before giving first dose. Begin therapy while awaiting results.
- Never give undiluted as a bolus.
- For infusion, dilute each 300 mg in 50 ml solution and give over 10 to 60 minutes at no more than 30 mg/minute.
- Check site daily for phlebitis and irritation.
- **Incompatibilities:** Allopurinol, aminophylline, ampicillin, azithromycin, barbiturates, calcium gluconate, ceftriaxone, ciprofloxacin hydrochloride, doxapram, filgrastim, fluconazole, gentamicin sulfate with cefazolin sodium, idarubicin, magnesium sulfate, phenytoin sodium, ranitidine, rubber closures such as those on I.V. tubing, tobramycin sulfate.

I.M.
- Obtain specimen for culture and sensitivity tests before giving first dose. Begin therapy while awaiting results.
- Inject deep into muscle. Rotate sites. Don't exceed 600 mg per injection.

ACTION

Inhibits bacterial protein synthesis by binding to the 50S subunit of the ribosome.

Route	Onset	Peak	Duration
P.O.	Unknown	45–60 min	Unknown
I.V.	Immediate	Immediate	Unknown
I.M.	Unknown	3 hr	Unknown

Half-life: 2½ to 3 hours.

ADVERSE REACTIONS

CV: thrombophlebitis.
GI: *nausea, **pseudomembranous colitis,*** abdominal pain, diarrhea, vomiting.
Hematologic: ***thrombocytopenia, transient leukopenia,*** eosinophilia.
Hepatic: jaundice.
Skin: maculopapular rash, urticaria.
Other: ***anaphylaxis.***

INTERACTIONS

Drug-drug. *Erythromycin:* May block access of clindamycin to its site of action. Avoid using together.
Kaolin: May decrease absorption of oral clindamycin. Separate dosage times.
Neuromuscular blockers: May increase neuromuscular blockade. Monitor patient closely.
Drug-food. *Diet foods with sodium cyclamate:* May decrease drug level. Discourage patient from eating these foods.

EFFECTS ON LAB TEST RESULTS

- May increase alkaline phosphatase, AST, and bilirubin levels.
- May increase eosinophil count. May decrease platelet and WBC counts.

CONTRAINDICATIONS & CAUTIONS

- Contraindicated in patients hypersensitive to drug or lincomycin.
- Use cautiously in neonates and patients with renal or hepatic disease, asthma, history of GI disease, or significant allergies.

NURSING CONSIDERATIONS

- I.M. injection may raise CK level in response to muscle irritation.
- Monitor renal, hepatic, and hematopoietic functions during prolonged therapy.
- Observe patient for signs and symptoms of superinfection.
- ***Alert:*** Don't give opioid antidiarrheals to treat drug-induced diarrhea; they may prolong and worsen this condition.

• Drug doesn't penetrate blood-brain barrier.

PATIENT TEACHING
• Advise patient to take capsule form with a full glass of water to prevent esophageal irritation.
• Warn patient that I.M. injection may be painful.
• Tell patient to report discomfort at I.V. insertion site.
• Instruct patient to notify prescriber of adverse reactions (especially diarrhea). Warn him not to treat diarrhea himself because drug may cause life-threatening colitis.

clonidine hydrochloride

KLOE-ni-deen

Catapres, Catapres-TTS, Dixarit†, Duraclon

Pharmacologic class: centrally acting alpha agonist
Pregnancy risk category C

AVAILABLE FORMS
Transdermal: TTS-1 (releases 0.1 mg/24 hours), TTS-2 (releases 0.2 mg/24 hours), TTS-3 (releases 0.3 mg/24 hours)
Injection for epidural use: 100 mcg/ml
Injection for epidural use, concentrate: 500 mcg/ml
Tablets: 0.025 mg†, 0.1 mg, 0.2 mg, 0.3 mg

INDICATIONS & DOSAGES
➤ **Essential and renal hypertension**
Adults and children age 12 and older: Initially, 0.1 mg P.O. b.i.d.; then increased by 0.1 to 0.2 mg daily on a weekly basis. Usual range is 0.2 to 0.6 mg daily in divided doses; infrequently, dosages as high as 2.4 mg daily are used.

Or, apply transdermal patch once every 7 days, starting with 0.1-mg system and adjusted with another 0.1-mg or larger system.

➤ **Severe cancer pain unresponsive to epidural or spinal opiate analgesia or other more conventional methods of analgesia**
Adults: Initially, 30 mcg/hour by continuous epidural infusion. Experience with rates greater than 40 mcg/hour is limited.
Children: Initially, 0.5 mcg/kg/hour by epidural infusion. Dosage should be cautiously adjusted, based on response.
➤ **Pheochromocytoma diagnosis ♦**
Adults: 0.3 mg P.O. for a single dose.
➤ **Migraine prophylaxis ♦**
Adults: 0.025 mg P.O. two to four times daily or up to 0.15 mg P.O. daily in divided doses.
➤ **Dysmenorrhea ♦**
Adults: 0.025 mg P.O. b.i.d. for 14 days before and during menses.
➤ **Vasomotor symptoms of menopause ♦**
Adults: 0.025 to 0.2 mg P.O. b.i.d. or 0.1-mg/24-hour patch applied once every 7 days.
➤ **Opiate dependence ♦**
Adults: Initially, 0.005 or 0.006 mg/kg test dose, followed by 0.017 mg/kg P.O. daily in three or four divided doses for 10 days. Or, initially, 0.1 mg P.O. three or four times daily, with dosage adjusted by 0.1 to 0.2 mg daily. Dosage range is 0.3 to 1.2 mg P.O. daily. Stop drug gradually. Follow protocols.
➤ **Alcohol withdrawal ♦**
Adults: 300 to 600 mcg every 6 hours.
➤ **Smoking cessation ♦**
Adults: Initially, 0.1 mg P.O. b.i.d., beginning on or shortly before the day of smoking cessation. Increase dosage every 7 days by 0.1 mg daily, if needed. Or, 0.1-mg/24-hour transdermal patch applied every 7 days. Therapy should begin on or shortly before the day of smoking cessation. Increase dosage by 0.1 mg/24 hours at weekly intervals, if needed.
➤ **Attention deficit hyperactivity disorder ♦**
Children: Initially, 0.05 mg P.O. at bedtime. May increase dosage cautiously over 2 to 4 weeks. Maintenance dosage is 0.05 to 0.4 mg P.O. daily.

ADMINISTRATION
P.O.
• Give last dose immediately before bedtime.

Transdermal
• Apply patch to nonhairy area of intact skin on upper arm or torso.

ACTION

Unknown. Thought to stimulate alpha$_2$ receptors and inhibit the central vasomotor centers, decreasing sympathetic outflow to the heart, kidneys, and peripheral vasculature, and lowering peripheral vascular resistance, blood pressure, and heart rate.

Route	Onset	Peak	Duration
P.O.	30–60 min	2–4 hr	12–24 hr
Trans-dermal	2–3 days	2–3 days	7–8 days
Epidural	Unknown	30–60 min	Unknown

Half-life: 6 to 20 hours.

ADVERSE REACTIONS

CNS: *drowsiness, dizziness, sedation, weakness,* fatigue, malaise, agitation, depression.
CV: ***bradycardia, severe rebound hypertension,*** orthostatic hypotension.
GI: *constipation, dry mouth,* nausea, vomiting, anorexia.
GU: urine retention, impotence.
Metabolic: weight gain.
Skin: *pruritus, dermatitis with transdermal patch,* rash.
Other: loss of libido.

INTERACTIONS

Drug-drug. *Amitriptyline, amoxapine, clomipramine, desipramine, doxepin, imipramine, nortriptyline, protriptyline, trimipramine:* May cause loss of blood pressure control with life-threatening elevations in blood pressure. Avoid using together.
CNS depressants: May increase CNS depression. Use together cautiously.
Digoxin, verapamil: May cause AV block and severe hypotension. Monitor blood pressure and ECG.
Diuretics, other antihypertensives: May increase hypotensive effect. Monitor patient closely.
Beta blockers: May cause life-threatening hypertension. Closely monitor blood pressure.
Levodopa: May reduce effectiveness of levodopa. Monitor patient.
MAO inhibitors, prazosin: May decrease antihypertensive effect. Use together cautiously.
Propranolol, other beta blockers: May cause paradoxical hypertensive response. Monitor patient carefully.
Drug-herb. *Capsicum:* May reduce antihypertensive effectiveness. Discourage use together.
Ma huang: May decrease antihypertensive effects. Discourage use together.

EFFECTS ON LAB TEST RESULTS

• May decrease urinary excretion of vanillylmandelic acid and catecholamines. May cause a weakly positive Coombs' test result.

CONTRAINDICATIONS & CAUTIONS

• Contraindicated in patients hypersensitive to drug.
• Transdermal form is contraindicated in patients hypersensitive to any component of the adhesive layer of transdermal system.
• Epidural form is contraindicated in patients receiving anticoagulant therapy, in those with bleeding diathesis, in those with an injection site infection, and in those who are hemodynamically unstable or have severe CV disease.
• Use cautiously in patients with severe coronary insufficiency, conduction disturbances, recent MI, cerebrovascular disease, chronic renal failure, or impaired liver function.

NURSING CONSIDERATIONS

• Drug may be given to lower blood pressure rapidly in some hypertensive emergencies.
• Monitor blood pressure and pulse rate frequently. Dosage is usually adjusted to patient's blood pressure and tolerance.
• Elderly patients may be more sensitive than younger ones to drug's hypotensive effects.
• Observe patient for tolerance to drug's therapeutic effects, which may require increased dosage.
• Noticeable antihypertensive effects of transdermal clonidine may take 2 to

3 days. Oral antihypertensive therapy may have to be continued in the interim.
- ***Alert:*** Remove transdermal patch before defibrillation to prevent arcing.
- Stop drug gradually by reducing dosage over 2 to 4 days to avoid rapid rise in blood pressure, agitation, headache, and tremor. When stopping therapy in patients receiving both clonidine and a beta blocker, gradually withdraw the beta blocker several days before gradually stopping clonidine to minimize adverse reactions.
- Don't stop drug before surgery.
- ***Look alike–sound alike:*** Don't confuse clonidine with quinidine or clomiphene; or Catapres with Cetapred or Combipres.
- ***Alert:*** The injection form is for epidural use only.
- The injection form concentrate containing 500 mcg/ml must be diluted before use in normal saline injection to yield 100 mcg/ml.
- When drug is given epidurally, carefully monitor infusion pump, and inspect catheter tubing for obstruction or dislodgment.

PATIENT TEACHING
- Instruct patient to take drug exactly as prescribed.
- Advise patient that stopping drug abruptly may cause severe rebound high blood pressure. Tell him dosage must be reduced gradually over 2 to 4 days, as instructed by prescriber.
- Tell patient to take the last dose immediately before bedtime.
- Reassure patient that the transdermal patch usually remains attached despite showering and other routine daily activities. Instruct him on the use of the adhesive overlay to provide additional skin adherence, if needed. Also tell him to place patch at a different site each week.
- Caution patient that drug may cause drowsiness but that this adverse effect usually diminishes over 4 to 6 weeks.
- Inform patient that dizziness upon standing can be minimized by rising slowly from a sitting or lying position and avoiding sudden position changes.

clopidogrel bisulfate
cloe-PID-oh-grel

Plavix

Pharmacologic class: inhibitor of adenosine diphosphate-induced platelet aggregation
Pregnancy risk category B

AVAILABLE FORMS
Tablets: 75 mg

INDICATIONS & DOSAGES
➤ **To reduce thrombotic events in patients with atherosclerosis documented by recent stroke, MI, or peripheral arterial disease**
Adults: 75 mg P.O. daily.
➤ **To reduce thrombotic events in patients with acute coronary syndrome (unstable angina and non–Q-wave MI), including those receiving drugs and those having percutaneous coronary intervention (with or without stent) or coronary artery bypass graft**
Adults: Initially, a single 300-mg P.O. loading dose; then 75 mg P.O. once daily. Start and continue aspirin (75 to 325 mg once daily) with clopidogrel.
➤ **ST-segment elevation acute MI**
Adults: 75 mg P.O. once daily, with aspirin, with or without thrombolytics. A 300-mg loading dose is optional.

ADMINISTRATION
P.O.
- Give drug without regard to meals.

ACTION
Inhibits the binding of adenosine diphosphate (ADP) to its platelet receptor, impeding ADP-mediated activation and subsequent platelet aggregation, and irreversibly modifies the platelet ADP receptor.

Route	Onset	Peak	Duration
P.O.	2 hr	Unknown	5 days

Half-life: 8 hours.

ADVERSE REACTIONS

CNS: depression, dizziness, fatigue, headache, pain.
CV: edema, hypertension.
EENT: epistaxis, rhinitis.
GI: ***hemorrhage,*** abdominal pain, constipation, diarrhea, dyspepsia, gastritis, ulcers.
GU: UTI.
Hematologic: purpura.
Musculoskeletal: arthralgia.
Respiratory: bronchitis, coughing, dyspnea, upper respiratory tract infection.
Skin: *rash,* pruritus.
Other: flulike syndrome.

INTERACTIONS

Drug-drug. *Aspirin, NSAIDs:* May increase risk of GI bleeding. Monitor patient.
Heparin, warfarin: Safety hasn't been established. Use together cautiously.
Salicylates: May increase the risk of serious bleeding in patients with TIA or ischemic stroke. Avoid use together.
Drug-herb. *Red clover:* May increase risk of bleeding. Discourage use together.

EFFECTS ON LAB TEST RESULTS

- May decrease platelet count.

CONTRAINDICATIONS & CAUTIONS

- Contraindicated in patients hypersensitive to drug or its components and in those with pathologic bleeding (such as peptic ulcer or intracranial hemorrhage).
- Use cautiously in patients at risk for increased bleeding from trauma, surgery, or other pathologic conditions and in those with renal or hepatic impairment.

NURSING CONSIDERATIONS

- Platelet aggregation won't return to normal for at least 5 days after drug has been stopped.
- ***Alert:*** Drug may cause fatal thrombotic thrombocytopenic purpura (thrombocytopenia, hemolytic anemia, neurologic findings, renal dysfunction, and fever) that requires urgent treatment, including plasmapheresis.
- ***Look alike–sound alike:*** Don't confuse Plavix with Paxil.

PATIENT TEACHING

- Advise patient it may take longer than usual to stop bleeding. Tell him to refrain from activities in which trauma and bleeding may occur, and encourage him to wear a seat belt when in a car.
- Instruct patient to notify prescriber if unusual bleeding or bruising occurs.
- Tell patient to inform all health care providers, including dentists, before undergoing procedures or starting new drug therapy, that he is taking drug.
- Inform patient that drug may be taken without regard to meals.

colesevelam hydrochloride

koe-leh-SEVE-eh-lam

WelChol

Pharmacologic class: bile acid sequestrant
Pregnancy risk category B

AVAILABLE FORMS

Tablets: 625 mg

INDICATIONS & DOSAGES

➤ **Adjunct to diet and exercise, either alone or with an HMG-CoA reductase inhibitor, to reduce elevated LDL cholesterol in patients with primary hypercholesterolemia (Fredrickson type IIa)**
Adults: 3 tablets (1,875 mg) P.O. b.i.d. with meals and liquid, or 6 tablets (3,750 mg) once daily with a meal and liquid. Maximum dosage is 7 tablets (4,375 mg) daily.

ADMINISTRATION

P.O.

- Give drug with a meal and plenty of fluids.
- Store tablets at room temperature and protect them from moisture.

ACTION

Binds bile acids in the intestinal tract, impeding their absorption and causing their elimination in feces. In response to this bile acid depletion, LDL cholesterol levels decrease as the liver uses LDL cholesterol to replenish reduced bile acid stores.

Route	Onset	Peak	Duration
P.O.	Unknown	2 wk	Unknown

Half-life: Unknown.

ADVERSE REACTIONS

CNS: *headache,* asthenia, pain.
EENT: pharyngitis, rhinitis, sinusitis.
GI: *constipation, flatulence,* abdominal pain, diarrhea, dyspepsia, nausea.
Musculoskeletal: back pain, myalgia.
Respiratory: increased cough.
Other: *infection,* accidental injury, flulike syndrome.

INTERACTIONS

None reported.

EFFECTS ON LAB TEST RESULTS

None reported.

CONTRAINDICATIONS & CAUTIONS

- Contraindicated in patients hypersensitive to drug or any of its components and in patients with bowel obstruction.
- Use cautiously in patients susceptible to vitamin K or fat-soluble vitamin deficiencies and in patients with swallowing disorders, severe GI motility disorders, or major GI tract surgery.
- Use cautiously in patients with triglyceride levels greater than 300 mg/dl.

NURSING CONSIDERATIONS

- Before starting drug, assess patient for underlying causes of hypercholesterolemia, such as poorly controlled diabetes, hypothyroidism, nephrotic syndrome, dysproteinemias, obstructive liver disease, other drug therapy, and alcoholism.
- Monitor patient's bowel habits. If severe constipation develops, decrease dosage, add a stool softener, or stop drug.
- Monitor the effects of patient's other drugs to identify drug interactions.
- Monitor total and LDL cholesterol and triglyceride levels periodically during therapy.
- Use only when clearly needed in breast-feeding women because it isn't known if drug appears in breast milk.

PATIENT TEACHING

- Instruct patient to take drug with a meal and plenty of fluids.
- Teach patient to monitor bowel habits. Encourage a diet high in fiber and fluids. Instruct patient to notify prescriber promptly if severe constipation develops.
- Encourage patient to follow prescribed diet, exercise, and monitoring of cholesterol and triglyceride levels.
- Tell patient to notify prescriber if she's pregnant or breast-feeding.

SAFETY ALERT!

dalteparin sodium

DAHL-tep-ah-rin

Fragmin

Pharmacologic class:
low–molecular-weight heparin
Pregnancy risk category B

AVAILABLE FORMS

Injection: 2,500 antifactor Xa international units/0.2 ml syringe, 5,000 antifactor Xa international units/0.2 ml syringe, 7,500 antifactor Xa international units/0.3 ml syringe, 10,000 antifactor Xa international units/ml syringe, 10,000 antifactor Xa international units/ml in 9.5-ml multidose vial, 25,000 antifactor Xa international units/ml in 3.8-ml multidose vial. Each multidose vial contains 14 mg/ml of benzyl alcohol.

INDICATIONS & DOSAGES

➤ **To prevent deep vein thrombosis (DVT) in patients undergoing abdominal surgery who are at moderate to high risk for thromboembolic complications**

Adults: 2,500 international units subcutaneously daily, starting 1 to 2 hours before surgery and repeated once daily for 5 to 10 days postoperatively. Or, for patients at high risk, give 5,000 international units subcutaneously the evening before surgery,

then once daily postoperatively for 5 to 10 days.
➤ **To prevent DVT in patients undergoing hip replacement surgery**
Adults: 2,500 international units subcutaneously within 2 hours before surgery and second dose 2,500 international units subcutaneously in the evening after surgery (at least 6 hours after first dose). If surgery is performed in the evening, omit second dose on day of surgery. Starting on first postoperative day, give 5,000 international units subcutaneously once daily for 5 to 10 days. Or, give 5,000 international units subcutaneously on the evening before surgery; then 5,000 international units subcutaneously once daily starting in the evening of surgery for 5 to 10 days postoperatively.
➤ **Unstable angina non–Q-wave MI**
Adults: 120 international units/kg subcutaneously every 12 hours with aspirin (75 to 165 mg daily) P.O., unless contraindicated. Maximum dose, 10,000 international units. Treatment usually lasts 5 to 8 days.
➤ **To prevent DVT in patients at risk for thromboembolic complications because of severely restricted mobility during acute illness**
Adults: 5,000 international units subcutaneously once daily for 12 to 14 days.
✱ ***NEW INDICATION:*** **Symptomatic venous thromboembolism in cancer patients**
Adults: Initially, 200 international units/kg (maximum, 18,000 international units) subcutaneously daily for 30 days; then 150 international units/kg (maximum, 18,000 international units) subcutaneously daily months 2 through 6.
Adjust-a-dose: In patients with platelet count 50,000 to 100,000/mm^3, reduce dose by 2,500 international units until platelet count exceeds 100,000/mm^3. In patients with platelet count less than 50,000/mm^3, stop drug until platelet count exceeds 50,000/mm^3. For patients with creatinine clearance of 30 ml/minute or less, monitor anti-Xa levels to determine appropriate dose. Target anti-Xa range is 0.5 to 1.5 international units/ml. Draw anti-Xa 4 to 6 hours after dose and only after the patient has received three to four doses.

ADMINISTRATION

Subcutaneous

- Before giving injection, obtain complete list of all prescribed and OTC medications, and supplements, including herbs.
- Have patient sit or lie supine when giving drug.
- Injection sites include a U-shaped area around the navel, upper outer side of thigh, and upper outer quadrangle of buttock. Rotate sites daily.
- When area around the navel or thigh is used, use thumb and forefinger to lift up a fold of skin while giving injection.
- Give subcutaneous injection deeply, inserting the entire length of needle at a 45- to 90-degree angle.

ACTION

Enhances inhibition of factor Xa and thrombin by antithrombin.

Route	Onset	Peak	Duration
Subcut.	Unknown	4 hr	Unknown

Half-life: 3 to 5 hours.

ADVERSE REACTIONS

CNS: fever.
GU: hematuria.
Hematologic: ***thrombocytopenia, hemorrhage,*** ecchymoses, bleeding complications.
Skin: pruritus, rash, *hematoma at injection site,* injection site pain.
Other: ***anaphylaxis.***

INTERACTIONS

Drug-drug. *Antiplatelet drugs (aspirin, NSAIDs, clopidogrel, dipyridamole, ticlodipine), oral anticoagulants, thrombolytics:* May increase risk of bleeding. Use together cautiously.
Drug-herb. *Angelica (dong quai), boldo, bromelains, capsicum, chamomile, dandelion, danshen, devil's claw, fenugreek, feverfew, garlic, ginger, ginkgo, ginseng, horse chestnut, licorice, meadowsweet, onion, passion flower, red clover, willow:* May increase risk of bleeding. Discourage use together.

EFFECTS ON LAB TEST RESULTS

- May increase ALT and AST levels.
- May decrease platelet count.

CONTRAINDICATIONS & CAUTIONS

- Contraindicated in patients hypersensitive to drug, heparin, or pork products; in those with active major bleeding; and in those with thrombocytopenia and antiplatelet antibodies in presence of drug.
- Contraindicated in patients with unstable angina or non-Q-wave MI who are undergoing regional anesthesia because of an increased risk of bleeding associated with the dose of dalteparin recommended for these indications.
- Use with caution in patients with history of heparin-induced thrombocytopenia and in patients at increased risk for hemorrhage, such as those with severe uncontrolled hypertension, bacterial endocarditis, congenital or acquired bleeding disorders, active ulceration, angiodysplastic GI disease, or hemorrhagic stroke; also use with caution shortly after brain, spinal, or ophthalmic surgery. Monitor vital signs.
- Use with caution in patients with bleeding diathesis, thrombocytopenia, platelet defects, severe hepatic or renal insufficiency, hypertensive or diabetic retinopathy, or recent GI bleeding.

NURSING CONSIDERATIONS

- ***Alert:*** Patients who have received epidural or spinal anesthesia are at increased risk for developing an epidural or spinal hematoma, which may result in long-term or permanent paralysis. Monitor these patients closely for neurologic impairment.
- DVT is a risk factor in patients who are candidates for therapy, including those older than age 40, those who are obese, those undergoing surgery under general anesthesia lasting longer than 30 minutes, and those who have additional risk factors (such as malignancy or history of DVT or pulmonary embolism).
- Never give drug I.M.
- Don't mix with other injections or infusions unless specific compatibility data support such mixing.
- Multidose vial shouldn't be used in pregnant women because of benzyl alcohol content. Benzyl alcohol has been associated with fatal "gasping syndrome" in premature neonates.
- ***Alert:*** Drug isn't interchangeable (unit for unit) with unfractionated heparin or other low–molecular-weight heparin.
- Periodic, routine CBC and fecal occult blood tests are recommended during therapy. Patients don't need regular monitoring of PT or activated PTT.
- Monitor patient closely for thrombocytopenia.
- Stop drug if a thromboembolic event occurs despite dalteparin prophylaxis. May use alternative therapy, or may have been inadequate dose.
- Obtain a complete list of patient's prescription and OTC drugs and supplements, including herbs.

PATIENT TEACHING

- Instruct patient and family to watch for and report signs of bleeding (bruising and blood in stools).
- Tell patient to avoid OTC drugs containing aspirin or other salicylates unless ordered by prescriber.
- Advise patient to consult with prescriber prior to initiating any herbal therapy; many herbs have anticoagulant, antiplatelet, and fibrinolytic properties.
- Tell patient to use a soft toothbrush and electric razor during treatment.

SAFETY ALERT!

digoxin

di-JOX-in

Digitek, Digoxin, Lanoxicaps, Lanoxin*

Pharmacologic class: cardiac glycoside
Pregnancy risk category C

AVAILABLE FORMS

Capsules: 0.05 mg, 0.1 mg, 0.2 mg
Elixir: 0.05 mg/ml (pediatric)
Injection: 0.05 mg/ml†, 0.1 mg/ml (pediatric), 0.25 mg/ml
Tablets: 0.125 mg, 0.25 mg

INDICATIONS & DOSAGES

➤ Heart failure, paroxysmal supraventricular tachycardia, atrial fibrillation and flutter

Capsules

Adults: For rapid digitalization, give 0.4 to 0.6 mg P.O. initially, followed by 0.1 to 0.3 mg every 6 to 8 hours, as needed and tolerated, for 24 hours. For slow digitalization, give 0.05 to 0.35 mg daily in two divided doses. Therapeutic levels are reached in 7 to 22 days. Maintenance dose is 0.05 to 0.35 mg daily in one or two divided doses.
Children: Digitalizing dose is based on child's age and is given in three or more divided doses over the first 24 hours. First dose is 50% of the total dose; subsequent doses are given as 25% of total dose for two doses every 6 to 8 hours as needed and tolerated.
Children age 10 and older: For rapid digitalization, give 8 to 12 mcg/kg P.O. over 24 hours, divided as described previously. Maintenance dose is 25% to 35% of total digitalizing dose, given daily as a single dose.
Children ages 5 to 10: For rapid digitalization, give 15 to 30 mcg/kg P.O. over 24 hours, divided as described previously. Maintenance dose is 25% to 35% of total digitalizing dose, divided and given in two or three equal portions daily.
Children ages 2 to 5: For rapid digitalization, give 25 to 35 mcg/kg P.O. over 24 hours, divided as described previously. Maintenance dose is 25% to 35% of total digitalizing dose, divided and given in two or three equal portions daily.

Elixir, tablets

Adults: For rapid digitalization, give 0.75 to 1.25 mg P.O. over 24 hours in two or more divided doses every 6 to 8 hours. For slow digitalization, give 0.0625 to 0.5 mg daily. Titrate every 2 weeks as needed. Maintenance dose is 0.0625 to 0.5 mg daily.
Children age 10 and older: 10 to 15 mcg/kg P.O. over 24 hours in two or more divided doses every 6 to 8 hours. Maintenance dose is 25% to 35% of total digitalizing dose.
Children ages 5 to 10: 20 to 35 mcg/kg P.O. over 24 hours in two or more divided doses every 6 to 8 hours. Maintenance dose is 25% to 35% of total digitalizing dose.
Children ages 2 to 5: 30 to 40 mcg/kg P.O. over 24 hours in two or more divided doses every 6 to 8 hours. Maintenance dose is 25% to 35% of total digitalizing dose.
Infants ages 1 month to 2 years: 35 to 60 mcg/kg P.O. over 24 hours in two or more divided doses every 6 to 8 hours. Maintenance dose is 25% to 35% of total digitalizing dose.
Neonates: 25 to 35 mcg/kg P.O. over 24 hours in two or more divided doses every 6 to 8 hours. Maintenance dose is 25% to 35% of total digitalizing dose.
Premature infants: 20 to 30 mcg/kg P.O. over 24 hours in two or more divided doses every 6 to 8 hours. Maintenance dose is 20% to 30% of total digitalizing dose.

Injection

Adults: For rapid digitalization, give 0.4 to 0.6 mg I.V. initially, followed by 0.1 to 0.3 mg I.V. every 6 to 8 hours, as needed and tolerated, for 24 hours. For slow digitalization, give appropriate daily maintenance dose for 7 to 22 days until therapeutic levels are reached. Maintenance dose is 0.075 to 0.35 mg I.V. daily in one or two divided doses.
Children: Digitalizing dose is based on child's age; give in three or more divided doses over the first 24 hours. First dose is 50% of total dose; subsequent doses are given every 6 to 8 hours as needed and tolerated.
Children age 10 and older: For rapid digitalization, give 8 to 12 mcg/kg I.V. over 24 hours, divided as described previously. Maintenance dose is 25% to 35% of total digitalizing dose, given daily as a single dose.
Children ages 5 to 10: For rapid digitalization, give 15 to 30 mcg/kg I.V. over 24 hours, divided as described previously. Maintenance dose is 25% to 35% of total digitalizing dose, divided and given in two or three equal portions daily.
Children ages 2 to 5: For rapid digitalization, give 25 to 35 mcg/kg I.V. over 24 hours, divided as described previously. Maintenance dose is 25% to 35% of total digitalizing dose, divided and given in two or three equal portions daily.

Infants ages 1 month to 2 years: For rapid digitalization, give 30 to 50 mcg/kg I.V. over 24 hours, divided as described previously. Maintenance dose is 25% to 35% of total digitalizing dose, divided and given in two or three equal portions daily.
Neonates: For rapid digitalization, give 20 to 30 mcg/kg I.V. over 24 hours, divided as described previously. Maintenance dose is 25% to 35% of the total digitalizing dose, divided and given in two or three equal portions daily.
Premature infants: For rapid digitalization, give 15 to 25 mcg/kg I.V. over 24 hours, divided as described previously. Maintenance dose is 20% to 30% of the total digitalizing dose, divided and given in two or three equal portions daily.
Adjust-a-dose: For patients with impaired renal function, give smaller loading and maintenance doses; extended dosing intervals may be needed.

ADMINISTRATION

P.O.

- Before giving loading dose, obtain baseline data (heart rate and rhythm, blood pressure, and electrolytes) and ask patient about use of cardiac glycosides within the previous 2 to 3 weeks.
- Before giving drug, take apical-radial pulse for 1 minute. Record and notify prescriber of significant changes (sudden increase or decrease in pulse rate, pulse deficit, irregular beats and, particularly, regularization of a previously irregular rhythm). If these occur, check blood pressure and obtain a 12-lead ECG.

I.V.

- Before giving loading dose, obtain baseline data (heart rate and rhythm, blood pressure, and electrolytes) and ask patient about use of cardiac glycosides within the previous 2 to 3 weeks.
- Before giving drug, take apical-radial pulse for 1 minute. Record and notify prescriber of significant changes (sudden increase or decrease in pulse rate, pulse deficit, irregular beats and, particularly, regularization of a previously irregular rhythm). If these occur, check blood pressure and obtain a 12-lead ECG.
- Dilute fourfold with D_5W, normal saline solution, or sterile water for injection to reduce the chance of precipitation.
- Infuse drug slowly over at least 5 minutes.
- Protect solution from light.
- **Incompatibilities:** Amiodarone, amphotericin B cholesteryl sulfate complex, dobutamine, doxapram, fluconazole, foscarnet, propofol, remifentanil. Mixing with other drugs isn't recommended.

ACTION

Inhibits sodium-potassium–activated adenosine triphosphatase, promoting movement of calcium from extracellular to intracellular cytoplasm and strengthening myocardial contraction. Also acts on CNS to enhance vagal tone, slowing conduction through the SA and AV nodes.

Route	Onset	Peak	Duration
P.O.	30–120 min	2–6 hr	3–4 days
I.V.	5–30 min	1–4 hr	3–4 days

Half-life: 30 to 40 hours.

ADVERSE REACTIONS

CNS: *agitation, fatigue, generalized muscle weakness, hallucinations,* dizziness, headache, malaise, paresthesia, stupor, vertigo.
CV: ***arrhythmias, heart block.***
EENT: blurred vision, diplopia, light flashes, photophobia, yellow-green halos around visual images.
GI: *anorexia, nausea,* diarrhea, vomiting.

INTERACTIONS

Drug-drug. *Amiloride:* May decrease digoxin effect and increase renal clearance of digoxin. Monitor patient for altered digoxin effect.
Amiodarone, *diltiazem, indomethacin, nifedipine,* ***quinidine, verapamil:*** May increase digoxin level. Monitor patient for toxicity.
Amphotericin B, carbenicillin, corticosteroids, ***diuretics (such as chlorthalidone, loop diuretics, metolazone, thiazides),*** *ticarcillin:* May cause hypokalemia, predisposing patient to digitalis toxicity. Monitor potassium level.

Antacids, kaolin-pectin: May decrease absorption of oral digoxin. Separate doses as much as possible.
Antibiotics (azole antifungals, macrolides, telithromycin, tetracyclines), propafenone, ritonavir: May increase risk of toxicity. Monitor patient for toxicity.
Anticholinergics: May increase digoxin absorption of oral digoxin tablets. Monitor drug level and observe for toxicity.
Beta blockers, calcium channel blockers: May have additive effects on AV node conduction causing advanced or complete heart block. Use cautiously.
Cholestyramine, colestipol, metoclopramide: May decrease absorption of oral digoxin. Monitor patient for decreased digoxin level and effect. Give digoxin 1½ hours before or 2 hours after other drugs.
Parenteral calcium, thiazides: May cause hypercalcemia and hypomagnesemia, predisposing patient to digitalis toxicity. Monitor calcium and magnesium levels.
Drug-herb. *Betel palm, Foxglove, fumitory, goldenseal, hawthorn, lily of the valley, motherwort, rue, shepherd's purse:* May increase cardiac effects. Discourage use together.
Gossypol, horsetail, licorice, oleander, Siberian ginseng, squill: May increase toxicity. Monitor patient closely.
Plantain, St. John's wort: May decrease effectiveness of drug. Discourage use together.

EFFECTS ON LAB TEST RESULTS

- May prolong PR interval or depress ST segment.

CONTRAINDICATIONS & CAUTIONS

- Contraindicated in patients hypersensitive to drug and in those with digitalis-induced toxicity, ventricular fibrillation, or ventricular tachycardia unless caused by heart failure.
- Don't use in patients with Wolff-Parkinson-White syndrome unless the conduction accessory pathway has been pharmacologically or surgically disabled.
- Use with extreme caution in elderly patients and in those with acute MI, incomplete AV block, sinus bradycardia, PVCs, chronic constrictive pericarditis, hypertrophic cardiomyopathy, renal insufficiency, severe pulmonary disease, or hypothyroidism.

NURSING CONSIDERATIONS

- Drug-induced arrhythmias may increase the severity of heart failure and hypotension.
- In children, cardiac arrhythmias, including sinus bradycardia, are usually early signs of toxicity.
- Patients with hypothyroidism are extremely sensitive to cardiac glycosides and may need lower doses.
- Loading dose is usually divided over the first 24 hours with about half the loading dose given in the first dose.
- Toxic effects on the heart may be life-threatening and require immediate attention.
- Absorption of digoxin from liquid-filled capsules is superior to absorption from tablets or elixir. Expect dosage reduction of 20% to 25% when changing from tablets or elixir to liquid-filled capsules or parenteral therapy.
- Monitor digoxin level. Therapeutic level ranges from 0.8 to 2 ng/ml. Obtain blood for digoxin level at least 6 to 8 hours after last oral dose, preferably just before next scheduled dose.
- ***Alert:*** Excessively slow pulse rate (60 beats/minute or less) may be a sign of digoxin toxicity. Withhold drug and notify prescriber.
- Monitor potassium level carefully. Take corrective action before hypokalemia occurs. Hyperkalemia may result from digoxin toxicity.
- Reduce drug dose for 1 or 2 days before elective cardioversion. Adjust dosage after cardioversion.
- ***Look alike–sound alike:*** Don't confuse digoxin with doxepin.

PATIENT TEACHING

- Teach patient and a responsible family member about drug action, dosage regimen, how to take pulse, reportable signs, and follow-up care.
- Tell patient to report pulse less than 60 beats/minute or more than 110 beats/minute, or skipped beats or other rhythm changes.

• Instruct patient to report adverse reactions promptly. Nausea, vomiting, diarrhea, appetite loss, and visual disturbances may be indicators of toxicity.
• Encourage patient to eat a consistent amount of potassium-rich foods.
• Tell patient not to substitute one brand for another.
• Advise patient to avoid the use of herbal drugs or to consult his prescriber before taking one.

diltiazem hydrochloride

dil-TYE-a-zem

Apo-Diltiaz†, Cardizem, Cardizem CD, Cardizem LA, Cartia XT, Dilacor XR, Diltia XT, Dilt-XR, Nu-Diltiaz†, Nu-Diltiaz CD†, Taztia XT, Tiazac, Tiazac XC†

Pharmacologic class: calcium channel blocker
Pregnancy risk category C

AVAILABLE FORMS

Capsules (extended-release): 120 mg, 180 mg, 240 mg, 300 mg, 360 mg, 420 mg
Injection: 5 mg/ml in 5-, 10-, 25-ml vials
Powder for injection: 25 mg
Tablets: 30 mg, 60 mg, 90 mg, 120 mg
Tablets (extended-release): 120 mg, 180 mg, 240 mg, 300 mg, 360 mg, 420 mg

INDICATIONS & DOSAGES

➤ To manage Prinzmetal's or variant angina or chronic stable angina pectoris
Adults: 30 mg P.O. q.i.d. before meals and at bedtime. Increase dose gradually to maximum of 360 mg/day divided into three or four doses, as indicated. Or, give 120- or 180-mg extended-release capsule or 180-mg extended-release tablet P.O. once daily. Adjust over a 7- to 14-day period as needed and tolerated up to a maximum dose of 360 mg/day (Cardizem LA), 480 mg/day (Cardizem CD, Cartia XT, Dilacor XR, Dilacor XT), or 540 mg/day (Tiazac).

➤ Hypertension
Adults: 180- to 240-mg extended-release capsule P.O. once daily. Adjust dosage based on patient response to a maximum dose of 480 mg/day. Or, 120 to 240 mg P.O. (Cardizem LA) once daily. Dosage can be adjusted about every 2 weeks to a maximum of 540 mg daily.

➤ Atrial fibrillation or flutter; paroxysmal supraventricular tachycardia
Adults: 0.25 mg/kg I.V. as a bolus injection over 2 minutes. Repeat after 15 minutes if response isn't adequate with a dose of 0.35 mg/kg I.V. over 2 minutes. Follow bolus with continuous I.V. infusion at 5 to 15 mg/hour (for up to 24 hours).

ADMINISTRATION

P.O.
• Don't crush or allow patient to chew extended-release tablets; they should be swallowed whole.
• Tiazac extended-release capsules can be opened and the contents sprinkled onto a spoonful of applesauce. The applesauce must be eaten immediately and without chewing, followed by a glass of cool water.

I.V.
• For 100-mg Cardizem Monovials, reconstitute according to manufacturer's directions.
• For direct injection, you need not dilute the 5 mg/ml injection.
• For continuous infusion, add 25 ml of drug to 100 ml solution, 50 ml of drug to 250 ml solution, or 50 ml of drug to 500 ml solution of 5 mg/ml injection to yield 1 mg/ml, 0.83 mg/ml, or 0.45 mg/ml, respectively. Compatible solutions include normal saline solution, D_5W, or 5% dextrose and half-normal saline solution.
• For direct injection or continuous infusion; give slowly while monitoring ECG and blood pressure continuously.
• Don't infuse for longer than 24 hours.
• **Incompatibilities:** Acetazolamide, acyclovir, aminophylline, ampicillin, ampicillin sodium and sulbactam sodium, cefoperazone, diazepam, furosemide, heparin, hydrocortisone, insulin, methylprednisolone, nafcillin, phenytoin, rifampin, sodium bicarbonate, thiopental.

ACTION

A calcium channel blocker that inhibits calcium ion influx across cardiac and smooth-muscle cells, decreasing myocardial contractility and oxygen demand. Drug also dilates coronary arteries and arterioles.

Route	Onset	Peak	Duration
P.O.	30–60 min	2–3 hr	6–8 hr
P.O. (extended-release capsule)	2–3 hr	10–14 hr	12–24 hr
P.O. (Cardizem LA)	3–4 hr	11–18 hr	6–9 hr
I.V.	< 3 min	2–7 min	1–10 hr

Half-life: 3 to 9 hours.

ADVERSE REACTIONS

CNS: *headache,* dizziness, asthenia, somnolence.
CV: *edema,* ***arrhythmias, AV block, bradycardia, heart failure,*** flushing, hypotension, conduction abnormalities, abnormal ECG.
GI: nausea, constipation, abdominal discomfort.
Hepatic: ***acute hepatic injury.***
Skin: rash.

INTERACTIONS

Drug-drug. *Anesthetics:* May increase effects of anesthetics. Monitor patient.
Carbamazepine: May increase level of carbamazepine. Monitor carbamazepine level, and watch for signs and symptoms of toxicity.
Cimetidine: May inhibit diltiazem metabolism, increasing additive AV node conduction slowing. Monitor patient for toxicity.
Cyclosporine: May increase cyclosporine level, possibly by decreasing its metabolism, leading to increased risk of cyclosporine toxicity. Monitor cyclosporine level with each dosage change.
Diazepam, midazolam, triazolam: May increase CNS depression and prolonged effects of these drugs. Use lower dose of these benzodiazepines.
Digoxin: May increase digoxin level. Monitor patient for digoxin toxicity.
Furosemide: May form a precipitate when mixed with diltiazem injection. Give through separate I.V. lines.
Lithium: May reduce lithium levels, causing loss of mania control, and neurotoxic and psychotic symptoms. Monitor patient for signs of neurotoxicity.
Propranolol, other beta blockers: May precipitate heart failure or prolong conduction time. Use together cautiously.
Sirolimus, tacrolimus: May increase level of these drugs. Monitor drug level and patient for toxicity.
Theophylline: May enhance action of theophylline, causing intoxication. Monitor theophylline levels.

EFFECTS ON LAB TEST RESULTS

None reported.

CONTRAINDICATIONS & CAUTIONS

- Contraindicated in patients hypersensitive to drug and in those with sick sinus syndrome or second- or third-degree AV block in the absence of an artificial pacemaker, cardiogenic shock, ventricular tachycardia, systolic blood pressure below 90 mm Hg, acute MI, or pulmonary congestion (documented by X-ray).
- Contraindicated in I.V. form for patients who have atrial fibrillation or flutter with an accessory bypass tract, as in Wolff-Parkinson-White syndrome or short PR interval syndrome.
- Use cautiously in elderly patients and in those with heart failure or impaired hepatic or renal function.

NURSING CONSIDERATIONS

- Patients controlled on drug alone or with other drugs may be switched to Cardizem LA tablets once a day at the nearest equivalent total daily dose.
- Monitor blood pressure and heart rate when starting therapy and during dosage adjustments.
- Maximal antihypertensive effect may not be seen for 14 days.
- If systolic blood pressure is below 90 mm Hg or heart rate is below 60 beats/minute, withhold dose and notify prescriber.

PATIENT TEACHING

- Instruct patient to take drug as prescribed, even when he feels better.
- Advise patient to avoid hazardous activities during start of therapy.
- If nitrate therapy is prescribed during dosage adjustment, stress patient compliance. Tell patient that S.L. nitroglycerin may be taken with drug, as needed, when angina symptoms are acute.
- ***Alert:*** Tell patient to swallow extended-release tablets whole, and not to crush or chew them.
- If patient is taking Tiazac extended-release capsules, inform him that these capsules can be opened and the contents sprinkled onto a spoonful of applesauce. He must eat the applesauce immediately and without chewing, and then drink a glass of cool water.

dipyridamole

dye-peer-IH-duh-mohl

Persantine

Pharmacologic class: pyrimidine analogue
Pregnancy risk category B

AVAILABLE FORMS

Injection: 5 mg/ml in 2- and 10-ml vials
Tablets: 25 mg, 50 mg, 75 mg

INDICATIONS & DOSAGES

➤ **To inhibit platelet adhesion in prosthetic heart valves (given together with warfarin)**
Adults: 75 to 100 mg P.O. q.i.d.

➤ **Alternative to exercise in evaluation of coronary artery disease (CAD) during thallium myocardial perfusion scintigraphy**
Adults: 0.57 mg/kg as an I.V. infusion at a constant rate over 4 minutes (0.142 mg/kg/minute).

ADMINISTRATION

P.O.

- If GI distress develops, give drug 1 hour before meals or with meals.

I.V.

- For use as a diagnostic drug, dilute in half-normal or normal saline solution or D_5W in at least a 1:2 ratio for a total volume of 20 to 50 ml.
- Inject thallium-201 within 5 minutes after completing the 4-minute dipyridamole infusion.
- Don't mix in same syringe or infusion container with other drugs.
- **Incompatibilities:** Other drugs.

ACTION

May involve drug's ability to increase adenosine, which is a coronary vasodilator and platelet aggregation inhibitor.

Route	Onset	Peak	Duration
P.O.	Unknown	75 min	Unknown
I.V.	Unknown	2 min	Unknown

Half-life: 1 to 12 hours.

ADVERSE REACTIONS

CNS: *dizziness, headache,* syncope.
CV: *angina pectoris, chest pain,* ***ECG abnormalities,*** blood pressure lability, flushing, hypertension, hypotension.
GI: *nausea,* abdominal distress, diarrhea, vomiting.

INTERACTIONS

Drug-drug. *Adenosine:* May increase levels and cardiac effects of adenosine. Adjust adenosine dose as needed.
Cholinesterase inhibitors: May counteract anticholinesterase effects and aggravate myasthenia gravis. Monitor patient.
Heparin: May increase risk of bleeding. Monitor patient closely.
Theophylline: May prevent coronary vasodilation by I.V. dipyridamole, causing a false-negative thallium-imaging result. Avoid using together.

EFFECTS ON LAB TEST RESULTS

- May increase liver enzyme levels.

CONTRAINDICATIONS & CAUTIONS

- Contraindicated in patients hypersensitive to drug.
- Use cautiously in patients with hypotension and those with severe CAD.

NURSING CONSIDERATIONS
• Observe for adverse reactions, especially with large doses. Monitor blood pressure.
• Observe for signs and symptoms of bleeding; note prolonged bleeding time (especially with large doses or long-term therapy).
• The value of drug as part of an antithrombotic regimen is controversial; its use may not provide significantly better results than aspirin alone.
• ***Look alike–sound alike:*** Don't confuse dipyridamole with disopyramide. Don't confuse Persantine with Periactin or Bosentan.
• Persantine may contain tartrazine.

PATIENT TEACHING
• Instruct patient to take drug exactly as prescribed.
• Tell patient to report adverse reactions promptly.
• Tell patient receiving drug I.V. to report discomfort at insertion site.

disopyramide
dye-soe-PEER-a-mide

Rythmodan†

disopyramide phosphate
Norpace, Norpace CR, Rythmodan-LA†

Pharmacologic class: pyridine derivative
Pregnancy risk category C

AVAILABLE FORMS
disopyramide
Capsules: 100 mg†, 150 mg†
disopyramide phosphate
Capsules: 100 mg, 150 mg
Capsules (controlled-release): 100 mg, 150 mg
Tablets (sustained-release): 250 mg†

INDICATIONS & DOSAGES
➤ **Ventricular tachycardia and life-threatening ventricular arrhythmias**
Adults who weigh more than 50 kg (110 lb): 150 mg P.O. every 6 hours with regular-release formulation or 300 mg every 12 hours with extended-release preparations.
Adults who weigh 50 kg or less: 100 mg P.O. every 6 hours with regular-release formulation or 200 mg P.O. every 12 hours with extended-release preparations.
Children ages 12 to 18 years: 6 to 15 mg/kg P.O. daily, divided into four doses (every 6 hours).
Children ages 4 to 12 years: 10 to 15 mg/kg P.O. daily, divided into four doses (every 6 hours).
Children ages 1 to 4 years: 10 to 20 mg/kg P.O. daily, divided into four doses (every 6 hours).
Children younger than age 1 year: 10 to 30 mg/kg P.O. daily, divided into four doses (every 6 hours).
Adjust-a-dose: If creatinine clearance is 30 to 40 ml/minute, give 100 mg every 8 hours; if clearance is 15 to 30 ml/minute, give 100 mg every 12 hours; if clearance is less than 15 ml/minute, give 100 mg every 24 hours. All dosages are for immediate-release form.

Don't use extended-release capsules in patients with a creatinine clearance less than or equal to 40 ml/minute. For patients with creatinine clearance greater than 40 ml/minute or patients with hepatic insufficiency, give 400 mg/day in divided doses (100 mg every 6 hours with immediate-release form or 200 mg every 12 hours with controlled-release form).

ADMINISTRATION
P.O.
• Correct electrolyte abnormalities before starting therapy.
• Check apical pulse before giving drug. Notify prescriber if pulse rate is slower than 60 beats/minute or faster than 120 beats/minute.
• Don't use sustained- or controlled-release preparations to control ventricular arrhythmias when therapeutic drug level must be rapidly attained, in patients with cardiomyopathy or possible cardiac decompensation, or in those with severe renal impairment.
• ***Alert:*** Don't open the extended-release capsules.
• For use in young children, pharmacist may prepare disopyramide suspension

using 100-mg capsules and cherry syrup. Pharmacist should dispense suspension in amber glass bottles. Protect suspension from light.

ACTION

A class IA antiarrhythmic that depresses phase 0, prolongs the action potential, and has membrane-stabilizing effects.

Route	Onset	Peak	Duration
P.O.	½–3½ hr	2–2½ hr	1½ –8½ hr

Half-life: 7 hours.

ADVERSE REACTIONS

CNS: *agitation,* dizziness, depression, fatigue, headache, nervousness, acute psychosis, syncope.
CV: *hypotension,* ***heart failure, heart block, arrhythmias,*** edema, shortness of breath, chest pain.
EENT: blurred vision, dry eyes or nose.
GI: *dry mouth, constipation,* nausea, vomiting, anorexia, bloating, gas, weight gain, abdominal pain, diarrhea.
GU: *urinary hesitancy,* urine retention, urinary frequency, urinary urgency, impotence.
Hepatic: cholestatic jaundice.
Musculoskeletal: muscle weakness, aches, pain.
Skin: rash, pruritus, dermatosis.

INTERACTIONS

Drug-drug. *Antiarrhythmics:* May increase QRS complex or QT interval, which may lead to other arrhythmias. Monitor ECG closely.
Macrolides and related antibiotics (azithromycin, clarithromycin, erythromycin, telithromycin): May prolong the QT interval. Use with caution. Avoid use with telithromycin.
Phenytoin: May increase metabolism of disopyramide. Watch for decreased antiarrhythmic effect.
Quinidine: May increase disopyramide levels and decrease quinidine levels. Monitor patient closely.
Quinolones: May cause life-threatening arrhythmias, including torsades de pointes. Avoid using together.
Rifampin: May decrease disopyramide level. Monitor patient for lack of effect.
Thioridazine: May cause life-threatening arrhythmias, including torsades de pointes. Avoid using together.
Verapamil: May cause additive effects and impairment of left ventricular function. Don't give disopyramide 48 hours before starting verapamil or 24 hours after verapamil is stopped.
Drug-herb. *Jimsonweed:* May adversely affect CV function. Discourage use together.

EFFECTS ON LAB TEST RESULTS

None reported.

CONTRAINDICATIONS & CAUTIONS

- Contraindicated in patients hypersensitive to drug.
- Contraindicated with sparfloxacin, thioridazine, or ziprasidone because of increased risk of life-threatening arrhythmias.
- Contraindicated in those with sick sinus syndrome, cardiogenic shock, congenital QT interval prolongation, or second- or third-degree heart block in the absence of an artificial pacemaker.
- Use cautiously, or avoid if possible, in patients with heart failure.
- Use cautiously in patients with underlying conduction abnormalities, urinary tract diseases (especially prostatic hyperplasia), hepatic or renal impairment, myasthenia gravis, or acute angle-closure glaucoma.

NURSING CONSIDERATIONS

- Digitalize patients with atrial fibrillation or flutter before starting disopyramide because of the risk of enhancing AV conduction.
- Watch for recurrence of arrhythmias and check for adverse reactions; notify prescriber if any occur.
- Stop drug if heart block develops, if QRS complex widens by more than 25%, or if QT interval lengthens by more than 25% above baseline.
- ***Look alike–sound alike:*** Don't confuse disopyramide with desipramine or dipyridamole.

PATIENT TEACHING

- Teach patient importance of taking drug on time and exactly as prescribed.
- If transferring patient from immediate-release to sustained-release capsules, advise him to take the first sustained-release capsule 6 hours after taking the last immediate-release capsule.
- Tell patient not to crush or chew sustained-release capsules or tablets.
- If not contraindicated, advise patient to chew gum or hard candy to relieve dry mouth and to increase fiber and fluid intake to relieve constipation.

SAFETY ALERT!

dobutamine hydrochloride

DOE-byoo-ta-meen

Pharmacologic class: adrenergic, $beta_1$ agonist
Pregnancy risk category B

AVAILABLE FORMS

Injection: 12.5 mg/ml in 20-ml vials (parenteral)
Dobutamine in 5% dextrose: 0.5 mg/ml (125 or 250 mg); 1 mg/ml (250 or 500 mg); 2 mg/ml (500 mg); 4 mg/ml (1,000 mg)

INDICATIONS & DOSAGES

➤ Increased cardiac output in short-term treatment of cardiac decompensation caused by depressed contractility, such as during refractory heart failure; adjunctive therapy in cardiac surgery

Adults: 0.5 to 1 mcg/kg/minute I.V. infusion, titrating to optimum dosage of 2 to 20 mcg/kg/minute. Usual effective range to increase cardiac output is 2.5 to 10 mcg/kg/minute. Rarely, rates up to 40 mcg/kg/minute may be needed.

ADMINISTRATION

I.V.

- Before starting therapy, give a plasma volume expander to correct hypovolemia and a cardiac glycoside.
- Dilute concentrate before injecting. Compatible solutions include D_5W, $D_{10}W$, half-normal or normal saline solution for injection, lactated Ringer's injection, Isolyte-M with D_5W, Normosol-M in D_5W, and 20% Osmitrol.
- Diluting one vial (250 mg) with 1,000 ml of solution yields 250 mcg/ml. Diluting with 500 ml yields 500 mcg/ml. Diluting with 250 ml yields 1,000 mcg/ml.
- Oxidation may slightly discolor admixture. This doesn't indicate a significant loss of potency, provided drug is used within 24 hours of reconstitution.
- Give through a central venous catheter or large peripheral vein using an infusion pump.
- Titrate rate according to patient's condition. Don't exceed 5 mg/ml.
- Infusions lasting up to 72 hours produce no more adverse effects than shorter infusions.
- Watch for irritation and infiltration; extravasation can cause tissue damage and necrosis. Change I.V. sites regularly to avoid phlebitis.
- Solution remains stable for 24 hours. Don't freeze.
- **Incompatibilities:** Acyclovir, alkaline solutions, alteplase, aminophylline, bretylium, bumetanide, calcium chloride, calcium gluconate, cefamandole, cefazolin, cefepime, diazepam, digoxin, ethacrynate, furosemide, heparin, hydrocortisone sodium succinate, indomethacin, insulin, magnesium sulfate, midazolam, penicillin, phenytoin, phytonadione, piperacillin with tazobactam, potassium chloride, sodium bicarbonate, thiopental, verapamil, warfarin. Don't give through same line with other drugs.

ACTION

Stimulates heart's $beta_1$ receptors to increase myocardial contractility and stroke volume. At therapeutic dosages, drug increases cardiac output by decreasing peripheral vascular resistance, reducing ventricular filling pressure, and facilitating AV node conduction.

Route	Onset	Peak	Duration
I.V.	1–2 min	10 min	< 5 min after infusion

Half-life: 2 minutes.

ADVERSE REACTIONS
CNS: headache.
CV: *hypertension, increased heart rate,* angina, PVCs, phlebitis, nonspecific chest pain, palpitations, ventricular ectopy, hypotension.
GI: nausea, vomiting.
Respiratory: ***asthma attack,*** shortness of breath.
Other: ***anaphylaxis,*** hypersensitivity reactions.

INTERACTIONS
Drug-drug. *Beta blockers:* May antagonize dobutamine effects. Avoid using together.
Bretylium: May increase risk of arrhythmias. Monitor ECG.
General anesthetics: May have greater risk of ventricular arrhythmias. Monitor ECG closely.
Guanethidine, oxytocic drugs: May increase pressor response, causing severe hypertension. Monitor blood pressure closely.
Tricyclic antidepressants: May potentiate pressor response and cause arrhythmias. Use together cautiously.
Drug-herb. *Rue:* May increase inotropic potential. Discourage use together.

EFFECTS ON LAB TEST RESULTS
- May decrease potassium level.
- May decrease platelet count.

CONTRAINDICATIONS & CAUTIONS
- Contraindicated in patients hypersensitive to drug or its components and in those with idiopathic hypertrophic subaortic stenosis.
- Use cautiously in patients with history of hypertension because drug may increase pressor response.
- Use cautiously after acute MI.
- Use cautiously in patients with history of sulfite sensitivity.

NURSING CONSIDERATIONS
- Because drug increases AV node conduction, patients with atrial fibrillation may develop a rapid ventricular rate.
- Continuously monitor ECG, blood pressure, pulmonary artery wedge pressure, cardiac output, and urine output.
- Monitor electrolyte levels. Drug may lower potassium level.
- ***Look alike–sound alike:*** Don't confuse dobutamine with dopamine.

PATIENT TEACHING
- Tell patient to report adverse reactions promptly, especially labored breathing and drug-induced headache.
- Instruct patient to report discomfort at I.V. insertion site.

dofetilide
doe-FE-ti-lyed

Tikosyn

Pharmacologic class: antiarrhythmic
Pregnancy risk category C

AVAILABLE FORMS
Capsules: 125 mcg, 250 mcg, 500 mcg

INDICATIONS & DOSAGES
➤ **To maintain normal sinus rhythm in patients with symptomatic atrial fibrillation or atrial flutter lasting longer than 1 week who have been converted to normal sinus rhythm; to convert atrial fibrillation and atrial flutter to normal sinus rhythm**
Adults: Individualized dosage based on creatinine clearance and baseline QTc interval (or QT interval if heart rate is below 60 beats/minute), determined before first dose; usually 500 mcg P.O. b.i.d. for patients with creatinine clearance greater than 60 ml/minute.
Adjust-a-dose: If creatinine clearance is 40 to 60 ml/minute, starting dose is 250 mcg P.O. b.i.d.; if clearance is 20 to 39 ml/minute, starting dose is 125 mcg P.O. b.i.d. Don't use drug at all if clearance is less than 20 ml/minute.

Determine QTc interval 2 to 3 hours after first dose. If QTc interval has increased by more than 15% above baseline or if it's more than 500 msec (550 msec in patients with ventricular conduction abnormalities), adjust dosage as follows: If starting dose based on creatinine clearance was 500 mcg P.O. b.i.d., give 250 mcg P.O. b.i.d. If starting dose based on clearance was 250 mcg b.i.d., give 125 mcg b.i.d. If starting dose based on clearance was 125 mcg b.i.d., give 125 mcg once a day.

Determine QTc interval 2 to 3 hours after each subsequent dose while patient is in hospital. If at any time after second dose the QTc interval exceeds 500 msec (550 msec in patients with ventricular conduction abnormalities), stop drug.

ADMINISTRATION

P.O.

- Give drug without regard for food or antacid administration.
- Don't give drug with grapefruit juice.

ACTION

Prolongs repolarization without affecting conduction velocity. Drug doesn't affect sodium channels, alpha-adrenergic receptors, or beta-adrenergic receptors.

Route	Onset	Peak	Duration
P.O.	Unknown	2–3 hr	Unknown

Half-life: 10 hours.

ADVERSE REACTIONS

CNS: *headache,* ***stroke,*** dizziness, insomnia, anxiety, migraine, cerebral ischemia, asthenia, paresthesia, syncope.
CV: *chest pain,* ***ventricular fibrillation, ventricular tachycardia, torsades de pointes, AV block, heart block, bradycardia, cardiac arrest, MI,*** bundle-branch block, angina, atrial fibrillation, hypertension, palpitations, edema.
GI: nausea, diarrhea, abdominal pain.
GU: UTI.
Hepatic: liver damage.
Musculoskeletal: back pain, arthralgia, facial paralysis.
Respiratory: respiratory tract infection, dyspnea, increased cough.
Skin: rash, sweating.
Other: ***angioedema,*** flu syndrome, peripheral edema.

INTERACTIONS

Drug-drug. *Antiarrhythmics (classes I and III):* May increase dofetilide level. Withhold other antiarrhythmics for at least three plasma half-lives before giving dofetilide.
Drugs secreted by renal tubular cationic transport (amiloride, metformin, triamterene): May increase dofetilide level. Use together cautiously; monitor patient for adverse effects.
Drugs that prolong QT interval: May increase risk of QT interval prolongation. Avoid using together.
Inhibitors of CYP3A4 (amiodarone), ***azole antifungals,*** *cannabinoids, diltiazem,* ***macrolides,*** *nefazodone, norfloxacin, protease inhibitors, quinine, SSRIs, zafirlukast:* May decrease metabolism and increase dofetilide level. Use together cautiously.
Inhibitors of renal cationic secretion (cimetidine, ketoconazole, megestrol, prochlorperazine, trimethoprim with or without sulfamethoxazole), verapamil: May increase dofetilide level. Use together is contraindicated.
Potassium-depleting diuretics: May increase risk of hypokalemia or hypomagnesemia. Monitor potassium and magnesium levels.
Thiazide diuretics: May cause hypokalemia and arrhythmias. Use together is contraindicated.
Drug-food. *Grapefruit juice:* May decrease hepatic metabolism and increase drug level. Discourage use together.

EFFECTS ON LAB TEST RESULTS

None reported.

CONTRAINDICATIONS & CAUTIONS

- Contraindicated in patients hypersensitive to drug, in those with congenital or acquired long QT interval syndromes or with baseline QTc interval greater than 440 msec (500 msec in patients with ventricular conduction abnormalities), and in those with creatinine clearance less than 20 ml/minute.
- Contraindicated for use with verapamil and with cation transport system inhibitors (cimetidine, ketoconazole, megestrol, prochlorperazine, trimethoprim with or without sulfamethoxazole).
- Use cautiously in patients with severe hepatic impairment.

NURSING CONSIDERATIONS

- Provide continuous ECG monitoring for at least 3 days.
- Don't discharge patient within 12 hours of conversion to normal sinus rhythm.
- Monitor patient for prolonged diarrhea, sweating, and vomiting. Report these signs to prescriber because electrolyte imbalance may increase potential for arrhythmia development.
- Monitor renal function and QTc interval every 3 months.
- Use of potassium-depleting diuretics may cause hypokalemia and hypomagnesemia, increasing the risk of torsades de pointes. Give dofetilide after potassium level reaches and stays in normal range.
- If patient doesn't convert to normal sinus rhythm within 24 hours of starting dofetilide, consider electrical conversion.
- Before starting dofetilide, stop previous antiarrhythmics while carefully monitoring patient for a minimum of three plasma half-lives. Don't give drug after amiodarone therapy until amiodarone level falls below 0.3 mcg/ml or until amiodarone has been stopped for at least 3 months.
- If dofetilide must be stopped to allow dosing with interacting drugs, allow at least 2 days before starting other drug therapy.

PATIENT TEACHING

- Tell patient to report any change in OTC or prescription drug use, or supplement or herb use.
- Inform patient that drug can be taken without regard to meals or antacid administration.
- Tell patient to immediately report excessive or prolonged diarrhea, sweating, vomiting, or loss of appetite or thirst.
- Advise patient not to take drug with grapefruit juice.
- Advise patient to use antacids, such as Zantac 75 mg, Pepcid, Prilosec, Axid, or Prevacid, instead of Tagamet HB if needed for ulcers or heartburn.
- Instruct patient to tell prescriber if she becomes pregnant.
- Advise patient not to breast-feed while taking dofetilide because drug appears in breast milk.
- If a dose is missed, tell patient not to double a dose but to skip that dose and take the next regularly scheduled dose.

SAFETY ALERT!

dopamine hydrochloride

DOE-pa-meen

Pharmacologic class: adrenergic
Pregnancy risk category C

AVAILABLE FORMS

Injection: 40 mg/ml, 80 mg/ml, 160 mg/ml parenteral concentrate for injection for I.V. infusion; 0.8 mg/ml (200 or 400 mg) in D_5W; 1.6 mg/ml (400 or 800 mg) in D_5W; 3.2 mg/ml (800 mg) in D_5W parenteral injection for I.V. infusion

INDICATIONS & DOSAGES

➤ **To treat shock and correct hemodynamic imbalances; to improve perfusion to vital organs; to increase cardiac output; to correct hypotension**

Adults: Initially, 2 to 5 mcg/kg/minute by I.V. infusion. Titrate dosage to desired hemodynamic or renal response. Increase by 1 to 4 mcg/kg/minute at 10- to 30-minute intervals. In seriously ill patients, start with 5 mcg/kg/minute and increase gradually in increments of 5 to 10 mcg/kg/minute to a rate of 20 to 50 mcg/kg/minute, as needed.
Adjust-a-dose: In patients with occlusive vascular disease, initial dose is 1 mcg/kg/minute or less.

ADMINISTRATION

I.V.

- Dilute with D_5W, normal saline solution, D_5W in normal saline or 0.45% saline, lactated Ringer's, or D_5W in lactated Ringer's. Mix just before use.
- Use a central line or large vein, as in the antecubital fossa, to minimize risk of extravasation.
- Use a continuous infusion pump to regulate flow rate.
- Watch infusion site carefully for extravasation; if it occurs, stop infusion immediately and call prescriber. You may

need to infiltrate area with 5 to 10 mg phentolamine in 10 to 15 ml normal saline solution.
• Because solution will deteriorate rapidly, discard after 24 hours or earlier if it's discolored.
• **Incompatibilities:** Acyclovir sodium, additives with a dopamine and dextrose solution, alteplase, amphotericin B, cefepime, furosemide, gentamicin, indomethacin sodium trihydrate, iron salts, insulin, oxidizing agents, penicillin G potassium, sodium bicarbonate or other alkaline solutions, thiopental. Don't mix other drugs in I.V. container with dopamine.

ACTION
Stimulates dopaminergic and alpha and beta receptors of the sympathetic nervous system resulting in a positive inotropic effect and increased cardiac output. Action is dose-related; large doses cause mainly alpha stimulation.

Route	Onset	Peak	Duration
I.V.	5 min	Unknown	< 10 min after infusion

Half-life: 2 minutes.

ADVERSE REACTIONS
CNS: headache, anxiety.
CV: *hypotension,* ***ventricular arrhythmias (high doses),*** ectopic beats, tachycardia, angina, palpitations, vasoconstriction.
GI: nausea, vomiting.
Metabolic: azotemia, hyperglycemia.
Respiratory: ***asthmatic episodes,*** dyspnea.
Skin: necrosis and tissue sloughing with extravasation, piloerection.
Other: ***anaphylactic reactions.***

INTERACTIONS
Drug-drug. *Alpha and beta blockers:* May antagonize dopamine effects. Monitor patient closely.
Ergot alkaloids: May cause extremely high blood pressure. Avoid using together.
Inhaled anesthetics: May increase risk of arrhythmias or hypertension. Monitor patient closely.
MAO inhibitors (phenelzine, tranylcypromine): May cause fever, hypertensive crisis, or severe headache. Avoid using together; if patient received an MAO inhibitor in the past 2 to 3 weeks, initial dopamine dose is less than or equal to 10% of the usual dose.
Oxytocics: May cause severe, persistent hypertension. Use together cautiously.
Phenytoin: May cause severe hypotension, bradycardia, and cardiac arrest. Monitor patient carefully.
Tricyclic antidepressants: May decrease pressor response. Monitor patient closely.

EFFECTS ON LAB TEST RESULTS
• May increase catecholamine, glucose, and urine urea levels.

CONTRAINDICATIONS & CAUTIONS
• Contraindicated in patients with uncorrected tachyarrhythmias, pheochromocytoma, or ventricular fibrillation.
• Use cautiously in patients with occlusive vascular disease, cold injuries, diabetic endarteritis, and arterial embolism; in pregnant or breast-feeding women; in those with a history of sulfite sensitivity; and in those taking MAO inhibitors.

NURSING CONSIDERATIONS
• Most patients receive less than 20 mcg/kg/minute. Doses of 0.5 to 2 mcg/kg/minute mainly stimulate dopamine receptors and dilate the renal vasculature. Doses of 2 to 10 mcg/kg/minute stimulate beta receptors for a positive inotropic effect. Higher doses also stimulate alpha receptors, constricting blood vessels and increasing blood pressure.
• Drug isn't a substitute for blood or fluid volume deficit. If deficit exists, replace fluid before giving vasopressors.
• During infusion, frequently monitor ECG, blood pressure, cardiac output, central venous pressure, pulmonary artery wedge pressure, pulse rate, urine output, and color and temperature of limbs.
• If diastolic pressure rises disproportionately with a significant decrease in pulse pressure, decrease infusion rate, and watch carefully for further evidence of predominant vasoconstrictor activity, unless such an effect is desired.

• Observe patient closely for adverse reactions; dosage may need to be adjusted or drug stopped.
• Check urine output often. If urine flow decreases without hypotension, notify prescriber because dosage may need to be reduced.
• ***Alert:*** After drug is stopped, watch closely for sudden drop in blood pressure. Taper dosage slowly to evaluate stability of blood pressure.
• Acidosis decreases effectiveness of drug.
• ***Look alike–sound alike:*** Don't confuse dopamine with dobutamine.

PATIENT TEACHING
• Tell patient to report adverse reactions promptly.
• Instruct patient to report discomfort at I.V. insertion site.

doxazosin mesylate
dox-AY-zo-sin

Cardura, Cardura XL

Pharmacologic class: alpha blocker
Pregnancy risk category C

AVAILABLE FORMS
Tablets: 1 mg, 2 mg, 4 mg, 8 mg
Tablets (extended-release): 4 mg, 8 mg

INDICATIONS & DOSAGES
➤ Essential hypertension
Adults: Initially, 1 mg P.O. daily; determine effect on standing and supine blood pressure at 2 to 6 hours and 24 hours after dose. May increase at 2-week intervals to 2 mg and, thereafter, 4 mg and 8 mg once daily, if needed. Maximum daily dose is 16 mg, but doses over 4 mg daily increase the risk of adverse reactions.
➤ BPH
Adults: Initially, 1 mg P.O. once daily in the morning or evening; may increase at 1- or 2-week intervals to 2 mg and, thereafter, 4 mg and 8 mg once daily, if needed.

ADMINISTRATION
P.O.
• Swallow extended-release tablets whole; don't chew, divide, cut, or crush.
• Give extended-release tablet with breakfast.
• Don't give evening dose the night before switching to extended-release from immediate-release formula.

ACTION
An alpha blocker that acts on the peripheral vasculature to reduce peripheral vascular resistance and produce vasodilation. Drug also decreases smooth muscle tone in the prostate and bladder neck.

Route	Onset	Peak	Duration
P.O.	1–2 hr	2–3 hr	24 hr

Half-life: 19 to 22 hours.

ADVERSE REACTIONS
CNS: *dizziness, asthenia, headache,* vertigo, somnolence, drowsiness, pain.
CV: *orthostatic hypotension,* ***arrhythmias,*** hypotension, edema, palpitations, tachycardia.
EENT: rhinitis, pharyngitis, abnormal vision.
GI: nausea, vomiting, diarrhea, constipation.
Hematologic: ***leukopenia, neutropenia.***
Musculoskeletal: arthralgia, myalgia.
Respiratory: dyspnea.
Skin: rash, pruritus.

INTERACTIONS
Drug-drug. *Midodrine:* May decrease the effectiveness of midodrine. Monitor patient for therapeutic effect.
Drug-herb. *Butcher's broom:* May decrease effect of doxazosin. Discourage use together.
Ma huang: May decrease antihypertensive effects. Discourage use together.

EFFECTS ON LAB TEST RESULTS
• May decrease WBC and neutrophil counts.

CONTRAINDICATIONS & CAUTIONS
• Contraindicated in patients hypersensitive to drug and quinazoline derivatives (including prazosin and terazosin).
• Use cautiously in patients with impaired hepatic function.

NURSING CONSIDERATIONS

- Monitor blood pressure closely.
- If syncope occurs, place patient in a recumbent position and treat supportively. A transient hypotensive response isn't considered a contraindication to continued therapy.
- Initial extended-release dose is 4 mg. If patient stops medication briefly, he should resume at 4-mg dose and titrate back to 8 mg if appropriate.
- Wait 3 to 4 weeks before increasing extended-release dose.
- ***Look alike–sound alike:*** Don't confuse doxazosin with doxapram, doxorubicin, or doxepin. Don't confuse Cardura with Coumadin, K-Dur, Cardene, or Cordarone.

PATIENT TEACHING

- Instruct patient to take drug exactly as prescribed.
- ***Alert:*** Advise patient that he is susceptible to a first-dose effect (marked low blood pressure on standing up with dizziness or fainting). This is most common after first dose but also can occur during dosage adjustment or interruption of therapy.
- Advise patient to consult prescriber if dizziness or palpitations are bothersome.
- Advise patient to rise slowly from sitting or lying position.
- Advise patient to avoid driving and other hazardous activities until drug's effects are known.

---

enalaprilat

eh-NAH-leh-prel-at

enalapril maleate

Vasotec

Pharmacologic class: ACE inhibitor
Pregnancy risk category C; D in 2nd and 3rd trimesters

AVAILABLE FORMS

enalaprilat
Injection: 1.25 mg/ml
enalapril maleate
Tablets: 2.5 mg, 5 mg, 10 mg, 20 mg

INDICATIONS & DOSAGES

➤ Hypertension
Adults: In patients not taking diuretics, initially, 5 mg P.O. once daily; then adjusted based on response. Usual dosage range is 10 to 40 mg daily as a single dose or two divided doses. Or, 1.25 mg I.V. infusion over 5 minutes every 6 hours.
Children ages 1 month to 16 years: 0.08 mg/kg (up to 5 mg) P.O. once daily; dosage should be adjusted as needed up to 0.58 mg/kg (maximum 40 mg). Don't use if creatinine clearance is less than 30 ml/minute.
Adjust-a-dose: If patient is taking diuretics or creatinine clearance is 30 ml/minute or less, initially, 2.5 mg P.O. once daily. Or, 0.625 mg I.V. over 5 minutes, and repeat in 1 hour, if needed; then 1.25 mg I.V. every 6 hours.

➤ To convert from I.V. therapy to oral therapy
Adults: Initially, 2.5 mg P.O. once daily; if patient was receiving 0.625 mg I.V. every 6 hours, then 2.5 mg P.O. once daily. Adjust dosage based on response.

➤ To convert from oral therapy to I.V. therapy
Adults: 1.25 mg I.V. over 5 minutes every 6 hours. Higher dosages aren't more effective.
Adjust-a-dose: If creatinine level is more than 1.6 mg/dl or sodium level below 130 mEq/L, initially, 2.5 mg P.O. daily and adjust slowly.

➤ To manage symptomatic heart failure
Adults: Initially, 2.5 mg P.O. daily or b.i.d., increased gradually over several weeks. Maintenance is 5 to 20 mg daily in two divided doses. Maximum daily dose is 40 mg in two divided doses.

➤ Asymptomatic left ventricular dysfunction
Adults: Initially, 2.5 mg P.O. b.i.d. Increase as tolerated to target daily dose of 20 mg P.O. in divided doses.

ADMINISTRATION

P.O.

- Give drug without regard for food.
- Request oral suspension for patient who has difficulty swallowing.

I.V.
• Compatible solutions include D_5W, normal saline solution for injection, dextrose 5% in lactated Ringer injection, dextrose 5% in normal saline solution for injection, and Isolyte E.
• Inject drug slowly over at least 5 minutes, or dilute in 50 ml of a compatible solution and infuse over 15 minutes.
• **Incompatibilities:** Amphotericin B, cefepime hydrochloride, phenytoin sodium.

ACTION
May inhibit ACE, preventing conversion of angiotensin I to angiotensin II, a potent vasoconstrictor. Less angiotensin II decreases peripheral arterial resistance, decreasing aldosterone secretion, reducing sodium and water retention, and lowering blood pressure.

Route	Onset	Peak	Duration
P.O.	1 hr	4–6 hr	24 hr
I.V.	15 min	1–4 hr	6 hr

Half-life: 12 hours.

ADVERSE REACTIONS
CNS: *asthenia,* headache, dizziness, fatigue, vertigo, syncope.
CV: hypotension, chest pain, angina pectoris.
GI: diarrhea, nausea, abdominal pain, vomiting.
GU: decreased renal function (in patients with bilateral renal artery stenosis or heart failure).
Hematologic: bone marrow depression.
Respiratory: *dry, persistent, tickling, nonproductive cough,* dyspnea.
Skin: rash.
Other: ***angioedema.***

INTERACTIONS
Drug-drug. *Azathioprine:* May increase risk of anemia or leukopenia. Monitor hematologic study results if used together.
Diuretics: May excessively reduce blood pressure. Use together cautiously.
Insulin, oral antidiabetics: May cause hypoglycemia, especially at start of enalapril therapy. Monitor patient closely.
Lithium: May cause lithium toxicity. Monitor lithium level.
NSAIDs: May reduce antihypertensive effect. Monitor blood pressure.
Potassium-sparing diuretics, potassium supplements: May cause hyperkalemia. Avoid using together unless hypokalemia is confirmed.
Drug-herb. *Capsaicin:* May cause cough. Discourage use together.
Ma huang: May decrease antihypertensive effects. Discourage use together.
Drug-food. *Salt substitutes containing potassium:* May cause hyperkalemia. Monitor patient closely.

EFFECTS ON LAB TEST RESULTS
• May increase bilirubin, BUN, creatinine, and potassium levels. May decrease sodium and hemoglobin levels and hematocrit.
• May increase liver function test values.

CONTRAINDICATIONS & CAUTIONS
• Contraindicated in patients hypersensitive to drug and in those with a history of angioedema related to previous treatment with an ACE inhibitor.
• Use cautiously in renally impaired patients or those with aortic stenosis or hypertrophic cardiomyopathy.

NURSING CONSIDERATIONS
• Closely monitor blood pressure response to drug.
• ***Look alike–sound alike:*** Similar packaging and labeling of enalaprilat injection and pancuronium, a neuromuscular-blocking drug, could result in a fatal medication error. Check all labels carefully.
• Monitor CBC with differential counts before and during therapy.
• Diabetic patients, those with impaired renal function or heart failure, and those receiving drugs that can increase potassium level may develop hyperkalemia. Monitor potassium intake and potassium level.
• ***Look alike–sound alike:*** Don't confuse enalapril with Anafranil or Eldepryl.

PATIENT TEACHING
• Instruct patient to report breathing difficulty or swelling of face, eyes, lips, or tongue. Swelling of the face and throat

(including swelling of the larynx) may occur, especially after first dose.
• Advise patient to report signs of infection, such as fever and sore throat.
• Inform patient that light-headedness can occur, especially during first few days of therapy. Tell him to rise slowly to minimize this effect and to notify prescriber if symptoms develop. If he faints, he should stop taking drug and call prescriber immediately.
• Tell patient to use caution in hot weather and during exercise. Inadequate fluid intake, vomiting, diarrhea, and excessive perspiration can lead to light-headedness and fainting.
• Advise patient to avoid salt substitutes; these products may contain potassium, which can cause high potassium levels in patients taking this drug.
• Tell woman of childbearing age to notify prescriber if pregnancy occurs. Drug will need to be stopped.

SAFETY ALERT!

enoxaparin sodium

en-OCKS-a-par-in

Lovenox

Pharmacologic class:
low–molecular-weight heparin
Pregnancy risk category B

AVAILABLE FORMS

Syringes (graduated prefilled): 60 mg/0.6 ml, 80 mg/0.8 ml, 100 mg/ml, 120 mg/0.8 ml, 150 mg/ml
Syringes (prefilled): 30 mg/0.3 ml, 40 mg/0.4 ml
Vial (multidose): 300 mg/3 ml (contains 15 mg/ml of benzyl alcohol)

INDICATIONS & DOSAGES

➤ To prevent pulmonary embolism and deep vein thrombosis (DVT) after hip or knee replacement surgery
Adults: 30 mg subcutaneously every 12 hours for 7 to 10 days. Give initial dose between 12 and 24 hours postoperatively, as long as hemostasis has been established. Continue treatment during postoperative period until risk of DVT has diminished. Hip replacement patients may receive 40 mg subcutaneously 12 hours preoperatively. After initial phase of therapy, hip replacement patients should continue with 40 mg subcutaneously daily for 3 weeks.

➤ To prevent pulmonary embolism and DVT after abdominal surgery
Adults: 40 mg subcutaneously daily with initial dose 2 hours before surgery. Give subsequent dose, as long as hemostasis has been established, 24 hours after initial preoperative dose and continue once daily for 7 to 10 days. Continue treatment during postoperative period until risk of DVT has diminished.

➤ To prevent pulmonary embolism and DVT in patients with acute illness who are at increased risk because of decreased mobility
Adults: 40 mg once daily subcutaneously for 6 to 11 days. Treatment for up to 14 days has been well tolerated.
Adjust-a-dose: In patients with creatinine clearance less than 30 ml/minute receiving drug as prophylaxis after abdominal surgery or hip or knee replacement surgery, and in medical patients for prophylaxis during acute illness, give 30 mg subcutaneously once daily.

➤ To prevent ischemic complications of unstable angina and non–Q-wave MI with oral aspirin therapy
Adults: 1 mg/kg subcutaneously every 12 hours until clinical stabilization (minimum 2 days) with aspirin 100 to 325 mg P.O. once daily.

✶*NEW INDICATION:* Acute ST-segment elevation MI
Adults younger than age 75: 30 mg single I.V. bolus plus 1 mg/kg subcutaneously followed by 1 mg/kg subcutaneously every 12 hours (maximum of 100 mg for the first two doses only) with aspirin. When given with a thrombolytic, give enoxaparin from 15 minutes before to 30 minutes after the start of fibrinolytic therapy. For patients with percutaneous coronary intervention (PCI), if the last subcutaneous dose was given less than 8 hours before balloon inflation, no additional dose is needed. If the last dose was given more than 8 hours

before balloon inflation, give 0.3 mg/kg I.V. bolus.
Adults age 75 and older: 0.75 mg/kg subcutaneously every 12 hours (maximum 75 mg for the first two doses only).
Adjust-a-dose: In adults younger than age 75 with severe renal impairment, 30 mg single I.V. bolus plus 1 mg/kg subcutaneously followed by 1 mg/kg subcutaneously once daily. In adults age 75 and older with severe renal impairment, 1 mg/kg subcutaneously once daily with no initial bolus.

➤ Inpatient treatment of acute DVT with and without pulmonary embolism when given with warfarin sodium
Adults: 1 mg/kg subcutaneously every 12 hours. Or, 1.5 mg/kg subcutaneously once daily (at same time daily) for 5 to 7 days until therapeutic oral anticoagulant effect (INR 2 to 3) is achieved. Warfarin sodium therapy is usually started within 72 hours of enoxaparin injection.

➤ Outpatient treatment of acute DVT without pulmonary embolism when given with warfarin sodium
Adults: 1 mg/kg subcutaneously every 12 hours for 5 to 7 days until therapeutic oral anticoagulant effect (INR 2 to 3) is achieved. Warfarin sodium therapy usually is started within 72 hours of enoxaparin injection.
Adjust-a-dose: In patients with creatinine clearance less than 30 ml/minute receiving drug for acute DVT or prophylaxis of ischemic complications of unstable angina and non–Q-wave MI, give 1 mg/kg subcutaneously once daily.

ADMINISTRATION

Subcutaneous

- With patient lying down, give by deep subcutaneous injection, alternating doses between left and right anterolateral and posterolateral abdominal walls.
- Don't massage after subcutaneous injection. Watch for signs of bleeding at site. Rotate sites and keep record.

ACTION

Accelerates formation of antithrombin III–thrombin complex and deactivates thrombin, preventing conversion of fibrinogen to fibrin. Drug has a higher antifactor-Xa-to-antifactor-IIa activity ratio than heparin.

Route	Onset	Peak	Duration
Subcut.	Unknown	4 hr	Unknown

Half-life: 4½ hours.

ADVERSE REACTIONS

CNS: confusion, fever, pain.
CV: edema, peripheral edema.
GI: nausea, diarrhea.
Hematologic: ***thrombocytopenia, hemorrhage,*** ecchymoses, bleeding complications, hypochromic anemia.
Skin: irritation, pain, hematoma, and erythema at injection site, *rash, urticaria.*
Other: ***angioedema, anaphylaxis.***

INTERACTIONS

Drug-drug. *Anticoagulants, antiplatelet drugs, NSAIDs:* May increase risk of bleeding. Use together cautiously. Monitor PT and INR.
Drug-herb. *Angelica (dong quai), boldo, bromelains, capsicum, chamomile, dandelion, danshen, devil's claw, fenugreek, feverfew, garlic, ginger, ginkgo, ginseng, horse chestnut, licorice, meadowsweet, onion, passion flower, red clover, willow:* May increase risk of bleeding. Discourage use together.

EFFECTS ON LAB TEST RESULTS

- May increase ALT and AST levels. May decrease hemoglobin level.
- May decrease platelet count.

CONTRAINDICATIONS & CAUTIONS

- Contraindicated in patients hypersensitive to drug, heparin, or pork products; in those with active major bleeding; and in those with thrombocytopenia and antiplatelet antibodies in presence of drug.
- Use cautiously in patients with history of heparin-induced thrombocytopenia, aneurysms, cerebrovascular hemorrhage, spinal or epidural punctures (as with anesthesia), uncontrolled hypertension, or threatened abortion.
- Use cautiously in elderly patients and in those with conditions that place them at increased risk for hemorrhage, such

as bacterial endocarditis, congenital or acquired bleeding disorders, ulcer disease, angiodysplastic GI disease, hemorrhagic stroke, or recent spinal, eye, or brain surgery.
• Use cautiously in patients with prosthetic heart valves, with regional or lumbar block anesthesia, blood dyscrasias, recent childbirth, pericarditis or pericardial effusion, renal insufficiency, or severe CNS trauma.

NURSING CONSIDERATIONS

• It's important to achieve hemostasis at the puncture site after PCI. The vascular access sheath for instrumentation should remain in place for 6 hours after a dose if manual compression method is used; give next dose no sooner than 6 to 8 hours after sheath removal. Monitor vital signs and site for hematoma and bleeding.
• Monitor pregnant women closely. Warn pregnant women and women of childbearing age about the potential risk of therapy to her and the fetus.
• Multidose vial shouldn't be used in pregnant women because of benzyl alcohol content.
• Monitor anti-Xa levels in pregnant women with mechanical heart valves.
• ***Alert:*** Patients who receive epidural or spinal anesthesia during therapy are at increased risk for developing an epidural or spinal hematoma, which may result in long-term or permanent paralysis. Monitor these patients closely for neurologic impairment.
• Draw blood to establish baseline coagulation parameters before therapy.
• Never give drug I.M.
• ***Alert:*** Don't try to expel the air bubble from the 30- or 40-mg prefilled syringes. This may lead to loss of drug and an incorrect dose.
• Avoid I.M. injections of other drugs to prevent or minimize hematoma.
• Monitor platelet counts regularly. Patients with normal coagulation won't need close monitoring of PT or PTT.
• Regularly inspect patient for bleeding gums, bruises on arms or legs, petechiae, nosebleeds, melena, tarry stools, hematuria, hematemesis.
• To treat severe overdose, give protamine sulfate (a heparin antagonist) by slow I.V. infusion at concentration of 1% to equal dose of drug injected.
• ***Alert:*** Drug isn't interchangeable with heparin or other low–molecular-weight heparins.

PATIENT TEACHING

• Instruct patient and family to watch for signs of bleeding or abnormal bruising and to notify prescriber immediately if any occur.
• Tell patient to avoid OTC drugs containing aspirin or other salicylates unless ordered by prescriber.
• Advise patient to consult with prescriber before initiating any herbal therapy; many herbs have anticoagulant, antiplatelet, or fibrinolytic properties.

SAFETY ALERT!

ephedrine sulfate

e-FED-rin

Pharmacologic class: adrenergic
Pregnancy risk category C

AVAILABLE FORMS

Capsules: 25 mg, 50 mg
Injection: 25 mg/ml, 50 mg/ml

INDICATIONS & DOSAGES

➤ Hypotension
Adults: 25 mg P.O. once daily to q.i.d. Or, 5 to 25 mg I.V., p.r.n., to maximum of 150 mg/24 hours. Or, 25 to 50 mg I.M. or subcutaneously.
Children: 3 mg/kg P.O. or 0.5 mg/kg or 16.7 mg/m^2 subcutaneously or I.M. every 4 to 6 hours.

➤ Bronchodilation
Adults and children older than age 12: 12.5 to 25 mg P.O. every 4 hours, as needed, not to exceed 150 mg in 24 hours.
Children age 2 to 12: 2 to 3 mg/kg or 100 mg/m^2 P.O. daily in four to six divided doses. Or, for children ages 6 to 12, 6.25 to 12.5 mg P.O. every 4 hours, not to exceed 75 mg in 24 hours.

ADMINISTRATION

P.O.

- Give last dose of the day at least 2 hours before bedtime, to prevent insomnia.

I.V.

- Drug is compatible with most common solutions.
- Give slowly by direct injection.
- If needed, repeat in 5 to 10 minutes.
- **Incompatibilities:** Fructose 10% in normal saline solution; hydrocortisone sodium succinate; Ionosol B, D-CM, and D solutions; pentobarbital sodium; phenobarbital sodium; thiopental.

I.M.

- Don't use solution with particulate matter or discoloration.
- Document injection site.

Subcutaneous

- Don't use solution with particulate matter or discoloration.
- Document injection site.

ACTION

Relaxes bronchial smooth muscle by stimulating $beta_2$ receptors; also stimulates alpha and beta receptors and is a direct- and indirect-acting sympathomimetic.

Route	Onset	Peak	Duration
P.O.	15–60 min	Unknown	3–5 hr
I.V.	5 min	Unknown	60 min
I.M., Subcut.	10–20 min	Unknown	30–60 min

Half-life: 3 to 6 hours.

ADVERSE REACTIONS

CNS: *insomnia, nervousness,* ***cerebral hemorrhage,*** dizziness, headache, muscle weakness, euphoria, confusion, delirium, tremor.
CV: *palpitations,* ***arrhythmias,*** tachycardia, hypertension, precordial pain.
EENT: dry nose and throat.
GI: nausea, vomiting, anorexia.
GU: urine retention, painful urination from visceral sphincter spasm.
Skin: diaphoresis.

INTERACTIONS

Drug-drug. *Acetazolamide:* May increase ephedrine level. Monitor patient for toxicity.
Alpha blockers: May reduce vasopressor response. Monitor patient closely.
Antihypertensives: May decrease effects. Monitor blood pressure.
Beta blockers: May block the effects of ephedrine. Monitor patient closely.
Cardiac glycosides, general anesthetics (halogenated hydrocarbons): May increase risk of ventricular arrhythmias. Monitor ECG closely.
Guanethidine: May decrease pressor effects of ephedrine. Monitor patient closely.
MAO inhibitors (phenelzine, tranylcypromine): May cause severe headache, hypertension, fever, and hypertensive crisis. Avoid using together.
Methyldopa, reserpine: May inhibit ephedrine effects. Use together cautiously.
Oxytocics: May cause severe hypertension. Avoid using together.
Tricyclic antidepressants: May decrease pressor response. Monitor patient closely.

EFFECTS ON LAB TEST RESULTS

None reported.

CONTRAINDICATIONS & CAUTIONS

- Contraindicated in patients hypersensitive to ephedrine and other sympathomimetics and in those with porphyria, severe coronary artery disease, arrhythmias, angle-closure glaucoma, psychoneurosis, angina pectoris, substantial organic heart disease, or CV disease.
- Contraindicated in those receiving MAO inhibitors or general anesthesia with cyclopropane or halothane.
- Use with caution in elderly patients and in those with hypertension, hyperthyroidism, nervous or excitable states, diabetes, or prostatic hyperplasia.

NURSING CONSIDERATIONS

- ***Alert:*** Hypoxia, hypercapnia, and acidosis must be identified and corrected before or during therapy because they may reduce effectiveness or increase adverse reactions.
- Drug isn't a substitute for blood or fluid volume replenishment. Volume deficit must be corrected before giving vasopressors.

• Effectiveness decreases after 2 to 3 weeks as tolerance develops. Prescriber may increase dosage. Drug isn't addictive.
• ***Look alike–sound alike:*** Don't confuse ephedrine with epinephrine.

PATIENT TEACHING
• Tell patient taking oral form of drug at home to take last dose of day at least 2 hours before bedtime to prevent insomnia.
• Warn patient not to take OTC drugs or herbs that contain ephedrine without consulting prescriber.

SAFETY ALERT!

epinephrine (adrenaline)
ep-i-NEF-rin

Primatene Mist ◊

epinephrine hydrochloride
Adrenalin Chloride, EpiPen, EpiPen Jr, microNefrin ◊, Nephron ◊

Pharmacologic class: adrenergic
Pregnancy risk category C

AVAILABLE FORMS
Aerosol inhaler: 220 mcg ◊
Injection: 0.1 mg/ml (1:10,000), 0.5 mg/ml (1:2,000), 1 mg/ml (1:1,000) parenteral
Nebulizer inhaler: 1% (1:100) ◊, 1.125% ◊

INDICATIONS & DOSAGES
➤ **Bronchospasm, hypersensitivity reactions, anaphylaxis**
Adults: 0.1 to 0.5 ml of 1:1,000 solution I.M. or subcutaneously. Repeat every 10 to 15 minutes as needed. Or, 0.1 to 0.25 ml of 1:1,000 solution I.V. slowly over 5 to 10 minutes (1 to 2.5 ml of a commercially available 1:10,000 injection or of a 1:10,000 dilution prepared by diluting 1 ml of a commercially available 1:1,000 injection with 10 ml of water for injection or normal saline solution for injection). May repeat every 5 to 15 minutes as needed, or follow with a continuous I.V. infusion, starting at 1 mcg/minute and increasing to 4 mcg/minute, as needed.
Children: 0.01 ml/kg (10 mcg) of 1:1,000 solution subcutaneously; repeat every 20 minutes to 4 hours, as needed. Maximum single dose shouldn't exceed 0.5 mg.
➤ **Hemostasis**
Adults: 1:50,000 to 1:1,000, sprayed or applied topically.
➤ **Acute asthma attacks**
Adults and children age 4 and older: One inhalation, repeated once if needed after at least 1 minute; don't give subsequent doses for at least 3 hours. Or, 1 to 3 deep inhalations using a hand-bulb nebulizer containing 1% (1:100) solution of epinephrine repeated every 3 hours, as needed.
➤ **To prolong local anesthetic effect**
Adults and children: With local anesthetics, may be used in concentrations of 1:500,000 to 1:50,000; most commonly, 1:200,000.
➤ **To restore cardiac rhythm in cardiac arrest**
Adults: 0.5 to 1 mg I.V., repeated every 3 to 5 minutes, if needed. A higher dose may be used if 1 mg fails: 3 to 5 mg (about 0.1 mg/kg); repeat every 3 to 5 minutes.
Children: 0.01 mg/kg (0.1 ml/kg of 1:10,000 injection) I.V. First endotracheal dose is 0.1 mg/kg (0.1 ml/kg of a 1:1,000 injection) diluted in 1 to 2 ml of half-normal or normal saline solution. Give subsequent I.V. or intratracheal doses from 0.1 to 0.2 mg/kg (0.1 to 0.2 ml/kg of a 1:1,000 injection), repeated every 3 to 5 minutes, if needed.

ADMINISTRATION
I.V.
• Keep solution in light-resistant container, and don't remove before use.
• Just before use, mix with D_5W, normal saline solution for injection, lactated Ringer's injection, or combinations of dextrose in saline solution.
• Monitor blood pressure, heart rate, and ECG when therapy starts and frequently thereafter.
• Discard solution if it's discolored or contains precipitate or after 24 hours.

• **Incompatibilities:** Aminophylline; ampicillin sodium; furosemide; hyaluronidase; Ionosol D-CM, PSL, and T solutions with D_5W; mephentermine; thiopental sodium. Compatible with most other I.V. solutions. Rapidly destroyed by alkalies or oxidizing drugs, including halogens, nitrates, nitrites, permanganates, sodium bicarbonate, and salts of easily reducible metals, such as iron, copper, and zinc. Don't mix with alkaline solutions.

I.M.

• Avoid I.M. use of parenteral suspension into buttocks. Gas gangrene may occur because drug reduces oxygen tension of the tissues, encouraging growth of contaminating organisms.

• Massage site after I.M. injection to counteract vasoconstriction. Repeated local injection can cause necrosis at injection site.

Subcutaneous

• Don't refrigerate and protect from light.

• Preferred route. Don't inject too deeply and enter muscle.

Inhalational

• Teach patient to perform oral inhalation correctly. See "Patient teaching" for complete instructions.

• Epinephrine 1:100 will turn from pink to brown if exposed to air, light, heat, alkalies, and some metals. Don't use solution that's discolored or has a precipitate.

ACTION

Relaxes bronchial smooth muscle by stimulating $beta_2$ receptors and alpha and beta receptors in the sympathetic nervous system.

Route	Onset	Peak	Duration
I.V.	Immediate	5 min	Short
I.M.	Variable	Unknown	1–4 hr
Subcut.	5–15 min	30 min	1–4 hr
Inhalation	1–5 min	Unknown	1–3 hr

Half-life: Unknown.

ADVERSE REACTIONS

CNS: *drowsiness, headache, nervousness, tremor,* ***cerebral hemorrhage, stroke,*** vertigo, pain, disorientation, agitation, fear, dizziness, weakness.

CV: *palpitations,* ***ventricular fibrillation, shock,*** widened pulse pressure, hypertension, tachycardia, anginal pain, altered ECG (including a decreased T-wave amplitude).

GI: *nausea, vomiting.*

Respiratory: dyspnea.

Skin: urticaria, hemorrhage at injection site, pallor.

Other: tissue necrosis.

INTERACTIONS

Drug-drug. *Alpha blockers:* May cause hypotension from unopposed beta-adrenergic effects. Avoid using together.

Antihistamines, thyroid hormones: When given with sympathomimetics, may cause severe adverse cardiac effects. Avoid using together.

Cardiac glycosides, general anesthetics (halogenated hydrocarbons): May increase risk of ventricular arrhythmias. Monitor ECG closely.

Carteolol, nadolol, penbutolol, pindolol, propranolol, timolol: May cause hypertension followed by bradycardia. Stop beta blocker 3 days before starting epinephrine.

Doxapram, methylphenidate: May enhance CNS stimulation or pressor effects. Monitor patient closely.

Ergot alkaloids: May decrease vasoconstrictor activity. Monitor patient closely.

Guanadrel, guanethidine: May enhance pressor effects of epinephrine. Monitor patient closely.

Levodopa: May enhance risk of arrhythmias. Monitor ECG closely.

MAO inhibitors: May increase risk of hypertensive crisis. Monitor blood pressure closely.

Tricyclic antidepressants: May potentiate the pressor response and cause arrhythmias. Use together cautiously.

EFFECTS ON LAB TEST RESULTS

• May increase BUN, glucose, and lactic acid levels.

CONTRAINDICATIONS & CAUTIONS

• Contraindicated in patients with angle-closure glaucoma, shock (other than anaphylactic shock), organic brain damage, cardiac dilation, arrhythmias, coronary insufficiency, or cerebral arteriosclerosis.

• Contraindicated in patients receiving general anesthesia with halogenated hydrocarbons or cyclopropane and in patients in labor (may delay second stage).
• Commercial products containing sulfites contraindicated in patients with sulfite allergies, except when epinephrine is being used to treat serious allergic reactions or other emergency situations.
• Contraindicated for use in fingers, toes, ears, nose, or genitalia when used with local anesthetic.
• Use cautiously in patients with long-standing bronchial asthma or emphysema who have developed degenerative heart disease.
• Use cautiously in elderly patients and in those with hyperthyroidism, CV disease, hypertension, psychoneurosis, and diabetes.

NURSING CONSIDERATIONS
• In patients with Parkinson disease, drug increases rigidity and tremor.
• Drug interferes with tests for urinary catecholamines.
• One mg equals 1 ml of 1:1,000 solution or 10 ml of 1:10,000 solution.
• Epinephrine is drug of choice in emergency treatment of acute anaphylactic reactions.
• Observe patient closely for adverse reactions. Notify prescriber if adverse reactions develop; adjusting dosage or stopping drug may be necessary.
• If blood pressure increases sharply, give rapid-acting vasodilators, such as nitrates and alpha blockers, to counteract the marked pressor effect of large doses.
• Drug is rapidly destroyed by oxidizing products, such as iodine, chromates, nitrites, oxygen, and salts of easily reducible metals (such as iron).
• When treating patient with reactions caused by other drugs given I.M. or subcutaneously, inject this drug into the site where the other drug was given to minimize further absorption.
• ***Look alike–sound alike:*** Don't confuse epinephrine with ephedrine or norepinephrine.

PATIENT TEACHING
• Teach patient to perform oral inhalation correctly. Give the following instructions for using a metered-dose inhaler:
– Shake canister.
– Clear nasal passages and throat.
– Breathe out, expelling as much air from lungs as possible.
– Place mouthpiece well into mouth, and inhale deeply as you release dose from inhaler. Or, hold inhaler about 1 inch (two fingerwidths) from open mouth, and inhale while releasing dose.
– Hold breath for several seconds, remove mouthpiece, and exhale slowly.
• If more than one inhalation is prescribed, advise patient to wait at least 2 minutes before repeating procedure.
• Tell patient that use of a spacer device may improve drug delivery to lungs.
• If patient is also using a corticosteroid inhaler, instruct him to use the bronchodilator first and then to wait about 5 minutes before using the corticosteroid. This lets the bronchodilator open the air passages for maximal effectiveness.
• Instruct patient to remove canister and wash inhaler with warm, soapy water at least once weekly.
• If patient has acute hypersensitivity reactions (such as to bee stings), you may need to teach him to self-inject drug.

eplerenone
ep-LER-eh-nown

Inspra

Pharmacologic class: selective aldosterone receptor antagonist
Pregnancy risk category B

AVAILABLE FORMS
Tablets: 25 mg, 50 mg

INDICATIONS & DOSAGES
➤ Hypertension
Adults: 50 mg P.O. once daily. If response is inadequate after 4 weeks, increase dosage to 50 mg P.O. b.i.d. Maximum daily dose, 100 mg.
Adjust-a-dose: In patients taking weak CYP3A4 inhibitors (erythromycin,

fluconazole, saquinavir, verapamil), reduce eplerenone starting dose to 25 mg P.O. once daily.

➤ **Heart failure after an MI**

Adults: Initially, 25 mg P.O. once daily. Increase within 4 weeks, as tolerated and according to potassium level, to 50 mg P.O. once daily.

Adjust-a-dose: If potassium level is less than 5 mEq/L, increase dosage from 25 mg every other day to 25 mg daily; or increase dosage from 25 mg daily to 50 mg daily. If potassium level is 5 to 5.4 mEq/L, don't adjust dosage. If potassium level is 5.5 to 5.9 mEq/L, decrease dosage from 50 mg daily to 25 mg daily; or decrease dosage from 25 mg daily to 25 mg every other day; or if dosage was 25 mg every other day, withhold drug. If potassium level is greater than 6 mEq/L,withhold drug. May restart drug at 25 mg every other day when potassium level is less than 5.5 mEq/L. In patients taking weak CYP3A4 inhibitors (erythromycin, fluconazole, saquinavir, verapamil), reduce eplerenone starting dose to 25 mg P.O. once daily.

ADMINISTRATION

P.O.

• Give drug without regard for meals.

ACTION

Binds to mineralocorticoid receptors and blocks aldosterone, which increases blood pressure through induction of sodium reabsorption and possibly other mechanisms.

Route	Onset	Peak	Duration
P.O.	Unknown	90 min	Unknown

Half-life: 4 to 6 hours.

ADVERSE REACTIONS

CNS: dizziness, fatigue.
GI: diarrhea, abdominal pain.
GU: albuminuria, abnormal vaginal bleeding.
Metabolic: ***hyperkalemia.***
Respiratory: cough.
Other: flulike syndrome, gynecomastia.

INTERACTIONS

Drug-drug. *ACE inhibitors, angiotensin II receptor antagonists:* May increase risk of hyperkalemia. Use together cautiously.
Azole antifungals (itraconazole, ketoconazole), macrolides (clarithromycin), nefazodone, protease inhibitors (nelfinavir, ritonavir): Inhibits the CYP3A4 metabolism of eplerenone. Use together is contraindicated.
Lithium: May increase risk of lithium toxicity. Monitor lithium level.
NSAIDs: May reduce the antihypertensive effect and cause severe hyperkalemia in patients with impaired renal function. Monitor blood pressure and potassium level.
Potassium supplements, potassium-sparing diuretics (amiloride, spironolactone, triamterene): May increase risk of hyperkalemia and sometimes-fatal arrhythmias. Use together is contraindicated.
Weak CYP3A4 inhibitors (erythromycin, fluconazole, saquinavir, verapamil): May increase eplerenone level. Reduce eplerenone starting dose to 25 mg P.O. once daily.
Drug-herb. *St. John's wort:* May decrease eplerenone level over time. Discourage use together.

EFFECTS ON LAB TEST RESULTS

• May increase ALT, BUN, cholesterol, creatinine, GGT, potassium, triglyceride, and uric acid levels. May decrease sodium level.

CONTRAINDICATIONS & CAUTIONS

• When used for hypertension, contraindicated in patients with type 2 diabetes with microalbuminuria, creatinine level greater than 2 mg/dl in men or greater than 1.8 mg/dl in women, or creatinine clearance less than 50 ml/minute and in patients taking potassium supplements or potassium-sparing diuretics (amiloride, spironolactone, or triamterene).
• Contraindicated in patients with potassium level greater than 5.5 mEq/ml or creatinine clearance 30 ml/minute or less and in patients taking strong CYP3A4 inhibitors, such as ketoconazole, clarithromycin, ritonavir, nelfinavir, nefazodone, or itraconazole.

• Use cautiously in patient with mild to moderate hepatic impairment.
• Use in pregnant woman only if the potential benefits justify the potential risk to the fetus. Use cautiously in breast-feeding women; it's unknown if drug appears in breast milk.

NURSING CONSIDERATIONS
• Drug may be used alone or with other antihypertensives.
• Full therapeutic effect of the drug occurs in 4 weeks.
• In patients with heart failure, measure potassium level at baseline, within the first week, at 1 month after starting therapy, and periodically thereafter.
• Monitor patient for signs and symptoms of hyperkalemia.
• ***Look alike–sound alike:*** Don't confuse Inspra with Spiriva.

PATIENT TEACHING
• Inform patient that drug may be taken with or without food.
• Advise patient to avoid potassium supplements and salt substitutes during treatment.
• Tell patient to report adverse reactions.

eprosartan mesylate
ep-row-SAR-tan

Teveten

Pharmacologic class: angiotensin II receptor antagonist
Pregnancy risk category C; D in 2nd and 3rd trimesters

AVAILABLE FORMS
Tablets: 400 mg, 600 mg

INDICATIONS & DOSAGES
➤ Hypertension (alone or with other antihypertensives)
Adults: Initially, 600 mg P.O. daily. Dosage ranges from 400 to 800 mg daily, given as single daily dose or two divided doses.

ADMINISTRATION
P.O.
• Give drug without regard for meals.

ACTION
An angiotensin II receptor antagonist that reduces blood pressure by blocking the vasoconstrictor and aldosterone-secreting effects of angiotensin II. Drug selectively blocks the binding of angiotensin II to its receptor sites found in many tissues, such as vascular smooth muscle and the adrenal gland.

Route	Onset	Peak	Duration
P.O.	1–2 hr	1–3 hr	24 hr

Half-life: 5 to 9 hours.

ADVERSE REACTIONS
CNS: depression, fatigue, headache, dizziness.
CV: chest pain, dependent edema.
EENT: pharyngitis, rhinitis, sinusitis.
GI: abdominal pain, dyspepsia, diarrhea.
GU: UTI.
Hematologic: ***neutropenia.***
Musculoskeletal: arthralgia, myalgia.
Respiratory: cough, upper respiratory tract infection, bronchitis.
Other: injury, viral infection.

INTERACTIONS
Drug-drug. *NSAIDs:* May decrease antihypertensive effects. Monitor blood pressure.
Drug-herb. *Ma huang:* May decrease antihypertensive effects. Discourage use together.

EFFECTS ON LAB TEST RESULTS
• May increase BUN and triglyceride levels.

CONTRAINDICATIONS & CAUTIONS
• Contraindicated in patients hypersensitive to eprosartan or its components.
• Use cautiously in patients with renal artery stenosis; in patients with an activated renin-angiotensin system, such as volume- or salt-depleted patients; and in patients whose renal function may depend on the renin-angiotensin-aldosterone

system, such as those with severe heart failure.
• Safety and effectiveness in children haven't been established.

NURSING CONSIDERATIONS
• Correct hypovolemia and hyponatremia before starting therapy to reduce risk of symptomatic hypotension.
• Monitor blood pressure closely for 2 hours at start of treatment. If hypotension occurs, place patient in a supine position and, if needed, give an I.V. infusion of normal saline solution.
• A transient episode of hypotension isn't a contraindication to continued treatment. Drug may be restarted once patient's blood pressure has stabilized.
• Drug may be used alone or with other antihypertensives, such as diuretics and calcium channel blockers. Maximal blood pressure response may take 2 or 3 weeks.
• Monitor patient for facial or lip swelling because angioedema has occurred with other angiotensin II antagonists.
• Closely observe infants exposed to eprosartan in utero for hypotension, oliguria, and hyperkalemia.

PATIENT TEACHING
• Advise woman of childbearing age to use a reliable form of contraception and to notify her prescriber immediately if pregnancy is suspected. Treatment may need to be stopped under medical supervision.
• Advise patient to report facial or lip swelling and signs and symptoms of infection, such as fever and sore throat.
• Tell patient to notify prescriber before taking OTC medication to treat a dry cough.
• Inform patient that drug may be taken without regard to meals.
• Advise breast-feeding woman to stop either therapy or breast-feeding because of potential for adverse reactions in infant.

eptifibatide
ep-tiff-IB-ah-tide

Integrilin

Pharmacologic class: glycoprotein IIb/IIIa (GP IIb/IIIa) inhibitor
Pregnancy risk category B

AVAILABLE FORMS
Injection: 10-ml (2 mg/ml), 100-ml (0.75 mg/ml and 2 mg/ml) vials

INDICATIONS & DOSAGES
➤ **Acute coronary syndrome (unstable angina or non–ST-segment elevation MI) in patients receiving drug therapy and in those having a percutaneous coronary intervention (PCI)**
Adults: 180 mcg/kg I.V. bolus as soon as possible after diagnosis, followed by a continuous I.V. infusion at a rate of 2 mcg/kg/minute until hospital discharge or start of coronary artery bypass graft (CABG) surgery, for up to 72 hours. If patient is having a PCI, continue infusion until hospital discharge or for 18 to 24 hours after the procedure, whichever comes first, for up to 96 hours. Patients who weigh more than 121 kg (266 lb) should receive a bolus not to exceed 22.6 mg, followed by a maximum infusion rate of 15 mg/hour.
Adjust-a-dose: If creatinine clearance is less than 50 ml/minute or creatinine level is greater than 2 mg/dl, give 180 mcg/kg I.V. bolus as soon as possible after diagnosis, followed by a continuous I.V. infusion at 1 mcg/kg/minute. Patients with this creatinine clearance who weigh more than 121 kg should receive a bolus not to exceed 22.6 mg, followed by a maximum infusion rate of 7.5 mg/hour.
➤ **PCI**
Adults: 180 mcg/kg I.V. bolus given just before the procedure, immediately followed by an infusion of 2 mcg/kg/minute and a second I.V. bolus of 180 mcg/kg given 10 minutes after the first bolus. Continue infusion until hospital discharge or for 18 to 24 hours, whichever comes first; the minimum duration of infusion is

12 hours. Patients weighing more than 121 kg should receive a bolus not to exceed 22.6 mg, followed by a maximum infusion rate of 15 mg/hour.
Adjust-a-dose: If creatinine clearance is less than 50 ml/minute or creatinine level is greater than 2 mg/dl, give 180 mcg/kg I.V. bolus just before the procedure, immediately followed by a continuous I.V. infusion at 1 mcg/kg/minute and a second bolus of 180 mcg/kg given 10 minutes after the first bolus. Patients with this creatinine clearance who weigh more than 121 kg should receive a bolus not to exceed 22.6 mg, followed by a maximum infusion rate of 7.5 mg/hour.

ADMINISTRATION

I.V.

- Inspect solution for particles before use; if they appear, drug may not be sterile. Discard it.
- Protect drug from light before giving.
- Drug may be given in same line with normal saline solution, D_5W, alteplase, atropine, dobutamine, heparin, lidocaine, meperidine, metoprolol, midazolam, morphine, nitroglycerin, or verapamil. Main infusion may also contain up to 60 mEq/L of potassium chloride.
- For I.V. push, withdraw bolus dose from 10-ml vial into a syringe and give over 1 or 2 minutes.
- For infusion, give undiluted drug directly from 100-ml vial using an infusion pump.
- If patient needs thrombolytics, stop infusion.
- Refrigerate vials at 36° to 46° F (2° to 8° C). Store vials at room temperature for no longer than 2 months; afterward, discard them.
- **Incompatibilities:** Furosemide.

ACTION

Reversibly binds to the GP IIb/IIIa receptor on human platelets and inhibits platelet aggregation.

Route	Onset	Peak	Duration
I.V.	Immediate	Immediate	4–6 hr

Half-life: 2½ hours.

ADVERSE REACTIONS

CV: hypotension.
GU: hematuria.
Hematologic: *bleeding,* ***thrombocytopenia.***
Other: bleeding at femoral artery access site.

INTERACTIONS

Drug-drug. *Clopidogrel, dipyridamole, NSAIDs, oral anticoagulants (warfarin), thrombolytics, ticlopidine:* May increase risk of bleeding. Monitor patient closely for signs of bleeding.
Other inhibitors of platelet receptor IIb/IIIa: May cause serious bleeding. Avoid using together.

EFFECTS ON LAB TEST RESULTS

- May decrease platelet count.

CONTRAINDICATIONS & CAUTIONS

- Contraindicated in patients hypersensitive to drug or its ingredients and in those with history of bleeding diathesis or evidence of active abnormal bleeding within previous 30 days; severe hypertension (systolic blood pressure higher than 200 mm Hg or diastolic blood pressure higher than 110 mm Hg) not adequately controlled with antihypertensives; major surgery within previous 6 weeks; history of stroke within 30 days or history of hemorrhagic stroke; current or planned use of another parenteral GP IIb/IIIa inhibitor; or platelet count less than 100,000/mm^3.
- Contraindicated in patients with creatinine level 4 mg/dl or higher and in patients dependent on renal dialysis.
- Use cautiously in patients at increased risk for bleeding, in those with platelet count less than 150,000/mm^3, in those with hemorrhagic retinopathy, and in those weighing more than 143 kg (315 lb).

NURSING CONSIDERATIONS

- Drug is intended for use with heparin and aspirin.
- At least 4 hours before hospital discharge, stop this drug and heparin and achieve sheath hemostasis by standard compressive techniques.

• Remove sheath during infusion only after heparin has been stopped and its effects largely reversed.
• If patient is to have a CABG, stop infusion before surgery.
• Minimize use of arterial and venous punctures, I.M. injections, urinary catheters, and nasotracheal and nasogastric tubes.
• When obtaining I.V. access, avoid use of noncompressible sites (such as subclavian or jugular veins).
• Monitor patient for bleeding.
• ***Alert:*** If patient's platelet count is less than 100,000/mm^3, stop this drug and heparin.
• Perform baseline laboratory tests before start of drug therapy; also determine hemoglobin level, hematocrit, PT, INR, activated PTT, platelet count, and creatinine level.

PATIENT TEACHING
• Explain that drug is a blood thinner used to prevent chest pain and heart attack.
• Explain that benefits of drug far outweigh risk of serious bleeding.
• Tell patient to report to prescriber chest discomfort or other adverse effects immediately.

SAFETY ALERT!

esmolol hydrochloride
ESS-moe-lol

Brevibloc

Pharmacologic class: beta blocker
Pregnancy risk category C

AVAILABLE FORMS
Injection: 10 mg/ml in 10-ml vials, 20 mg/ml in 5-ml vials, 250 mg/ml in 10-ml ampules
Premixed bags in sodium chloride: 10 mg/ml in 250-ml bags; 20 mg/ml in 100-ml bags

INDICATIONS & DOSAGES
➤ **Supraventricular tachycardia; postoperative tachycardia or hypertension; noncompensatory sinus tachycardias**
Adults: 500 mcg/kg/minute as loading dose by I.V. infusion over 1 minute; then 4-minute maintenance infusion of 50 mcg/kg/minute. If adequate response doesn't occur within 5 minutes, repeat loading dose and follow with maintenance infusion of 100 mcg/kg/minute for 4 minutes. Repeat loading dose and increase maintenance infusion by increments of 50 mcg/kg/minute. Maximum maintenance infusion for tachycardia is 200 mcg/kg/minute.
➤ **Intraoperative tachycardia or hypertension**
Adults: For intraoperative treatment of tachycardia or hypertension, 80 mg (about 1 mg/kg) I.V. bolus over 30 seconds; then 150 mcg/kg/minute I.V. infusion, if needed. Titrate infusion rate, as needed, to maximum of 300 mcg/kg/minute.
➤ **Unstable angina ♦**
Adults ♦: 2 to 24 mg/minute by continuous I.V. infusion.

ADMINISTRATION
I.V.
• Don't dilute 10-mg/ml single-dose, ready-to-use vials.
• Before infusion, dilute 250-mg/ml injection concentrate to maximum of 10 mg/ml. Remove and discard 20 ml from 500-ml bag of D_5W, lactated Ringer's solution, or half-normal or normal saline solution, and add two ampules of esmolol to the bag. The final concentration is 10 mg/ml.
• Give with an infusion-control device rather than by I.V. push.
• If concentration exceeds 10 mg/ml, give drug through a central line.
• Don't use for longer than 48 hours. Watch infusion site carefully for signs of extravasation; if they occur, stop infusion immediately and call prescriber.
• **Incompatibilities:** Amphotericin B cholesteryl sulfate complex, diazepam, furosemide, procainamide, sodium bicarbonate 5%, thiopental sodium, warfarin sodium.

ACTION
A class II antiarrhythmic and ultra–short-acting selective beta blocker that decreases heart rate, contractility, and blood pressure.

Route	Onset	Peak	Duration
I.V.	Immediate	30 min	30 min after infusion

Half-life: About 9 minutes.

ADVERSE REACTIONS
CNS: anxiety, depression, dizziness, somnolence, headache, agitation, fatigue, confusion.
CV: *hypotension,* peripheral ischemia.
GI: nausea, vomiting.
Skin: inflammation or induration at infusion site.

INTERACTIONS
Drug-drug. *Digoxin:* May increase digoxin level by 10% to 20%. Monitor digoxin level.
Morphine: May increase esmolol level. Adjust esmolol dosage carefully.
Prazosin: May increase risk of orthostatic hypotension. Help patient to stand slowly until effects are known.
Reserpine, other catecholamine-depleting drugs: May increase bradycardia and hypotension. Adjust esmolol dosage carefully.
Succinylcholine: May prolong neuromuscular blockade. Monitor patient closely.
Verapamil: May increase the effects of both drugs. Monitor cardiac function closely and decrease dosages as necessary.

EFFECTS ON LAB TEST RESULTS
None reported.

CONTRAINDICATIONS & CAUTIONS
- Contraindicated in patients with sinus bradycardia, second- or third-degree heart block, cardiogenic shock, or overt heart failure.
- Use cautiously in patients with renal impairment, diabetes, or bronchospasm.

NURSING CONSIDERATIONS
- Dosage for postoperative treatment of tachycardia and hypertension is same as for supraventricular tachycardia.
- ***Alert:*** Monitor ECG and blood pressure continuously during infusion. Nearly half of patients will develop hypotension. Diaphoresis and dizziness may accompany hypotension. Monitor patient closely, especially if he had low blood pressure before treatment.
- Hypotension can usually be reversed within 30 minutes by decreasing the dose or, if needed, by stopping the infusion. Notify prescriber if this becomes necessary.
- If a local reaction develops at the infusion site, change to another site. Avoid using butterfly needles.
- When patient's heart rate becomes stable, replace drug with an alternative antiarrhythmic, such as propranolol, digoxin, or verapamil. Reduce infusion rate by half, 30 minutes after the first dose of the new drug. Monitor patient response and, if heart rate is controlled for 1 hour after administration of the second dose of the replacement drug, stop esmolol infusion.

PATIENT TEACHING
- Instruct patient to report adverse reactions promptly.
- Tell patient to report discomfort at I.V. site.

ethacrynate sodium
eth-uh-KRIH-nayt

Edecrin Sodium

ethacrynic acid
Edecrin

Pharmacologic class: loop diuretic
Pregnancy risk category B

AVAILABLE FORMS
ethacrynate sodium
Injection: 50 mg
ethacrynic acid
Tablets: 25 mg, 50 mg

INDICATIONS & DOSAGES
➤ Acute pulmonary edema
Adults: 50 mg or 0.5 to 1 mg/kg I.V. Usually only one dose is needed, although a second dose may be needed.

➤ **Edema**
Adults: 50 to 200 mg P.O. daily. May increase to 200 mg b.i.d. for desired effect.
Children: First dose is 25 mg P.O., increase cautiously by 25 mg daily until desired effect is achieved. Dosage for infants hasn't been established.
Adjust-a-dose: If added to an existing diuretic regimen, first dose is 25 mg and dosage adjustments are made in 25-mg increments.

ADMINISTRATION

P.O.
- Give drug in morning to prevent nocturia.

I.V.
- Add to vial 50 ml of D_5W or normal saline solution.
- Don't use cloudy or opalescent solution.
- Give over several minutes through tubing of running infusion.
- If more than one I.V. dose is needed, use a new injection site to avoid thrombophlebitis.
- Discard unused solution after 24 hours.
- **Incompatibilities:** Hydralazine, Normosol-M, procainamide, ranitidine, reserpine, solutions or drugs with pH below 5, tolazoline, triflupromazine, whole blood, and its derivatives.

ACTION

Potent loop diuretic; inhibits sodium and chloride reabsorption at the proximal and distal tubules and the ascending loop of Henle.

Route	Onset	Peak	Duration
P.O.	30 min	2 hr	6–8 hr
I.V.	5 min	15–30 min	2 hr

ADVERSE REACTIONS

CNS: malaise, confusion, fatigue, vertigo, headache, nervousness, fever.
CV: orthostatic hypotension.
EENT: transient or permanent deafness with over-rapid I.V. injection, blurred vision, tinnitus, hearing loss.
GI: cramping, diarrhea, anorexia, nausea, vomiting, GI bleeding, ***pancreatitis.***
GU: oliguria, hematuria, nocturia, polyuria, frequent urination.
Hematologic: ***agranulocytosis, neutropenia, thrombocytopenia,*** azotemia.
Metabolic: asymptomatic hyperuricemia, hypokalemia, hypochloremic alkalosis, fluid and electrolyte imbalances, including dilutional hyponatremia, hypocalcemia and hypomagnesemia, hyperglycemia and impaired glucose tolerance, volume depletion and dehydration.
Skin: rash.
Other: chills.

INTERACTIONS

Drug-drug. *Aminoglycoside antibiotics:* May increase ototoxic adverse reactions of both drugs. Use together cautiously.
Antidiabetics: May decrease hypoglycemic effects. Monitor glucose level.
Antihypertensives: May increase risk of hypotension. Use together cautiously.
Cardiac glycosides: May increase risk of digoxin toxicity from ethacrynate-induced hypokalemia. Monitor potassium and digoxin levels.
Chlorothiazide, chlorthalidone, hydrochlorothiazide, indapamide, metolazone: May cause excessive diuretic response, causing serious electrolyte abnormalities or dehydration. Adjust doses carefully, and monitor patient closely for signs and symptoms of excessive diuretic response.
Cisplatin: May increase risk of ototoxicity. Avoid using together.
Lithium: May decrease lithium clearance, increasing risk of lithium toxicity. Monitor lithium level.
Neuromuscular blockers: May enhance neuromuscular blockade. Monitor patient closely.
NSAIDs: May decrease diuretic effect. Use together cautiously.
Other potassium-wasting drugs (amphotericin B, corticosteroids): May increase risk of hypocalcemia. Use together cautiously.
Probenecid: May decrease diuretic effect. Avoid using together.
Warfarin: May increase anticoagulant effect. Use together cautiously.
Drug-herb. *Dandelion:* May interfere with diuretic activity. Discourage use together.
Licorice: May cause unexpected rapid potassium loss. Discourage use together.

EFFECTS ON LAB TEST RESULTS

- May increase glucose and uric acid levels. May decrease calcium, magnesium, potassium, and sodium levels.
- May decrease granulocyte, neutrophil, and platelet counts.

CONTRAINDICATIONS & CAUTIONS

- Contraindicated in infants, patients hypersensitive to drug, and patients with anuria.
- Use cautiously in patients with electrolyte abnormalities or hepatic impairment.

NURSING CONSIDERATIONS

- Monitor fluid intake and output, weight, blood pressure, and electrolyte levels.
- Watch for signs of hypokalemia, such as muscle weakness and cramps.
- Monitor glucose level in diabetic patients.
- Consult prescriber and dietitian about providing a high-potassium diet. Foods rich in potassium include citrus fruits, tomatoes, bananas, dates, and apricots. Potassium chloride and sodium supplements may be needed.
- Drug may increase risk of gastric hemorrhage caused by steroid treatment.
- Monitor elderly patients, who are especially susceptible to excessive diuresis.
- Monitor uric acid level, especially in patients with history of gout.
- ***Alert:*** If patient develops severe diarrhea, stop drug. Patient shouldn't receive drug again after diarrhea has resolved.

PATIENT TEACHING

- Instruct patient to take drug with food to minimize GI upset.
- Advise patient to take drug in morning to avoid need to urinate at night; if patient needs second dose, have him take it in early afternoon.
- Advise patient to avoid sudden posture changes and to rise slowly to avoid dizziness upon standing quickly.
- Tell patient to notify prescriber about muscle weakness, cramps, nausea, or dizziness.
- Caution patient not to perform hazardous activities if drug causes drowsiness.
- Advise diabetic patient to closely monitor glucose level.

ezetimibe

ee-ZET-ah-mibe

Zetia

Pharmacologic class: selective cholesterol absorption inhibitor
Pregnancy risk category C

AVAILABLE FORMS

Tablets: 10 mg

INDICATIONS & DOSAGES

➤ **Adjunct to diet and exercise to reduce total-cholesterol (C), LDL-C, and apolipoprotein B (Apo B) levels in patients with primary hypercholesterolemia, alone or combined with HMG-CoA reductase inhibitors (statins) or bile acid sequestrants; adjunct to other lipid-lowering drugs (combined with atorvastatin or simvastatin) in patients with homozygous familial hypercholesterolemia; adjunct to diet in patients with homozygous sitosterolemia to reduce sitosterol and campesterol levels; adjunct to fenofibrate and diet to reduce total-C, LDL-C, Apo B, and non–HDL-C levels in patients with mixed hyperlipidemia**

Adults and children age 10 and older: 10 mg P.O. daily.

ADMINISTRATION

P.O.

- Give drug without regard for meals.

ACTION

Inhibits absorption of cholesterol by the small intestine, unlike other drugs used for cholesterol reduction; causes reduced hepatic cholesterol stores and increased cholesterol clearance from the blood.

Route	Onset	Peak	Duration
P.O.	Unknown	4–12 hr	Unknown

Half-life: 22 hours.

ADVERSE REACTIONS

CNS: dizziness, fatigue, headache.
CV: chest pain.
EENT: pharyngitis, sinusitis.
GI: abdominal pain, diarrhea.
Musculoskeletal: arthralgia, back pain, myalgia.
Respiratory: *upper respiratory tract infection,* cough.
Other: viral infection.

INTERACTIONS

Drug-drug. *Bile acid sequestrant (cholestyramine):* May decrease ezetimibe level. Give ezetimibe at least 2 hours before or 4 hours after cholestyramine.
Cyclosporine, fenofibrate, gemfibrozil: May increase ezetimibe level. Monitor patient for adverse reactions.
Fibrates: May increase excretion of cholesterol into the gallbladder bile. Avoid using together.

EFFECTS ON LAB TEST RESULTS

- May increase liver function test values.

CONTRAINDICATIONS & CAUTIONS

- Contraindicated in patients allergic to any component of the drug.
- Contraindicated with HMG-CoA reductase inhibitor in pregnant or breast-feeding women and in patients with active hepatic disease or unexplained increased transaminase level.
- Use cautiously in elderly patients.

NURSING CONSIDERATIONS

- Before starting treatment, assess patient for underlying causes of dyslipidemia.
- Obtain baseline triglyceride and total, LDL, and HDL cholesterol levels.
- Using drug with an HMG-CoA reductase inhibitor significantly decreases total and LDL cholesterol, Apo B, and triglyceride levels and (except with pravastatin) increases HDL cholesterol level more than use of an HMG-CoA reductase inhibitor alone. Check liver function test values when therapy starts and thereafter according to the HMG-CoA reductase inhibitor manufacturer's recommendations.
- Patient should maintain a cholesterol-lowering diet during treatment.

PATIENT TEACHING

- Emphasize importance of following a cholesterol-lowering diet during drug therapy.
- Tell patient he may take drug without regard for meals.
- Advise patient to notify prescriber of unexplained muscle pain, weakness, or tenderness.
- Urge patient to tell his prescriber about any herbal or dietary supplements he's taking.
- Advise patient to visit his prescriber for routine follow-ups and blood tests.
- Tell woman to notify prescriber if she becomes pregnant.

felodipine

fell-OH-di-peen

Plendil, Renedil†

Pharmacologic class: calcium channel blocker
Pregnancy risk category C

AVAILABLE FORMS

Tablets (extended-release): 2.5 mg, 5 mg, 10 mg

INDICATIONS & DOSAGES

➤ Hypertension

Adults: Initially, 5 mg P.O. daily. Adjust dosage based on patient response, usually at intervals not less than 2 weeks. Usual dose is 2.5 to 10 mg daily; maximum dosage is 10 mg daily.
Elderly patients: 2.5 mg P.O. daily; adjust dosage as for adults. Maximum dosage is 10 mg daily.
Adjust-a-dose: For patients with impaired hepatic function, 2.5 mg P.O. daily; adjust dosage as for adults. Maximum daily dose is 10 mg.

ADMINISTRATION

P.O.

- Give drug whole; don't crush or cut tablets.
- Give drug without food or with a light meal.
- Don't give drug with grapefruit juice.

ACTION
Unknown. A dihydropyridine-derivative calcium channel blocker that prevents entry of calcium ions into vascular smooth muscle and cardiac cells; shows some selectivity for smooth muscle compared with cardiac muscle.

Route	Onset	Peak	Duration
P.O.	2–5 hr	2½–5 hr	24 hr

Half-life: 11 to 16 hours.

ADVERSE REACTIONS
CNS: *headache,* dizziness, paresthesia, asthenia.
CV: *peripheral edema,* chest pain, palpitations, flushing.
EENT: rhinorrhea, pharyngitis.
GI: abdominal pain, nausea, constipation, diarrhea.
Musculoskeletal: muscle cramps, back pain.
Respiratory: upper respiratory tract infection, cough.
Skin: rash.

INTERACTIONS
Drug-drug. *Anticonvulsants:* May decrease felodipine level. Avoid using together.
CYP3A4 inhibitors such as azole antifungals, cimetidine, erythromycin: May decrease clearance of felodipine. Reduce doses of felodipine; monitor patient for toxicity.
Metoprolol: May alter pharmacokinetics of metoprolol. Monitor patient for adverse reactions.
NSAIDs: May decrease antihypertensive effects. Monitor blood pressure.
Tacrolimus: May increase tacrolimus level. Monitor patient closely.
Theophylline: May slightly decrease theophylline level. Monitor patient response closely.
Drug-herb. *Ma huang:* May decrease antihypertensive effects. Discourage use together.
Drug-food. *Grapefruit, lime:* May increase drug level and adverse effects. Discourage use together.

EFFECTS ON LAB TEST RESULTS
None reported.

CONTRAINDICATIONS & CAUTIONS
- Contraindicated in patients hypersensitive to drug.
- Use cautiously in patients with heart failure, particularly those receiving beta blockers, and in patients with impaired hepatic function.

NURSING CONSIDERATIONS
- Monitor blood pressure for response.
- Monitor patient for peripheral edema, which appears to be both dose- and age-related. It's more common in patients taking higher doses, especially those older than age 60.
- ***Look alike–sound alike:*** Don't confuse Plendil with pindolol.

PATIENT TEACHING
- Tell patient to swallow tablets whole and not to crush or chew them.
- Tell patient to take drug without food or with a light meal.
- Advise patient not to take drug with grapefruit juice.
- Advise patient to continue taking drug even when he feels better, to watch his diet, and to check with prescriber or pharmacist before taking other drugs, including OTC drugs, nutritional supplements, or herbal remedies.
- Advise patient to observe good oral hygiene and to see a dentist regularly; use of drug may cause mild gum problems.

fenofibrate
fee-no-FYE-brate

Antara, Lipofen, Lofibra, TriCor, Triglide

Pharmacologic class: fibric acid derivative
Pregnancy risk category C

AVAILABLE FORMS
Capsules: 50 mg, 100 mg, 150 mg
Capsules (micronized): 43 mg, 67 mg, 130 mg, 134 mg, 200 mg

Tablets: 48 mg, 50 mg, 54 mg, 145 mg, 160 mg

INDICATIONS & DOSAGES

➤ Hypertriglyceridemia (Fredrickson types IV and V hyperlipidemia) in patients who don't respond adequately to diet alone

Adults: For Antara, initial dose is 43 to 130 mg P.O. daily. Maximum dose, 130 mg daily. For Lipofen, initial dose is 50 to 150 mg daily. Maximum dose, 150 mg daily. For Lofibra capsules, initial dose is 67 to 200 mg daily. Maximum dose, 200 mg daily. For Lofibra tablets, initial dose is 54 to 160 mg daily. Maximum dose, 160 mg daily. For TriCor, initial dose is 48 to 145 mg daily. Maximum dose, 145 mg daily. For Triglide, initial dose is 50 to 160 mg daily. Maximum dose, 160 mg daily. For all forms, adjust dose based on patient response and repeat lipid determinations every 4 to 8 weeks.

➤ Primary hypercholesterolemia or mixed dyslipidemia (Fredrickson types IIa and IIb) in patients who don't respond adequately to diet alone

Adults: For Antara, initial dose is 130 mg P.O. daily. For Lipofen, initial dose is 150 mg daily. For Lofibra, initial dose is 200 mg (capsules) or 160 mg (tablets) daily. For TriCor, initial dose is 145 mg daily. For Triglide, initial dose is 160 mg daily. May reduce dose if lipid levels fall significantly below the target range.

Adjust-a-dose: If creatinine clearance is less than 50 ml/minute or in elderly patients, initially 43 mg daily for Antara, 50 mg daily for Lipofen, 67 mg daily for Lofibra capsules or 54 mg daily for Lofibra tablets, 48 mg daily for TriCor, or 50 mg daily for Triglide. Increase only after evaluating effects on renal function and triglyceride level at this dose.

ADMINISTRATION

P.O.

- Give Lipofen or Lofibra capsules with food to enhance absorption; give other preparations without regard for food.

ACTION

May lower triglyceride levels by inhibiting triglyceride synthesis with less very–low-density lipoproteins released into circulation. Drug may also stimulate breakdown of triglyceride-rich protein.

Route	Onset	Peak	Duration
P.O.	Unknown	6–8 hr	Unknown

Half-life: 20 hours.

ADVERSE REACTIONS

CNS: *dizziness, headache,* asthenia, fatigue, insomnia, localized pain, paresthesia.
CV: ***arrhythmias.***
EENT: blurred vision, conjunctivitis, earache, eye discomfort, eye floaters, rhinitis, sinusitis.
GI: abdominal pain, constipation, diarrhea, dyspepsia, eructation, flatulence, increased appetite, nausea, vomiting.
GU: polyuria, vaginitis.
Musculoskeletal: arthralgia.
Respiratory: cough.
Skin: pruritus, rash.
Other: *infection,* decreased libido, flulike syndrome, hypersensitivity reactions.

INTERACTIONS

Drug-drug. *Bile-acid sequestrants:* May bind and inhibit absorption of fenofibrate. Give drug 1 hour before or 4 to 6 hours after bile-acid sequestrants.
Coumarin-type anticoagulants: May potentiate anticoagulant effect, prolonging PT and INR. Monitor PT and INR closely. May need to reduce anticoagulant dosage.
Cyclosporine, immunosuppressants, nephrotoxic drugs: May induce renal dysfunction that may affect fenofibrate elimination. Use together cautiously.
HMG-CoA reductase inhibitors: May increase risk of adverse musculoskeletal effects. Avoid using together, unless potential benefit outweighs risk.
Drug-food. *Any food:* May increase capsule absorption. Advise patient to take capsule with meals.
Drug-lifestyle. *Alcohol use:* May increase triglyceride levels. Discourage use together.

EFFECTS ON LAB TEST RESULTS
- May increase ALT, AST, BUN, CK, and creatinine levels. May decrease uric acid and hemoglobin levels and hematocrit.
- May decrease WBC count.

CONTRAINDICATIONS & CAUTIONS
- Contraindicated in patients hypersensitive to drug and in those with gallbladder disease, hepatic dysfunction, primary biliary cirrhosis, severe renal dysfunction, or unexplained persistent liver function abnormalities.
- Use cautiously in patients with a history of pancreatitis.

NURSING CONSIDERATIONS
- Obtain baseline lipid levels and liver function test results before therapy, and monitor liver function periodically during therapy. Stop drug if enzyme levels persist above three times normal.
- Watch for signs and symptoms of pancreatitis, myositis, rhabdomyolysis, cholelithiasis, and renal failure. Monitor patient for muscle pain, tenderness, or weakness, especially with malaise or fever.
- If an adequate response isn't obtained after 2 months of treatment with maximum daily dose, stop therapy.
- Drug lowers uric acid level by increasing uric acid excretion in patients with or without hyperuricemia.
- Beta blockers, estrogens, and thiazide diuretics may increase triglyceride levels; evaluate need for continued use of these drugs.
- Hemoglobin level, hematocrit, and WBC count may decrease when therapy starts but will stabilize with long-term administration.

PATIENT TEACHING
- Inform patient that drug therapy doesn't reduce need for following a triglyceride-lowering diet.
- Advise patient to promptly report unexplained muscle weakness, pain, or tenderness, especially with malaise or fever.
- Tell patient to take capsules with meals for best drug absorption.
- Advise patient to continue weight control measures, including diet and exercise, and to limit alcohol before therapy.
- Instruct patient who is also taking a bile-acid resin to take fenofibrate 1 hour before or 4 to 6 hours after resin.
- Advise patient about risk of tumor growth.
- Tell breast-feeding woman to either stop breast-feeding or stop taking drug.

flecainide acetate
FLEH-kay-nighd

Tambocor

Pharmacologic class: benzamide derivative
Pregnancy risk category C

AVAILABLE FORMS
Tablets: 50 mg, 100 mg, 150 mg

INDICATIONS & DOSAGES
➤ **Paroxysmal supraventricular tachycardia, including AV nodal reentrant tachycardia and AV reentrant tachycardia or paroxysmal atrial fibrillation or flutter in patients without structural heart disease; life-threatening ventricular arrhythmias such as sustained ventricular tachycardia**

Adults: For paroxysmal supraventricular tachycardia, 50 mg P.O. every 12 hours. Increase in increments of 50 mg b.i.d. every 4 days. Maximum dose is 300 mg/day. For life-threatening ventricular arrhythmias, 100 mg P.O. every 12 hours. Increase in increments of 50 mg b.i.d. every 4 days until desired effect occurs. Maximum dose for most patients is 400 mg/day.
Adjust-a-dose: If creatinine clearance is 35 ml/minute or less, first dose is 100 mg P.O. once daily or 50 mg P.O. b.i.d.

ADMINISTRATION
P.O.
- Give drug exactly as prescribed.
- Give drug without regard for food.

ACTION
A class IC antiarrhythmic that decreases excitability, conduction velocity, and automaticity by slowing atrial, AV node, His-Purkinje system, and intraventricular conduction; prolongs refractory periods in these tissues.

Route	Onset	Peak	Duration
P.O.	Unknown	2–3 hr	Unknown

Half-life: 12 to 27 hours.

ADVERSE REACTIONS
CNS: *dizziness, headache, light-headedness, syncope,* fatigue, fever, tremor, anxiety, insomnia, depression, malaise, paresthesia, ataxia, vertigo, asthenia.
CV: ***new or worsened arrhythmias, heart failure, cardiac arrest,*** chest pain, palpitations, edema, flushing.
EENT: *blurred vision and other visual disturbances,* eye pain, eye irritation.
GI: nausea, constipation, abdominal pain, dyspepsia, vomiting, diarrhea, anorexia.
Respiratory: *dyspnea.*
Skin: rash.

INTERACTIONS
Drug-drug. *Amiodarone, cimetidine:* May increase level of flecainide. Watch for toxicity. In the presence of amiodarone, reduce usual flecainide dose by 50% and monitor the patient for adverse effects.
Digoxin: May increase digoxin level by 15% to 25%. Monitor digoxin level.
Disopyramide, verapamil: May increase negative inotropic properties. Avoid using together.
Propranolol, other beta blockers: May increase flecainide and propranolol levels by 20% to 30%. Watch for propranolol and flecainide toxicity.
Ritonavir: May significantly increase flecainide levels and toxicity. Use together is contraindicated.
Urine-acidifying and urine-alkalinizing drugs: May cause extremes of urine pH, which may alter flecainide excretion. Monitor patient for flecainide toxicity or decreased effectiveness.
Drug-lifestyle. *Smoking:* May decrease flecainide level. Monitor patient closely.

EFFECTS ON LAB TEST RESULTS
None reported.

CONTRAINDICATIONS & CAUTIONS
- Contraindicated in patients hypersensitive to drug and in those with second- or third-degree AV block or right bundle-branch block with a left hemiblock (in the absence of an artificial pacemaker), recent MI, or cardiogenic shock, and in patients taking ritonavir.
- Use cautiously in patients with heart failure, cardiomyopathy, severe renal or hepatic disease, prolonged QT interval, sick sinus syndrome, or blood dyscrasia.

NURSING CONSIDERATIONS
- When used to prevent ventricular arrhythmias, reserve drug for patients with documented life-threatening arrhythmias.
- Check that pacing threshold was determined 1 week before and after starting therapy in a patient with a pacemaker; flecainide can alter endocardial pacing thresholds.
- Correct hypokalemia or hyperkalemia before giving flecainide because these electrolyte disturbances may alter drug's effect.
- Monitor ECG rhythm for proarrhythmic effects.
- Most patients can be adequately maintained on an every-12-hours dosing schedule, but some need to receive flecainide every 8 hours.
- Adjust dosage only once every 3 to 4 days.
- Monitor flecainide level, especially if patient has renal or heart failure. Therapeutic flecainide levels range from 0.2 to 1 mcg/ml. Risk of adverse effects increases when trough blood level exceeds 1 mcg/ml.

PATIENT TEACHING
- Stress importance of taking drug exactly as prescribed.
- Instruct patient to report adverse reactions promptly and to limit fluid and sodium intake to minimize fluid retention.

fluvastatin sodium
flue-va-STA-tin

Lescol, Lescol XL

Pharmacologic class: HMG-CoA reductase inhibitor
Pregnancy risk category X

AVAILABLE FORMS
Capsules: 20 mg, 40 mg
Tablets (extended-release): 80 mg

INDICATIONS & DOSAGES
➤ **To reduce LDL and total cholesterol levels in patients with primary hypercholesterolemia (types IIa and IIb); to slow progression of coronary atherosclerosis in patients with coronary artery disease; elevated triglyceride and apolipoprotein B levels in patients with primary hypercholesterolemia and mixed dyslipidemia whose response to dietary restriction and other nonpharmacologic measures has been inadequate**
Adults: Initially, 20 to 40 mg P.O. at bedtime, increasing if needed to maximum of 80 mg daily in divided doses or 80 mg Lescol XL P.O. at bedtime.
➤ **To reduce risk of undergoing coronary revascularization procedures**
Adults: In patients who must reduce LDL cholesterol level by at least 25%, initially, 40 mg P.O. once daily or b.i.d.; or one 80-mg extended-release tablet as a single dose in the evening. In patients who must reduce LDL cholesterol level by less than 25%, initially, 20 mg P.O. daily. Dosages range from 20 to 80 mg daily.

ADMINISTRATION
P.O.
- Give drug without regard for meals.
- For once-daily dosage, give immediate-release capsules in the evening.
- Don't crush or break tablets; don't open capsules.

ACTION
Inhibits HMG-CoA reductase, an early (and rate-limiting) step in the synthetic pathway of cholesterol.

Route	Onset	Peak	Duration
P.O.	Unknown	1 hr	Unknown

Half-life: Less than 1 hour.

ADVERSE REACTIONS
CNS: dizziness, fatigue, headache, insomnia.
EENT: pharyngitis, rhinitis, sinusitis.
GI: abdominal pain, constipation, diarrhea, dyspepsia, flatulence, nausea, vomiting.
Hematologic: ***leukopenia, thrombocytopenia,*** hemolytic anemia.
Musculoskeletal: ***rhabdomyolysis,*** arthralgia, back pain, myalgia.
Respiratory: *upper respiratory tract infection,* bronchitis, cough.
Other: hypersensitivity reactions.

INTERACTIONS
Drug-drug. *Cholestyramine, colestipol:* May bind with fluvastatin in the GI tract and decrease absorption. Separate doses by at least 4 hours.
Cimetidine, omeprazole, ranitidine: May decrease fluvastatin metabolism. Monitor patient for enhanced effects.
Cyclosporine and other immunosuppressants, erythromycin, gemfibrozil, niacin: May increase risk of polymyositis and rhabdomyolysis. Avoid using together.
Digoxin: May alter digoxin pharmacokinetics. Monitor digoxin level carefully.
Fluconazole, itraconazole, ketoconazole: May increase fluvastatin level and adverse effects. Use cautiously together, or, if given together, reduce dose of fluvastatin.
Glyburide: May increase levels of both drugs. Monitor serum glucose and signs and symptoms of toxicity.
Phenytoin: May increase phenytoin levels. Monitor phenytoin levels.
Rifampin: May enhance fluvastatin metabolism and decrease levels. Monitor patient for lack of effect.
Warfarin: May increase anticoagulant effect with bleeding. Monitor PT and INR.

Drug-herb. *Eucalyptus, jin bu huan, kava:* May increase risk of hepatotoxicity. Discourage use together.
Red yeast rice: May increase risk of adverse reactions because herb contains compounds similar to those in drug. Discourage use together.
Drug-lifestyle. *Alcohol use:* May increase risk of hepatotoxicity. Discourage use together.

EFFECTS ON LAB TEST RESULTS

- May increase ALT, AST, and CK levels. May decrease hemoglobin level and hematocrit.
- May decrease platelet and WBC counts.

CONTRAINDICATIONS & CAUTIONS

- Contraindicated in patients hypersensitive to drug and in those with active liver disease or unexplained persistent elevations of transaminase levels; also contraindicated in pregnant and breast-feeding women and in women of childbearing age.
- Use cautiously in patients with severe renal impairment and history of liver disease or heavy alcohol use.

NURSING CONSIDERATIONS

- Patient should follow a diet restricted in saturated fat and cholesterol during therapy.
- Test liver function at start of therapy, at 12 weeks after start of therapy, 12 weeks after an increase in dose, and then periodically. Stop drug if there is a persistent increase in ALT or AST levels of at least three times the upper limit of normal.
- Watch for signs of myositis.
- ***Look alike–sound alike:*** Don't confuse fluvastatin with fluoxetine.

PATIENT TEACHING

- Tell patient that drug may be taken without regard for meals; if taken once daily, immediate-release capsules are taken in the evening.
- Advise patient who is also taking a bile-acid resin such as cholestyramine to take fluvastatin at bedtime, at least 4 hours after taking the resin.
- Teach patient about proper dietary management, weight control, and exercise. Explain their importance in controlling elevated cholesterol and triglyceride levels.
- Warn patient to avoid alcohol.
- Tell patient to notify prescriber of adverse reactions, especially muscle aches and pains.
- Advise patient that it may take up to 4 weeks for the drug to be completely effective.
- ***Alert:*** Tell woman of childbearing age to stop drug and notify prescriber immediately if she is or may be pregnant or if she's breast-feeding.

SAFETY ALERT!

fondaparinux sodium

fon-dah-PEAR-ah-nucks

Arixtra

Pharmacologic class: activated factor X inhibitor
Pregnancy risk category B

AVAILABLE FORMS

Injection: 2.5 mg/0.5 ml, 5 mg/0.4 ml, 7.5 mg/0.6 ml, 10 mg/0.8 ml single-dose prefilled syringe

INDICATIONS & DOSAGES

➤ **To prevent deep vein thrombosis (DVT), which may lead to pulmonary embolism, in patients undergoing surgery for hip fracture, hip replacement, knee replacement, or abdominal surgery**
Adults who weigh 50 kg (110 lb) or more: 2.5 mg subcutaneously once daily for 5 to 9 days. Give first dose after hemostasis is established, 6 to 8 hours after surgery. Giving the dose earlier than 6 hours after surgery increases the risk of major bleeding. Patients undergoing hip fracture surgery should receive an extended prophylaxis course of up to 24 additional days; a total of 32 days (perioperative and extended prophylaxis) has been tolerated.
➤ **Acute DVT (with warfarin); acute pulmonary embolism (with warfarin) when treatment is started in the hospital**

Adults who weigh more than 100 kg (220 lb): Give 10 mg subcutaneously daily for 5 to 9 days, and until INR level is 2 to 3. Begin warfarin therapy as soon as possible, usually within 72 hours.
Adults who weigh 50 to 100 kg: Give 7.5 mg subcutaneously daily for 5 to 9 days, and until INR level is 2 to 3. Begin warfarin therapy as soon as possible, usually within 72 hours.
Adults who weigh less than 50 kg: Give 5 mg subcutaneously daily for 5 to 9 days, and until INR level is 2 to 3. Begin warfarin therapy as soon as possible, usually within 72 hours.

ADMINISTRATION

Subcutaneous

• Give subcutaneously only, never I.M. Inspect the single-dose, prefilled syringe for particulate matter and discoloration before giving.
• Give drug in fatty tissue, rotating injection sites. If drug has been properly injected, the needle will pull back into the syringe security sleeve and the white safety indicator will appear above the blue upper body. A soft click may be heard or felt when the syringe plunger is fully released. After injection of syringe contents, the plunger automatically rises while the needle withdraws from the skin and retracts into the security sleeve. Don't recap the needle.
• **Incompatibilities:** Other injections or infusions.

ACTION

Binds to antithrombin III (AT-III) and potentiates the neutralization of factor Xa by AT-III, which interrupts coagulation and inhibits formation of thrombin and blood clots.

Route	Onset	Peak	Duration
Subcut.	Unknown	2–3 hr	Unknown

Half-life: 17 to 21 hours.

ADVERSE REACTIONS

CNS: *fever,* insomnia, dizziness, confusion, headache, pain.
CV: hypotension, edema.
GI: *nausea,* constipation, vomiting, diarrhea, dyspepsia.
GU: UTI, urine retention.
Hematologic: ***hemorrhage,*** *anemia,* hematoma, ***postoperative hemorrhage, thrombocytopenia.***
Metabolic: hypokalemia.
Skin: mild local irritation (injection site bleeding, rash, pruritus), bullous eruption, purpura, rash, increased wound drainage.

INTERACTIONS

Drug-drug. *Drugs that increase risk of bleeding (NSAIDs, platelet inhibitors, anticoagulants):* May increase risk of hemorrhage. Stop these drugs before starting fondaparinux. If use together is unavoidable, monitor patient closely.
Drug-herb. *Angelica (dong quai), boldo, bromelains, capsicum, chamomile, dandelion, danshen, devil's claw, fenugreek, feverfew, garlic, ginger, ginkgo, ginseng, horse chestnut, licorice, meadowsweet, onion, passion flower, red clover, willow:* May increase risk of bleeding. Discourage use together.

EFFECTS ON LAB TEST RESULTS

• May increase AST, ALT, and bilirubin levels. May decrease potassium and hemoglobin levels and hematocrit.
• May decrease platelet count.

CONTRAINDICATIONS & CAUTIONS

• Contraindicated in patients with creatinine clearance less than 30 ml/minute and in those who are hypersensitive to the drug.
• Contraindicated for prophylaxis in patients who weigh less than 50 kg who are undergoing hip fracture, hip replacement, knee replacement, or abdominal surgery.
• Contraindicated in patients with active major bleeding, bacterial endocarditis, or thrombocytopenia with a positive test result for antiplatelet antibody after taking fondaparinux.
• Use cautiously in patients being treated with platelet inhibitors; in those at increased risk for bleeding, such as congenital or acquired bleeding disorders; in those with active ulcerative and angiodysplastic GI disease; in those with hemorrhagic

stroke; and in patients shortly after brain, spinal, or ophthalmologic surgery.
• Use cautiously in patients who have had epidural or spinal anesthesia or spinal puncture; they are at increased risk for developing an epidural or spinal hematoma (which may cause paralysis).
• Use cautiously in elderly patients, in patients with creatinine clearance of 30 to 50 ml/minute, and in those with a history of heparin-induced thrombocytopenia, a bleeding diathesis, uncontrolled arterial hypertension, or a history of recent GI ulceration, diabetic retinopathy, or hemorrhage.

NURSING CONSIDERATIONS
• Don't use interchangeably with heparin, low–molecular-weight heparins, or heparinoids.
• ***Alert:*** To avoid loss of drug, don't expel air bubble from the syringe.
• ***Alert:*** Patients who receive epidural or spinal anesthesia are at increased risk for developing an epidural or spinal hematoma, which may result in long-term or permanent paralysis. Monitor these patients closely for neurologic impairment.
• Monitor renal function periodically and stop drug in patients who develop unstable renal function or severe renal impairment while receiving therapy.
• Routinely assess patient for signs and symptoms of bleeding, and regularly monitor CBC, platelet count, creatinine level, and stool occult blood test results. Stop use if platelet count is less than 100,000/mm^3.
• Anticoagulant effects may last for 2 to 4 days after stopping drug in patients with normal renal function.
• PT and activated PTT aren't suitable monitoring tests to measure drug activity. If coagulation parameters change unexpectedly or patient develops major bleeding, stop drug.

PATIENT TEACHING
• Tell patient to report signs and symptoms of bleeding.
• Instruct patient to avoid OTC products that contain aspirin or other salicylates.
• Advise patient to consult with prescriber before starting herbal therapy; many herbs have anticoagulant, antiplatelet, or fibrinolytic properties.
• Teach patient the correct technique for subcutaneous use, if needed.

fosinopril sodium
foh-SIN-oh-pril

Monopril

Pharmacologic class: ACE inhibitor
Pregnancy risk category C; D in 2nd and 3rd trimesters

AVAILABLE FORMS
Tablets: 10 mg, 20 mg, 40 mg

INDICATIONS & DOSAGES
➤ Hypertension
Adults: Initially, 10 mg P.O. daily; adjust dosage based on blood pressure response at peak and trough levels. Usual dosage is 20 to 40 mg daily; maximum is 80 mg daily. Dosage may be divided.
➤ Heart failure
Adults: Initially, 10 mg P.O. once daily. Increase dosage over several weeks to a maximum of 40 mg P.O. daily, if needed.
Adjust-a-dose: For patients with moderate to severe renal failure or vigorous diuresis, start with 5 mg P.O. once daily.

ADMINISTRATION
P.O.
• Give drug without regard for meals.

ACTION
Inhibits ACE, preventing conversion of angiotensin I to angiotensin II, a potent vasoconstrictor. Less angiotensin II decreases peripheral arterial resistance, thus decreasing aldosterone secretion, which reduces sodium and water retention and lowers blood pressure.

Route	Onset	Peak	Duration
P.O.	1 hr	3 hr	24 hr

Half-life: 11½ hours.

ADVERSE REACTIONS
CNS: *dizziness,* ***stroke,*** headache, fatigue, syncope, paresthesia, sleep disturbance.

CV: ***MI,*** chest pain, angina pectoris, rhythm disturbances, palpitations, hypotension, orthostatic hypotension.
EENT: tinnitus, sinusitis.
GI: ***pancreatitis,*** nausea, vomiting, diarrhea, dry mouth, abdominal distention, abdominal pain, constipation.
GU: sexual dysfunction, renal insufficiency.
Hepatic: ***hepatitis.***
Metabolic: ***hyperkalemia.***
Musculoskeletal: arthralgia, musculoskeletal pain, myalgia.
Respiratory: *dry, persistent, tickling, nonproductive cough,* ***bronchospasm.***
Skin: urticaria, rash, photosensitivity reactions, pruritus.
Other: ***angioedema,*** decreased libido, gout.

INTERACTIONS

Drug-drug. *Antacids:* May impair absorption. Separate dosage times by at least 2 hours.
Azathioprine: May increase risk of anemia or leukopenia. Monitor hematologic studies if used together.
Diuretics, other antihypertensives: May cause excessive hypotension. Stop diuretic or lower fosinopril dosage.
Lithium: May increase lithium level and lithium toxicity. Monitor lithium level.
Nesiritide: May increase hypotensive effects. Monitor blood pressure.
NSAIDs: May decrease antihypertensive effects. Monitor blood pressure.
Potassium-sparing diuretics, potassium supplements: May cause risk of hyperkalemia. Monitor patient closely.
Drug-herb. *Capsaicin:* May cause cough. Discourage use together.
Ma huang: May decrease antihypertensive effects. Discourage use together.
Drug-food. *Salt substitutes containing potassium:* May cause hyperkalemia. Discourage use together.

EFFECTS ON LAB TEST RESULTS

- May increase BUN, creatinine, potassium, and hemoglobin levels and hematocrit.
- May increase liver function test values.
- May cause falsely low digoxin level with the Digi-Tab radioimmunoassay kit for digoxin.

CONTRAINDICATIONS & CAUTIONS

- Contraindicated in patients hypersensitive to drug or other ACE inhibitors and in breast-feeding women.
- Use cautiously in patients with impaired renal or hepatic function.

NURSING CONSIDERATIONS

- Monitor blood pressure for drug effect.
- Although ACE inhibitors reduce blood pressure in all races, they reduce it less in blacks taking the ACE inhibitor alone. Black patients should take drug with a thiazide diuretic for a more favorable response.
- ACE inhibitors appear to cause a higher risk of angioedema in black patients.
- Monitor potassium intake and potassium level. Diabetic patients, those with impaired renal function, and those receiving drugs that can increase potassium level may develop hyperkalemia.
- Other ACE inhibitors may cause agranulocytosis and neutropenia. Monitor CBC with differential counts before therapy and periodically thereafter.
- Assess renal and hepatic function before and periodically throughout therapy.
- ***Look alike–sound alike:*** Don't confuse fosinopril with lisinopril. Don't confuse Monopril with Monurol.

PATIENT TEACHING

- Tell patient to avoid salt substitutes; these products may contain potassium, which can cause high potassium level in patients taking drug.
- Instruct patient to contact prescriber if light-headedness or fainting occurs.
- Advise patient to report evidence of infection, such as fever and sore throat.
- Instruct patient to call prescriber if he develops easy bruising or bleeding; swelling of tongue, lips, face, eyes, mucous membranes, arms, or legs; difficulty swallowing or breathing; and hoarseness.
- Urge patient to use caution in hot weather and during exercise. Inadequate fluid intake, vomiting, diarrhea,

and excessive perspiration can lead to light-headedness and fainting.
- Tell woman of childbearing age to notify prescriber if pregnancy occurs. Drug will need to be stopped.

furosemide

fur-OH-se-mide

Furosemide Special†, Lasix*, Novo-semide†

Pharmacologic class: loop diuretic
Pregnancy risk category C

AVAILABLE FORMS

Injection: 10 mg/ml
Oral solution: 10 mg/ml, 40 mg/5 ml
Tablets: 20 mg, 40 mg, 80 mg, 500 mg†

INDICATIONS & DOSAGES

➤ **Acute pulmonary edema**
Adults: 40 mg I.V. injected slowly over 1 to 2 minutes; then 80 mg I.V. in 60 to 90 minutes if needed.

➤ **Edema**
Adults: 20 to 80 mg P.O. daily in the morning. If response is inadequate, give a second dose, and each succeeding dose, every 6 to 8 hours. Carefully increase dose in 20- to 40-mg increments up to 600 mg daily. Once effective dose is attained, may give once or twice daily. Or, 20 to 40 mg I.V. or I.M., increased by 20 mg every 2 hours until desired effect achieved.
Infants and children: 2 mg/kg P.O. daily, increased by 1 to 2 mg/kg in 6 to 8 hours if needed; carefully adjusted up to 6 mg/kg daily if needed.

➤ **Hypertension**
Adults: 40 mg P.O. b.i.d. Dosage adjusted based on response. May be used as adjunct to other antihypertensives if needed.
Children ♦: 0.5 to 2 mg/kg P.O. once or twice daily. Increase dose as needed up to 6 mg/kg daily.

ADMINISTRATION

P.O.
- To prevent nocturia, give in the morning. Give second dose if ordered in early afternoon, 6 to 8 hours after morning dose.
- Give drug with food to prevent GI upset.
- Store tablets in light-resistant container to prevent discoloration (doesn't affect potency). Refrigerate oral solution to ensure drug stability.

I.V.
- If discolored yellow, don't use.
- For direct injection, give over 1 to 2 minutes.
- For infusion, dilute with D_5W, normal saline solution, or lactated Ringer's solution.
- To avoid ototoxicity, infuse no more than 4 mg/minute.
- Use prepared infusion solution within 24 hours.
- **Incompatibilities:** Acidic solutions, aminoglycosides, amiodarone, ascorbic acid, azithromycin, bleomycin, buprenorphine, chlorpromazine, ciprofloxacin, diazepam, diltiazem, dobutamine, doxapram, doxorubicin, droperidol, epinephrine, erythromycin, esmolol, filgrastim, fluconazole, fructose 10% in water, gentamicin, hydralazine, idarubicin, invert sugar 10% in electrolyte #2, isoproterenol, levofloxacin, mannitol, meperidine, methocarbamol, metoclopramide, midazolam, milrinone, morphine, netilmicin, norepinephrine, ondansetron, oxytetracycline, prochlorperazine, promethazine, protamine, quinidine, tetracycline, thiamine, vinblastine, vincristine, vitamins B and C.

I.M.
- To prevent nocturia, give in the morning. Give second dose if ordered in early afternoon, 6 to 8 hours after morning dose.
- Record administration site.

ACTION

Inhibits sodium and chloride reabsorption at the proximal and distal tubules and the ascending loop of Henle.

Route	Onset	Peak	Duration
P.O.	20–60 min	1–2 hr	6–8 hr
I.V.	Within 5 min	30 min	2 hr
I.M.	Unknown	30 min	2 hr

Half-life: 30 minutes.

ADVERSE REACTIONS

CNS: vertigo, headache, dizziness, paresthesia, weakness, restlessness, fever.

CV: orthostatic hypotension, thrombophlebitis with I.V. administration.
EENT: transient deafness, blurred or yellowed vision, tinnitus.
GI: abdominal discomfort and pain, diarrhea, anorexia, nausea, vomiting, constipation, ***pancreatitis.***
GU: azotemia, nocturia, polyuria, frequent urination, oliguria.
Hematologic: ***agranulocytosis, aplastic anemia, leukopenia, thrombocytopenia,*** anemia.
Hepatic: hepatic dysfunction, jaundice.
Metabolic: volume depletion and dehydration, asymptomatic hyperuricemia, impaired glucose tolerance, hypokalemia, hypochloremic alkalosis, hyperglycemia, dilutional hyponatremia, hypocalcemia, hypomagnesemia.
Musculoskeletal: muscle spasm.
Skin: dermatitis, purpura, photosensitivity reactions, transient pain at I.M. injection site.
Other: gout.

INTERACTIONS

Drug-drug. *Aminoglycoside antibiotics, cisplatin:* May increase ototoxicity. Use together cautiously.
Amphotericin B, corticosteroids, corticotropin, metolazone: May increase risk of hypokalemia. Monitor potassium level closely.
Antidiabetics: May decrease hypoglycemic effects. Monitor glucose level.
Antihypertensives: May increase risk of hypotension. Use together cautiously. Decrease antihypertensive dose if needed.
Cardiac glycosides, neuromuscular blockers: May increase toxicity of these drugs from furosemide-induced hypokalemia. Monitor potassium level.
Chlorothiazide, chlorthalidone, hydrochlorothiazide, indapamide, metolazone: May cause excessive diuretic response, causing serious electrolyte abnormalities or dehydration. Adjust doses carefully, and monitor patient closely for signs and symptoms of excessive diuretic response.
Ethacrynic acid: May increase risk of ototoxicity. Avoid using together.
Lithium: May decrease lithium excretion, resulting in lithium toxicity. Monitor lithium level.
NSAIDs: May inhibit diuretic response. Use together cautiously.
Phenytoin: May decrease diuretic effects of furosemide. Use together cautiously.
Propranolol: May increase propranolol level. Monitor patient closely.
Salicylates: May cause salicylate toxicity. Use together cautiously.
Sucralfate: May reduce diuretic and antihypertensive effect. Separate doses by 2 hours.
Drug-herb. *Aloe:* May increase drug effect. Discourage use together.
Dandelion: May interfere with drug activity. Discourage use together.
Ginseng: May decrease drug effect. Discourage use together.
Licorice: May cause unexpected rapid potassium loss. Discourage use together.
Drug-lifestyle. *Sun exposure:* May increase risk of photosensitivity reactions. Advise patient to avoid excessive sunlight exposure.

EFFECTS ON LAB TEST RESULTS

• May increase cholesterol, glucose, BUN, creatinine, and uric acid levels. May decrease calcium, hemoglobin, magnesium, potassium, and sodium levels.
• May decrease granulocyte, platelet, and WBC counts.

CONTRAINDICATIONS & CAUTIONS

• Contraindicated in patients hypersensitive to drug and in those with anuria.
• Use cautiously in patients with hepatic cirrhosis and in those allergic to sulfonamides. Use during pregnancy only if potential benefits to mother clearly outweigh risks to fetus.

NURSING CONSIDERATIONS

• ***Alert:*** Monitor weight, blood pressure, and pulse rate routinely with long-term use and during rapid diuresis. Use can lead to profound water and electrolyte depletion.
• If oliguria or azotemia develops or increases, drug may need to be stopped.
• Monitor fluid intake and output and electrolyte, BUN, and carbon dioxide levels frequently.

• Watch for signs of hypokalemia, such as muscle weakness and cramps.
• Consult prescriber and dietitian about a high-potassium diet or potassium supplements. Foods rich in potassium include citrus fruits, tomatoes, bananas, dates, and apricots.
• Monitor glucose level in diabetic patients.
• Drug may not be well absorbed orally in patient with severe heart failure. Drug may need to be given I.V. even if patient is taking other oral drugs.
• Monitor uric acid level, especially in patients with a history of gout.
• Monitor elderly patients, who are especially susceptible to excessive diuresis, because circulatory collapse and thromboembolic complications are possible.
• ***Look alike–sound alike:*** Don't confuse furosemide with torsemide or Lasix with Lonox, Lidex, or Luvox.

PATIENT TEACHING

• Advise patient to take drug with food to prevent GI upset, and to take drug in morning to prevent need to urinate at night. If patient needs second dose, tell him to take it in early afternoon, 6 to 8 hours after morning dose.
• Inform patient of possible need for potassium or magnesium supplements.
• Instruct patient to stand slowly to prevent dizziness and to limit alcohol intake and strenuous exercise in hot weather to avoid worsening dizziness upon standing quickly.
• Advise patient to immediately report ringing in ears, severe abdominal pain, or sore throat and fever; these symptoms may indicate toxicity.
• ***Alert:*** Discourage patient from storing different types of drugs in the same container, increasing the risk of drug errors. The most popular strengths of this drug and digoxin are white tablets about equal in size.
• Tell patient to check with prescriber or pharmacist before taking OTC drugs.
• Teach patient to avoid direct sunlight and to use protective clothing and a sunblock because of risk of photosensitivity reactions.

gemfibrozil
jem-FI-broe-zil

Lopid

Pharmacologic class: fibric acid derivative
Pregnancy risk category C

AVAILABLE FORMS

Tablets: 600 mg

INDICATIONS & DOSAGES

➤ **Types IV and V hyperlipidemia unresponsive to diet and other drugs; to reduce risk of coronary heart disease in patients with type IIb hyperlipidemia who can't tolerate or who are refractory to treatment with bile-acid sequestrants or niacin**
Adults: 1,200 mg P.O. daily in two divided doses, 30 minutes before morning and evening meals.

ADMINISTRATION

P.O.
• Give drug 30 minutes before breakfast and dinner.

ACTION

Inhibits peripheral lipolysis and reduces triglyceride synthesis in the liver; lowers triglyceride levels and increases HDL cholesterol levels.

Route	Onset	Peak	Duration
P.O.	2–5 days	4 wk	Unknown

Half-life: 1¼ hours.

ADVERSE REACTIONS

CNS: fatigue, headache, vertigo.
CV: atrial fibrillation.
GI: *abdominal and epigastric pain, dyspepsia,* acute appendicitis, constipation, diarrhea, nausea, vomiting.
Hematologic: ***leukopenia, thrombocytopenia,*** anemia, eosinophilia.
Hepatic: bile duct obstruction.
Metabolic: hypokalemia.
Skin: dermatitis, eczema, pruritus, rash.

INTERACTIONS

Drug-drug. *Cyclosporine:* May decrease cyclosporine levels. Monitor cyclosporine levels and adjust dose as needed.
Glyburide: May increase hypoglycemic effects. Monitor glucose level, and watch for signs of hypoglycemia.
HMG-CoA reductase inhibitors: May cause myopathy with rhabdomyolysis. Avoid using together.
Oral anticoagulants: May enhance effects of oral anticoagulants. Monitor patient closely.
Repaglinide: May increase repaglinide level. Avoid using together if possible. If already taking both drugs, monitor glucose levels and adjust repaglinide dosage.

EFFECTS ON LAB TEST RESULTS

- May increase ALT, AST, and CK levels. May decrease potassium and hemoglobin levels and hematocrit.
- May decrease eosinophil, WBC, and platelet counts.

CONTRAINDICATIONS & CAUTIONS

- Contraindicated in patients hypersensitive to drug and in those with hepatic or severe renal dysfunction (including primary biliary cirrhosis) or gallbladder disease.

NURSING CONSIDERATIONS

- Check CBC and test liver function periodically during the first 12 months of therapy.
- If drug has no benefits after 3 months of therapy, stop drug.
- Patient shouldn't take drug together with repaglinide or itraconazole.

PATIENT TEACHING

- Instruct patient to take drug 30 minutes before breakfast and dinner.
- Teach patient about proper dietary management of cholesterol and triglycerides. When appropriate, recommend weight control, exercise, and smoking cessation programs.
- Because of possible dizziness and blurred vision, advise patient to avoid driving and other hazardous activities until effects of drug are known.
- Tell patient to observe bowel movements and to report evidence of excess fat in feces or other signs of bile duct obstruction.
- Advise patient to report muscle pain to prescriber if it occurs during therapy.

gentamicin sulfate

jen-ta-MYE-sin

Pharmacologic class:
aminoglycoside
Pregnancy risk category D

AVAILABLE FORMS

Injection: 40 mg/ml (adults), 10 mg/ml (children)
I.V. infusion (premixed): 60 mg, 70 mg, 80 mg, 90 mg, 100 mg, in normal saline solution

INDICATIONS & DOSAGES

➤ **Serious infections caused by sensitive strains of *Pseudomonas aeruginosa, Escherichia coli, Proteus, Klebsiella, Serratia,* or *Staphylococcus***
Adults: 3 mg/kg daily in three divided doses I.M. or I.V. infusion every 8 hours. For life-threatening infections, may give up to 5 mg/kg daily in three or four divided doses; reduce dosage to 3 mg/kg daily as soon as patient improves.
Children: 2 to 2.5 mg/kg every 8 hours I.M. or by I.V. infusion.
Neonates older than 1 week and infants: 2.5 mg/kg every 8 hours I.M. or by I.V. infusion.
Neonates younger than 1 week and preterm infants: 2.5 mg/kg every 12 hours I.M. or by I.V. infusion.
➤ **To prevent endocarditis before GI or GU procedure or surgery**
Adults: 1.5 mg/kg I.M. or I.V. 30 minutes before procedure or surgery. Maximum dose is 80 mg. Give with ampicillin (vancomycin in penicillin-allergic patients).
Children: 2 mg/kg I.M. or I.V. 30 minutes before procedure or surgery. Maximum dose is 80 mg. Give with ampicillin (vancomycin in penicillin-allergic patients).
Adjust-a-dose: For adults with impaired renal function, doses and frequency are

determined by drug level and renal function. To maintain therapeutic levels, adults should receive 1 to 1.7 mg/kg I.M. or by I.V. infusion after each dialysis session, and children should receive 2 to 2.5 mg/kg I.M. or by I.V. infusion after each dialysis session.

ADMINISTRATION

I.V.

- Obtain specimen for culture and sensitivity tests before giving. Begin therapy while awaiting results.
- For intermittent infusion, dilute with 50 to 200 ml of D_5W or normal saline solution for injection.
- Infuse over 30 minutes to 2 hours.
- After completing infusion, flush the line with normal saline solution or D_5W.
- **Incompatibilities:** Allopurinol, amphotericin B, ampicillin, azithromycin, cefazolin, cefepime, cefotaxime, ceftazidime, ceftriaxone sodium, cefuroxime, certain parenteral nutrition formulations, cytarabine, dopamine, fat emulsions, furosemide, heparin, hetastarch, idarubicin, indomethacin sodium trihydrate, nafcillin, propofol, ticarcillin, warfarin.

I.M.

- Obtain specimen for culture and sensitivity tests before giving. Begin therapy while awaiting results.
- Obtain blood for peak level 1 hour after I.M. injection or 30 minutes after I.V. infusion finishes; for trough levels, draw blood just before next dose. Don't collect blood in a heparinized tube; heparin is incompatible with aminoglycosides.

ACTION

Inhibits protein synthesis by binding directly to the 30S ribosomal subunit; bactericidal.

Route	Onset	Peak	Duration
I.V.	Immediate	30–90 min	Unknown
I.M.	Unknown	30–90 min	Unknown

Half-life: 2 to 3 hours.

ADVERSE REACTIONS

CNS: ***encephalopathy, seizures,*** fever, headache, lethargy, confusion, dizziness, numbness, peripheral neuropathy, vertigo, ataxia, tingling.
CV: hypotension.
EENT: *ototoxicity,* blurred vision, tinnitus.
GI: vomiting, nausea.
GU: ***nephrotoxicity,*** possible increase in urinary excretion of casts.
Hematologic: ***agranulocytosis, leukopenia, thrombocytopenia,*** anemia, eosinophilia.
Musculoskeletal: muscle twitching, myasthenia gravis–like syndrome.
Respiratory: ***apnea.***
Skin: rash, urticaria, pruritus, injection site pain.
Other: ***anaphylaxis.***

INTERACTIONS

Drug-drug. *Acyclovir, amphotericin B, cephalosporins, cidofovir, cisplatin, methoxyflurane, vancomycin, other aminoglycosides:* May increase ototoxicity and nephrotoxicity. Monitor hearing and renal function test results.
Atracurium, pancuronium, rocuronium, vecuronium: May increase effects of nondepolarizing muscle relaxants, including prolonged respiratory depression. Use together only when necessary, and expect to reduce dosage of nondepolarizing muscle relaxant.
Dimenhydrinate: May mask ototoxicity symptoms. Monitor patient's hearing.
General anesthetics: May increase neuromuscular blockade. Monitor patient closely.
Indomethacin: May increase peak and trough levels of gentamicin. Monitor gentamicin level.
I.V. loop diuretics (such as furosemide): May increase risk of ototoxicity. Monitor patient's hearing.
Parenteral penicillins (such as ampicillin and ticarcillin): May inactivate gentamicin in vitro. Don't mix together.

EFFECTS ON LAB TEST RESULTS

- May increase ALT, AST, bilirubin, BUN, creatinine, LDH, and nonprotein nitrogen levels. May decrease hemoglobin level.
- May increase eosinophil count. May decrease granulocyte, platelet, and WBC counts.

CONTRAINDICATIONS & CAUTIONS

- Contraindicated in patients hypersensitive to drug or other aminoglycosides.
- Use cautiously in neonates, infants, elderly patients, and patients with impaired renal function or neuromuscular disorders.

NURSING CONSIDERATIONS

- ***Alert:*** Evaluate patient's hearing before and during therapy. Notify prescriber if patient complains of tinnitus, vertigo, or hearing loss.
- Weigh patient and review renal function studies before therapy begins.
- ***Alert:*** Use preservative-free form when intrathecal route is used adjunctively for serious CNS infections, such as meningitis and ventriculitis.
- Maintain peak levels at 4 to 12 mcg/ml and trough levels at 1 to 2 mcg/ml. The maximum peak level is usually 8 mcg/ml, except in patients with cystic fibrosis, who need increased lung penetration. Prolonged peak levels of 10 to 12 mcg/ml or prolonged trough levels greater than 2 mcg/ml may increase risk of toxicity.
- ***Alert:*** Monitor renal function: urine output, specific gravity, urinalysis, BUN and creatinine levels, and creatinine clearance. Report to prescriber evidence of declining renal function.
- Hemodialysis for 8 hours may remove up to 50% of drug from blood.
- Watch for signs and symptoms of superinfection (especially of upper respiratory tract), such as continued fever, chills, and increased pulse rate.
- Therapy usually continues for 7 to 10 days. If no response occurs in 3 to 5 days, stop therapy and obtain new specimens for culture and sensitivity testing.

PATIENT TEACHING

- Instruct patient to promptly report adverse reactions, such as dizziness, vertigo, unsteady gait, ringing in the ears, hearing loss, numbness, tingling, or muscle twitching.
- Encourage patient to drink plenty of fluids.
- Warn patient to avoid hazardous activities if adverse CNS reactions occur.

guanfacine hydrochloride

GWAHN-fa-seen

Tenex

Pharmacologic class: centrally acting antiadrenergic
Pregnancy risk category B

AVAILABLE FORMS

Tablets: 1 mg, 2 mg

INDICATIONS & DOSAGES

➤ **Hypertension**

Adults: Initially, 1 mg P.O. once daily at bedtime. If response isn't adequate after 3 to 4 weeks, increase dosage to 2 mg daily. Dosage may be further increased to 3 mg P.O. after an additional 3 to 4 weeks.

➤ **To relieve symptoms of heroin withdrawal ♦**

Adults: 0.03 mg to 1.5 mg P.O. once daily.

➤ **Migraine ♦**

Adults: 1 mg P.O. once daily for 12 weeks.

ADMINISTRATION

P.O.

- When given with another antihypertensive, give dose at bedtime to reduce somnolence.

ACTION

Reduces sympathetic outflow from the vasomotor center to the heart and blood vessels, resulting in a decrease in peripheral vascular resistance and a reduction in heart rate.

Route	Onset	Peak	Duration
P.O.	Unknown	1–4 hr	24 hr

Half-life: About 17 hours.

ADVERSE REACTIONS

CNS: *dizziness, somnolence,* fatigue, headache, insomnia, asthenia.
CV: ***bradycardia.***
GI: *constipation, dry mouth,* diarrhea, nausea.
GU: impotence.
Skin: dermatitis, pruritus.

INTERACTIONS

Drug-drug. *CNS depressants:* May increase sedation. Use together cautiously.
Tricyclic antidepressants: May inhibit antihypertensive effects. Monitor blood pressure.
Drug-lifestyle. *Alcohol:* May increase sedation. Discourage alcohol use.

EFFECTS ON LAB TEST RESULTS

None reported.

CONTRAINDICATIONS & CAUTIONS

- Contraindicated in patients hypersensitive to drug.
- Use cautiously in patients with severe coronary insufficiency, recent MI, cerebrovascular disease, or chronic renal or hepatic insufficiency.

NURSING CONSIDERATIONS

- Monitor blood pressure frequently.
- Risk and severity of adverse reactions increase with higher dosages.
- Drug may be used alone or with a diuretic.
- Rebound hypertension may occur and, if it occurs, will be noticeable within 2 to 4 days after therapy ends.
- ***Look alike–sound alike:*** Don't confuse guanfacine with guanidine, guaifenesin, or guanabenz. Don't confuse Tenex with Xanax, Entex, or Ten-K.

PATIENT TEACHING

- Tell patient not to stop therapy abruptly. Rebound high blood pressure may occur but is less common than that which occurs with similar drugs.
- Advise patient to avoid activities that require alertness before drug's effects are known; drowsiness may occur.
- Warn patient that he may have a lower tolerance to alcohol and other CNS depressants during therapy.

SAFETY ALERT!

heparin sodium

HEP-ah-rin

Hepalean†, Heparin Lock Flush Solution (with Tubex), Heparin Sodium Injection, Hep-Lock, Hep-Pak

Pharmacologic class: anticoagulant
Pregnancy risk category C

AVAILABLE FORMS

Products are derived from beef lung or pork intestinal mucosa.
heparin sodium
Carpuject: 5,000 units/ml
Premixed I.V. solutions: 1,000 units in 500 ml of normal saline solution; 2,000 units in 1,000 ml of normal saline solution; 12,500 units in 250 ml of half-normal saline solution; 25,000 units in 250 ml of half-normal saline solution; 25,000 units in 500 ml of half-normal saline solution; 10,000 units in 100 ml of D_5W; 12,500 units in 250 ml of D_5W; 20,000 units in 500 ml of D_5W; 25,000 units in 250 ml D_5W; 25,000 units in 500 ml D_5W
Single-dose ampules and vials: 1,000 units/ml, 5,000 units/ml, 10,000 units/ml, 20,000 units/ml, 40,000 units/ml
Syringes: 1,000 units/ml, 2,500 units/ml, 5,000 units/ml, 7,500 units/ml, 10,000 units/ml, 20,000 units/ml
Unit-dose vials: 1,000 units/ml, 2,500 units/ml, 5,000 units/ml, 7,500 units/ml, 10,000 units/ml, 20,000 units/ml
Vials (multidose): 1,000 units/ml, 2,000 units/ml, 2,500 units/ml, 5,000 units/ml, 10,000 units/ml, 20,000 units/ml, 40,000 units/ml
heparin sodium flush
Syringes: 10 units/ml, 100 units/ml
Vials: 10 units/ml, 100 units/ml

INDICATIONS & DOSAGES

➤ Full-dose continuous I.V. infusion therapy for deep vein thrombosis (DVT), MI, pulmonary embolism

Adults: Initially, 5,000 units by I.V. bolus; then 750 to 1,500 units/hour by I.V. infusion with pump. Titrate hourly rate based on PTT results (every 4 to 6 hours in the early stages of treatment).
Children: Initially, 50 units/kg I.V.; then 25 units/kg/hour or 20,000 units/m^2 daily by I.V. infusion pump. Titrate dosage based on PTT.

➤ **Full-dose subcutaneous therapy for DVT, MI, pulmonary embolism**
Adults: Initially, 5,000 units I.V. bolus and 10,000 to 20,000 units in a concentrated solution subcutaneously; then 8,000 to 10,000 units subcutaneously every 8 hours or 15,000 to 20,000 units in a concentrated solution every 12 hours.

➤ **Full-dose intermittent I.V. therapy for DVT, MI, pulmonary embolism**
Adults: Initially, 10,000 units by I.V. bolus; then titrated according to PTT, and 5,000 to 10,000 units I.V. every 4 to 6 hours.
Children: Initially, 100 units/kg by I.V. bolus; then 50 to 100 units/kg every 4 hours.

➤ **Fixed low-dose therapy for prevention of venous thrombosis, pulmonary embolism, embolism associated with atrial fibrillation, and postoperative DVT**
Adults: 5,000 units subcutaneously every 12 hours. In surgical patients, give first dose 1 to 2 hours before procedure; then 5,000 units subcutaneously every 8 to 12 hours for 5 to 7 days or until patient can walk.

➤ **Consumptive coagulopathy (such as disseminated intravascular coagulation)**
Adults: 50 to 100 units/kg by I.V. bolus or continuous I.V. infusion every 4 hours.
Children: 25 to 50 units/kg by I.V. bolus or continuous I.V. infusion every 4 hours. If no improvement within 4 to 8 hours, stop heparin.

➤ **Open-heart surgery**
Adults: For total body perfusion, 150 to 400 units/kg continuous I.V. infusion.

➤ **Patency maintenance of I.V. indwelling catheters**
Adults: 10 to 100 units I.V. flush. Use sufficient volume to fill device. Not intended for therapeutic use.

ADMINISTRATION

I.V.

- Draw blood to establish baseline coagulation parameters before therapy.
- Use an infusion pump to provide maximum safety. Check constant infusions regularly, even when pumps are in good working order, to ensure correct dosing. Place notice above patient's bed to caution I.V. team or laboratory personnel to apply pressure dressings after taking blood.
- During intermittent infusion, always draw blood 30 minutes before next scheduled dose to avoid falsely elevated PTT. Blood for PTT may be drawn 4 hours after continuous I.V. heparin therapy starts. Never draw blood for PTT from the tubing of the heparin infusion or from the infused vein because falsely elevated PTT will result. Always draw blood from the opposite arm.
- Don't skip a dose or try to "catch up" with a solution containing heparin. If solution runs out, restart it as soon as possible, and reschedule bolus dose immediately. Monitor PTT.
- Concentrated heparin solutions (more than 100 units/ml) can irritate blood vessels.
- Never piggyback other drugs into an infusion line while heparin infusion is running. Never mix another drug and heparin in same syringe when giving a bolus.
- **Incompatibilities:** Alteplase; amikacin; amiodarone; amphotericin B cholesteryl; ampicillin sodium; atracurium; caspofungin; chlorpromazine; ciprofloxacin; codeine phosphate; cytarabine; dacarbazine; dantrolene; daunorubicin; dextrose 4.3% in sodium chloride solution 0.18%; diazepam; diltiazem; dobutamine; doxorubicin; doxycycline hyclate; droperidol; ergotamine; erythromycin gluceptate or lactobionate; filgrastim; gentamicin; haloperidol lactate; hydrocortisone sodium succinate; hydroxyzine hydrochloride; idarubicin; kanamycin; labetalol; levofloxacin; levorphanol; meperidine; methadone; methylprednisolone sodium succinate; morphine sulfate; nesiritide; netilmicin; nicardipine; penicillin G potassium; penicillin G sodium; pentazocine lactate; phenytoin sodium; polymyxin

B sulfate; prochlorperazine edisylate; promethazine hydrochloride; quinidine gluconate; reteplase; 1/6 M sodium lactate; solutions containing a phosphate buffer, sodium carbonate, or sodium oxalate; streptomycin; sulfamethoxazole and trimethoprim; tobramycin sulfate; trifluoperazine; triflupromazine; vancomycin; vinblastine; warfarin.

Subcutaneous

- Give low-dose injections sequentially between iliac crests in lower abdomen deep into subcutaneous fat. Inject drug subcutaneously slowly into fat pad.
- Don't massage injection site; watch for signs of bleeding there.
- Alternate sites every 12 hours—right for morning, left for evening. Record location.

ACTION

Accelerates formation of antithrombin III-thrombin complex and deactivates thrombin, preventing conversion of fibrinogen to fibrin.

Route	Onset	Peak	Duration
I.V.	Immediate	Unknown	Variable
Subcut.	20–60 min	2–4 hr	Variable

Half-life: 1 to 2 hours. Half-life is dose-dependent and nonlinear and may be disproportionately prolonged at higher doses.

ADVERSE REACTIONS

CNS: fever.
EENT: rhinitis.
Hematologic: ***hemorrhage, overly prolonged clotting time, thrombocytopenia, white clot syndrome.***
Metabolic: ***hyperkalemia,*** hypoaldosteronism.
Skin: irritation, mild pain, hematoma, ulceration, cutaneous or subcutaneous necrosis, pruritus, urticaria.
Other: hypersensitivity reactions, including chills, ***anaphylactoid reactions.***

INTERACTIONS

Drug-drug. *Antihistamines, digoxin, quinine, tetracycline:* May interfere with anticoagulant effect of heparin. Monitor patient for therapeutic effect.
Antiplatelet drugs, salicylates: May increase anticoagulant effect. Use together cautiously. Monitor coagulation studies and patient closely.
Cephalosporins, penicillins: May increase risk of bleeding. Monitor patient closely.
Nitroglycerin: May decrease effects of heparin. Monitor patient closely.
Oral anticoagulants: May increase additive anticoagulation. Monitor PT, INR, and PTT.
Thrombolytics: May increase risk of hemorrhage. Monitor patient closely.
Drug-herb. *Angelica (dong quai), boldo, bromelains, capsicum, chamomile, dandelion, danshen, devil's claw, fenugreek, feverfew, garlic, ginger, ginkgo, ginseng, horse chestnut, licorice, meadowsweet, motherwort, onion, passion flower, red clover, white willow:* May increase risk of bleeding. Discourage herb use.
Drug-lifestyle. *Smoking:* May interfere with anticoagulant effect of heparin. Discourage smoking.

EFFECTS ON LAB TEST RESULTS

- May increase ALT, AST, and potassium levels.
- May increase INR, PT, and PTT. May decrease platelet count.
- Drug may cause false elevations in some tests for thyroxine level.

CONTRAINDICATIONS & CAUTIONS

- Contraindicated in patients hypersensitive to drug. Conditionally contraindicated in patients with active bleeding, blood dyscrasia, or bleeding tendencies, such as hemophilia, thrombocytopenia, or hepatic disease with hypoprothrombinemia; suspected intracranial hemorrhage; suppurative thrombophlebitis; inaccessible ulcerative lesions (especially of GI tract) and open ulcerative wounds; extensive denudation of skin; ascorbic acid deficiency and other conditions that cause increased capillary permeability.
- Conditionally contraindicated during or after brain, eye, or spinal cord surgery; during spinal tap or spinal anesthesia; during continuous tube drainage of stomach or small intestine; and in subacute bacterial endocarditis, shock, advanced renal

disease, threatened abortion, or severe hypertension.
• Use cautiously in women during menses or after childbirth and in patients with mild hepatic or renal disease, alcoholism, occupations with high risk of physical injury, or history of allergies, asthma, or GI ulcerations.

NURSING CONSIDERATIONS

• Although heparin use is clearly hazardous in certain conditions, its risks and benefits must be evaluated.
• If a woman needs anticoagulation during pregnancy, most prescribers use heparin.
• Some commercially available heparin injections contain benzyl alcohol. Avoid using these products in neonates and pregnant women if possible.
• Drug requirements are higher in early phases of thrombogenic diseases and febrile states; they are lower when patient's condition stabilizes.
• Elderly patients should usually start at lower dosage.
• Check order and vial carefully; heparin comes in various concentrations.
• ***Alert:*** USP and international units aren't equivalent for heparin.
• ***Alert:*** Heparin, low–molecular-weight heparins, and danaparoid aren't interchangeable.
• ***Alert:*** Don't change concentrations of infusions unless absolutely necessary. This is a common source of dosage errors.
• ***Alert:*** There is the potential for delayed onset of heparin-induced thrombocytopenia (HIT), a serious antibody-mediated reaction resulting from irreversible aggregation of platelets. HIT may progress to the development of venous and arterial thromboses, a condition referred to as heparin-induced thrombocytopenia and thrombosis (HITT). Thrombotic events may be the initial presentation for HITT, which can occur up to several weeks after stopping heparin therapy. Evaluate patients presenting with thrombocytopenia or thrombosis after stopping heparin for HIT and HITT.
• Draw blood for PTT 4 to 6 hours after dose given subcutaneously.
• Avoid I.M. injections of other drugs to prevent or minimize hematoma.
• Measure PTT carefully and regularly. Anticoagulation is present when PTT values are 1½ to 2 times the control values.
• Monitor platelet count regularly. When new thrombosis accompanies thrombocytopenia (white clot syndrome), stop heparin.
• Regularly inspect patient for bleeding gums, bruises on arms or legs, petechiae, nosebleeds, melena, tarry stools, hematuria, and hematemesis.
• Monitor vital signs.
• ***Alert:*** To treat severe overdose, use protamine sulfate, a heparin antagonist. Dosage is based on the dose of heparin, its route of administration, and the time since it was given. Generally, 1 to 1.5 mg of protamine per 100 units of heparin is given if only a few minutes have elapsed; 0.5 to 0.75 mg protamine per 100 units heparin, if 30 to 60 minutes have elapsed; and 0.25 to 0.375 mg protamine per 100 units heparin, if 2 hours or more have elapsed. Don't give more than 50 mg protamine in a 10-minute period.
• Abrupt withdrawal may cause increased coagulability; warfarin therapy usually overlaps heparin therapy for continuation of prophylaxis or treatment.
• ***Look alike–sound alike:*** Don't confuse heparin with Hespan.
• ***Look alike–sound alike:*** Don't confuse heparin sodium injection 10,000 units/ml and Hep-Lock 10 units/ml.

PATIENT TEACHING

• Instruct patient and family to watch for signs of bleeding or bruising and to notify prescriber immediately if any occur.
• Tell patient to avoid OTC drugs containing aspirin, other salicylates, or drugs that may interact with heparin unless ordered by prescriber.
• Advise patient to consult with prescriber before starting herbal therapy; many herbs have anticoagulant, antiplatelet, or fibrinolytic properties.

hydralazine hydrochloride
hye-DRAL-a-zeen

Apresoline, Novo-Hylazin†

Pharmacologic class: peripheral dilator
Pregnancy risk category C

AVAILABLE FORMS
Injection: 20 mg/ml in 1-ml vial
Tablets: 10 mg, 25 mg, 50 mg, 100 mg

INDICATIONS & DOSAGES
➤ **Hypertension**
Adults: Initially, 10 mg P.O. q.i.d.; gradually increase over 2 weeks to 50 mg q.i.d., based on patient tolerance and response. Once stabilized, maintenance dosage can be divided b.i.d. Recommended range is 12.5 to 50 mg b.i.d.
Children: Initially, 0.75 mg/kg daily P.O. divided into four doses; gradually increased over 3 to 4 weeks to maximum of 7.5 mg/kg or 200 mg daily. Maximum first P.O. dose is 25 mg.

Or, 0.1 to 0.2 mg/kg I.V. every 4 to 6 hours, p.r.n. Maximum first parenteral dose is 20 mg.
➤ **Hypertensive crisis**
Adults: 10 to 20 mg I.V. slowly or 10 to 50 mg I.M.; repeat as needed. Switch to oral form as soon as possible.
➤ **Preeclampsia, eclampsia**
Adults: Initially, 5 to 10 mg I.V., followed by 5- to 10-mg I.V. doses (range 5 to 20 mg) every 20 to 30 minutes, as needed; or, 0.5 to 10 mg/hour I.V. infusion.
➤ **Severe heart failure ♦**
Adults: Initially, 50 to 75 mg P.O. daily. Maintenance doses range from 200 to 600 mg P.O. daily in divided doses every 6 to 12 hours.

ADMINISTRATION
P.O.
- Give drug with food to increase absorption.

I.V.
- Give drug slowly and repeat p.r.n., generally every 4 to 6 hours. Hydralazine changes color in most infusion solutions; these color changes don't indicate loss of potency.
- Drug is compatible with normal saline, Ringer's, lactated Ringer's, and several other common I.V. solutions.
- Replace parenteral therapy with oral therapy as soon as possible.
- **Incompatibilities:** Aminophylline, ampicillin sodium, chlorothiazide, D_5W, dextrose 10% in lactated Ringer's solution, dextrose 10% in normal saline solution, diazoxide, doxapram, edetate calcium disodium, ethacrynate, fructose 10% in normal saline solution, fructose 10% in water, furosemide, hydrocortisone sodium succinate, mephentermine, metaraminol bitartrate, methohexital, nitroglycerin, phenobarbital sodium, verapamil.

I.M.
- Switch to oral form as soon as possible.

ACTION
Unknown. A direct-acting peripheral vasodilator that relaxes arteriolar smooth muscle.

Route	Onset	Peak	Duration
P.O.	20–30 min	1–2 hr	2–4 hr
I.V.	5–20 min	10–80 min	2–6 hr
I.M.	10–30 min	1 hr	2–6 hr

Half-life: 3 to 7 hours.

ADVERSE REACTIONS
CNS: *headache,* peripheral neuritis, dizziness.
CV: *angina pectoris, palpitations, tachycardia,* orthostatic hypotension, edema, flushing.
EENT: nasal congestion.
GI: *nausea, vomiting, diarrhea, anorexia,* constipation.
Hematologic: ***neutropenia, leukopenia, agranulocytopenia, agranulocytosis, thrombocytopenia with or without purpura.***
Skin: rash.
Other: *lupuslike syndrome.*

INTERACTIONS
Drug-drug. *Diazoxide, MAO inhibitors:* May cause severe hypotension. Use together cautiously.

Diuretics, other hypotensive drugs: May cause excessive hypotension. Dosage adjustment may be needed.
Indomethacin: May decrease effects of hydralazine. Monitor blood pressure.
Metoprolol, propranolol: May increase levels and effects of these beta blockers. Monitor patient closely. May need to adjust dosage of either drug.

EFFECTS ON LAB TEST RESULTS
- May decrease hemoglobin level.
- May decrease neutrophil, WBC, granulocyte, platelet, and RBC counts.
- May cause positive ANA titers.

CONTRAINDICATIONS & CAUTIONS
- Contraindicated in patients hypersensitive to drug.
- Contraindicated in those with coronary artery disease or mitral valvular rheumatic heart disease.
- Use cautiously in patients with suspected cardiac disease, stroke, or severe renal impairment and in those taking other antihypertensives.

NURSING CONSIDERATIONS
- Monitor patient's blood pressure, pulse rate, and body weight frequently. Drug may be given with diuretics and beta blockers to decrease sodium retention and tachycardia and to prevent angina attacks.
- Elderly patients may be more sensitive to drug's hypotensive effects.
- Monitor CBC, lupus erythematosus cell preparation, and antinuclear antibody titer determination before therapy and periodically during long-term therapy.
- ***Alert:*** Monitor patient closely for signs and symptoms of lupuslike syndrome (sore throat, fever, muscle and joint aches, rash), and notify prescriber immediately if they develop.
- Improve patient compliance by giving drug b.i.d. Check with prescriber.
- ***Look alike–sound alike:*** Don't confuse hydralazine with hydroxyzine or Apresoline with Apresazide.
- Apresoline may contain tartrazine.

PATIENT TEACHING
- Instruct patient to take oral form with meals to increase absorption.
- Inform patient that low blood pressure and dizziness upon standing can be minimized by rising slowly and avoiding sudden position changes.
- Tell woman of childbearing age to notify prescriber if she suspects pregnancy. Drug will need to be stopped.
- Tell patient to notify prescriber of unexplained prolonged general tiredness or fever, muscle or joint aching, or chest pain.

hydrochlorothiazide
hye-droe-klor-oh-THYE-a-zide

Apo-Hydro†, Esidrix, Ezide, Hydro-Par, Microzide, Novo-Hydrazide†, Nu-hydro†, Oretic, Urozide†

Pharmacologic class: thiazide diuretic
Pregnancy risk category B

AVAILABLE FORMS
Capsules: 12.5 mg
Oral solution: 50 mg/5 ml
Tablets: 25 mg, 50 mg, 100 mg

INDICATIONS & DOSAGES
➤ **Edema**
Adults: 25 to 100 mg P.O. daily or intermittently; up to 200 mg initially for several days until nonedematous weight is attained.
➤ **Hypertension**
Adults: 12.5 to 50 mg P.O. once daily. Increase or decrease daily dose based on blood pressure.
Children ages 6 months to 12 years: 1 to 2 mg/kg P.O. daily in a single dose or two divided doses. The total daily dose shouldn't exceed 37.5 mg for children up to age 2 or 100 mg in children ages 2 to 12.
Children younger than age 6 months: Up to 3 mg/kg P.O. daily in two divided doses.
Adjust-a-dose: In patients older than age 65, initially 12.5 mg daily. Adjust in increments of 12.5 mg, if needed.

ADMINISTRATION
P.O.
- Give drug with food to minimize GI upset.

• To prevent nocturia, give drug in morning. If second dose is needed, give in early afternoon.

ACTION

Increases sodium and water excretion by inhibiting sodium and chloride reabsorption in distal segment of the nephron.

Route	Onset	Peak	Duration
P.O.	2 hr	4–6 hr	6–12 hr

Half-life: 5½ to 15 hours.

ADVERSE REACTIONS

CNS: dizziness, vertigo, headache, paresthesia, weakness, restlessness.
CV: orthostatic hypotension, allergic myocarditis, vasculitis.
GI: ***pancreatitis,*** anorexia, nausea, epigastric distress, vomiting, abdominal pain, diarrhea, constipation.
GU: ***renal failure,*** polyuria, frequent urination, interstitial nephritis.
Hematologic: ***aplastic anemia, agranulocytosis, leukopenia, thrombocytopenia,*** hemolytic anemia.
Hepatic: jaundice.
Metabolic: asymptomatic hyperuricemia, hypokalemia, hyperglycemia and impaired glucose tolerance, fluid and electrolyte imbalances, including dilutional hyponatremia and hypochloremia, metabolic alkalosis, hypercalcemia, volume depletion and dehydration.
Musculoskeletal: muscle cramps.
Respiratory: ***respiratory distress,*** pneumonitis.
Skin: dermatitis, photosensitivity reactions, rash, purpura, alopecia.
Other: ***anaphylactic reactions,*** hypersensitivity reactions, gout.

INTERACTIONS

Drug-drug. *Amphotericin B, corticosteroids:* May increase risk of hypokalemia. Monitor potassium level closely.
Antidiabetics: May decrease hypoglycemic effects. Adjust dosage if needed. Monitor glucose level.
Antihypertensives: May have additive antihypertensive effect. Use together cautiously.
Barbiturates, opioids: May increase orthostatic hypotensive effect. Monitor patient closely.
Bumetanide, ethacrynic acid, furosemide, torsemide: May cause excessive diuretic response, causing serious electrolyte abnormalities or dehydration. Adjust doses carefully, and monitor patient closely for signs and symptoms of excessive diuretic response.
Cardiac glycosides: May increase risk of digoxin toxicity from diuretic-induced hypokalemia. Monitor potassium and digoxin levels.
Cholestyramine, colestipol: May decrease intestinal absorption of thiazides. Separate doses by 2 hours.
Diazoxide: May increase antihypertensive, hyperglycemic, and hyperuricemic effects. Use together cautiously.
Lithium: May decrease lithium excretion, increasing risk of lithium toxicity. Monitor lithium level.
NSAIDs: May increase risk of renal failure. May decrease diuretic and antihypertensive effects. Monitor renal function and blood pressure.
Drug-herb. *Dandelion:* May interfere with diuretic activity. Discourage use together.
Licorice: May cause unexpected rapid potassium loss. Discourage use together.
Drug-lifestyle. *Alcohol use:* May increase orthostatic hypotensive effect. Discourage use together.

EFFECTS ON LAB TEST RESULTS

• May increase glucose, cholesterol, triglyceride, calcium, and uric acid levels. May decrease potassium, sodium, chloride, and hemoglobin levels.
• May decrease granulocyte, WBC, and platelet counts.

CONTRAINDICATIONS & CAUTIONS

• Contraindicated in patients with anuria and patients hypersensitive to other thiazides or other sulfonamide derivatives.
• Use cautiously in children and in patients with severe renal disease, impaired hepatic function, or progressive hepatic disease.

NURSING CONSIDERATIONS

• Monitor fluid intake and output, weight, blood pressure, and electrolyte levels.

• Watch for signs and symptoms of hypokalemia, such as muscle weakness and cramps.
• Drug may be used with potassium-sparing diuretic to prevent potassium loss.
• Consult prescriber and dietitian about a high-potassium diet or potassium supplement. Foods rich in potassium include citrus fruits, tomatoes, bananas, dates, and apricots.
• Monitor creatinine and BUN levels regularly. Cumulative effects of drug may occur with impaired renal function.
• Monitor uric acid level, especially in patients with history of gout.
• Monitor glucose level, especially in diabetic patients.
• Monitor elderly patients, who are especially susceptible to excessive diuresis.
• Stop thiazides and thiazide-like diuretics before parathyroid function tests.
• In patients with hypertension, therapeutic response may be delayed several weeks.

PATIENT TEACHING

• Instruct patient to take drug with food to minimize GI upset.
• Advise patient to take drug in morning to avoid need to urinate at night; if patient needs second dose, have him take it in early afternoon.
• Advise patient to avoid sudden posture changes and to rise slowly to avoid dizziness upon standing quickly.
• Encourage patient to use a sunblock to prevent photosensitivity reactions.
• Tell patient to check with prescriber or pharmacist before using OTC drugs.

SAFETY ALERT!

ibutilide fumarate

eye-BYOO-ti-lyed

Corvert

Pharmacologic class: methanesulfonanilide derivative
Pregnancy risk category C

AVAILABLE FORMS

Injection: 0.1 mg/ml in 10-ml vials

INDICATIONS & DOSAGES

➤ **Rapid conversion of recent onset atrial fibrillation or atrial flutter to sinus rhythm**

Adults who weigh 60 kg (132 lb) or more: 1 mg I.V. infusion over 10 minutes. May repeat dose if arrhythmia doesn't respond 10 minutes after completing first dose.
Adults who weigh less than 60 kg: 0.01 mg/kg I.V. infusion over 10 minutes. May repeat dose if arrhythmia doesn't respond 10 minutes after completing first dose.

ADMINISTRATION

I.V.

• Give drug undiluted or diluted in 50 ml of diluent, and add to normal saline solution for injection or D_5W before infusion. Add contents of 10-ml vial (0.1 mg/ml) to 50-ml infusion bag to form admixture of about 0.017 mg/ml ibutilide. Use drug with polyvinyl chloride plastic bags or polyolefin bags.
• Give drug over 10 minutes.
• Stop infusion if arrhythmia is terminated or patient develops ventricular tachycardia or marked prolongation of QT or QTc interval. If arrhythmia doesn't respond 10 minutes after infusion ends, may repeat dose.
• Admixtures with approved diluents are stable for 24 hours at room temperature; 48 hours if refrigerated.
• Don't infuse parenteral products that contain particulate matter or are discolored.
• **Incompatibilities:** None reported.

ACTION

Prolongs action potential in isolated cardiac myocyte and increases atrial and ventricular refractoriness, namely class III electrophysiologic effects.

Route	Onset	Peak	Duration
I.V.	Unknown	Unknown	Unknown

Half-life: Averages about 6 hours.

ADVERSE REACTIONS

CNS: headache.
CV: ***sustained polymorphic ventricular tachycardia, AV block, bradycardia,***

heart failure, ventricular extrasystoles, ***nonsustained ventricular tachycardia,*** hypotension, bundle-branch block, hypertension, ***prolonged QT interval,*** palpitations, tachycardia.
GI: nausea.

INTERACTIONS
Drug-drug. *Class IA antiarrhythmics (disopyramide, procainamide, quinidine), other class III drugs (amiodarone, sotalol):* May increase potential for prolonged refractoriness. Don't give these drugs for at least five half-lives before and 4 hours after ibutilide dose.
Digoxin: Supraventricular arrhythmias may mask cardiotoxicity from excessive digoxin level. Use with caution in patients who may have an increased digoxin therapeutic range.
H_1-receptor antagonist antihistamines, phenothiazines, tetracyclic antidepressants, tricyclic antidepressants, other drugs that prolong QT interval: May increase risk of proarrhythmia. Monitor patient closely.

EFFECTS ON LAB TEST RESULTS
None reported.

CONTRAINDICATIONS & CAUTIONS
- Contraindicated in patients hypersensitive to drug or its components.
- Contraindicated in patients with history of polymorphic ventricular tachycardia. Use not recommended in breast-feeding women.
- Use cautiously in patients with hepatic or renal dysfunction.
- Safety and effectiveness of drug haven't been established in children.

NURSING CONSIDERATIONS
- Only skilled personnel should give drug. Cardiac monitor, intracardiac pacing, cardioverter or defibrillator, and drugs to treat sustained ventricular tachycardia must be available.
- Before therapy, correct hypokalemia and hypomagnesemia to reduce risk of proarrhythmia. Patients with atrial fibrillation lasting longer than 2 to 3 days must be adequately anticoagulated, generally over at least 2 weeks.
- Monitor ECG continuously during administration and for at least 4 hours afterward or until QTc interval returns to baseline; drug can induce or worsen ventricular arrhythmias. Longer monitoring is required if ECG shows arrhythmia or patient has hepatic insufficiency.
- Don't give class IA or other class III antiarrhythmics with infusion or for 4 hours afterward.

PATIENT TEACHING
- Tell patient to report adverse reactions promptly.
- Instruct patient to alert nurse of discomfort at injection site.

iloprost
EYE-loe-prost

Ventavis

Pharmacologic class: prostacyclin analog
Pregnancy risk category C

AVAILABLE FORMS
Inhalation solution: 10 mcg/ml in 1- and 2-ml single-dose ampules

INDICATIONS & DOSAGES
➤ **Pulmonary arterial hypertension in patients with New York Heart Association Class III or IV symptoms**
Adults: Initially, 2.5 mcg inhaled using the I-neb or the Prodose Adaptive Aerosol Delivery (AAD) systems. As tolerated, increase to 5 mcg inhaled six to nine times daily while patient is awake, as needed, but to no more than every 2 hours. Maximum, 5 mcg nine times daily.

ADMINISTRATION
Inhalational
- Use only I-neb AAD or Prodose AAD delivery devices, per manufacturer's instructions.

ACTION
Lowers pulmonary arterial pressure by dilating systemic and pulmonary arterial beds. Drug also affects platelet

aggregation, although effect in pulmonary hypertension treatment isn't known.

Route	Onset	Peak	Duration
Inhalation	Unknown	Unknown	30–60 min

Half-life: 20 to 30 minutes.

ADVERSE REACTIONS

CNS: *headache,* insomnia, syncope.
CV: *hypotension, vasodilation, chest pain,* ***heart failure, supraventricular tachycardia,*** palpitations, peripheral edema.
GI: *nausea,* tongue pain, vomiting.
GU: ***renal failure.***
Musculoskeletal: *trismus,* back pain, muscle cramps.
Respiratory: *cough,* dyspnea, hemoptysis, pneumonia.
Other: *flulike syndrome.*

INTERACTIONS

Drug-drug. *Anticoagulants:* May increase risk of bleeding. Monitor patient closely.
Antihypertensives, vasodilators: May increase effects of these drugs. Monitor patient's blood pressure.

EFFECTS ON LAB TEST RESULTS

- May increase alkaline phosphatase and GGT levels.

CONTRAINDICATIONS & CAUTIONS

- No contraindications known. Avoid using in patients whose systolic blood pressure is less than 85 mm Hg.
- Use cautiously in elderly patients, patients with hepatic or renal impairment, and patients with COPD, severe asthma, or acute pulmonary infection.

NURSING CONSIDERATIONS

- Keep drug away from skin and eyes.
- The 2-ml ampule must be used with the Prodose AAD System and may be used with the I-neb AAD System. The 1-ml ampule must be used only with the I-neb AAD System.
- Take care not to inhale drug while providing treatment.
- Monitor patient's vital signs carefully at start of treatment.
- Watch for syncope.
- If patient develops evidence of pulmonary edema, stop treatment immediately.

PATIENT TEACHING

- Advise patient to take drug exactly as prescribed and using Prodose AAD or I-neb AAD.
- Urge patient to follow manufacturer's instructions for preparing and inhaling drug.
- Advise patient to keep a backup Prodose AAD or I-neb AAD in case the original malfunctions.
- Tell patient to keep drug away from skin and eyes and to rinse the area immediately if contact occurs.
- Caution patient not to ingest drug solution.
- Inform patient that drug may cause dizziness and fainting. Urge him to stand up slowly from a sitting or lying position and to report to prescriber worsening of symptoms.
- Tell patient to take drug before physical exertion but no more than every 2 hours.
- Tell patient not to expose others, especially pregnant women and infants, to drug.
- Teach patient how to clean equipment and safely dispose of used ampules after each treatment. Caution patient not to save or use leftover solution.

SAFETY ALERT!

inamrinone lactate

in-AM-ri-none

Pharmacologic class: bipyridine phosphodiesterase inhibitor
Pregnancy risk category C

AVAILABLE FORMS

Injection: 5 mg/ml in 20-ml ampules

INDICATIONS & DOSAGES

➤ Short-term management of heart failure

Adults: Initially, 0.75 mg/kg I.V. bolus over 2 to 3 minutes. Then begin maintenance infusion of 5 to 10 mcg/kg/minute. May give additional bolus of 0.75 mg/kg after 30 minutes. Don't exceed total daily dose of 10 mg/kg.

ADMINISTRATION

I.V.

- Give drug with an infusion pump. Use drug as supplied or dilute in half-normal saline solution or normal saline solution to a concentration of 1 to 3 mg/ml. Use diluted solution within 24 hours.
- Don't dilute with solutions containing dextrose because a slow chemical reaction occurs over 24 hours. Inamrinone can be injected into free-flowing dextrose infusions through a Y-connector or directly into tubing.
- Monitor blood pressure and heart rate throughout the infusion. If patient's blood pressure falls, slow or stop infusion and notify prescriber.
- **Incompatibilities:** Bicarbonate, dextrose-containing solutions such as D_5W, furosemide, glucose, procainamide, sodium bicarbonate, torsemide.

ACTION

Produces inotropic action by increasing cellular levels of cAMP. Produces vasodilation through a direct relaxant effect on vascular smooth muscle.

Route	Onset	Peak	Duration
I.V.	2–5 min	10 min	30–120 min

Half-life: About 4 hours.

ADVERSE REACTIONS

CNS: fever.
CV: ***arrhythmias,*** chest pain, hypotension.
GI: abdominal pain, anorexia, nausea, vomiting.
Hematologic: ***thrombocytopenia.***
Hepatic: ***hepatotoxicity.***
Metabolic: hypokalemia.
Skin: burning at injection site.
Other: hypersensitivity reactions.

INTERACTIONS

Drug-drug. *Cardiac glycosides:* May increase inotropic effect, which is a beneficial drug interaction. Monitor patient.
Disopyramide: May cause excessive hypotension. Monitor blood pressure.

EFFECTS ON LAB TEST RESULTS

- May increase liver enzyme level. May decrease potassium level.
- May increase sedimentation rate. May decrease platelet count.

CONTRAINDICATIONS & CAUTIONS

- Contraindicated in patients hypersensitive to inamrinone or bisulfites.
- Contraindicated in patients with severe aortic or pulmonic valvular disease in place of surgery or during acute phase of MI.
- Use cautiously in patients with hypertrophic cardiomyopathy.
- Safety and effectiveness haven't been established in children, although drug has been used in preterm infants for heart failure.

NURSING CONSIDERATIONS

- Drug is prescribed primarily for patients who haven't responded to cardiac glycosides, diuretics, and vasodilators.
- Dosage depends on clinical response, including assessment of pulmonary wedge pressure and cardiac output, as well as lessening of dyspnea, orthopnea, and fatigue.
- In patients with atrial fibrillation and flutter, drug may be added to cardiac glycoside therapy because it slightly enhances AV conduction and increases ventricular response rate.
- Correct hypokalemia before or during therapy.
- Monitor platelet count. If it falls below 150,000/mm^3, decrease dosage or stop drug if risk outweighs benefit.
- Monitor patient for hypersensitivity reactions, such as pericarditis, ascites, myositis, vasculitis, and pleuritis.
- Monitor intake and output and daily weight.
- Patients with end-stage cardiac disease may receive home treatment while awaiting heart transplantation.
- ***Look alike–sound alike:*** Because of confusion with amiodarone, "amrinone" was changed to "inamrinone."

PATIENT TEACHING

- Warn patient that burning may occur at injection site.
- Instruct home care patient and family about drug administration; tell them to report adverse reactions promptly.

indapamide

in-DAP-a-mide

Lozide†, Lozol

Pharmacologic class: thiazide-like diuretic
Pregnancy risk category B

AVAILABLE FORMS

Tablets: 1.25 mg, 2.5 mg

INDICATIONS & DOSAGES

➤ Edema

Adults: Initially, 2.5 mg P.O. daily in the morning. Increased to 5 mg daily after 1 week, if needed.

➤ Hypertension

Adults: Initially, 1.25 mg P.O. daily in the morning. Increased to 2.5 mg daily after 4 weeks, if needed. Increased to 5 mg daily after 4 more weeks, if needed. If response is inadequate, a second antihypertensive, given at 50% of the usual starting dose, may be needed.

ADMINISTRATION

P.O.

- Give drug with food to minimize GI upset.
- To prevent nocturia, give drug in the morning.

ACTION

Enhances excretion of sodium chloride and water by interfering with sodium transport in the distal tubule.

Route	Onset	Peak	Duration
P.O.	1–2 hr	Within 2 hr	Up to 36 hr

Half-life: About 14 hours.

ADVERSE REACTIONS

CNS: headache, nervousness, dizziness, light-headedness, weakness, vertigo, restlessness, drowsiness, fatigue, anxiety, depression, numbness of limbs, irritability, agitation, lethargy.
CV: orthostatic hypotension, palpitations, PVCs, irregular heartbeat, vasculitis, flushing.
EENT: rhinorrhea, blurred vision.
GI: anorexia, nausea, epigastric distress, vomiting, abdominal pain or cramps, diarrhea, constipation.
GU: nocturia, polyuria, frequent urination, impotence.
Metabolic: asymptomatic hyperuricemia, fluid and electrolyte imbalances, including dilutional hyponatremia, hypochloremia, metabolic alkalosis and hypokalemia, weight loss, volume depletion and dehydration, hyperglycemia.
Musculoskeletal: muscle cramps and spasms.
Skin: rash, pruritus, urticaria.
Other: gout.

INTERACTIONS

Drug-drug. *Amphotericin B, corticosteroids:* May increase risk of hypokalemia. Monitor potassium level closely.
Antidiabetics: May decrease hypoglycemic effect of sulfonylureas, causing elevated glucose levels. Adjust dosage, if needed. Monitor glucose level.
Barbiturates, opioids: May increase orthostasis. Monitor patient closely.
Bumetanide, ethacrynic acid, furosemide, torsemide: May cause excessive diuretic response, causing serious electrolyte abnormalities or dehydration. Adjust doses carefully, and monitor patient closely for signs and symptoms of excessive diuretic response.
Cardiac glycosides: May increase risk of digoxin toxicity from indapamide-induced hypokalemia. Monitor potassium and digoxin levels.
Cholestyramine, colestipol: May decrease absorption of thiazides. Separate doses by 2 hours.
Diazoxide: May increase antihypertensive, hyperglycemic, and hyperuricemic effects. Use together cautiously.
Lithium: May decrease lithium clearance that may increase lithium toxicity. Avoid using together.
NSAIDs: May increase risk of NSAID-induced renal failure. Monitor patient for signs and symptoms of renal failure.
Drug-herb. *Dandelion:* May interfere with drug activity. Discourage use together.
Licorice: May cause unexpected rapid potassium loss. Discourage use together.

Drug-lifestyle. *Alcohol use:* May increase orthostatic hypotensive effect. Discourage use together.

EFFECTS ON LAB TEST RESULTS
- May increase BUN, creatinine, glucose, cholesterol, triglyceride, calcium, and uric acid levels. May decrease potassium, sodium, phosphate, and chloride levels.

CONTRAINDICATIONS & CAUTIONS
- Contraindicated in patients hypersensitive to other sulfonamide-derived drugs and in those with anuria.
- Use cautiously in patients with severe renal disease, impaired hepatic function, or progressive hepatic disease.

NURSING CONSIDERATIONS
- Monitor fluid intake and output, weight, blood pressure, and electrolyte levels.
- Watch for signs of hypokalemia, such as muscle weakness and cramps. Drug may be used with potassium-sparing diuretic to prevent potassium loss.
- Consult prescriber and dietitian about a high-potassium diet or potassium supplement. Foods rich in potassium include citrus fruits, tomatoes, bananas, dates, and apricots.
- Monitor creatinine and BUN levels regularly. Cumulative effects of drug may occur in patients with impaired renal function.
- Monitor uric acid level, especially in patients with history of gout.
- Monitor glucose level, especially in diabetic patients.
- Monitor elderly patients, who are especially susceptible to excessive diuresis.
- Stop thiazides and thiazide-like diuretics before parathyroid function tests.
- Therapeutic response may be delayed several weeks in hypertensive patients.

PATIENT TEACHING
- Instruct patient to take drug in morning to prevent need to urinate at night.
- Tell patient to take drug with food to minimize GI upset.
- Advise patient to avoid sudden posture changes and to rise slowly to avoid dizziness upon standing quickly.

indomethacin
in-doe-METH-a-sin

Indocid†, Indocid SR†, Indocin, Indocin SR, Novo-Methacin†

indomethacin sodium trihydrate
Indocin I.V, Novo-Methacin†

Pharmacologic class: NSAID
Pregnancy risk category B; D in 3rd trimester

AVAILABLE FORMS
indomethacin
Capsules: 25 mg, 50 mg
Capsules (sustained-release): 75 mg
Oral suspension: 25 mg/5 ml
Suppositories: 50 mg
indomethacin sodium trihydrate
Injection: 1-mg vials

INDICATIONS & DOSAGES
➤ **Moderate to severe rheumatoid arthritis or osteoarthritis, ankylosing spondylitis**
Adults: 25 mg P.O. or P.R. b.i.d. or t.i.d. with food or antacids; increase daily dose by 25 or 50 mg every 7 days, up to 200 mg daily. Or, 75 mg sustained-release capsules P.O. to start, in morning or at bedtime, followed by 75 mg sustained-release capsules b.i.d. if needed.
➤ **Acute gouty arthritis**
Adults: 50 mg P.O. t.i.d. Reduce dose as soon as possible; then stop therapy. Don't use sustained-release form.
➤ **Acute painful shoulders (bursitis or tendinitis)**
Adults: 75 to 150 mg P.O. daily in divided doses t.i.d. or q.i.d. for 7 to 14 days.
➤ **To close a hemodynamically significant patent ductus arteriosus in premature neonates**
Neonates older than age 7 days: 0.2 mg/kg I.V.; then two doses of 0.25 mg/kg at 12- to 24-hour intervals.
Neonates ages 2 to 7 days: 0.2 mg/kg I.V.; then two doses of 0.2 mg/kg at 12- to 24-hour intervals.

Neonates younger than age 48 hours: 0.2 mg/kg I.V.; then two doses of 0.1 mg/kg at 12- to 24-hour intervals.

ADMINISTRATION

P.O.

- Give drug with food, milk, or antacid.

I.V.

- Reconstitute powder for injection with sterile water or normal saline solution. For each 1-mg vial, add 1 or 2 ml of diluent for a solution containing 1 mg/ml or 0.5 mg/ml, respectively. Give over 20 to 30 minutes.
- Use only preservative-free sterile saline solution or sterile water to prepare. Never use diluents containing benzyl alcohol because it has been linked to toxicity in newborns.
- Because injection contains no preservatives, reconstitute drug immediately before use and discard unused solution.
- If anuria or marked oliguria is evident, withhold administration of second or third scheduled I.V. dose and notify prescriber.
- Watch carefully for bleeding and for reduced urine output.
- **Incompatibilities:** Amino acid injection, calcium gluconate, cimetidine, dextrose injection, dobutamine, dopamine, gentamicin, levofloxacin, solutions with pH less than 6, tobramycin sulfate, tolazoline.

Rectal

- If suppository is too soft, place in refrigerator for 15 minutes or run under cold water in wrapper.

ACTION

May inhibit prostaglandin synthesis, to produce anti-inflammatory, analgesic, and antipyretic effects.

Route	Onset	Peak	Duration
P.O.	30 min	1–4 hr	4–6 hr
I.V.	Immediate	Immediate	4–6 hr
P.R.	Unknown	Unknown	4–6 hr

Half-life: 4¼ hours.

ADVERSE REACTIONS

P.O. and P.R.

CNS: *headache,* confusion, dizziness, depression, drowsiness, fatigue, peripheral neuropathy, psychic disturbances, somnolence, syncope, vertigo.
CV: edema, hypertension.
EENT: hearing loss, tinnitus.
GI: ***pancreatitis,*** abdominal pain, anorexia, constipation, diarrhea, dyspepsia, ***GI bleeding,*** nausea, peptic ulceration.
GU: hematuria.
Hematologic: iron deficiency anemia.
Metabolic: ***hyperkalemia.***
Skin: ***Stevens-Johnson syndrome,*** pruritus, urticaria.
Other: hypersensitivity reactions.

I.V.

GU: hematuria, interstitial nephritis, proteinuria.

INTERACTIONS

Drug-drug. *Aminoglycosides, cyclosporine, methotrexate:* May enhance toxicity of these drugs. Avoid using together.
Anticoagulants: May cause bleeding. Monitor patient closely.
Antihypertensives: May decrease antihypertensive effect. Monitor patient closely.
Antihypertensives, furosemide, thiazide diuretics: May impair response to both drugs. Avoid using together, if possible.
Aspirin: May decrease level of indomethacin. Avoid using together.
Aspirin, corticosteroids: May increase risk of GI toxicity. Avoid using together.
Bisphosphonates: May increase risk of gastric ulceration. Monitor patient for symptoms of gastric irritation or GI bleeding.
Diflunisal, probenecid: May decrease indomethacin excretion. Watch for increased indomethacin adverse reactions.
Digoxin: May prolong half-life of digoxin. Use together cautiously.
Dipyridamole: May enhance fluid retention. Avoid using together.
Lithium: May increase lithium level. Monitor patient for toxicity.
Penicillamine: May increase bioavailability of penicillamine. Monitor patient closely.
Phenytoin: May increase phenytoin level. Monitor patient closely.
Triamterene: May cause nephrotoxicity. Avoid using together.

Drug-herb. *Dong quai, feverfew, garlic, ginger, horse chestnut, red clover:* May cause bleeding. Discourage use together.
Senna: May inhibit diarrheal effects. Discourage use together.
White willow: Herb and drug contain similar components. Discourage use together.
Drug-lifestyle. *Alcohol use:* May cause GI toxicity. Discourage use together.

EFFECTS ON LAB TEST RESULTS

- May increase potassium level. May decrease hemoglobin level and hematocrit.
- May increase liver function test values.

CONTRAINDICATIONS & CAUTIONS

- Contraindicated in patients hypersensitive to drug and in those with a history of aspirin- or NSAID-induced asthma, rhinitis, or urticaria.
- Contraindicated in pregnant or breastfeeding women and in neonates with untreated infection, active bleeding, coagulation defects or thrombocytopenia, congenital heart disease needing patency of the ductus arteriosus, necrotizing enterocolitis, or significant renal impairment. Suppositories are contraindicated in patients with history of proctitis or recent rectal bleeding.
- Contraindicated in pregnant women.
- Use cautiously in elderly patients, those with history of GI disease, and those with epilepsy, parkinsonism, hepatic or renal disease, CV disease, infection, and mental illness or depression.

NURSING CONSIDERATIONS

- Because of the high risk of adverse effects from long-term use, drug shouldn't be used routinely as an analgesic or antipyretic.
- Sustained-release capsules shouldn't be used for acute gouty arthritis.
- If ductus arteriosus reopens, a second course of one to three doses may be given. If ineffective, surgery may be needed.
- Watch for bleeding in patients receiving anticoagulants, patients with coagulation defects, and neonates.
- Because NSAIDs impair synthesis of renal prostaglandins, they can decrease renal blood flow and lead to reversible renal impairment, especially in patients with renal failure, heart failure, or liver dysfunction; in elderly patients; and in those taking diuretics. Monitor these patients closely.
- Drug causes sodium retention; watch for weight gain (especially in elderly patients) and increased blood pressure in patients with hypertension.
- Monitor patient for rash and respiratory distress, which may indicate a hypersensitivity reaction.
- Because of their antipyretic and anti-inflammatory actions, NSAIDs may mask signs and symptoms of infection.
- Serious GI toxicity (including peptic ulcers and bleeding) can occur in patient taking NSAIDs, despite lack of symptoms.
- NSAIDs may cause increased risk of thrombotic events, MI, and stroke. Risk may be increased with duration of use and in patients with history of CV disease or risk factors of CV disease.
- Monitor patient on long-term oral therapy for toxicity by conducting regular eye examinations, hearing tests, CBCs, and kidney function tests.

PATIENT TEACHING

- Tell patient to take oral dose with food, milk, or antacid to prevent GI upset.
- Alert patient that using oral form with aspirin, alcohol, other NSAIDs, or corticosteroids may increase risk of adverse GI reactions.
- Teach patient signs and symptoms of GI bleeding, including blood in vomit, urine, or stool; coffee-ground vomit; and black, tarry stool. Tell him to notify prescriber immediately if any of these occurs.
- Tell patient to immediately report signs or symptoms of cardiac events, such as chest pain, shortness of breath, weakness, and slurred speech.
- Warn patient to avoid hazardous activities that require mental alertness until CNS effects are known.
- Tell patient to notify prescriber immediately if visual or hearing changes occur.

irbesartan

er-bah-SAR-tan

Avapro

Pharmacologic class: angiotensin II receptor antagonist
Pregnancy risk category C; D in 2nd and 3rd trimesters

AVAILABLE FORMS

Tablets: 75 mg, 150 mg, 300 mg

INDICATIONS & DOSAGES

➤ Hypertension
Adults and children age 13 and older: Initially, 150 mg P.O. daily, increased to maximum of 300 mg daily, if needed.
Children ages 6 to 12: Initially, 75 mg P.O. once daily, increased to maximum of 150 mg daily, if needed.
Adjust-a-dose: For volume- and sodium-depleted patients, initially, 75 mg P.O. daily.

➤ Nephropathy in patients with type 2 diabetes
Adults: Target maintenance dose is 300 mg P.O. once daily.

ADMINISTRATION

P.O.
- Give drug without regard for meals.

ACTION

Produces antihypertensive effect by competitive antagonist activity at the angiotensin II receptor.

Route	Onset	Peak	Duration
P.O.	Unknown	$^1/_2$–2 hr	24 hr

Half-life: 11 to 15 hours.

ADVERSE REACTIONS

CNS: fatigue, anxiety, dizziness, headache.
CV: chest pain, edema, tachycardia.
EENT: pharyngitis, rhinitis, sinus abnormality.
GI: diarrhea, dyspepsia, abdominal pain, nausea, vomiting.
GU: UTI.
Musculoskeletal: musculoskeletal trauma or pain.
Respiratory: upper respiratory tract infection, cough.
Skin: rash.

INTERACTIONS

None reported.

EFFECTS ON LAB TEST RESULTS

None reported.

CONTRAINDICATIONS & CAUTIONS

- Contraindicated in patients hypersensitive to drug or its components.
- Use cautiously in patients with impaired renal function, heart failure, and renal artery stenosis and in breast-feeding women.
- ***Alert:*** Use during pregnancy can cause injury and death to the developing fetus. When pregnancy is detected, stop drug as soon as possible.

NURSING CONSIDERATIONS

- Drug may be given with a diuretic or other antihypertensive, if needed, for control of hypertension.
- Symptomatic hypotension may occur in volume- or sodium-depleted patients (vigorous diuretic use or dialysis). Correct the cause of volume depletion before administration or before a lower dose is used.
- If hypotension occurs, place patient in a supine position and give an I.V. infusion of normal saline solution, if needed. Once blood pressure has stabilized after a transient hypotensive episode, drug may be continued.
- Dizziness and orthostatic hypotension may occur more frequently in patients with type 2 diabetes and renal disease.

PATIENT TEACHING

- Warn woman of childbearing age of consequences of drug exposure to fetus. Tell her to call prescriber immediately if pregnancy is suspected.
- Tell patient that drug may be taken without regard for food.

isoproterenol hydrochloride
eye-soe-proe-TER-e-nole

Isuprel

Pharmacologic class: nonselective beta-adrenergic agonist
Pregnancy risk category C

AVAILABLE FORMS
Injection: 20 mcg/ml in 10-ml prefilled syringes, 200 mcg/ml in 1- and 5-ml ampules and 5- and 10-ml vials

INDICATIONS & DOSAGES
➤ **Bronchospasm during anesthesia**
Adults: Dilute 1 ml of a 1:5,000 solution with 10 ml of normal saline or D_5W. Give 0.01 to 0.02 mg I.V. and repeat as necessary. Or, give 1:50,000 solution undiluted using same dose.
➤ **Heart block, ventricular arrhythmias**
Adults: Initially, 0.02 to 0.06 mg I.V.; then 0.01 to 0.2 mg I.V. or 5 mcg/minute I.V. Or, initially, 0.2 mg I.M.; then 0.02 to 1 mg I.M., as needed.
Children: Initial I.V. infusion of 0.1 mcg/kg/minute. Adjust dosage based on patient's response. Usual dosage range is 0.1 to 1 mcg/kg/minute.
➤ **Shock**
Adults and children: 0.5 to 5 mcg/minute isoproterenol hydrochloride by continuous I.V. infusion. Usual concentration is 1 mg or 5 ml in 500 ml D_5W. Titrate infusion rate according to heart rate, central venous pressure, blood pressure, and urine flow.
➤ **Postoperative cardiac patients with bradycardia ♦**
Children: I.V. infusion of 0.029 mcg/kg/minute.
➤ **As an aid in diagnosing the cause of mitral regurgitation ♦**
Adults: 4 mcg/minute I.V. infusion.
➤ **As an aid in diagnosing coronary artery disease or lesions ♦**
Adults: 1 to 3 mcg/minute I.V. infusion.

ADMINISTRATION
I.V.
- For infusion, dilute with most common I.V. solutions, but don't use with sodium bicarbonate injection; drug decomposes rapidly in alkaline solutions.
- Don't use solution if it's discolored or contains precipitate.
- Give by direct injection or I.V. infusion.
- For shock, closely monitor blood pressure, central venous pressure, ECG, arterial blood gas measurements, and urine output. Carefully titrate infusion rate according to these measurements. Use a continuous infusion pump to regulate flow rate.
- Store at room temperature. Protect from light.
- **Incompatibilities:** Alkalies, aminophylline, furosemide, metals, sodium bicarbonate.

ACTION
Relaxes bronchial smooth muscle by stimulating $beta_2$ receptors. As a cardiac stimulant, acts on $beta_1$ receptors in the heart.

Route	Onset	Peak	Duration
I.V.	Immediate	Unknown	< 60 min

Half-life: Unknown.

ADVERSE REACTIONS
CNS: headache, mild tremor, weakness, dizziness, nervousness, insomnia, anxiety.
CV: *palpitations, rapid rise and fall in blood pressure, tachycardia, angina,* ***arrhythmias, cardiac arrest.***
GI: nausea, vomiting.
Metabolic: hyperglycemia.
Skin: diaphoresis.
Other: swelling of parotid glands with prolonged use.

INTERACTIONS
Drug-drug. *Epinephrine, other sympathomimetics:* May increase risk of arrhythmias. Use together cautiously. If used together, give at least 4 hours apart.
Halogenated general anesthetics or cyclopropane: May increase risk of arrhythmias. Avoid using together.
Propranolol, other beta blockers: May block bronchodilating effect of isoproterenol. Monitor patient carefully.

EFFECTS ON LAB TEST RESULTS
- May increase glucose level.

CONTRAINDICATIONS & CAUTIONS
- Contraindicated in patients with tachycardia or AV block caused by digoxin intoxication, arrhythmias other than those that may respond to drug, angina pectoris, or angle-closure glaucoma.
- Contraindicated when used with general anesthetics with halogenated drugs or cyclopropane.
- Use cautiously in elderly patients and in those with renal or CV disease, coronary insufficiency, diabetes, hyperthyroidism, or history of sensitivity to sympathomimetic amines.

NURSING CONSIDERATIONS
- Correct volume deficit before giving vasopressors.
- ***Alert:*** If heart rate exceeds 110 beats/minute during I.V. infusion, notify prescriber. Doses that increase the heart rate to more than 130 beats/minute may induce ventricular arrhythmias.
- Drug may cause a slight increase in systolic blood pressure and a slight to marked decrease in diastolic blood pressure.
- Monitor patient for adverse reactions.
- ***Look alike–sound alike:*** Don't confuse Isuprel with Isordil.

PATIENT TEACHING
- Tell patient to report chest pain, fluttering in chest, or other adverse reactions.
- Remind patient to report pain at the I.V. injection site.

isosorbide dinitrate
eye-soe-SOR-bide

Apo-ISDN†, Cedocard SR†, Dilatrate-SR, Isordil, Isordil Titradose

isosorbide mononitrate
Apo-ISMN†, Imdur, ISMO, Monoket

Pharmacologic class: nitrate
Pregnancy risk category C; B for mononitrate

AVAILABLE FORMS
isosorbide dinitrate
Capsules (sustained-release): 40 mg
Tablets: 5 mg, 10 mg, 20 mg, 30 mg, 40 mg
Tablets (S.L.): 2.5 mg, 5 mg
Tablets (sustained-release): 40 mg
isosorbide mononitrate
Tablets: 10 mg, 20 mg
Tablets (extended-release): 30 mg, 60 mg, 120 mg

INDICATIONS & DOSAGES
➤ **Acute anginal attacks (S.L. isosorbide dinitrate only); to prevent situations that may cause anginal attacks**
Adults: 2.5 to 5 mg S.L. tablets for prompt relief of angina, repeated every 5 to 10 minutes (maximum of three doses for each 30-minute period). For prevention, 2.5 to 10 mg every 2 to 3 hours. Or, 5 to 40 mg isosorbide dinitrate P.O. b.i.d. or t.i.d. for prevention only (use smallest effective dose). Or, 30 to 60 mg Imdur P.O. once daily on arising; increase to 120 mg once daily after several days, if needed. Or, 20 mg ISMO or Monoket b.i.d. with the two doses given 7 hours apart.

ADMINISTRATION
P.O.
- Give patient S.L. tablet at first sign of attack. Tell him to wet tablet with saliva and place under his tongue until absorbed. Dose may be repeated every 10 to 15 minutes for a maximum of three doses.
- Tell patient taking P.O. form of isosorbide dinitrate to swallow oral tablet whole on an empty stomach either 30 minutes before or 1 to 2 hours after meals.
- Store drug in a cool place, in a tightly closed container, and away from light.

ACTION
Thought to reduce cardiac oxygen demand by decreasing preload and afterload. Drug also may increase blood flow through the collateral coronary vessels.

Route	Onset	Peak	Duration
P.O.	15–40 min	Unknown	4–8 hr
P.O. (extended-release)	½–4 hr	Unknown	6–12 hr
P.O. (S.L.)	2–5 min	Unknown	1–4 hr

Half-life: dinitrate P.O., 5 to 6 hours; S.L., 2 hours; mononitrate, about 5 hours.

ADVERSE REACTIONS

CNS: *headache,* dizziness, weakness.
CV: *orthostatic hypotension, tachycardia, palpitations, ankle edema, flushing,* fainting.
EENT: S.L. burning.
GI: nausea, vomiting.
Skin: cutaneous vasodilation, rash.

INTERACTIONS

Drug-drug. *Antihypertensives:* May increase hypotensive effects. Monitor patient closely during initial therapy.
Sildenafil, tadalafil, vardenafil: May cause life-threatening hypotension. Use of nitrates in any form with these drugs is contraindicated.
Drug-lifestyle. *Alcohol use:* May increase hypotension. Discourage use together.

EFFECTS ON LAB TEST RESULTS

- May falsely reduce value in cholesterol tests using the Zlatkis-Zak color reaction.

CONTRAINDICATIONS & CAUTIONS

- Contraindicated in patients with hypersensitivity or idiosyncrasy to nitrates and in those with severe hypotension, angle-closure glaucoma, increased intracranial pressure, shock, or acute MI with low left ventricular filling pressure.
- Use cautiously in patients with blood volume depletion (such as from diuretic therapy) or mild hypotension.

NURSING CONSIDERATIONS

- To prevent tolerance, a nitrate-free interval of 10 to 14 hours per day is recommended. The regimen for isosorbide mononitrate (1 tablet on awakening with the second dose in 7 hours, or 1 extended-release tablet daily) is intended to minimize nitrate tolerance by providing a substantial nitrate-free interval.
- Monitor blood pressure and intensity and duration of drug response.
- Drug may cause headaches, especially at beginning of therapy. Dosage may be reduced temporarily, but tolerance usually develops. Treat headache with aspirin or acetaminophen.
- Methemoglobinemia has been seen with nitrates. Symptoms are those of impaired oxygen delivery despite adequate cardiac output and adequate arterial partial pressure of oxygen.
- ***Look alike–sound alike:*** Don't confuse Isordil with Isuprel or Inderal.

PATIENT TEACHING

- Caution patient to take drug regularly, as prescribed, and to keep it accessible at all times.
- ***Alert:*** Advise patient that stopping drug abruptly may cause spasm of the coronary arteries with increased angina symptoms and potential risk of heart attack.
- Tell patient to take S.L. tablet at first sign of attack. He should wet tablet with saliva and place under his tongue until absorbed; he should sit down and rest. Dose may be repeated every 10 to 15 minutes for a maximum of three doses. If drug doesn't provide relief, tell patient to seek medical help promptly.
- Advise patient who complains of tingling sensation with S.L. drug to try holding tablet in cheek.
- Warn patient not to confuse S.L. with P.O. form.
- Advise patient taking P.O. form of isosorbide dinitrate to take oral tablet on an empty stomach either 30 minutes before or 1 to 2 hours after meals and to swallow oral tablets whole.
- Tell patient to minimize dizziness upon standing up by changing to upright position slowly. Advise him to go up and down stairs carefully and to lie down at first sign of dizziness.
- Caution patient to avoid alcohol because it may worsen low blood pressure effects.
- Advise patient that use of sildenafil, tadalafil, or vardenafil with any nitrate may cause severe low blood pressure. Patient should talk to his prescriber before using these drugs together.
- Instruct patient to store drug in a cool place, in a tightly closed container, and away from light.

SAFETY ALERT!

labetalol hydrochloride
la-BET-ah-loll

Trandate

Pharmacologic class: alpha and beta blocker
Pregnancy risk category C

AVAILABLE FORMS
Injection: 5 mg/ml in 20- and 40-ml multiple-dose vials
Tablets: 100 mg, 200 mg, 300 mg

INDICATIONS & DOSAGES
➤ **Hypertension**
Adults: 100 mg P.O. b.i.d. with or without a diuretic. If needed, dosage is increased to 200 mg b.i.d. after 2 days. Further increases may be made every 2 to 3 days until optimal response is reached. Usual maintenance dosage is 100 to 400 mg b.i.d. Maximum dose is 2.4 g daily in two divided doses given alone or with a diuretic.
➤ **Severe hypertension, hypertensive emergencies**
Adults: 200 mg diluted in 160 ml of D_5W, infused at 2 mg/minute until satisfactory response is obtained; then infusion is stopped. May be repeated every 6 to 12 hours.

Or, give by repeated I.V. injection: initially, 20 mg I.V. slowly over 2 minutes. Repeat injections of 40 to 80 mg every 10 minutes until maximum dose of 300 mg is reached, as needed.

ADMINISTRATION
P.O.
- When switching from I.V. to P.O. form, begin P.O. regimen at 200 mg after blood pressure begins to rise; repeat dose with 200 to 400 mg in 6 to 12 hours. Adjust dosage according to blood pressure response.
- If dizziness occurs, give dose at bedtime or in smaller doses t.i.d.

I.V.
- Give by slow, direct I.V. injection over 2 minutes at 10-minute intervals.
- For I.V. infusion, prepare by diluting with D_5W or normal saline solutions; for example, 200 mg of drug to 160 ml D_5W to yield 1 mg/ml.
- Give labetalol infusion with an infusion-control device.
- Monitor blood pressure closely every 5 minutes for 30 minutes; then every 30 minutes for 2 hours. Then, monitor hourly for 6 hours.
- Patient should remain supine for 3 hours after infusion. When given I.V. for hypertensive emergencies, drug produces a rapid, predictable fall in blood pressure within 5 to 10 minutes.
- Store at room temperature. Protect from light.
- **Incompatibilities:** Alkali solutions, amphotericin B, cefoperazone, ceftriaxone, furosemide, heparin, nafcillin, sodium bicarbonate, thiopental, warfarin.

ACTION
May be related to reduced peripheral vascular resistance, as a result of alpha and beta blockade.

Route	Onset	Peak	Duration
P.O.	20 min	2–4 hr	8–12 hr
I.V.	2–5 min	5 min	2–4 hr

Half-life: About 5½ hours after I.V. use; 6 to 8 hours after P.O. use.

ADVERSE REACTIONS
CNS: *dizziness,* vivid dreams, fatigue, headache, paresthesia, transient scalp tingling, syncope.
CV: *orthostatic hypotension,* ***ventricular arrhythmias.***
EENT: nasal congestion.
GI: nausea, vomiting.
GU: sexual dysfunction, urine retention.
Respiratory: ***bronchospasm,*** dyspnea.
Skin: rash.

INTERACTIONS
Drug-drug. *Beta agonists:* May blunt bronchodilator effect of these drugs in patients with bronchospasm. May need to increase dosages of these drugs.
Cimetidine: May enhance labetalol's effect. Use together cautiously.

Halothane: May increase hypotensive effect. Monitor blood pressure closely.
Insulin, oral antidiabetics: May alter dosage requirements in previously stabilized diabetic patient. Monitor patient closely.
Nitroglycerin: May blunt reflex tachycardia produced by nitroglycerin but not the hypotension. Monitor BP if used together.
NSAIDs: May decrease antihypertensive effects. Monitor blood pressure.
Tricyclic antidepressants: May increase incidence of tremor. Monitor patient for tremor.
Drug-herb. *Ma huang:* May decrease antihypertensive effects. Discourage use together.

EFFECTS ON LAB TEST RESULTS
- May increase transaminase and urea levels.
- May cause false-positive increase of urine free and total catecholamine levels when measured by a nonspecific trihydroxyindole fluorometric method. May cause false-positive test result for amphetamines when screening urine for drugs.

CONTRAINDICATIONS & CAUTIONS
- Contraindicated in patients hypersensitive to drug and in those with bronchial asthma, overt cardiac failure, greater than first-degree heart block, cardiogenic shock, severe bradycardia, and other conditions that may cause severe and prolonged hypotension.
- Use cautiously in patients with heart failure, hepatic failure, chronic bronchitis, emphysema, peripheral vascular disease, and pheochromocytoma.

NURSING CONSIDERATIONS
- Monitor blood pressure frequently. Drug masks common signs and symptoms of shock.
- In diabetic patients, monitor glucose level closely because beta blockers may mask certain signs and symptoms of hypoglycemia.
- ***Look alike–sound alike:*** Don't confuse Trandate with Trental or Tridrate.

PATIENT TEACHING
- ***Alert:*** Tell patient that stopping drug abruptly can worsen chest pain and trigger a heart attack.
- Advise patient that dizziness is the most troublesome adverse reaction and tends to occur in the early stages of treatment, in patients taking diuretics, and with higher dosages. Inform patient that dizziness can be minimized by rising slowly and avoiding sudden position changes.
- Warn patient that occasional, harmless scalp tingling may occur, especially when therapy begins.

SAFETY ALERT!

lidocaine hydrochloride (lignocaine hydrochloride)
LYE-doe-kane

LidoPen Auto-Injector, Xylocaine, Xylocard†

Pharmacologic class: amide derivative
Pregnancy risk category B

AVAILABLE FORMS
Infusion (premixed): 0.2% (2 mg/ml), 0.4% (4 mg/ml), 0.8% (8 mg/ml)
Injection (for direct I.V. use): 1% (10 mg/ml), 2% (20 mg/ml)
Injection (for I.M. use): 300 mg/3 ml automatic injection device
Injection (for I.V. admixtures): 4% (40 mg/ml), 10% (100 mg/ml), 20% (200 mg/ml)

INDICATIONS & DOSAGES
➤ **Ventricular arrhythmias caused by MI, cardiac manipulation, or cardiac glycosides**
Adults: 50 to 100 mg (1 to 1.5 mg/kg) by I.V. bolus at 25 to 50 mg/minute. Bolus dose is repeated every 3 to 5 minutes until arrhythmias subside or adverse reactions develop. Don't exceed 300-mg total bolus during a 1-hour period. Simultaneously, constant infusion of 20 to 50 mcg/kg/minute (1 to 4 mg/minute)

is begun. If single bolus has been given, smaller bolus dose may be repeated 15 to 20 minutes after start of infusion to maintain therapeutic level. Or, 200 to 300 mg I.M.; then second I.M. dose 60 to 90 minutes later, if needed.
Children: 1 mg/kg by I.V. or intraosseous bolus. If no response, start infusion of 20 to 50 mcg/kg/minute. Give an additional bolus dose of 0.5 to 1 mg/kg if delay of greater than 15 minutes between initial bolus and starting the infusion. Bolus doses shouldn't exceed 3 to 5 mg/kg.
Elderly patients: Reduce dosage and rate of infusion by 50%.
Adjust-a-dose: For patients with heart failure, with renal or liver disease, or who weigh less than 50 kg (110 lb), reduce dosage.

ADMINISTRATION

I.V.

• Injections (additive syringes and single-use vials) containing 40, 100, or 200 mg/ml are for the preparation of I.V. infusion solutions only and must be diluted before use.
• Prepare I.V. infusion by adding 1 g (using 25 ml of 4% or 5 ml of 20% injection) to 1 L of D_5W injection to provide a solution containing 1 mg/ml.
• Use a more concentrated solution of up to 8 mg/ml in fluid-restricted patient.
• Patients receiving infusions must be on a cardiac monitor and must be attended at all times. Use an infusion control device for giving infusion precisely. Don't exceed 4 mg/minute; faster rate greatly increases risk of toxicity.
• Avoid giving injections containing preservatives.
• **Incompatibilities:** Amphotericin, ampicillin, cefazolin, ceftriaxone, fentanyl citrate (higher pH brands), methohexital sodium, phenytoin sodium, sodium bicarbonate, thiopental sodium.

I.M.

• Give I.M. injections in the deltoid muscle only.
• Drug may cause soreness at injection site.

ACTION

A class IB antiarrhythmic that decreases the depolarization, automaticity, and excitability in the ventricles during the diastolic phase by direct action on the tissues, especially the Purkinje network.

Route	Onset	Peak	Duration
I.V.	Immediate	Immediate	10–20 min
I.M.	5–15 min	10 min	2 hr

Half-life: 1½ to 2 hours (may be prolonged in patients with heart failure or hepatic disease).

ADVERSE REACTIONS

CNS: *confusion, tremor, stupor, restlessness, light-headedness,* ***seizures,*** lethargy, somnolence, anxiety, hallucinations, nervousness, paresthesia, muscle twitching.
CV: *hypotension,* ***bradycardia, new or worsened arrhythmias, cardiac arrest.***
EENT: *tinnitus, blurred or double vision.*
GI: vomiting.
Respiratory: ***respiratory depression and arrest.***
Skin: soreness at injection site.
Other: ***anaphylaxis,*** sensation of cold.

INTERACTIONS

Drug-drug. *Atenolol, metoprolol, nadolol, pindolol, propranolol:* May reduce hepatic metabolism of lidocaine, increasing the risk of toxicity. Give bolus doses of lidocaine at a slower rate, and monitor lidocaine level and patient closely.
Cimetidine: May decrease clearance of lidocaine, increasing the risk of toxicity. Consider using a different H_2 receptor antagonist if possible. Monitor lidocaine level closely.
Ergot-type oxytocic drugs: May cause severe, persistent hypertension or stroke. Avoid using together.
Mexiletine: May increase pharmacologic effects. Avoid using together.
Phenytoin, procainamide, propranolol, quinidine: May increase cardiac depressant effects. Monitor patient closely.
Succinylcholine: May prolong neuromuscular blockade. Monitor patient closely.

Drug-herb. *Pareira:* May increase the effects of neuromuscular blockade. Discourage use together.
Drug-lifestyle. *Smoking:* May increase metabolism of lidocaine. Monitor patient closely.

EFFECTS ON LAB TEST RESULTS
• May increase CK levels with I.M. use.

CONTRAINDICATIONS & CAUTIONS
• Contraindicated in patients hypersensitive to the amide-type local anesthetics.
• Contraindicated in those with Adams-Stokes syndrome, Wolff-Parkinson-White syndrome, and severe degrees of SA, AV, or intraventricular block in the absence of an artificial pacemaker.
• Use cautiously and at reduced dosages in patients with complete or second-degree heart block or sinus bradycardia, in elderly patients, in those with heart failure or renal or hepatic disease, and in those who weigh less than 50 kg (110 lb).

NURSING CONSIDERATIONS
• Monitor isoenzymes when using I.M. drug for suspected MI. A patient who has received I.M. lidocaine will show a sevenfold increase in CK level. Such an increase originates in the skeletal muscle, not the heart.
• Monitor drug level. Therapeutic levels are 2 to 5 mcg/ml.
• ***Alert:*** Monitor patient for toxicity. In many severely ill patients, seizures may be the first sign of toxicity, but severe reactions are usually preceded by somnolence, confusion, tremors, and paresthesia. If signs of toxicity occur, stop drug at once and notify prescriber. Continuing could lead to seizures and coma. Give oxygen through a nasal cannula if not contraindicated. Keep oxygen and cardiopulmonary resuscitation equipment available.
• Monitor patient's response, especially blood pressure and electrolytes, BUN, and creatinine levels. Notify prescriber promptly if abnormalities develop.
• If arrhythmias worsen or ECG changes (for example, QRS complex widens or PR interval substantially prolongs), stop infusion and notify prescriber.

PATIENT TEACHING
• For I.M. form, tell patient that drug may cause soreness at injection site. Tell him to report discomfort at the site.
• Tell patient to report adverse reactions promptly because toxicity can occur.

lisinopril
lye-SIN-oh-pril

Prinivil, Zestril

Pharmacologic class: ACE inhibitor
Pregnancy risk category C; D in 2nd and 3rd trimesters

AVAILABLE FORMS
Tablets: 2.5 mg, 5 mg, 10 mg, 20 mg, 30 mg, 40 mg

INDICATIONS & DOSAGES
➤ **Hypertension**
Adults: Initially, 10 mg P.O. daily for patients not taking a diuretic. Most patients are well controlled on 20 to 40 mg daily as a single dose. For patients taking a diuretic, initially, 5 mg P.O. daily.
Children age 6 and older: Initially, 0.07 mg/kg (up to 5 mg) P.O. once daily. Increase dosage based on patient response and tolerance. Maximum dose, 0.61 mg/kg (don't exceed 40 mg). Don't use in children with a creatinine clearance less than 30 ml/minute.
Adjust-a-dose: In adults, if creatinine clearance is 10 to 30 ml/minute, give 5 mg P.O. daily; if clearance is less than 10 ml/minute, give 2.5 mg P.O. daily.
➤ **Adjunct treatment (with diuretics and cardiac glycosides) for heart failure**
Adults: Initially, 5 mg P.O. daily; increased as needed to maximum of 20 mg P.O. daily.
Adjust-a-dose: If sodium level is less than 130 mEq/L or creatinine clearance less than 30 ml/minute, start treatment at 2.5 mg daily.

➤ Hemodynamically stable patients within 24 hours of acute MI to improve survival
Adults: Initially, 5 mg P.O.; then 5 mg after 24 hours, 10 mg after 48 hours, followed by 10 mg once daily for 6 weeks.
Adjust-a-dose: For patients with systolic blood pressure 120 mm Hg or less when treatment is started or during first 3 days after an infarct, decrease dosage to 2.5 mg P.O. If systolic blood pressure drops to 100 mm Hg or less, reduce daily maintenance dose of 5 mg to 2.5 mg, if needed. If prolonged systolic blood pressure stays under 90 mm Hg for longer than 1 hour, withdraw drug.
➤ Hypertension in children
Children ages 6 to 16: Initially, 0.07 mg/kg P.O. once daily (up to 5 mg total). Adjust dosage according to blood pressure response. Doses above 0.61 mg/kg (or above 40 mg) haven't been studied in children.

ADMINISTRATION

P.O.

- Give drug without regard for food.
- If made into a suspension by pharmacist, shake before each use.

ACTION

Causes decreased production of angiotensin II and suppression of the renin-angiotensin-aldosterone system.

Route	Onset	Peak	Duration
P.O.	1 hr	7 hr	24 hr

Half-life: 12 hours.

ADVERSE REACTIONS

CNS: *dizziness,* headache, fatigue, paresthesia.
CV: *orthostatic hypotension,* hypotension, chest pain.
EENT: *nasal congestion.*
GI: *diarrhea,* nausea, dyspepsia.
GU: impaired renal function, impotence.
Metabolic: ***hyperkalemia.***
Respiratory: dyspnea, dry, persistent, tickling, nonproductive cough.
Skin: rash.

INTERACTIONS

Drug-drug. *Allopurinol:* May cause hypersensitivity reaction. Use together cautiously.
Azathioprine: May increase risk of anemia or leukopenia. Monitor hematologic studies if used together.
Diuretics, thiazide diuretics: May cause excessive hypotension with diuretics. Monitor blood pressure closely.
Indomethacin, NSAIDs: May reduce hypotensive effects of drug. Adjust dose as needed.
Insulin, oral antidiabetics: May cause hypoglycemia, especially at start of lisinopril therapy. Monitor glucose level.
Lithium: May cause lithium toxicity. Monitor lithium levels.
Phenothiazines: May increase hypotensive effects. Monitor blood pressure closely.
Potassium-sparing diuretics, potassium supplements: May cause hyperkalemia. Monitor laboratory values.
Tizanidine: May cause severe hypotension. Monitor patient.
Drug-herb. *Capsaicin:* May cause ACE inhibitor-induced cough. Discourage use together.
Ma huang: May decrease antihypertensive effects. Discourage use together.
Drug-food. *Potassium-containing salt substitutes:* May cause hyperkalemia. Monitor laboratory values.

EFFECTS ON LAB TEST RESULTS

- May increase BUN, creatinine, potassium, and bilirubin levels.
- May increase liver function test values.

CONTRAINDICATIONS & CAUTIONS

- Contraindicated in patients hypersensitive to ACE inhibitors and in those with a history of angioedema related to previous treatment with ACE inhibitor.
- Use cautiously in patients with impaired renal function; adjust dosage.
- Use cautiously in patients at risk for hyperkalemia and in those with aortic stenosis or hypertrophic cardiomyopathy. The safety and efficacy of lisinopril on blood pressure in children younger than age 6 or in children with GFR less than 30 ml/minute hasn't been established.

NURSING CONSIDERATIONS

- When using drug in acute MI, give patient the appropriate and standard recommended treatment, such as thrombolytics, aspirin, and beta blockers.
- Although ACE inhibitors reduce blood pressure in all races, blood pressure reduction is less in blacks taking the ACE inhibitor alone. Black patients should take drug with a thiazide diuretic for a more favorable response.
- ACE inhibitors appear to increase risk of angioedema in black patients.
- Monitor blood pressure frequently. If drug doesn't adequately control blood pressure, diuretics may be added.
- Monitor WBC with differential counts before therapy, every 2 weeks for first 3 months of therapy, and periodically thereafter.
- ***Look alike–sound alike:*** Don't confuse lisinopril with fosinopril or Lioresal. Don't confuse Zestril with Zostrix, Zetia, Zebeta, or Zyrtec. Don't confuse Prinivil with Proventil or Prilosec.

PATIENT TEACHING

- ***Alert:*** Rarely, facial and throat swelling (including swelling of the larynx) may occur, especially after first dose. Advise patient to report signs or symptoms of breathing problems or swelling of face, eyes, lips, or tongue.
- Inform patient that light-headedness can occur, especially during first few days of therapy. Tell him to rise slowly to minimize this effect and to report symptoms to prescriber. If he faints, advise patient to stop taking drug and call prescriber immediately.
- If unpleasant adverse reactions occur, tell patient not to stop drug suddenly but to notify prescriber.
- Advise patient to report signs and symptoms of infection, such as fever and sore throat.
- Tell woman of childbearing age to notify prescriber if pregnancy occurs. Drug will need to be stopped.
- Instruct patient not to use salt substitutes that contain potassium without first consulting prescriber.

losartan potassium

low-SAR-tan

Cozaar

Pharmacologic class: angiotensin II receptor antagonist
Pregnancy risk category C; D in 2nd and 3rd trimesters

AVAILABLE FORMS

Tablets: 25 mg, 50 mg, 100 mg

INDICATIONS & DOSAGES

➤ Hypertension

Adults: Initially, 25 to 50 mg P.O. daily. Maximum daily dose is 100 mg in one or two divided doses.
Children age 6 and older: 0.7 mg/kg (up to 50 mg) P.O. daily, adjust as needed up to 1.4 mg/kg/day (maximum 100 mg).
Adjust-a-dose: For adults who are hepatically impaired or intravascularly volume depleted (such as those taking diuretics), initially, 25 mg.

➤ Nephropathy in type 2 diabetic patients

Adults: 50 mg P.O. once daily. Increase dosage to 100 mg once daily based on blood pressure response.

➤ To reduce risk of stroke in patients with hypertension and left ventricular hypertrophy

Adults: Initially, 50 mg P.O. once daily. Adjust dosage based on blood pressure response, adding hydrochlorothiazide 12.5 mg once daily, increasing losartan to 100 mg daily, or both. If further adjustments are required, may increase the daily dosage of hydrochlorothiazide to 25 mg.

ADMINISTRATION

P.O.

- Give drug without regard for meals.
- If made into suspension by pharmacist, store in refrigerator and shake well before each use.

ACTION

Inhibits vasoconstrictive and aldosterone-secreting action of angiotensin II by blocking angiotensin II receptor on the surface of vascular smooth muscle and other tissue cells.

Route	Onset	Peak	Duration
P.O.	Unknown	1 hr	Unknown

Half-life: 2 hours.

ADVERSE REACTIONS

Patients with hypertension or left ventricular hypertrophy

CNS: dizziness, asthenia, fatigue, headache, insomnia.
CV: edema, chest pain.
EENT: nasal congestion, sinusitis, pharyngitis, sinus disorder.
GI: abdominal pain, nausea, diarrhea, dyspepsia.
Musculoskeletal: muscle cramps, myalgia, back or leg pain.
Respiratory: cough, upper respiratory infection.
Other: ***angioedema.***

Patients with nephropathy

CNS: *asthenia, fatigue,* fever, hypesthesia.
CV: *chest pain,* hypotension, orthostatic hypotension.
EENT: sinusitis, cataract.
GI: *diarrhea,* dyspepsia, gastritis.
GU: *UTI.*
Hematologic: *anemia.*
Metabolic: ***hyperkalemia, hypoglycemia,*** weight gain.
Musculoskeletal: *back pain,* leg or knee pain, muscle weakness.
Respiratory: *cough, bronchitis.*
Skin: cellulitis.
Other: *flulike syndrome,* ***diabetic vascular disease, angioedema,*** infection, trauma, diabetic neuropathy.

INTERACTIONS

Drug-drug. *Lithium:* May increase lithium level. Monitor lithium level and patient for toxicity.
NSAIDs: May decrease antihypertensive effects. Monitor blood pressure.
Potassium-sparing diuretics, potassium supplements: May cause hyperkalemia. Monitor patient closely.
Drug-herb. *Ma huang:* May decrease antihypertensive effects. Discourage use together.
Drug-food. *Salt substitutes containing potassium:* May cause hyperkalemia. Monitor patient closely.

EFFECTS ON LAB TEST RESULTS

None reported.

CONTRAINDICATIONS & CAUTIONS

- Contraindicated in patients hypersensitive to drug. Breast-feeding isn't recommended during losartan therapy.
- Use cautiously in patients with impaired renal or hepatic function.
- Drugs that act directly on the renin-angiotensin system (such as losartan) can cause fetal and neonatal morbidity and death when given to women in the second or third trimester of pregnancy. These problems haven't been detected when exposure was limited to the first trimester. If pregnancy is suspected, notify prescriber because drug should be stopped.

NURSING CONSIDERATIONS

- Drug can be used alone or with other antihypertensives.
- If antihypertensive effect is inadequate using once-daily doses, a twice-daily regimen using the same or increased total daily dose may give a more satisfactory response.
- Monitor patient's blood pressure closely to evaluate effectiveness of therapy. When used alone, drug has less of an effect on blood pressure in black patients than in patients of other races.
- Monitor patients who are also taking diuretics for symptomatic hypotension.
- Regularly assess the patient's renal function (via creatinine and BUN levels).
- Patients with severe heart failure whose renal function depends on the angiotensin-aldosterone system may develop acute renal failure during therapy. Closely monitor patient, especially during first few weeks of therapy.
- ***Look alike–sound alike:*** Don't confuse Cozaar with Zocor.

PATIENT TEACHING

- Tell patient to avoid salt substitutes; these products may contain potassium, which can cause high potassium level in patients taking losartan.

• Inform woman of childbearing age about consequences of second and third trimester exposure to drug. Prescriber should be notified immediately if pregnancy is suspected.
• Advise patient to immediately report swelling of face, eyes, lips, or tongue or any breathing difficulty.

lovastatin (mevinolin)

loe-va-STA-tin

Altoprev, Mevacor

Pharmacologic class: HMG-CoA reductase inhibitor
Pregnancy risk category X

AVAILABLE FORMS

Tablets: 10 mg, 20 mg, 40 mg
Tablets (extended-release): 10 mg, 20 mg, 40 mg, 60 mg

INDICATIONS & DOSAGES

➤ **To prevent and treat coronary heart disease; hyperlipidemia**
Adults: Initially, 20 mg P.O. once daily with evening meal. Recommended range is 10 to 80 mg as a single dose or in two divided doses; maximum daily recommended dose is 80 mg.

Or, 20 to 60 mg extended-release tablets P.O. at bedtime. Starting dose of 10 mg can be used for patients requiring smaller reductions; usual dosage range is 10 to 60 mg daily.

➤ **Heterozygous familial hypercholesterolemia in adolescents**
Adolescents ages 10 to 17: Give 10 to 40 mg daily P.O. with evening meal. Patients requiring reductions in LDL cholesterol level of 20% or more should start with 20 mg daily.
Adjust-a-dose: For patients also taking cyclosporine, give 10 mg P.O. daily, not to exceed 20 mg daily. Avoid use of lovastatin with fibrates or niacin; if combined with either, the dosage of lovastatin shouldn't exceed 20 mg daily. For patients also taking amiodarone or verapamil, the dosage of lovastatin shouldn't exceed 40 mg daily. For patients with creatinine clearance less than 30 ml/minute, carefully consider dosage increase greater than 20 mg daily and implement cautiously if necessary.

ADMINISTRATION

P.O.
• Give drug with evening meal, which improves absorption and cholesterol biosynthesis.
• Don't crush or split extended-release tablets.

ACTION

Inhibits HMG-CoA reductase, an early (and rate-limiting) step in cholesterol biosynthesis.

Route	Onset	Peak	Duration
P.O.	Unknown	2 hr	Unknown
P.O. (extended-release)	Unknown	14 hr	Unknown

Half-life: 3 hours.

ADVERSE REACTIONS

CNS: *headache,* dizziness, insomnia, peripheral neuropathy.
CV: chest pain.
EENT: blurred vision.
GI: abdominal pain or cramps, constipation, diarrhea, dyspepsia, flatulence, heartburn, nausea, vomiting.
Musculoskeletal: muscle cramps, myalgia, myositis, ***rhabdomyolysis.***
Skin: alopecia, rash, pruritus.

INTERACTIONS

Drug-drug. *Amiodarone,* ***verapamil:*** May cause myopathy and rhabdomyolysis. Don't exceed 40 mg lovastatin daily.
Azole antifungals, ***protease inhibitors:*** May cause myopathy and rhabdomyolysis. Avoid using together.
Cyclosporine, *danazol, gemfibrozil or other fibrates, niacin:* May cause myopathy and rhabdomyolysis. Don't exceed 20 mg lovastatin daily.
Diltiazem, macrolides (azithromycin, clarithromycin, erythromycin, telithromycin), nefazodone: May decrease metabolism of HMG-CoA reductase inhibitor, increasing toxicity. Monitor patient for adverse effects and report unexplained muscle pain.

Oral anticoagulants: May increase oral anticoagulant effect. Monitor patient closely.
Drug-herb. *Eucalyptus, jin bu huan, kava:* May increase risk of hepatotoxicity. Discourage use together.
Pectin: May decrease drug effect. Discourage use together.
Red yeast rice: May increase risk of adverse reactions because herb contains compounds similar to those in drug. Discourage use together.
Drug-food. *Grapefruit juice:* May increase drug level, increasing risk of adverse effects. Discourage use together.
Drug-lifestyle. *Alcohol use:* May increase risk of hepatotoxicity. Discourage use together.

EFFECTS ON LAB TEST RESULTS

- May increase ALT, AST, and CK levels.

CONTRAINDICATIONS & CAUTIONS

- Contraindicated in patients hypersensitive to drug and in those with active liver disease or unexplained persistently increased transaminase level.
- Contraindicated in pregnant and breast-feeding women and in women of child-bearing age.
- Use cautiously in patients who consume substantial quantities of alcohol or have a history of liver disease.

NURSING CONSIDERATIONS

- Have patient follow a diet restricted in saturated fat and cholesterol during therapy.
- Obtain liver function test results at the start of therapy, at 6 and 12 weeks after the start of therapy, and when increasing dose; then monitor results periodically.
- Heterozygous familial hypercholesterolemia can be diagnosed in adolescent boys and in girls who are at least 1 year postmenarche and are 10 to 17 years old; or, if after an adequate trial of diet therapy LDL cholesterol level remains over 189 mg/dl or LDL cholesterol over 160 mg/dl and patient has a positive family history of premature CV disease or two or more other CV disease risk factors.
- ***Look alike–sound alike:*** Don't confuse lovastatin with Lotensin, Leustatin, or Livostin. Don't confuse Mevacor with Mivacron.

PATIENT TEACHING

- Instruct patient to take drug with the evening meal.
- Teach patient about proper dietary management of cholesterol and triglycerides. When appropriate, recommend weight control, exercise, and smoking cessation programs.
- Advise patient to have periodic eye examinations; related compounds cause cataracts.
- Instruct patient to store tablets at room temperature in a light-resistant container.
- Advise patient to promptly report unexplained muscle pain, tenderness, or weakness, particularly when accompanied by malaise or fever.
- ***Alert:*** Tell woman to stop drug and notify prescriber immediately if she is or may be pregnant or if she's breast-feeding.
- ***Alert:*** Advise patient not to crush or chew extended-release tablets.

SAFETY ALERT!

magnesium sulfate

mag-NEE-zee-um

Pharmacologic class: mineral; electrolyte
Pregnancy risk category A

AVAILABLE FORMS

Injection: 4%, 8%, 10%, 12.5%, 25%, 50%
Injection solution: 1% in D_5W, 2% in D_5W

INDICATIONS & DOSAGES

➤ To prevent or control seizures in preeclampsia or eclampsia
Women: Initially, 4 g I.V. in 250 ml D_5W or normal saline and 4 to 5 g deep I.M. into each buttock; then 4 to 5 g deep I.M. into alternate buttock every 4 hours, as needed. Or, 4 g I.V. loading dose; then 1 to 3 g hourly as I.V. infusion. Total dose shouldn't exceed 30 or 40 g daily.
➤ Hypomagnesemia
Adults: For mild deficiency, 1 g I.M. every 6 hours for four doses; for severe

deficiency, 5 g in 1,000 ml D_5W or normal saline solution infused over 3 hours.

➤ **Seizures, hypertension, and encephalopathy with acute nephritis in children**

Children: 20 to 40 mg/kg I.M. as needed to control seizures. Dilute the 50% concentration to a 20% solution and give 0.1 to 0.2 ml/kg of the 20% solution.

➤ **To manage paroxysmal atrial tachycardia**

Adults: 3 to 4 g I.V. over 30 seconds, with extreme caution.

➤ **To manage life-threatening ventricular arrhythmias, such as sustained ventricular tachycardia or torsades de pointes ♦**

Adults: 1 to 6 g I.V. over several minutes; then continuous I.V. infusion of 3 to 20 mg/minute for 5 to 48 hours. Base dosage and duration of therapy on patient response and magnesium level.

➤ **To manage preterm labor ♦**

Adults: 4 to 6 g I.V. over 20 minutes, followed by 2 to 4 g/hour I.V. infusion for 12 to 24 hours, as tolerated, after contractions have stopped.

ADMINISTRATION

I.V.

- If necessary, dilute to maximum level of 20%. Infuse no faster than 150 mg/minute (1.5 ml/minute of a 10% solution or 0.75 ml/minute of a 20% solution). Drug is compatible with D_5W and normal saline solution.
- Maximum infusion rate is 150 mg/minute. Too-rapid infusion produces uncomfortable feeling of heat.
- Monitor vital signs every 15 minutes when giving drug I.V.
- **Incompatibilities:** Alkali carbonates and bicarbonates, amiodarone, amphotericin B, calcium gluconate, cefepime, ciprofloxacin, clindamycin, cyclosporine, dobutamine, heavy metals, I.V. fat emulsion 10%, polymyxin B, procaine, salicylates, sodium bicarbonate, soluble phosphates.

I.M.

- For adults, give undiluted 50% concentration by deep injection.
- For children, dilute to concentration of 20% or less with D_5W or normal saline for injection.

ACTION

May decrease acetylcholine released by nerve impulses, but anticonvulsant mechanism is unknown.

Route	Onset	Peak	Duration
I.V.	1–2 min	Rapid	30 min
I.M.	1 hr	Unknown	3–4 hr

Half-life: Unknown.

ADVERSE REACTIONS

CNS: *depressed reflexes,* drowsiness, flaccid paralysis, hypothermia.
CV: *flushing, hypotension,* ***bradycardia, circulatory collapse,*** depressed cardiac function.
EENT: diplopia.
Metabolic: hypocalcemia.
Respiratory: ***respiratory paralysis.***
Skin: diaphoresis.

INTERACTIONS

Drug-drug. *Anesthetics, CNS depressants:* May cause additive CNS depression. Use together cautiously.
Cardiac glycosides: May worsen arrhythmias. Use together cautiously.
Neuromuscular blockers: May cause increased neuromuscular blockade. Use together cautiously.

EFFECTS ON LAB TEST RESULTS

- May increase magnesium level. May decrease calcium level.

CONTRAINDICATIONS & CAUTIONS

- Parenteral administration contraindicated in patients with heart block or myocardial damage.
- Contraindicated in patients with toxemia of pregnancy during 2 hours preceding delivery.
- Use cautiously in patients with impaired renal function.
- Use cautiously in pregnant women during labor.

NURSING CONSIDERATIONS

- If used to treat seizures, take appropriate seizure precautions.
- ***Alert:*** Watch for respiratory depression and signs and symptoms of heart block.
- Keep I.V. calcium gluconate available to reverse magnesium intoxication, but use cautiously in digitalized patients because of danger of arrhythmias.
- Check magnesium level after repeated doses. Disappearance of knee-jerk and patellar reflexes is sign of impending magnesium toxicity.
- Signs of hypermagnesemia begin to appear at levels of 4 mEq/L.
- Effective anticonvulsant level ranges from 2.5 to 7.5 mEq/L.
- Monitor fluid intake and output. Make sure urine output is 100 ml or more in 4-hour period before each dose.
- Observe neonates for signs of magnesium toxicity, including neuromuscular or respiratory depression, when giving I.V. form of drug to toxemic mothers within 24 hours before delivery.
- ***Look alike–sound alike:*** Don't confuse magnesium sulfate with manganese sulfate.

PATIENT TEACHING

- Inform patient of short-term need for drug and answer any questions and address concerns.
- Review potential adverse reactions and instruct patient to promptly report any occurrences. Reassure patient that, although adverse reactions can occur, vital signs, reflexes, and drug level will be monitored frequently to ensure safety.

mannitol

MAN-i-tole

Osmitrol

Pharmacologic class: osmotic diuretic
Pregnancy risk category B

AVAILABLE FORMS

Injection: 5%, 10%, 15%, 20%, 25%

INDICATIONS & DOSAGES

➤ **Test dose for marked oliguria or suspected inadequate renal function**
Adults and children older than age 12: 200 mg/kg or 12.5 g as a 15% to 20% I.V. solution over 3 to 5 minutes. Response is adequate if 30 to 50 ml of urine/hour is excreted over 2 to 3 hours; if response is inadequate, a second test dose is given. If still no response after second dose, stop drug.

➤ **Oliguria**
Adults and children older than age 12: 50 to 100 g I.V. as a 15% to 25% solution over 90 minutes to several hours.

➤ **To prevent oliguria or acute renal failure**
Adults and children older than age 12: 50 to 100 g I.V. of a 5% to 25% solution. Determine exact concentration by fluid requirements.

➤ **To reduce intraocular or intracranial pressure or cerebral edema**
Adults and children older than age 12: 1.5 to 2 g/kg as a 15%, 20%, or 25% I.V. solution over 30 to 60 minutes. For maximum intraocular pressure reduction before surgery, give 60 to 90 minutes preoperatively.

➤ **Diuresis in drug intoxication**
Adults and children older than age 12: 5% to 25% solution continuously up to 200 g I.V., while maintaining 100 to 500 ml urine output/hour and a positive fluid balance.

➤ **Irrigating solution during transurethral resection of prostate gland**
Adults: 2.5% to 5% solution.

ADMINISTRATION

I.V.

- Change I.V. administration apparatus every 24 hours.
- To redissolve crystallized solution (crystallization occurs at low temperatures or in concentrations higher than 15%), warm bottle or bag in a hot water bath with occasional shaking. Cool to body temperature before giving. Don't use solution with undissolved crystals.
- Give as intermittent or continuous infusion at prescribed rate, using an inline filter

and an infusion pump. Don't give as direct injection.
• Check patency at infusion site before and during administration.
• Monitor patient for signs and symptoms of infiltration; if it occurs, watch for inflammation, edema, and necrosis.
• **Incompatibilities:** Blood products, cefepime, doxorubicin liposomal, filgrastim, imipenem-cilastatin, meropenem, potassium chloride, sodium chloride, strongly acidic or alkaline solutions.

ACTION

Increases osmotic pressure of glomerular filtrate, thus inhibiting tubular reabsorption of water and electrolytes. Drug elevates plasma osmolality and increases water flow into extracellular fluid.

Route	Onset	Peak	Duration
I.V.	30–60 min	1 hr	6–8 hr

Half-life: About 1½ hours.

ADVERSE REACTIONS

CNS: ***seizures,*** dizziness, headache, fever.
CV: edema, thrombophlebitis, hypotension, hypertension, ***heart failure,*** tachycardia, angina-like chest pain, vascular overload.
EENT: blurred vision, rhinitis.
GI: thirst, dry mouth, nausea, vomiting, *diarrhea.*
GU: urine retention.
Metabolic: dehydration.
Skin: local pain, urticaria.
Other: chills, thirst.

INTERACTIONS

Drug-drug. *Lithium:* May increase urinary excretion of lithium. Monitor lithium level closely.

EFFECTS ON LAB TEST RESULTS

• May increase or decrease electrolyte levels.
• May interfere with tests for inorganic phosphorus or ethylene glycol level.

CONTRAINDICATIONS & CAUTIONS

• Contraindicated in patients hypersensitive to drug.
• Contraindicated in patients with anuria; severe pulmonary congestion; frank pulmonary edema; active intracranial bleeding (except during craniotomy); severe dehydration; metabolic edema; previous progressive renal disease or dysfunction after starting drug, including increasing azotemia and oliguria; or previous progressive heart failure or pulmonary congestion after drug.

NURSING CONSIDERATIONS

• Monitor vital signs, including central venous pressure and fluid intake and output hourly. Report increasing oliguria. Check weight, renal function, fluid balance, and serum and urine sodium and potassium levels daily.
• In comatose or incontinent patient, use urinary catheter because therapy is based on strict evaluation of fluid intake and output. If patient has urinary catheter, use an hourly urometer collection bag to evaluate output accurately and easily.
• To relieve thirst, give frequent mouth care or fluids.
• Drug is commonly used in chemotherapy regimens to enhance diuresis of renally toxic drugs.
• Don't give electrolyte-free solutions with blood. If blood is given simultaneously, add at least 20 mEq of sodium chloride to each liter of drug solution to avoid pseudoagglutination.

PATIENT TEACHING

• Tell patient that he may feel thirsty or have a dry mouth, and emphasize importance of drinking only the amount of fluids ordered.
• Instruct patient to promptly report adverse reactions and discomfort at I.V. site.

SAFETY ALERT!

methyldopa

meth-ill-DOE-pa

Novo-Medopa†, Nu-Medopa†

methyldopate hydrochloride

Pharmacologic class: centrally acting antiadrenergic
Pregnancy risk category B; for P.O.; C for I.V.

AVAILABLE FORMS

methyldopa
Tablets: 250 mg, 500 mg
methyldopate hydrochloride
Injection: 50 mg/ml

INDICATIONS & DOSAGES

➤ **Hypertension, hypertensive crisis**
Adults: Initially, 250 mg P.O. b.i.d. to t.i.d. in first 48 hours. Increase if needed every 2 days. May give entire daily dose in evening or at bedtime. Adjust dosages if other antihypertensives are added to or deleted from therapy. Maintenance dosage is 500 mg to 2 g daily in two to four divided doses. Maximum recommended daily dose is 3 g. Or, 250 to 500 mg I.V. every 6 hours. Maximum dosage is 1 g every 6 hours. Switch to oral antihypertensives as soon as possible.
Children: Initially, 10 mg/kg P.O. daily in two to four divided doses; or, 20 to 40 mg/kg I.V. daily in four divided doses. Increase dose daily until desired response occurs. Maximum daily dose is 65 mg/kg or 3 g, whichever is less.

ADMINISTRATION

P.O.
- If unpleasant adverse reactions occur, patient shouldn't suddenly stop taking drug but should notify his prescriber.

I.V.
- Dilute appropriate dose in 100 ml D_5W. Infuse slowly over 30 to 60 minutes.
- **Incompatibilities:** Amphotericin B; drugs with poor solubility in acidic media, such as barbiturates and sulfonamides; methohexital; some total parenteral nutrition solutions.

ACTION

May inhibit the central vasomotor centers, decreasing sympathetic outflow to the heart, kidneys, and peripheral vasculature.

Route	Onset	Peak	Duration
P.O.	4–6 hr	Unknown	12–48 hr
I.V.	4–6 hr	Unknown	10–16 hr

Half-life: About 2 hours.

ADVERSE REACTIONS

CNS: *decreased mental acuity, sedation, headache,* weakness, dizziness, paresthesia, parkinsonism, involuntary choreoathetoid movements, psychic disturbances, depression, nightmares.
CV: *orthostatic hypotension, edema,* ***bradycardia, myocarditis,*** aggravated angina.
EENT: *nasal congestion.*
GI: *dry mouth,* ***pancreatitis,*** nausea, vomiting, diarrhea, constipation.
GU: galactorrhea.
Hematologic: ***thrombocytopenia, leukopenia, bone marrow depression,*** hemolytic anemia.
Hepatic: ***hepatic necrosis, hepatitis.***
Musculoskeletal: arthralgia.
Skin: rash.
Other: drug-induced fever, gynecomastia.

INTERACTIONS

Drug-drug. *Amphetamines, nonselective beta blockers, norepinephrine, phenothiazines, tricyclic antidepressants:* May cause hypertensive effects. Monitor patient closely.
Anesthetics: May need lower doses of anesthetics. Use together cautiously.
Barbiturates: May decrease actions of methyldopa. Monitor patient closely.
Ferrous sulfate: May decrease bioavailability of methyldopa. Separate doses.
Haloperidol: May increase antipsychotic effects of haloperidol or cause psychosis. Use together cautiously.
Levodopa: May increase hypotensive effects, which may increase adverse CNS reactions. Monitor patient closely.
Lithium: May increase lithium level. Watch for increased lithium level and signs and symptoms of toxicity.

MAO inhibitors: May cause excessive sympathetic stimulation. Avoid using together.
Tolbutamide: May impair metabolism of tolbutamide. Monitor patient for hypoglycemic effect.
Drug-herb. *Capsicum:* May reduce antihypertensive effect. Discourage use together.

EFFECTS ON LAB TEST RESULTS

- May increase creatinine level. May decrease hemoglobin level and hematocrit.
- May increase liver function test values. May decrease platelet and WBC counts.
- May interfere with results of urinary uric acid testing, serum creatinine test, and AST test. May cause positive Coombs' test result. May falsely increase urine catecholamine level, interfering with the diagnosis of pheochromocytoma.

CONTRAINDICATIONS & CAUTIONS

- Contraindicated in patients hypersensitive to drug and in those with active hepatic disease (such as acute hepatitis) or active cirrhosis.
- Contraindicated in those whose previous methyldopa therapy caused liver problems and in those taking MAO inhibitors.
- Use cautiously in patients with history of impaired hepatic function or sulfite sensitivity and in breast-feeding women.

NURSING CONSIDERATIONS

- Monitor patient's blood pressure regularly. Elderly patients are more likely to experience hypotension and sedation.
- Occasionally, tolerance may occur, usually between the second and third months of therapy. Adding a diuretic or adjusting dosage may be needed. If patient's response changes significantly, notify prescriber.
- After dialysis, monitor patient for hypertension and notify prescriber, if needed. Patient may need an extra dose of drug.
- Monitor CBC with differential counts before therapy and periodically thereafter.
- Patients who need blood transfusions should have direct and indirect Coombs' tests to prevent crossmatching problems.
- Monitor patient's Coombs' test results. In patients who have received drug for several months, positive reaction to direct Coombs' test indicates hemolytic anemia.
- Report involuntary choreoathetoid movements. Drug may be stopped.
- ***Look alike–sound alike:*** Don't confuse Aldomet with Anzemet.

PATIENT TEACHING

- If unpleasant adverse reactions occur, advise patient not to suddenly stop taking drug but to notify prescriber.
- Instruct patient to report signs and symptoms of infection.
- Tell patient to check his weight daily and to notify prescriber if he gains 2 or more pounds in 1 day or 5 pounds in 1 week. Sodium and water retention may occur but can be relieved with diuretics.
- Warn patient that, particularly at the start of therapy, drug may impair ability to perform tasks that require mental alertness. A once-daily dose at bedtime minimizes daytime drowsiness.
- Inform patient that low blood pressure and dizziness upon rising can be minimized by rising slowly and avoiding sudden position changes and that dry mouth can be relieved by chewing gum or sucking on hard candy or ice chips.
- Tell patient that urine may turn dark if left sitting in toilet bowl or if toilet bowl has been treated with bleach.

metolazone

me-TOLE-a-zone

Zaroxolyn

Pharmacologic class: thiazide-like diuretic
Pregnancy risk category B

AVAILABLE FORMS

Tablets (extended-release): 2.5 mg, 5 mg, 10 mg

INDICATIONS & DOSAGES

➤ **Edema in heart failure or renal disease**
Adults: 5 to 20 mg P.O. once daily.
➤ **Hypertension**
Adults: 2.5 to 5 mg P.O. once daily. Base maintenance dosage on blood pressure.

ADMINISTRATION

P.O.

- Give drug without regard for meals.
- To prevent nocturia, give drug in the morning.

ACTION

Increases sodium and water excretion by inhibiting sodium reabsorption in ascending loop of Henle.

Route	Onset	Peak	Duration
P.O.	1 hr	2–8 hr	12–24 hr

Half-life: About 14 hours.

ADVERSE REACTIONS

CNS: *dizziness,* headache, fatigue, vertigo, paresthesia, weakness, restlessness, drowsiness, anxiety, depression, nervousness, blurred vision.
CV: orthostatic hypotension, palpitations, vasculitis.
GI: ***pancreatitis,*** anorexia, nausea, epigastric distress, vomiting, abdominal pain, diarrhea, constipation, dry mouth.
GU: nocturia, polyuria, impotence.
Hematologic: ***aplastic anemia, agranulocytosis, leukopenia,*** purpura.
Hepatic: jaundice, ***hepatitis.***
Metabolic: hyperglycemia and impaired glucose tolerance, fluid and electrolyte imbalances, including hypokalemia, hypomagnesemia, dilutional hyponatremia and hypochloremia, metabolic alkalosis, and hypercalcemia, volume depletion and dehydration.
Musculoskeletal: muscle cramps.
Skin: dermatitis, photosensitivity reactions, rash, pruritus, urticaria.

INTERACTIONS

Drug-drug. *Amphotericin B, corticosteroids:* May increase risk of hypokalemia. Monitor potassium level closely.
Anticoagulants: May decrease anticoagulant response. Monitor PT and INR.
Antidiabetics: May alter glucose level and require dosage adjustment of antidiabetics. Monitor glucose level.
Barbiturates, opioids: May increase orthostatic hypotensive effect. Monitor patient closely.
Bumetanide, ethacrynic acid, furosemide, torsemide: May cause excessive diuretic response, causing serious electrolyte abnormalities or dehydration. Adjust doses carefully, and monitor patient closely for signs and symptoms of excessive diuretic response.
Cardiac glycosides: May increase risk of digoxin toxicity from metolazone-induced hypokalemia. Monitor potassium and digoxin levels.
Cholestyramine, colestipol: May decrease intestinal absorption of thiazides. Separate doses.
Diazoxide: May increase antihypertensive, hyperglycemic, and hyperuricemic effects. Use together cautiously.
Lithium: May decrease lithium clearance, increasing risk of lithium toxicity. Monitor lithium level.
NSAIDs: May increase risk of renal failure. May decrease diuretic and antihypertensive effects. Monitor renal function and blood pressure.
Other antihypertensives: May have additive effects. Use together cautiously.
Drug-herb. *Dandelion:* May interfere with diuretic activity. Discourage use together.
Licorice: May cause unexpected rapid potassium loss. Discourage use together.
Drug-lifestyle. *Alcohol use:* May increase orthostatic hypotensive effect. Discourage use together.
Sun exposure: May increase risk for photosensitivity reaction. Advise patient to avoid excessive sunlight exposure.

EFFECTS ON LAB TEST RESULTS

- May increase glucose, calcium, cholesterol, and triglyceride levels. May decrease potassium, sodium, magnesium, chloride, and hemoglobin levels.
- May decrease granulocyte and WBC counts.

CONTRAINDICATIONS & CAUTIONS

- Contraindicated in patients hypersensitive to thiazides or other sulfonamide-derived drugs and in those with anuria, hepatic coma, or precoma.
- Use cautiously in patients with impaired renal or hepatic function.

NURSING CONSIDERATIONS

- Monitor fluid intake and output, weight, blood pressure, and electrolyte levels.
- Watch for signs and symptoms of hypokalemia, such as muscle weakness and cramps. Drug may be used with potassium-sparing diuretic to prevent potassium loss.
- Consult prescriber and dietitian about a high-potassium diet. Foods rich in potassium include citrus fruits, tomatoes, bananas, dates, and apricots.
- Monitor glucose level, especially in diabetic patients.
- Monitor uric acid level, especially in patients with history of gout.
- Monitor elderly patients, who are especially susceptible to excessive diuresis.
- In hypertensive patients, therapeutic response may be delayed several weeks.
- Monitor blood pressure. If response is inadequate, another antihypertensive may be added.
- Metolazone and furosemide may be used together to enhance diuretic effect.
- Unlike thiazide diuretics, metolazone is effective in patients with decreased renal function.
- Stop thiazides and thiazide-like diuretics before parathyroid function tests.
- ***Look alike–sound alike:*** Don't confuse Zaroxolyn with Zarontin.

PATIENT TEACHING

- Tell patient to take drug in morning to prevent need to urinate at night.
- Advise patient to avoid sudden posture changes and to rise slowly to avoid effects of dizziness upon standing quickly.
- Instruct patient to use a sunblock to prevent photosensitivity reactions.

metoprolol succinate

meh-TOH-pruh-lol

Toprol-XL

metoprolol tartrate

Betaloc Durules†, Lopresor†, Lopresor SR†, Lopressor, Novo-Metoprol†, Nu-Metop†

Pharmacologic class: beta blocker
Pregnancy risk category C

AVAILABLE FORMS

metoprolol succinate
Tablets (extended-release): 25 mg, 50 mg, 100 mg, 200 mg
metoprolol tartrate
Injection: 1 mg/ml in 5-ml ampules
Tablets: 50 mg, 100 mg
Tablets (extended-release): 100 mg†, 200 mg†

INDICATIONS & DOSAGES

➤ Hypertension
Adults: Initially, 50 mg P.O. b.i.d. or 100 mg P.O. once daily; then up to 100 to 450 mg daily in two or three divided doses. Or, 50 to 100 mg of extended-release tablets (tartrate equivalent) once daily. Adjust dosage as needed and tolerated at intervals of not less than 1 week to maximum of 400 mg daily.

➤ Early intervention in acute MI
Adults: 5 mg metoprolol tartrate I.V. bolus every 2 minutes for three doses. Then, 15 minutes after the last I.V. dose, give 25 to 50 mg P.O. every 6 hours for 48 hours. Maintenance dosage is 100 mg P.O. b.i.d.

➤ Angina pectoris
Adults: Initially, 100 mg P.O. daily as a single dose or in two equally divided doses; increased at weekly intervals until an adequate response or a pronounced decrease in heart rate is seen. Effects of daily dose beyond 400 mg aren't known. Or, give 100 mg of extended-release tablets (tartrate equivalent) once daily. Adjust dosage as needed and tolerated at intervals of not less than 1 week to maximum of 400 mg daily.

➤ **Stable symptomatic heart failure (New York Heart Association class II) resulting from ischemia, hypertension, or cardiomyopathy**
Adults: 25 mg Toprol-XL P.O. once daily for 2 weeks. Double the dose every 2 weeks, as tolerated, to a maximum of 200 mg daily.
Adjust-a-dose: In patients with more severe heart failure, start with 12.5 mg Toprol-XL P.O. once daily for 2 weeks.

ADMINISTRATION

P.O.
• Give drug with or immediately after meal.
I.V.
• Give drug undiluted by direct injection.
• Although best avoided, drug can be mixed with meperidine hydrochloride or morphine sulfate or given with an alteplase infusion at a Y-site connection.
• Store drug at room temperature and protect from light. Discard solution if it's discolored or contains particles.
• **Incompatibilities:** Amphotericin B.

ACTION

Unknown. A selective beta blocker that selectively blocks $beta_1$ receptors; decreases cardiac output, peripheral resistance, and cardiac oxygen consumption; and depresses renin secretion.

Route	Onset	Peak	Duration
P.O.	15 min	1 hr	6–12 hr
P.O. (extended-release)	15 min	6–12 hr	24 hr
I.V.	5 min	20 min	5–8 hr

Half-life: 3 to 7 hours.

ADVERSE REACTIONS

CNS: *fatigue, dizziness,* depression.
CV: *hypotension,* ***bradycardia, heart failure, AV block,*** edema.
GI: nausea, diarrhea.
Respiratory: dyspnea.
Skin: rash.

INTERACTIONS

Drug-drug. *Amobarbital, butabarbital, butalbital, pentobarbital, phenobarbital, primidone, secobarbital:* May reduce metoprolol effect. May need to increase metoprolol dose.
Cardiac glycosides, diltiazem: May cause excessive bradycardia and increased depressant effect on myocardium. Use together cautiously.
Catecholamine-depleting drugs such as MAO inhibitors, reserpine: May have additive effect. Monitor patient for hypotension and bradycardia.
Chlorpromazine: May decrease hepatic clearance. Watch for greater beta-blocking effect.
Cimetidine: May increase metoprolol effects. Give another H_2 agonist or decrease dose of metoprolol.
Fluoxetine, paroxetine, propafenone, quinidine: May increase metoprolol level. Monitor vital signs.
Hydralazine: May increase levels and effects of both drugs. Monitor patient closely. May need to adjust dosage.
Indomethacin, NSAIDs: May decrease antihypertensive effect. Monitor blood pressure and adjust dosage.
Insulin, oral antidiabetics: May alter dosage requirements in previously stabilized diabetic patients. Monitor patient closely.
I.V. lidocaine: May reduce hepatic metabolism of lidocaine, increasing risk of toxicity. Give bolus doses of lidocaine at a slower rate, and monitor lidocaine level closely.
Prazosin: May increase risk of orthostatic hypotension in the early phases of use together. Assist patient to stand slowly until effects are known.
Rifampin: May increase metoprolol metabolism. Watch for decreased effect.
Terbutaline: May antagonize bronchodilatory effects of terbutaline. Monitor patient.
Verapamil: May increase effects of both drugs. Monitor cardiac function closely, and decrease dosages as needed.
Drug-herb. *Ma huang:* May decrease antihypertensive effects. Discourage use together.
Drug-food. *Food:* May increase absorption. Encourage patient to take drug with food.

EFFECTS ON LAB TEST RESULTS
- May increase transaminase, alkaline phosphatase, LDH, and uric acid levels.

CONTRAINDICATIONS & CAUTIONS
- Contraindicated in patients hypersensitive to drug or other beta blockers.
- Contraindicated in patients with sinus bradycardia, greater than first-degree heart block, cardiogenic shock, or overt cardiac failure when used to treat hypertension or angina. When used to treat MI, drug is contraindicated in patients with heart rate less than 45 beats/minute, greater than first-degree heart block, PR interval of 0.24 second or longer with first-degree heart block, systolic blood pressure less than 100 mm Hg, or moderate to severe cardiac failure.
- Use cautiously in patients with heart failure, diabetes, or respiratory or hepatic disease.

NURSING CONSIDERATIONS
- Always check patient's apical pulse rate before giving drug. If it's slower than 60 beats/minute, withhold drug and call prescriber immediately.
- In diabetic patients, monitor glucose level closely because drug masks common signs and symptoms of hypoglycemia.
- Monitor blood pressure frequently; drug masks common signs and symptoms of shock.
- Beta blockers may mask tachycardia caused by hyperthyroidism. In patients with suspected thyrotoxicosis, taper off beta blocker to avoid thyroid storm.
- When stopping therapy, taper dose over 1 to 2 weeks.
- Beta selectivity is lost at higher doses. Watch for peripheral side effects.
- ***Look alike–sound alike:*** Don't confuse metoprolol with metaproterenol or metolazone. Don't confuse Toprol-XL with Topamax, Tegretol, or Tegretol-XR.

PATIENT TEACHING
- Instruct patient to take drug exactly as prescribed and with meals.
- Caution patient to avoid driving and other tasks requiring mental alertness until response to therapy has been established.
- Advise patient to inform dentist or prescriber about use of this drug before procedures or surgery.
- Tell patient to alert prescriber if shortness of breath occurs.
- Instruct patient not to stop drug suddenly but to notify prescriber about unpleasant adverse reactions. Inform him that drug must be withdrawn gradually over 1 or 2 weeks.
- Inform patient that use isn't advisable in breast-feeding women.

---

metronidazole
me-troe-NI-da-zole

Flagyl, Flagyl 375, Flagyl ER, Florazole ER†, Novo-Nidazol†

metronidazole hydrochloride
Flagyl IV RTU

Pharmacologic class: nitroimidazole
Pregnancy risk category B

AVAILABLE FORMS
Capsules: 375 mg
Injection: 500 mg/100 ml in vials or ready-to-use minibags
Powder for injection: 500-mg single-dose vials
Tablets: 250 mg, 500 mg
Tablets (extended-release): 750 mg

INDICATIONS & DOSAGES
➤ Amebic liver abscess
Adults: 500 to 750 mg P.O. t.i.d. for 5 to 10 days; or 2.4 g P.O. once daily for 1 to 2 days. Or, 500 mg I.V. every 6 hours for 10 days if patient can't tolerate P.O. route.
Children: 30 to 50 mg/kg daily in three divided doses for 10 days. Maximum, 750 mg/dose.
➤ Intestinal amebiasis
Adults: 750 mg P.O. t.i.d. for 5 to 10 days; then treat with a luminal amebicide, such as iodoquinol or paromomycin.
Children: 30 to 50 mg/kg daily in three divided doses for 10 days; then treat with a luminal amebicide, such as iodoquinol or paromomycin.

➤ Trichomoniasis
Adults: 250 mg P.O. t.i.d. for 7 days, or 500 mg P.O. b.i.d. for 7 days, or 2 g P.O. in single dose (may give the 2-g dose in two 1-g doses, both on the same day); wait 4 to 6 weeks before repeating course.
Children: 5 mg/kg P.O. t.i.d. for 7 days.
➤ Refractory trichomoniasis
Adults: 250 mg P.O. b.i.d. for 10 days. Or, 500 mg P.O. b.i.d. for 7 days.
➤ Bacterial infections caused by anaerobic microorganisms
Adults: Loading dose is 15 mg/kg I.V. infused over 1 hour. Maintenance dose is 7.5 mg/kg I.V. or P.O. every 6 hours. Give first maintenance dose 6 hours after loading dose. Maximum dose shouldn't exceed 4 g daily.
➤ To prevent postoperative infection in contaminated or potentially contaminated colorectal surgery
Adults: Infuse 15 mg/kg I.V. over 30 to 60 minutes and complete about 1 hour before surgery. Then, infuse 7.5 mg/kg I.V. over 30 to 60 minutes at 6 and 12 hours after first dose.
➤ Bacterial vaginosis
Adults: 750 mg Flagyl ER P.O. daily for 7 days.
➤ *Clostridium difficile*–associated diarrhea and colitis ♦
Adults: Usually 250 mg P.O. q.i.d. or 500 mg P.O. t.i.d. for 10 days. Or, 500 mg to 750 mg I.V. every 6 to 8 hours when P.O. route isn't practical.
Children: 30 to 50 mg/kg/day P.O. given in three to four equally divided doses for 7 to 10 days. Don't exceed adult dose.
➤ Pelvic inflammatory disease (PID) ♦
Adults: 500 mg I.V. every 8 hours with ofloxacin or with I.V. levofloxacin. For ambulatory patients, 500 mg P.O. b.i.d. with ofloxacin for 14 days.
➤ Bacterial vaginosis ♦
Nonpregnant women: 500 mg P.O. b.i.d. for 7 days. Or, 2 g P.O. as a single dose.
Pregnant women: 250 mg P.O. t.i.d. or 500 mg P.O. b.i.d. for 7 days.

ADMINISTRATION
P.O.
- Give drug with food.

I.V.
- Flagyl IV ready-to-use (RTU) minibags need no preparation.
- Don't use aluminum needles or hubs to reconstitute the drug or to transfer reconstituted drug. Equipment that contains aluminum will turn the solution orange; the potency isn't affected.
- To reconstitute lyophilized vials, add 4.4 ml of sterile water for injection, bacteriostatic water for injection, sterile normal saline solution for injection, or bacteriostatic normal saline solution for injection. Reconstituted drug contains 100 mg/ml. Add contents of vial to 100 ml of D_5W, lactated Ringer's injection, or normal saline solution to yield 5 mg/ml. Neutralize this highly acidic solution by carefully adding 5 mEq sodium bicarbonate to each 500 mg; the carbon dioxide gas that forms may need to be vented.
- Infuse drug over at least 1 hour. Don't give by I.V. push.
- Don't refrigerate the neutralized diluted solution; precipitation may occur. Refrigerated Flagyl IV RTU may form crystals, which disappear after the solution warms to room temperature.
- **Incompatibilities:** Aluminum, amino acid 10%, amoxicillin sodium and clavulanate potassium, amphotericin B, aztreonam, ceftriaxone, dopamine, filgrastim, meropenem, other I.V. drugs, warfarin.

ACTION
Direct-acting trichomonacide and amebicide that works inside and outside the intestines. It's thought to enter the cells of microorganisms that contain nitroreductase, forming unstable compounds that bind to DNA and inhibit synthesis, causing cell death.

Route	Onset	Peak	Duration
P.O.	Unknown	2 hr	Unknown
I.V.	Immediate	1 hr	Unknown

Half-life: 6 to 8 hours.

ADVERSE REACTIONS
CNS: *headache,* ***seizures,*** fever, vertigo, ataxia, dizziness, syncope, incoordination, confusion, irritability, depression, weakness, insomnia, peripheral neuropathy.

CV: flattened T wave, edema, flushing, thrombophlebitis after I.V. infusion.
EENT: rhinitis, sinusitis, pharyngitis.
GI: *nausea,* abdominal cramping or pain, stomatitis, epigastric distress, vomiting, anorexia, diarrhea, constipation, proctitis, dry mouth, metallic taste.
GU: *vaginitis,* darkened urine, polyuria, dysuria, cystitis, dyspareunia, dryness of vagina and vulva, vaginal candidiasis, genital pruritus.
Hematologic: ***transient leukopenia, neutropenia.***
Musculoskeletal: transient joint pains.
Respiratory: upper respiratory tract infection.
Skin: rash.
Other: decreased libido, overgrowth of nonsusceptible organisms, especially *Candida*.

INTERACTIONS

Drug-drug. ***Busulfan:*** May increase busulfan toxicity. Avoid using together.
Cimetidine: May increase risk of metronidazole toxicity because of inhibited hepatic metabolism. Monitor patient for toxicity.
Disulfiram: May cause acute psychosis and confusion. Avoid giving metronidazole within 2 weeks of disulfiram.
Lithium: May increase lithium level, which may cause toxicity. Monitor lithium level.
Phenobarbital, phenytoin: May decrease metronidazole effectiveness; may reduce total phenytoin clearance. Monitor patient.
Warfarin: May increase anticoagulant effects and risk of bleeding. Reduce warfarin as needed.
Drug-lifestyle. *Alcohol use:* May cause disulfiram-like reaction, including nausea, vomiting, headache, cramps, and flushing. Warn patient to avoid alcohol during and for 3 days after completing drug therapy.

EFFECTS ON LAB TEST RESULTS

- May decrease WBC and neutrophil counts.
- May falsely decrease triglyceride and aminotransferase levels.

CONTRAINDICATIONS & CAUTIONS

- Contraindicated in patients hypersensitive to drug or other nitroimidazole derivatives and in patients in first trimester of pregnancy.
- ***Alert:*** If drug must be given to a pregnant woman for trichomoniasis, use the 7-day regimen, not the 2-g single-dose regimen. The 2-g dose produces a high level that's more likely to reach fetal circulation.
- Use cautiously in patients with history of blood dyscrasia, CNS disorder, or retinal or visual field changes.
- Use cautiously in patients who take hepatotoxic drugs or have hepatic disease or alcoholism.

NURSING CONSIDERATIONS

- Monitor liver function test results carefully in elderly patients.
- Observe patient for edema, especially if he's receiving corticosteroids; Flagyl IV RTU may cause sodium retention.
- Record number and character of stools when drug is used to treat amebiasis. Give drug only after *Trichomonas vaginalis* infection is confirmed by wet smear or culture or *Entameba histolytica* is identified.
- Sexual partners of patients being treated for *T. vaginalis* infection, even if asymptomatic, must also be treated to avoid reinfection.

PATIENT TEACHING

- Instruct patient to take extended-release tablets at least 1 hour before or 2 hours after meals but to take all other oral forms with food to minimize GI upset.
- Inform patient of need for sexual partners to be treated simultaneously to avoid reinfection.
- Instruct patient in proper hygiene.
- Tell patient to avoid alcohol and alcohol-containing drugs during and for at least 3 days after treatment course.
- Tell patient he may experience a metallic taste and have dark or red-brown urine.
- Tell patient to report to prescriber symptoms of candidal overgrowth.
- Tell patient to report to prescriber immediately any neurologic symptoms (seizures, peripheral neuropathy).

mexiletine hydrochloride

mex-ILL-i-teen

Mexitil

Pharmacologic class: lidocaine analogue
Pregnancy risk category C

AVAILABLE FORMS

Capsules: 100 mg†, 150 mg, 200 mg, 250 mg

INDICATIONS & DOSAGES

➤ **Life-threatening ventricular arrhythmias, including ventricular tachycardia and PVCs**

Adults: Initially, 200 mg P.O. every 8 hours. If satisfactory control isn't obtained at this dosage, increase dosage by 50 to 100 mg every 2 to 3 days up to maximum of 400 mg every 8 hours. If rapid control of ventricular rate is desired, give a loading dose of 400 mg P.O., followed by 200 mg 8 hours later. Patients controlled on 300 mg or less every 8 hours can receive the total daily dose in evenly divided doses every 12 hours.

ADMINISTRATION

P.O.

- Give drug with meals or antacids to lessen GI distress.
- When changing from lidocaine to mexiletine, stop the lidocaine infusion when the first mexiletine dose is given. But keep the infusion line open until the arrhythmia is satisfactorily controlled.
- When switching to mexiletine from another oral class 1A antiarrhythmic, begin with a 200-mg dose 6 to 12 hours after the last dose of quinidine sulfate or disopyramide, 3 to 6 hours after the last dose of procainamide, or 8 to 12 hours after the last dose of tocainide.

ACTION

Blocks the fast sodium channel in cardiac tissues without involving the autonomic nervous system. Drug reduces rate of rise, amplitude, and duration of action potential, and automaticity and effective refractory period in the Purkinje fibers.

Route	Onset	Peak	Duration
P.O.	30–120 min	2–3 hr	Unknown

Half-life: 10 to 12 hours.

ADVERSE REACTIONS

CNS: *tremor, dizziness, light-headedness, incoordination, nervousness,* confusion, changes in sleep habits, paresthesia, weakness, fatigue, speech difficulties, depression, headache.
CV: NEW OR WORSENED ARRHYTHMIAS, palpitations, chest pain, nonspecific edema, angina.
EENT: blurred vision, diplopia, tinnitus.
GI: *nausea, vomiting, upper GI distress, heartburn,* diarrhea, constipation, dry mouth, changes in appetite, abdominal pain.
Skin: rash.

INTERACTIONS

Drug-drug. *Antacids, atropine, narcotics:* May slow mexiletine absorption. Monitor patient for effectiveness.
Cimetidine: May alter mexiletine level. Monitor patient.
Fluvoxamine: May decrease mexiletine clearance. Monitor patient for adverse effects and toxicity.
Methylxanthines (such as caffeine, theophylline): May reduce methylxanthine clearance, which may cause toxicity. Monitor drug level.
Metoclopramide: May speed up mexiletine absorption. Monitor patient for toxicity.
Phenobarbital, phenytoin, rifampin, urine acidifiers: May decrease mexiletine level. Monitor patient for effectiveness.
Urine alkalinizers: May increase mexiletine level. Monitor patient for adverse reactions.

EFFECTS ON LAB TEST RESULTS

- May increase AST level.

CONTRAINDICATIONS & CAUTIONS

- Contraindicated in patients with cardiogenic shock or second- or third-degree AV block in the absence of an artificial pacemaker.
- Use cautiously in patients with first-degree heart block, a ventricular

pacemaker, sinus node dysfunction, intraventricular conduction disturbances, hypotension, severe heart failure, liver disease, or seizure disorder.

NURSING CONSIDERATIONS

- If patient may be a good candidate for every-12-hours therapy, notify prescriber. Twice-daily dosage enhances compliance.
- Monitor therapeutic drug level, which may range from 0.5 to 2 mcg/ml.
- An early sign of mexiletine toxicity is tremor, usually a fine tremor of the hands, progressing to dizziness and then to ataxia and nystagmus as drug level in the blood increases. Watch for and ask patient about these symptoms.
- Monitor blood pressure and heart rate and rhythm frequently. Notify prescriber of significant change.

PATIENT TEACHING

- Tell patient to take drug exactly as prescribed.
- Instruct patient to take drug with food or an antacid if GI reactions occur.
- Instruct patient to report adverse reactions promptly.
- Advise patient to notify prescriber if he develops jaundice, fever, or general tiredness; these symptoms may indicate liver damage.

midodrine hydrochloride

MID-oh-dryn

ProAmatine

Pharmacologic class: synthetic sympathomimetic amine
Pregnancy risk category C

AVAILABLE FORMS

Tablets: 2.5 mg, 5 mg, 10 mg

INDICATIONS & DOSAGES

➤ Symptomatic orthostatic hypotension unresponsive to standard clinical care

Adults: 10 mg P.O. t.i.d. The patient takes the first dose upon arising in the morning, the second dose at noon, and the third dose in late afternoon but no later than 6 p.m. or 4 hours before bedtime.

Adjust-a-dose: For patients with renal impairment, initially, 2.5 mg.

ADMINISTRATION

P.O.

- Space doses at least 3 hours apart.
- Give drug during the day when patient can be upright and performing activities of daily living. Don't give drug after the evening meal or within 4 hours of bedtime to reduce risk of supine hypertension during sleep.

ACTION

Forms an active metabolite, desglymidodrine, which is an alpha$_1$ agonist. It increases blood pressure by activating alpha-adrenergic receptors in arteriolar and venous vasculature.

Route	Onset	Peak	Duration
P.O.	Unknown	1–2 hr	Unknown

Half-life: 3 to 4 hours.

ADVERSE REACTIONS

CNS: *paresthesia,* anxiety, confusion, headache.
CV: *vasodilation,* ***supine and sitting hypertension.***
GI: abdominal pain, dry mouth.
GU: *dysuria,* frequency and urgency, urine retention.
Skin: *piloerection, pruritus,* rash.
Other: chills, pain.

INTERACTIONS

Drug-drug. *Alpha agonists:* May enhance vasopressor effects. Monitor blood pressure closely.
Alpha blockers: May antagonize drug effects. Avoid using together.
Beta blockers, cardiac glycosides: May cause or worsen bradycardia, AV block, or arrhythmias. Avoid using together.
Fludrocortisone: May increase risk of supine hypertension and lead to increased intraocular pressure and worsened glaucoma. Monitor patient closely.

EFFECTS ON LAB TEST RESULTS

None reported.

CONTRAINDICATIONS & CAUTIONS

- Contraindicated in patients with severe organic heart disease, persistent and excessive supine hypertension, acute renal disease, urine retention, pheochromocytoma, or thyrotoxicosis.
- Use cautiously in patients with history of urine retention, visual problems, diabetes, or renal or hepatic impairment, and in breast-feeding women.
- Safety and effectiveness of drug in children haven't been established.
- Give drug to pregnant woman only if potential benefit outweighs fetal risk.

NURSING CONSIDERATIONS

- Perform renal and hepatic tests before and during drug therapy.
- Monitor supine and sitting blood pressures closely, and notify prescriber if supine blood pressure increases excessively.
- Monitor patient for signs and symptoms of bradycardia, such as slowed pulse, syncope or dizziness, especially after giving the drug.
- Continue drug only if symptoms improve during initial therapy.
- ***Look alike–sound alike:*** Don't confuse ProAmatine with protamine.

PATIENT TEACHING

- Instruct patient to separate doses by 3 to 4 hours; tell him to take last dose of the day 4 hours before bedtime.
- Instruct patient to stop drug and immediately notify prescriber about signs and symptoms of supine hypertension (cardiac awareness, pounding in ears, headache, blurred vision).
- Tell patient to consult prescriber before taking OTC drugs.

SAFETY ALERT!

milrinone lactate

MILL-ri-none

Primacor

Pharmacologic class: bipyridine phosphodiesterase inhibitor
Pregnancy risk category C

AVAILABLE FORMS

Injection: 1 mg/ml
Injection (premixed): 200 mcg/ml in D_5W

INDICATIONS & DOSAGES

➤ **Short-term treatment of acutely decompensated heart failure**

Adults: Give first loading dose of 50 mcg/kg I.V. slowly over 10 minutes; then give continuous I.V. infusion of 0.375 to 0.75 mcg/kg/minute. Titrate infusion dose based on clinical and hemodynamic responses. Don't exceed 1.13 mg/kg/day.

Adjust-a-dose: If creatinine clearance is 50 ml/minute, infusion rate is 0.43 mcg/kg/minute; if 40 ml/minute, infusion rate is 0.38 mcg/kg/minute; if 30 ml/minute, infusion rate is 0.33 mcg/kg/minute; if 20 ml/minute, infusion rate is 0.28 mcg/kg/minute; if 10 ml/minute,infusion rate is 0.23 mcg/kg/minute; and if 5 ml/minute, infusion rate is 0.2 mcg/kg/minute. Don't exceed 1.13 mg/kg/day.

ADMINISTRATION

I.V.

- Give loading dose undiluted as a direct injection over 10 minutes.
- Prepare I.V. infusion solution using half-normal saline solution, normal saline solution, or D_5W. Prepare the 100-mcg/ml solution by adding 180 ml of diluent per 20-mg (20-ml) vial, the 150-mcg/ml solution by adding 113 ml of diluent per 20-mg (20-ml) vial, and the 200-mcg/ml solution by adding 80 ml of diluent per 20-mg (20-ml) vial.

• **Incompatibilities:** Bumetanide, furosemide, imipenem and cilastatin sodium, procainamide, torsemide.

ACTION

Produces inotropic action by increasing cellular levels of cAMP and vasodilation by relaxing vascular smooth muscle.

Route	Onset	Peak	Duration
I.V.	5–15 min	1–2 hr	3–6 hr

Half-life: 2½ to 3¾ hours.

ADVERSE REACTIONS

CNS: headache.

CV: **VENTRICULAR ARRHYTHMIAS,** *ventricular ectopic activity,* ***sustained ventricular tachycardia, ventricular fibrillation,*** hypotension, nonsustained ventricular tachycardia.

INTERACTIONS

None significant.

EFFECTS ON LAB TEST RESULTS

• May cause abnormal liver function test results.

CONTRAINDICATIONS & CAUTIONS

• Contraindicated in patients hypersensitive to drug.
• Contraindicated for use in patients with severe aortic or pulmonic valvular disease in place of surgery and during acute phase of MI.
• Use cautiously in patients with atrial flutter or fibrillation because drug slightly shortens AV node conduction time and may increase ventricular response rate.

NURSING CONSIDERATIONS

• In patients with atrial flutter or fibrillation, give digoxin before milrinone therapy. Drug is typically given with digoxin and diuretics.
• Improved cardiac output may increase urine output. Reduce diuretic dosage when heart failure improves. Potassium loss may cause digitalis toxicity.
• Monitor fluid and electrolyte status, blood pressure, heart rate, and renal function during therapy. Excessive decrease in blood pressure requires stopping or slowing rate of infusion.
• Correct hypoxemia.

PATIENT TEACHING

• Instruct patient to report adverse reactions to prescriber promptly, especially angina.
• Tell patient that drug may cause headache, which can be treated with analgesics.
• Tell patient to report discomfort at I.V. insertion site.

minoxidil

mi-NOX-i-dill

Pharmacologic class: peripheral vasodilator
Pregnancy risk category C

AVAILABLE FORMS

Tablets: 2.5 mg, 10 mg

INDICATIONS & DOSAGES

➤ **Severe hypertension**

Adults and children older than age 12: Initially, 2.5 to 5 mg P.O. as a single dose. Effective dosage range is usually 10 to 40 mg daily. Maximum dose is 100 mg daily.
Children younger than age 12: Give 0.2 mg/kg P.O. (maximum 5 mg) as a single daily dose. Effective dosage range is usually 0.25 to 1 mg/kg daily. Maximum dose is 50 mg daily.

ADMINISTRATION

P.O.

• Give drug without regard for meals.

ACTION

Unknown. Predominantly produces direct arteriolar vasodilation.

Route	Onset	Peak	Duration
P.O.	30 min	2–3 hr	2–5 days

Half-life: Average, 4¼ hours.

ADVERSE REACTIONS
CV: *edema, tachycardia, pericardial effusion,* ***tamponade,*** *ECG changes,* ***heart failure,*** rebound hypertension.
GI: nausea, vomiting.
Metabolic: weight gain.
Skin: ***Stevens-Johnson syndrome,*** rash.
Other: *hypertrichosis,* breast tenderness.

INTERACTIONS
Drug-drug. *Antihypertensives:* May cause severe orthostatic hypotension. Advise patient to rise slowly.
NSAIDs: May decrease antihypertensive effects. Monitor blood pressure.
Drug-herb. *Ma huang:* May decrease antihypertensive effects. Discourage use together.

EFFECTS ON LAB TEST RESULTS
• May increase alkaline phosphatase, BUN, and creatinine levels. May decrease hemoglobin level and hematocrit.

CONTRAINDICATIONS & CAUTIONS
• Contraindicated in patients hypersensitive to drug and in those with pheochromocytoma. Also contraindicated in patients with acute MI or dissecting aortic aneurysm.
• Use cautiously in patients with impaired renal function and after recent MI (within past month).

NURSING CONSIDERATIONS
• Monitor blood pressure and pulse rate at beginning of therapy and periodically thereafter.
• Elderly patients may be more sensitive to drug's hypotensive effects.
• Initially, assess CBC, electrolytes, alkaline phosphatase, renal function, ECG, chest X-ray, and echocardiogram. Repeat tests that are abnormal at 1- to 3-month intervals and every 6 to 12 months when stabilized.
• Drug is removed by hemodialysis. Give dose after dialysis.
• Give with a thiazide or loop diuretic to prevent fluid retention and heart failure.
• Monitor fluid intake and urine output. Check for weight gain and edema.
• Monitor patient for elongated, thickened, and enhanced pigmentation of fine body hair.
• Minoxidil may elevate ANA titers.
• ***Look alike–sound alike:*** Don't confuse Loniten with Lotensin.

PATIENT TEACHING
• Make sure patient receives and reads manufacturer's patient package insert that describes the drug and its adverse reactions. Also provide an oral explanation.
• Tell patient not to suddenly stop taking drug but to notify prescriber if unpleasant adverse effects occur.
• Make sure patient understands importance of compliance with total treatment regimen. Drug is usually prescribed with a beta blocker to control rapid heart rate and a diuretic to counteract fluid retention.
• Teach patient how to take his own pulse and to notify prescriber of increases of more than 20 beats/minute.
• Tell patient to weigh himself at least weekly and to report weight gain of 2 or more pounds in 1 day or more than 5 pounds in 1 week.
• About 8 of 10 patients experience elongation, thickening, and enhanced pigmentation of fine body hair within 3 to 6 weeks of beginning treatment. Shaving or using a depilatory can control unwanted hair. Assure patient that extra hair disappears within 1 to 6 months of stopping minoxidil. Advise patient not to stop drug without prescriber's approval.
• Advise woman of childbearing age to discuss drug therapy with prescriber if considering pregnancy or currently breastfeeding.

SAFETY ALERT!

morphine hydrochloride
MOR-feen

Doloral†, M.O.S†, M.O.S.-S.R†

morphine sulfate
Astramorph PF, Avinza, DepoDur, Duramorph, Infumorph, Kadian, M-Eslon†, Morphine H.P†, MS Contin, MSIR, Oramorph SR, RMS Uniserts, Roxanol, Statex†

Pharmacologic class: opioid
Pregnancy risk category C
Controlled substance schedule II

AVAILABLE FORMS
morphine hydrochloride
Oral solution: 1 mg/ml†, 5 mg/ml†, 10 mg/ml†, 20 mg/ml†, 50 mg/ml†
Suppositories: 10 mg†, 20 mg†, 30 mg†
Syrup: 1 mg/ml†*, 5 mg/ml†*, 10 mg/ml†*, 20 mg/ml†*, 50 mg/ml†*
Tablets: 10 mg†, 20 mg†, 40 mg†, 60 mg†
Tablets (extended-release): 30 mg†, 60 mg†
morphine sulfate
Capsules: 15 mg, 30 mg
Capsules (extended-release beads): 30 mg, 60 mg, 90 mg, 120 mg
Capsules (extended-release pellets): 10 mg, 20 mg, 30 mg, 50 mg, 60 mg, 80 mg, 100 mg, 200 mg
Injection (with preservative): 0.5 mg/ml, 1 mg/ml, 2 mg/ml, 4 mg/ml, 5 mg/ml, 8 mg/ml, 10 mg/ml, 15 mg/ml, 25 mg/ml, 50 mg/ml
Injection (without preservative): 0.5 mg/ml, 1 mg/ml, 10 mg/ml, 15 mg/ml, 25 mg/ml
Oral solution: 10 mg/5 ml, 20 mg/5 ml, 20 mg/ml (concentrate), 100 mg/5 ml (concentrate)
Soluble tablets: 10 mg, 15 mg, 30 mg
Suppositories: 5 mg, 10 mg, 20 mg, 30 mg
Tablets: 15 mg, 30 mg
Tablets (extended-release): 15 mg, 30 mg, 60 mg, 100 mg, 200 mg

INDICATIONS & DOSAGES
➤ Severe pain
Adults: 5 to 20 mg subcutaneously or I.M. or 2.5 to 15 mg I.V. every 4 hours p.r.n. Or, 5 to 30 mg P.O. or 10 to 20 mg P.R. every 4 hours p.r.n.

For continuous I.V. infusion, give loading dose of 15 mg I.V.; then continuous infusion of 0.8 to 10 mg/hour.

For extended-release tablet, give 15 or 30 mg P.O., every 8 to 12 hours.

For extended-release Kadian capsules used as a first opioid, give 20 mg P.O. every 12 hours or 40 mg P.O. once daily; increase conservatively in opioid-naive patients.

For epidural injection, give 5 mg by epidural catheter; then, if pain isn't relieved adequately in 1 hour, give supplementary doses of 1 to 2 mg at intervals sufficient to assess effectiveness. Maximum total epidural dose shouldn't exceed 10 mg/24 hours.

For intrathecal injection, a single dose of 0.2 to 1 mg may provide pain relief for 24 hours (only in the lumbar area). Don't repeat injections.
Children: 0.1 to 0.2 mg/kg subcutaneously or I.M. every 4 hours. Maximum single dose, 15 mg.

➤ Moderate to severe pain requiring continuous, around-the-clock opioid
Adults: Individualize dosage of Avinza. For patients with no tolerance to opioids, begin with 30 mg Avinza P.O. daily; adjust dosage by no more than 30 mg every 4 days. When converting from another oral morphine form, individualize the dosage schedule according to patient's schedule.

➤ Single-dose, epidural extended pain relief after major surgery
Adults: Inject 10 to 15 mg (maximum 20 mg) DepoDur via lumbar epidural administration before surgery or after clamping of umbilical cord during cesarean section. May be injected undiluted or may be diluted up to 5 ml total volume with preservative-free normal saline solution.

ADMINISTRATION
P.O.
- Oral solutions of various concentrations and an intensified oral solution (20 mg/ml)

are available. Carefully note the strength given.
• Give morphine sulfate without regard to food.
• Oral capsules may be carefully opened and the entire contents poured into cool, soft foods, such as water, orange juice, applesauce, or pudding; patient should consume mixture immediately.
• Don't crush, break, or chew extended-release forms.
Sublingual
• For S.L. use, measure oral solution with tuberculin syringe. Give dose a few drops at a time to allow maximal S.L. absorption and minimize swallowing.
I.V.
• For direct injection, dilute 2.5 to 15 mg in 4 or 5 ml of sterile water for injection and give slowly over 4 to 5 minutes.
• For continuous infusion, mix drug with D_5W to yield 0.1 to 1 mg/ml, and give by a continuous infusion device.
• In adults with severe, chronic pain, maintenance I.V. infusion is 0.8 to 80 mg/hour; sometimes higher doses are needed.
• Don't mix DepoDur with other drugs. Once DepoDur is given, don't give any other drugs into epidural space for at least 48 hours. Don't use in-line filter during administration.
• Store DepoDur in refrigerator. Unopened vials can be stored at room temperature for up to 7 days. After drug is withdrawn from vial, it can be stored at room temperature for up to 4 hours before use.
• **Incompatibilities:** Aminophylline, amobarbital, cefepime, chlorothiazide, fluorouracil, haloperidol, heparin sodium, meperidine, pentobarbital, phenobarbital sodium, phenytoin sodium, prochlorperazine, promethazine hydrochloride, sodium bicarbonate, thiopental.
I.M.
• Document injection site.
• Store injection solution at room temperature and protect from light.
• Solution may darken with age. Don't use if injection is darker than pale yellow, discolored, or contains precipitate.
Subcutaneous
• Document injection site.
• Store injection solution at room temperature and protect from light.
• Solution may darken with age. Don't use if injection is darker than pale yellow, discolored, or contains precipitate.
Rectal
• Refrigeration of rectal suppository isn't needed.

ACTION
Unknown. Binds with opioid receptors in the CNS, altering perception of and emotional response to pain.

Route	Onset	Peak	Duration
P.O.	30 min	1–2 hr	4–12 hr
P.O. (extended-release)	1–2 hr	3–4 hr	12–24 hr
I.V.	5 min	20 min	4–5 hr
I.M.	10–30 min	30–60 min	4–5 hr
Subcut.	10–30 min	50–90 min	4–5 hr
P.R.	20–60 min	20–60 min	4–5 hr
Epidural	15–60 min	15–60 min	24 hr
Intrathecal	15–60 min	30–60 min	24 hr

Half-life: 2 to 3 hours.

ADVERSE REACTIONS
CNS: *dizziness, euphoria, light-headedness, nightmares, sedation, somnolence,* ***seizures,*** depression, hallucinations, nervousness, physical dependence, syncope.
CV: ***bradycardia, cardiac arrest, shock,*** hypertension, hypotension, tachycardia.
GI: *constipation, nausea, vomiting,* anorexia, biliary tract spasms, dry mouth, ileus.
GU: urine retention.
Hematologic: ***thrombocytopenia.***
Respiratory: ***apnea, respiratory arrest, respiratory depression.***
Skin: diaphoresis, edema, pruritus and skin flushing.
Other: decreased libido.

INTERACTIONS
Drug-drug. *Cimetidine:* May increase respiratory and CNS depression when given with morphine sulfate. Monitor patient closely.
CNS depressants, general anesthetics, hypnotics, MAO inhibitors, other opioid

analgesics, sedatives, tranquilizers, tricyclic antidepressants: May cause respiratory depression, hypotension, profound sedation, or coma. Use together with caution, reduce morphine dose, and monitor patient response.
Drug-lifestyle. *Alcohol use:* May cause additive CNS effects. Warn patient to avoid alcohol.

EFFECTS ON LAB TEST RESULTS

- May increase amylase level. May decrease hemoglobin level (morphine sulfate).
- May decrease platelet count.
- May cause abnormal liver function test values (morphine sulfate).

CONTRAINDICATIONS & CAUTIONS

- Contraindicated in patients hypersensitive to drug and in those with conditions that would preclude I.V. administration of opioids (acute bronchial asthma or upper airway obstruction).
- Contraindicated in patients with GI obstruction.
- Use with caution in elderly or debilitated patients and in those with head injury, increased intracranial pressure, seizures, chronic pulmonary disease, prostatic hyperplasia, severe hepatic or renal disease, acute abdominal conditions, hypothyroidism, Addison's disease, and urethral stricture.
- Use with caution in patients with circulatory shock, biliary tract disease, CNS depression, toxic psychosis, acute alcoholism, delirium tremens, and seizure disorders.

NURSING CONSIDERATIONS

- Reassess patient's level of pain at least 15 and 30 minutes after giving parenterally and 30 minutes after giving orally.
- Keep opioid antagonist (naloxone) and resuscitation equipment available.
- Monitor circulatory, respiratory, bladder, and bowel functions carefully. Drug may cause respiratory depression, hypotension, urine retention, nausea, vomiting, ileus, or altered level of consciousness regardless of the route. If respirations drop below 12 breaths/minute, withhold dose and notify prescriber.
- Preservative-free preparations are available for epidural and intrathecal use.
- When drug is given epidurally, monitor patient closely for respiratory depression up to 24 hours after the injection. Check respiratory rate and depth every 30 to 60 minutes for 24 hours. Watch for pruritus and skin flushing.
- Morphine is drug of choice in relieving MI pain; may cause transient decrease in blood pressure.
- An around-the-clock regimen best manages severe, chronic pain.
- Morphine may worsen or mask gallbladder pain.
- Constipation is commonly severe with maintenance dose. Ensure that stool softener and/or stimulant laxative is ordered.
- Taper morphine sulfate therapy gradually when stopping therapy.
- ***Look alike–sound alike:*** Don't confuse morphine with hydromorphone or Avinza with Invanz.

PATIENT TEACHING

- When drug is used after surgery, encourage patient to turn, cough, deep-breathe, and use incentive spirometer to prevent lung problems.
- Caution ambulatory patient about getting out of bed or walking. Warn outpatient to avoid driving and other potentially hazardous activities that require mental alertness until drug's adverse CNS effects are known.
- ***Alert:*** Drinking alcohol or taking drugs containing alcohol while taking extended-release capsules may cause additive CNS effects. Warn patient to read labels on OTC drugs carefully and not to use alcohol in any form.
- Tell patient to swallow morphine sulfate whole or to open capsule and sprinkle beads or pellets on a small amount of applesauce immediately before taking.
- ***Alert:*** Warn patient not to crush, break, or chew extended-release forms.

nadolol

nay-DOE-lol

Apo-Nadol†, Corgard

Pharmacologic class: nonselective beta blocker
Pregnancy risk category C

AVAILABLE FORMS

Tablets: 20 mg, 40 mg, 80 mg, 120 mg, 160 mg

INDICATIONS & DOSAGES

➤ **Angina pectoris**

Adults: 40 mg P.O. once daily. Increase in 40- to 80-mg increments at 3- to 7-day intervals until optimal response occurs. Usual maintenance dose is 40 to 80 mg once daily; up to 240 mg once daily may be needed.

➤ **Hypertension**

Adults: 40 mg P.O. once daily. Increase in 40- to 80-mg increments until optimal response occurs. Usual maintenance dose is 40 to 80 mg once daily. Doses of 320 mg may be needed.

Adjust-a-dose: If creatinine clearance is 31 to 50 ml/minute, change dosing interval to every 24 to 36 hours; if clearance is 10 to 30 ml/minute, every 24 to 48 hours; and if clearance is less than 10 ml/minute, every 40 to 60 hours.

ADMINISTRATION

P.O.

- Give drug without regard for food.
- Check apical pulse before giving drug. If slower than 60 beats/minute, withhold drug and call prescriber.
- ***Alert:*** Abruptly stopping drug may worsen angina and cause an MI. Reduce dosage gradually over 1 to 2 weeks.

ACTION

Reduces cardiac oxygen demand by blocking catecholamine-induced increases in heart rate, blood pressure, and force of myocardial contraction. Depresses renin secretion.

Route	Onset	Peak	Duration
P.O.	Unknown	2–4 hr	Unknown

Half-life: About 10 to 24 hours.

ADVERSE REACTIONS

CNS: fatigue, dizziness, fever.
CV: **BRADYCARDIA, HEART FAILURE,** *hypotension,* peripheral vascular disease, rhythm and conduction disturbances.
GI: nausea, vomiting, diarrhea, abdominal pain, constipation, anorexia.
Respiratory: *increased airway resistance.*
Skin: rash.

INTERACTIONS

Drug-drug. *Antihypertensives:* May increase antihypertensive effect. Monitor blood pressure closely.
Cardiac glycosides: May cause excessive bradycardia and additive effects on AV conduction. Use together cautiously.
Epinephrine: May decrease the patient response to epinephrine for treatment of an allergic reaction. Monitor patient closely for decreased clinical effect.
General anesthetics: May increase hypotensive effects. Consider stopping nadolol before surgery.
Insulin: May mask symptoms of hypoglycemia, as a result of beta blockade (such as tachycardia). Use with caution in patients with diabetes.
I.V. lidocaine: May reduce hepatic metabolism of lidocaine, increasing the risk of toxicity. Give bolus doses of lidocaine at a slower rate and monitor lidocaine level closely.
NSAIDs: May decrease antihypertensive effect. Monitor blood pressure and adjust dosage.
Oral antidiabetics: May alter dosage requirements in previously stabilized diabetic patients. Monitor glucose closely.
Phenothiazines: May increase hypotensive effects. Monitor blood pressure.
Prazosin: May increase risk of orthostatic hypotension in the early phases of use together. Assist patient to stand slowly until effects are known.

Reserpine: May increase hypotension or bradycardia. Monitor patient for adverse effects, such as dizziness, syncope, and postural hypotension.
Verapamil: May increase effects of both drugs. Monitor cardiac function closely and decrease dosages as necessary.

EFFECTS ON LAB TEST RESULTS
None reported.

CONTRAINDICATIONS & CAUTIONS
- Contraindicated in patients with bronchial asthma, sinus bradycardia and greater than first-degree heart block, cardiogenic shock, and overt heart failure.
- Use cautiously in patients with heart failure, chronic bronchitis, emphysema, or renal or hepatic impairment and in patients undergoing major surgery involving general anesthesia.
- Use cautiously in diabetic patients because beta blockers may mask certain signs and symptoms of hypoglycemia.

NURSING CONSIDERATIONS
- Monitor blood pressure frequently. If patient develops severe hypotension, give a vasopressor, as prescribed.
- Drug masks signs and symptoms of shock and hyperthyroidism.

PATIENT TEACHING
- Explain importance of taking drug as prescribed, even when patient feels well.
- Teach patient how to check pulse rate and tell him to check it before each dose. If pulse rate is below 60 beats/minute, tell patient to notify prescriber.
- Warn patient not to stop drug suddenly.

SAFETY ALERT!

nesiritide
neh-SIR-ih-tide

Natrecor

Pharmacologic class: human B-type natriuretic peptide
Pregnancy risk category C

AVAILABLE FORMS
Injection: Single-dose vials of 1.5 mg sterile, lyophilized powder

INDICATIONS & DOSAGES
➤ **Acutely decompensated heart failure in patients with dyspnea at rest or with minimal activity**
Adults: 2 mcg/kg by I.V. bolus over 60 seconds, followed by continuous infusion of 0.01 mcg/kg/minute.
Adjust-a-dose: If hypotension develops during administration, reduce dosage or stop drug. Restart drug at dosage reduced by 30% with no bolus doses.

ADMINISTRATION
I.V.
- Reconstitute one 1.5-mg vial with 5 ml of diluent (such as D_5W, normal saline solution, 5% dextrose and 0.2% saline solution injection, or 5% dextrose and half-normal saline solution) from a prefilled 250-ml I.V. bag.
- Gently rock (don't shake) vial until solution becomes clear and colorless.
- Withdraw contents of vial and add back to the 250-ml I.V. bag to yield 6 mcg/ml. Invert the bag several times to ensure complete mixing, and use the solution within 24 hours.
- Use the formulas below to calculate bolus volume (2 mcg/kg) and infusion flow rate (0.01 mcg/kg/minute):

$$\underset{\text{(ml)}}{\text{Bolus volume}} = 0.33 \times \underset{\text{(kg)}}{\text{patient weight}}$$

$$\underset{\text{(ml/hr)}}{\text{Infusion flow rate}} = 0.1 \times \underset{\text{(kg)}}{\text{patient weight}}$$

• Before giving bolus dose, prime the I.V. tubing. Withdraw the bolus and give over 60 seconds through an I.V. port in the tubing.
• Immediately after giving bolus, infuse drug at 0.1 ml/kg/hour to deliver 0.01 mcg/kg/minute.
• Store drug at 68° to 77° F (20° to 25° C).
• **Incompatibilities:** Bumetanide, enalaprilat, ethacrynate sodium, furosemide, heparin, hydralazine, insulin, sodium metabisulfite.

ACTION

Increases cyclic guanosine monophosphate (cGMP) level, relaxes smooth muscle, and dilates veins and arteries. Drug reduces pulmonary capillary wedge pressure and systemic arterial pressure in patients with heart failure.

Route	Onset	Peak	Duration
I.V.	15 min	1 hr	3 hr

Half-life: 18 minutes.

ADVERSE REACTIONS

CNS: anxiety, confusion, dizziness, fever, headache, insomnia, paresthesia, somnolence, tremor.
CV: *hypotension,* ***bradycardia, ventricular tachycardia,*** angina, atrial fibrillation, AV node conduction abnormalities, ventricular extrasystoles.
GI: abdominal pain, nausea, vomiting.
Hematologic: anemia.
Musculoskeletal: back pain, leg cramps.
Respiratory: ***apnea,*** cough.
Skin: injection site reactions, rash, pruritus, sweating.

INTERACTIONS

Drug-drug. *ACE inhibitors:* May increase hypotension symptoms. Monitor blood pressure closely.

EFFECTS ON LAB TEST RESULTS

• May increase creatinine level more than 0.5 mg/dl above baseline. May decrease hemoglobin level and hematocrit.

CONTRAINDICATIONS & CAUTIONS

• Contraindicated in patients hypersensitive to drug or its components.
• Contraindicated in patients with cardiogenic shock, systolic blood pressure below 90 mm Hg, low cardiac filling pressures, conditions in which cardiac output depends on venous return, or conditions that make vasodilators inappropriate, such as valvular stenosis, restrictive or obstructive cardiomyopathy, constrictive pericarditis, and pericardial tamponade.

NURSING CONSIDERATIONS

• Don't start drug at higher-than-recommended dosage because this may cause hypotension and may increase creatinine level.
• ***Alert:*** This drug may cause hypotension. Monitor patient's blood pressure closely, particularly if he also takes an ACE inhibitor.
• ***Alert:*** Drug binds to heparin, including the heparin lining of a coated catheter, decreasing the amount of nesiritide delivered. Don't give nesiritide through a central heparin-coated catheter.
• Drug may affect renal function. In patients with severe heart failure whose renal function depends on the renin-angiotensin-aldosterone system, treatment may lead to azotemia.
• Results of giving this drug for longer than 48 hours are unknown.

PATIENT TEACHING

• Tell patient to report discomfort at I.V. site.
• Urge patient to report to prescriber symptoms of hypotension, such as dizziness, light-headedness, blurred vision, or sweating.
• Tell patient to report to prescriber other adverse effects promptly.

niacin (nicotinic acid, vitamin B_3)

Niacor ◊, Niaspan ◊, Slo-Niacin ◊

niacinamide ◊ (nicotinamide ◊)

Pregnancy risk category A; C if dose exceeds RDA

AVAILABLE FORMS

niacin
Capsules (timed-release): 125 mg ◊, 250 mg ◊, 400 mg ◊, 500 mg
Tablets: 50 mg ◊, 100 mg ◊, 250 mg ◊, 500 mg
Tablets (extended-release): 250 mg ◊, 500 mg ◊, 750 mg ◊, 1,000 mg ◊
niacinamide
Tablets: 50 mg ◊, 100 mg ◊, 125 mg ◊, 250 mg ◊, 500 mg ◊

INDICATIONS & DOSAGES

➤ RDA
Adult men and boys ages 14 to 18: Give 16 mg.
Adult women and girls ages 14 to 18: Give 14 mg.
Children ages 9 to 13: Give 12 mg.
Children ages 4 to 8: Give 8 mg.
Children ages 1 to 3: Give 6 mg.
Infants ages 6 months to 1 year: 4 mg.
Neonates and infants younger than age 6 months: 2 mg.
Pregnant women: 18 mg.
Breast-feeding women: 17 mg.

➤ Pellagra
Adults: 300 to 500 mg P.O. daily in divided doses.
Children: 100 to 300 mg P.O. daily in divided doses.

➤ Hartnup disease
Adults: 50 to 200 mg P.O. daily.

➤ Niacin deficiency
Adults: Up to 100 mg P.O. daily.

➤ Hyperlipidemias, especially with hypercholesterolemia
Adults: 250 mg PO. daily at bedtime. Increase at 4- to 7-day intervals up to 1.5 to 2 g P.O. daily divided b.i.d. to t.i.d. Maximum 6 g daily. Or, 1 to 2 g extended-release tablets P.O. daily at bedtime.

nicardipine hydrochloride

nye-KAR-de-peen

Cardene, Cardene I.V., Cardene SR

Pharmacologic class: calcium channel blocker
Pregnancy risk category C

AVAILABLE FORMS

Capsules: 20 mg, 30 mg
Capsules (sustained-release): 30 mg, 45 mg, 60 mg
Injection: 2.5 mg/ml

INDICATIONS & DOSAGES

➤ Chronic stable angina (used alone or with other antianginals)
Adults: Initially, 20 mg immediate-release capsule P.O. t.i.d. Adjust dosage based on patient response every 3 days. Usual range, 20 to 40 mg t.i.d.

➤ Hypertension
Adults: Initially, 20 mg immediate-release capsule P.O. t.i.d.; range, 20 to 40 mg t.i.d. Or, 30 mg sustained-release capsule b.i.d.; range, 30 to 60 mg b.i.d. Increase dosage based on patient response. Or, for patient who can't take oral form, 5 mg/hour (50 ml/hour) I.V. infusion initially; then, increase by 2.5 mg/hour (25 ml/hour) every 15 minutes to maximum of 15 mg/hour (150 ml/hour).

ADMINISTRATION

P.O.
- Give drug with or without food, but avoid giving with high-fat meal.
- Don't break or crush sustained-release capsules; they must be swallowed whole.

I.V.
- Dilute to a concentration of 0.1 mg/ml with D_5W, dextrose 5% in normal saline solution or half-normal saline solution, and normal saline solution or half-normal saline solution.
- Give by slow infusion.
- Closely monitor blood pressure during and after completion of infusion.
- If hypotension or tachycardia occurs, titrate infusion rate.

• Change peripheral infusion site every 12 hours to minimize risk of venous irritation.
• When switching to oral form, give first dose of t.i.d. regimen 1 hour before stopping infusion. If using a different oral drug, start it when infusion ends.
• If solution is kept at room temperature, use within 24 hours.
• **Incompatibilities:** Ampicillin sodium, ampicillin and sulbactam sodium, cefoperazone, ceftazidime, furosemide, heparin sodium, lactated Ringer's solution, sodium bicarbonate, thiopental.

ACTION
Inhibits calcium ion influx across cardiac and smooth muscle cells but is more selective to vascular smooth muscle than cardiac muscle. Drug also dilates coronary arteries and arterioles.

Route	Onset	Peak	Duration
P.O. (immediate-release)	20 min	1–2 hr	Unknown
P.O. (sustained-release)	20 min	1–4 hr	12 hr
I.V.	Immediate	Immediate	Unknown

Half-life: 2 to 4 hours.

ADVERSE REACTIONS
CNS: *headache,* dizziness, lightheadedness, asthenia.
CV: *peripheral edema, palpitations, flushing,* angina, tachycardia.
GI: nausea, abdominal discomfort, dry mouth.
Skin: rash.

INTERACTIONS
Drug-drug. *Antihypertensives:* May increase antihypertensive effect. Monitor blood pressure closely.
Cimetidine: May decrease metabolism of calcium channel blockers. Monitor patient for increased pharmacologic effect.
Cyclosporine: May increase plasma level of cyclosporine. Monitor patient for toxicity.
Drug-food. *Grapefruit and grapefruit juice:* May increase bioavailability of nicardipine. Discourage use together.
High-fat foods: May decrease absorption of nicardipine. Discourage use together.

EFFECTS ON LAB TEST RESULTS
None reported.

CONTRAINDICATIONS & CAUTIONS
• Contraindicated in patients hypersensitive to drug and in those with advanced aortic stenosis.
• Use cautiously in patients with hypotension, heart failure, or impaired hepatic and renal function.

NURSING CONSIDERATIONS
• Measure blood pressure frequently during initial therapy. Maximal response occurs about 1 hour after giving the immediate-release form and 2 to 4 hours after giving the sustained-release form. Check for orthostatic hypotension. Because large swings in blood pressure may occur based on drug level, assess antihypertensive effect 8 hours after dosing.
• Extended-release form is preferred because of improved compliance, fewer fluctuations in blood pressure, and less risk of death than with shorter-acting drugs.
• ***Look alike–sound alike:*** Don't confuse Cardene with Cardura or codeine.

PATIENT TEACHING
• Tell patient to take oral form exactly as prescribed.
• Advise patient to report chest pain immediately. Some patients may experience increased frequency, severity, or duration of chest pain at beginning of therapy or during dosage adjustments.
• Tell patient to get up from a sitting or lying position slowly to avoid dizziness caused by a decrease in blood pressure.
• Tell patient drug may be taken with or without food but shouldn't be taken with high-fat foods.
• Tell patient to swallow sustained-release capsules whole; don't crush, break, or chew.

nifedipine

nye-FED-i-peen

Adalat CC, Adalat XL†, Apo-Nifed†, Nifedical XL, Nu-Nifed†, Procardia XL

Pharmacologic class: calcium channel blocker
Pregnancy risk category C

AVAILABLE FORMS

Capsules: 10 mg, 20 mg
Tablets (extended-release): 20 mg†, 30 mg, 60 mg, 90 mg

INDICATIONS & DOSAGES

➤ Vasospastic angina (Prinzmetal's or variant angina), classic chronic stable angina pectoris
Adults: Initially, 10 mg short-acting capsule P.O. t.i.d. Usual effective dosage range is 10 to 20 mg t.i.d. Some patients may require up to 30 mg q.i.d. Maximum daily dose is 180 mg. Adjust dosage over 7 to 14 days to evaluate response. Or, 30 to 60 mg (extended-release tablets, except Adalat CC) P.O. once daily. Maximum daily dose is 120 mg. Adjust dosage over 7 to 14 days to evaluate response.

➤ Hypertension
Adults: 30 or 60 mg P.O. extended-release tablet once daily. Adjusted over 7 to 14 days. Doses larger than 90 mg (Adalat CC) and 120 mg (Procardia XL) aren't recommended.

ADMINISTRATION

P.O.

- Don't give immediate-release capsules within 1 week of acute MI or in acute coronary syndrome.
- ***Alert:*** Don't use capsules S.L. to rapidly reduce severe high blood pressure because the result may be fatal.
- Give extended-release tablets whole; don't break or crush tablet.
- Don't give drug with grapefruit juice.
- Protect capsules from direct light and moisture and store at room temperature.

ACTION

Thought to inhibit calcium ion influx across cardiac and smooth muscle cells, decreasing contractility and oxygen demand. Drug may also dilate coronary arteries and arterioles.

Route	Onset	Peak	Duration
P.O.	20 min	30–60 min	4–8 hr
P.O. (extended)	20 min	6 hr	24 hr

Half-life: 2 to 5 hours.

ADVERSE REACTIONS

CNS: *dizziness, light-headedness, headache, weakness,* somnolence, syncope, nervousness.
CV: *flushing, peripheral edema,* ***heart failure, MI,*** hypotension, palpitations.
EENT: nasal congestion.
GI: *nausea,* diarrhea, constipation, abdominal discomfort.
Musculoskeletal: muscle cramps.
Respiratory: dyspnea, ***pulmonary edema,*** cough.
Skin: rash, pruritus.

INTERACTIONS

Drug-drug. *Antiretrovirals, cimetidine, verapamil:* May decrease nifedipine metabolism. Monitor blood pressure closely and adjust nifedipine dosage as needed.
Azole antifungals, dalfopristin, erythromycin, and quinupristin: May increase the effects of nifedipine. Monitor blood pressure closely and decrease nifedipine dosage as needed.
Digoxin: May cause elevated digoxin level. Monitor digoxin level.
Diltiazem: May increase the effects of nifedipine. Monitor patient closely.
Fentanyl: May cause severe hypotension. Monitor blood pressure.
Phenytoin: May reduce phenytoin metabolism. Monitor phenytoin level.
Propranolol, other beta blockers: May cause hypotension and heart failure. Use together cautiously.
Quinidine: May decrease levels and effects of quinidine while increasing effects of nifedipine. Monitor heart rate and adjust nifedipine dose as needed.

Rifamycins: May decrease nifedipine levels. Monitor patient.
Tacrolimus: May increase tacrolimus levels and risk for toxicity. Decrease tacrolimus dose as needed.
Drug-herb. *Ginkgo:* May increase effects of drug. Discourage use together.
Ginseng: May increase drug levels with possible toxicity. Discourage use together.
Melatonin, St. John's wort: May interfere with antihypertensive effect. Discourage use together.
Drug-food. *Grapefruit juice:* May increase bioavailability of drug. Discourage use together.

EFFECTS ON LAB TEST RESULTS

- May increase ALT, AST, alkaline phosphatase, and LDH levels.

CONTRAINDICATIONS & CAUTIONS

- Contraindicated in patients hypersensitive to drug.
- Use cautiously in patients with heart failure or hypotension and in elderly patients. Use extended-release tablets cautiously in patients with severe GI narrowing.

NURSING CONSIDERATIONS

- Monitor blood pressure regularly, especially in patients who take beta blockers or antihypertensives.
- Watch for symptoms of heart failure.
- ***Look alike–sound alike:*** Don't confuse nifedipine with nimodipine or nicardipine.

PATIENT TEACHING

- If patient is kept on nitrate therapy while nifedipine dosage is being adjusted, urge continued compliance. Patient may take S.L. nitroglycerin, as needed, for acute chest pain.
- Tell patient that chest pain may worsen briefly as therapy starts or dosage increases.
- Instruct patient to swallow extended-release tablets without breaking, crushing, or chewing them.
- Advise patient to avoid taking drug with grapefruit juice.
- Reassure patient taking the extended-release tablet that the wax mold may be passed in the stools. Assure him that drug has already been completely absorbed.
- Tell patient to protect capsules from direct light and moisture and to store at room temperature.

nimodipine

nye-MOE-dih-peen

Nimotop

Pharmacologic class: calcium channel blocker
Pregnancy risk category C

AVAILABLE FORMS

Capsules: 30 mg

INDICATIONS & DOSAGES

➤ **To improve neurologic deficits after subarachnoid hemorrhage from ruptured intracranial berry aneurysm**

Adults: 60 mg P.O. every 4 hours for 21 days. Begin therapy within 96 hours after subarachnoid hemorrhage.
Adjust-a-dose: For patients with hepatic failure, 30 mg P.O. every 4 hours for 21 days.

ADMINISTRATION

P.O.

- If drug needs to be given via nasogastric (NG) tube, make a hole in each end of capsule with an 18G needle and extract contents into syringe. Empty syringe into patient's NG tube. Flush tube with 30 ml of normal saline solution according to manufacturer's directions.
- ***Alert:*** If using a needle to extract contents of capsule, make sure that drug isn't then given I.V. instead of P.O. Label the syringe "for oral use only" before withdrawing the contents of the capsule.

ACTION

Inhibits calcium ion influx across cardiac and smooth-muscle cells, decreasing myocardial contractility and oxygen demand; also dilates coronary and cerebral arteries and arterioles.

Route	Onset	Peak	Duration
P.O.	Unknown	1 hr	Unknown

Half-life: 8 to 9 hours; may be 1 to 2 hours.

ADVERSE REACTIONS

CNS: headache, psychic disturbances.
CV: hypotension, flushing, edema, tachycardia.
GI: nausea, diarrhea, abdominal discomfort.
Musculoskeletal: muscle cramps.
Respiratory: dyspnea, wheezing.
Skin: dermatitis, rash.

INTERACTIONS

Drug-drug. *Antihypertensives:* May increase hypotensive effect. Monitor blood pressure.
Calcium channel blockers: May increase CV effects. Monitor patient closely.
Cimetidine: May increase nimodipine bioavailability. Monitor patient for adverse effects.
Drug-food. *Any food:* May decrease drug absorption. Advise patient to take drug on empty stomach.

EFFECTS ON LAB TEST RESULTS

None reported.

CONTRAINDICATIONS & CAUTIONS

- No known contraindications.
- Use cautiously in patients with hepatic failure.

NURSING CONSIDERATIONS

- Monitor blood pressure and heart rate in all patients, especially at start of therapy.

PATIENT TEACHING

- Explain use of drug and review administration schedule with patient and family. Stress importance of compliance for maximum drug effectiveness.
- Instruct patient to report persistent or severe adverse reactions promptly.
- Tell patient not to drink grapefruit juice while taking this drug.

nisoldipine

nye-SOHL-di-peen

Sular

Pharmacologic class: calcium channel blocker
Pregnancy risk category C

AVAILABLE FORMS

Tablets (extended-release): 10 mg, 20 mg, 30 mg, 40 mg

INDICATIONS & DOSAGES

➤ Hypertension

Adults: Initially, 20 mg P.O. once daily; increased by 10 mg/week or at longer intervals, as needed. Usual maintenance dose is 20 to 40 mg daily. Doses of more than 60 mg daily aren't recommended.
Patients older than age 65: Initially, 10 mg P.O. once daily; adjust dosage as for other adults.
Adjust-a-dose: For patients with impaired liver function, initially, 10 mg P.O. once daily; dosage is adjusted as for adults.

ADMINISTRATION

P.O.

- Give drug whole; don't crush or split tablet.
- Don't give with high-fat meal or grapefruit products.

ACTION

Prevents calcium ions from entering vascular smooth muscle cells, causing dilation of arterioles, which decreases peripheral vascular resistance.

Route	Onset	Peak	Duration
P.O.	Unknown	6–12 hr	24 hr

Half-life: 7 to 12 hours.

ADVERSE REACTIONS

CNS: *headache,* dizziness.
CV: *peripheral edema,* vasodilation, palpitations, chest pain.
EENT: sinusitis, pharyngitis.
GI: nausea.
Skin: rash.

INTERACTIONS

Drug-drug. *Cimetidine:* May increase bioavailability and peak nisoldipine level. Monitor blood pressure closely.
CYP3A4 inducers such as phenytoin: May decrease nisoldipine level. Avoid using together; consider alternative antihypertensive therapy.
Quinidine: May decrease bioavailability of nisoldipine. Adjust dosage accordingly.
Drug-herb. *Ma huang:* May decrease antihypertensive effects. Discourage use together.
Peppermint oil: May decrease drug effect. Discourage use together.
Drug-food. *Grapefruit products:* May increase drug level, increasing adverse reactions. Discourage use together.
High-fat foods: May increase peak drug level. Discourage use together.

EFFECTS ON LAB TEST RESULTS

None reported.

CONTRAINDICATIONS & CAUTIONS

- Contraindicated in patients hypersensitive to dihydropyridine calcium channel blockers.
- Contraindicated in breast-feeding women.
- Use cautiously in patients with heart failure or compromised ventricular function, particularly those receiving beta blockers and those with severe hepatic dysfunction.

NURSING CONSIDERATIONS

- Monitor frequency, duration, or severity of angina after starting calcium channel blocker therapy or at time of dosage increase. Report worsening of symptoms to prescriber immediately.
- Monitor blood pressure regularly, especially when starting therapy and during dosage adjustment.

PATIENT TEACHING

- Tell patient to take drug as prescribed, even if he feels better.
- Advise patient to swallow tablet whole and not to chew, divide, or crush it.
- Remind patient not to take drug with a high-fat meal or with grapefruit products. Both may increase drug level in the body beyond intended amount.

SAFETY ALERT!

nitroglycerin (glyceryl trinitrate)

nye-troe-GLIH-ser-in

Deponit, Minitran, Nitrek, Nitro-Bid, Nitro-Dur, Nitrogard, Nitrolingual, NitroQuick, Nitrostat, NitroTab, Nitro-Time, NTS, Trinipatch†

Pharmacologic class: nitrate
Pregnancy risk category C

AVAILABLE FORMS

Aerosol (translingual): 0.4 mg/metered spray
Capsules (sustained-release): 2.5 mg, 6.5 mg, 9 mg
Injection: 5 mg/ml; 100 mcg/ml, 200 mcg/ml, 400 mcg/ml
Tablets (S.L.): 0.3 mg (1/200 grain), 0.4 mg (1/150 grain), 0.6 mg (1/100 grain)
Tablets (sustained-release): 2.6 mg, 6.5 mg, 9 mg, 13 mg
Topical: 2% ointment
Transdermal: 0.1 mg/hour, 0.2 mg/hour, 0.3 mg/hour, 0.4 mg/hour, 0.6 mg/hour, 0.8 mg/hour release rate

INDICATIONS & DOSAGES

➤ To prevent chronic anginal attacks

Adults: 2.5 or 2.6 mg sustained-release capsule or tablet every 8 to 12 hours. Increase to an effective dose in 2.5- or 2.6-mg increments b.i.d. to q.i.d. Or, use 2% ointment: Start dosage with ½-inch ointment, increasing by ½-inch increments until desired results are achieved. Range of dosage with ointment is ½ to 5 inches. Usual dose is 1 to 2 inches every 6 to 8 hours. Or, transdermal patch 0.2 to 0.4 mg/hour once daily.

➤ Acute angina pectoris; to prevent or minimize anginal attacks before stressful events

Adults: 1 S.L. tablet (1/200 grain, 1/150 grain, 1/100 grain) dissolved under the tongue or in the buccal pouch as soon as angina begins. Repeat every 5 minutes, if needed, for 15 minutes. Or, one or two sprays Nitrolingual into mouth, preferably onto or under the tongue. Repeat every 3 to 5 minutes, if needed, to a maximum of three doses within a 15-minute period. Or, 1 to 3 mg transmucosally every 3 to 5 hours while awake.

➤ **Hypertension from surgery, heart failure after MI, angina pectoris in acute situations, to produce controlled hypotension during surgery (by I.V. infusion)**
Adults: Initially, infuse at 5 mcg/minute, increasing as needed by 5 mcg/minute every 3 to 5 minutes until response occurs. If a 20-mcg/minute rate doesn't produce a response, increase dosage by as much as 20 mcg/minute every 3 to 5 minutes. Up to 100 mcg/minute may be needed.

ADMINISTRATION

P.O.

- Give 30 minutes before or 1 to 2 hours after meals.
- Drug must be swallowed whole and not chewed.

I.V.

- Dilute with D_5W or normal saline solution for injection. Concentration shouldn't exceed 400 mcg/ml.
- Always give with an infusion control device and titrate to desired response.
- Regular polyvinyl chloride tubing can bind up to 80% of drug, making it necessary to infuse higher dosages. A special nonabsorbent polyvinyl chloride tubing is available from the manufacturer. Always mix in glass bottles and avoid using a filter.
- Use the same type of infusion set when changing lines.
- When changing the concentration of infusion, flush the administration set with 15 to 20 ml of the new concentration before use. This will clear the line of the old drug solution.
- **Incompatibilities:** Alteplase, bretylium, hydralazine, levofloxacin, phenytoin sodium.

Topical

- To apply ointment, measure the prescribed amount on the application paper; then place the paper on any nonhairy area. Don't rub in. Cover with plastic film to aid absorption and to protect clothing. Remove all excess ointment from previous site before applying the next dose. Avoid getting ointment on fingers.

Transdermal

- Patch can be applied to any nonhairy part of the skin except distal parts of the arms or legs. (Absorption won't be maximal at distal sites.) Patch may cause contact dermatitis.
- Remove patch before defibrillation. Because of the aluminum backing on the patch, the electric current may cause arcing that can damage the paddles and burn the patient.
- When stopping transdermal treatment of angina, gradually reduce the dosage and frequency of application over 4 to 6 weeks.

Sublingual

- Give tablet at first sign of attack. Patient should wet the tablet with saliva, place it under tongue until absorbed. Dose may be repeated every 5 minutes for a maximum of three doses. If drug doesn't provide relief, contact prescriber.

Buccal

- The tablet should be placed between the lip and gum above the incisors or between the cheek and gum. Tablets shouldn't be swallowed or chewed.

Translingual

- Patient using translingual aerosol form shouldn't inhale the spray but should release it onto or under the tongue. He should wait about 10 seconds or so before swallowing.

ACTION

A nitrate that reduces cardiac oxygen demand by decreasing left ventricular end-diastolic pressure (preload) and, to a lesser extent, systemic vascular resistance (afterload). Also increases blood flow through the collateral coronary vessels.

Route	Onset	Peak	Duration
P.O.	20–45 min	Unknown	3–8 hr
I.V.	Immediate	Immediate	3–5 min
Topical	30 min	Unknown	2–12 hr
Transdermal	30 min	Unknown	24 hr
S.L.	1–3 min	Unknown	30–60 min
Buccal	3 min	Unknown	3–5 hr
Translingual	2–4 min	Unknown	30–60 min

Half-life: About 1 to 4 minutes.

ADVERSE REACTIONS

CNS: *headache, dizziness,* syncope, weakness.
CV: *orthostatic hypotension, tachycardia, flushing, palpitations.*
EENT: S.L. burning.
GI: nausea, vomiting.
Skin: cutaneous vasodilation, contact dermatitis, rash.
Other: hypersensitivity reactions.

INTERACTIONS

Drug-drug. *Alteplase:* May decrease tissue plasminogen activator-antigen level. Avoid using together; if unavoidable, use lowest effective dose of nitroglycerin.
Antihypertensives: May increase hypotensive effect. Monitor blood pressure closely.
Heparin: I.V. nitroglycerin may interfere with anticoagulant effect of heparin. Monitor PTT.
Sildenafil, tadalafil, vardenafil: May cause severe hypotension. Use of nitrates in any form with these drugs is contraindicated.
Drug-lifestyle. *Alcohol use:* May increase hypotension. Discourage use together.

EFFECTS ON LAB TEST RESULTS

- May falsely decrease values in cholesterol determination tests using the Zlatkis-Zak color reaction.

CONTRAINDICATIONS & CAUTIONS

- Contraindicated in patients with early MI (oral and sublingual), severe anemia, increased intracranial pressure, angle-closure glaucoma, orthostatic hypotension, allergy to adhesives (transdermal), or hypersensitivity to nitrates.
- I.V. nitroglycerin is contraindicated in patients hypersensitive to I.V. form, with cardiac tamponade, restrictive cardiomyopathy, or constrictive pericarditis.
- Use cautiously in patients with hypotension or volume depletion.

NURSING CONSIDERATIONS

- Closely monitor vital signs during infusion, particularly blood pressure, especially in a patient with an MI. Excessive hypotension may worsen the MI.
- Monitor blood pressure and intensity and duration of drug response.
- Drug may cause headaches, especially at beginning of therapy. Dosage may be reduced temporarily, but tolerance usually develops. Treat headache with aspirin or acetaminophen.
- Tolerance to drug can be minimized with a 10- to 12-hour nitrate-free interval. To achieve this, remove the transdermal system in the early evening and apply a new system the next morning or omit the last daily dose of a buccal, sustained-release, or ointment form. Check with the prescriber for alterations in dosage regimen if tolerance is suspected.
- ***Look alike–sound alike:*** Don't confuse Nitro-Bid with Nicobid or nitroglycerin with nitroprusside.

PATIENT TEACHING

- Caution patient to take nitroglycerin regularly, as prescribed, and to have it accessible at all times.
- ***Alert:*** Advise patient that stopping drug abruptly causes spasm of the coronary arteries.
- Teach patient how to give the prescribed form of nitroglycerin.
- Tell patient to take S.L. tablet at first sign of attack. Patient should wet the tablet with saliva, place it under tongue until absorbed, and then sit down and rest. Dose may be repeated every 5 minutes for a maximum of three doses. If drug doesn't provide relief, he should obtain medical help promptly.
- Advise patient who complains of a tingling sensation with S.L. drug to try holding tablet in cheek.
- Tell patient to take oral tablets on an empty stomach either 30 minutes before or 1 to 2 hours after meals, to swallow oral tablets whole, and not to chew tablets.
- Remind patient using translingual aerosol form that he shouldn't inhale the spray but should release it onto or under the tongue. Tell him to wait about 10 seconds or so before swallowing.
- Tell patient to place the buccal tablet between the lip and gum above the incisors or between the cheek and gum. Tablets shouldn't be swallowed or chewed.
- Tell patient to take an additional dose before anticipated stress or at bedtime if chest pain occurs at night.

• Urge patient using skin patches to dispose of them carefully because enough medication remains after normal use to be hazardous to children and pets.
• Advise patient to avoid alcohol.
• To minimize dizziness when standing up, tell patient to rise slowly. Advise him to go up and down stairs carefully and to lie down at the first sign of dizziness.
• ***Alert:*** Advise patient that use of sildenafil, tadalafil, or vardenafil with any nitrate may cause life-threatening low blood pressure. Use together is contraindicated.
• Tell patient to store drug in cool, dark place in a tightly closed container. Tell him to remove cotton from container because it absorbs drug.
• Tell patient to store S.L. tablets in original container or other container specifically approved for this use and to carry the container in a jacket pocket or purse, not in a pocket close to the body.

SAFETY ALERT!

nitroprusside sodium
nye-troe-PRUSS-ide

Nipride†, Nitropress

Pharmacologic class: vasodilator
Pregnancy risk category C

AVAILABLE FORMS
Injection: 50 mg/vial in 2-ml and 5-ml vials

INDICATIONS & DOSAGES
➤ **To lower blood pressure quickly in hypertensive emergencies, to produce controlled hypotension during anesthesia, to reduce preload and afterload in cardiac pump failure or cardiogenic shock (may be used with or without dopamine)**
Adults and children: Begin infusion at 0.25 to 0.3 mcg/kg/minute I.V. and gradually titrate every few minutes to a maximum infusion rate of 10 mcg/kg/minute.
Adjust-a-dose: Patients also taking other antihypertensives are extremely sensitive to nitroprusside. Titrate dosage accordingly. Use with caution in patients with severe renal impairment or hepatic insufficiency; use minimum effective dose.

ADMINISTRATION
I.V.
• Prepare solution by dissolving 50 mg in 2 to 3 ml of D_5W injection or according to manufacturer's instructions. Further dilute concentration in 250, 500, or 1,000 ml of D_5W to provide solutions with 200, 100, or 50 mcg/ml, respectively. Reconstitute ADD-Vantage vials labeled as containing 50 mg of drug according to manufacturer's directions.
• Because drug is sensitive to light, wrap solution in foil or other opaque material; it's not necessary to wrap the tubing. Fresh solution has a faint brownish tint. Discard if highly discolored after 24 hours.
• Use an infusion pump. Drug is best given via piggyback through a peripheral line with no other drug. Don't titrate rate of main I.V. line while drug is being infused. Even a small bolus can cause severe hypotension.
• Check blood pressure every 5 minutes during titration at start of infusion and every 15 minutes thereafter.
• If severe hypotension occurs, stop infusion; effects of drug quickly reverse. Notify prescriber.
• If possible, start an arterial pressure line. Regulate drug flow to desired blood pressure response.
• **Incompatibilities:** Amiodarone, atracurium besylate, bacteriostatic water for injection, levofloxacin. Don't mix with other I.V. drugs or preservatives.

ACTION
Relaxes arteriolar and venous smooth muscle.

Route	Onset	Peak	Duration
I.V.	Immediate	1–2 min	10 min

Half-life: 2 minutes.

ADVERSE REACTIONS
CNS: *headache, dizziness,* ***increased intracranial pressure,*** loss of consciousness, apprehension, restlessness.
CV: ***bradycardia,*** hypotension, tachycardia, palpitations, ECG changes, flushing.

GI: *nausea, abdominal pain,* ileus.
Hematologic: ***methemoglobinemia.***
Metabolic: acidosis, hypothyroidism.
Musculoskeletal: *muscle twitching.*
Skin: *diaphoresis,* pink color, rash.
Other: ***thiocyanate toxicity, cyanide toxicity,*** venous streaking, irritation at infusion site.

INTERACTIONS

Drug-drug. *Antihypertensives:* May cause sensitivity to nitroprusside. Adjust dosage. *Ganglionic-blocking drugs, general anesthetics, negative inotropic drugs, other antihypertensives:* May cause additive effects. Monitor blood pressure closely. *Sildenafil, vardenafil:* May increase hypotensive effects. Avoid use together.

EFFECTS ON LAB TEST RESULTS

- May increase creatinine level.
- May decrease RBC and WBC counts.

CONTRAINDICATIONS & CAUTIONS

- Contraindicated in patients hypersensitive to drug.
- Contraindicated in those with compensatory hypertension (such as in arteriovenous shunt or coarctation of the aorta), inadequate cerebral circulation, acute heart failure with reduced peripheral vascular resistance, congenital optic atrophy, or tobacco-induced amblyopia.
- Use with extreme caution in patients with increased intracranial pressure.
- Use cautiously in patients with hypothyroidism, hepatic or renal disease, hyponatremia, or low vitamin B level.

NURSING CONSIDERATIONS

- Obtain baseline vital signs before giving drug; find out parameters prescriber wants to achieve.
- Keep patient in supine position when starting therapy or titrating drug.
- ***Alert:*** Giving excessive doses of 500 mcg/kg delivered faster than 2 mcg/kg/minute or using maximum infusion rate of 10 mcg/kg/minute for more than 10 minutes can cause cyanide toxicity. If patient is at risk, check thiocyanate level every 72 hours. Level higher than 100 mcg/ml may be toxic. If profound hypotension, metabolic acidosis, dyspnea, headache, loss of consciousness, ataxia, or vomiting occurs, stop drug immediately and notify prescriber.
- ***Look alike–sound alike:*** Don't confuse nitroprusside with nitroglycerin.

PATIENT TEACHING

- Instruct patient to report adverse reactions promptly.
- Tell patient to alert nurse if discomfort occurs at I.V. insertion site.

SAFETY ALERT!

norepinephrine bitartrate (levarterenol bitartrate, noradrenaline acid tartrate)

nor-ep-i-NEF-rin

Levophed

Pharmacologic class: direct-acting adrenergic
Pregnancy risk category C

AVAILABLE FORMS

Injection: 1 mg/ml

INDICATIONS & DOSAGES

➤ **To restore blood pressure in acute hypotension; severe hypotension during cardiac arrest**

Adults: Initially, 8 to 12 mcg/minute by I.V. infusion; then titrate to maintain systolic blood pressure at 80 to 100 mm Hg in previously normotensive patients and 30 to 40 mm Hg below preexisting systolic blood pressure in previously hypertensive patients. Average maintenance dose is 2 to 4 mcg/minute.

ADMINISTRATION

I.V.

- Use a central venous catheter or large vein, such as the antecubital fossa, to minimize risk of extravasation. Give in D_5W alone or D_5W in normal saline solution for injection. Use continuous infusion pump to regulate infusion flow rate and a piggyback setup so I.V. line stays open if norepinephrine is stopped.
- Never leave patient unattended during infusion. Check blood pressure every

2 minutes until stabilized; then check every 5 minutes.
• During infusion, frequently monitor ECG, cardiac output, central venous pressure, pulmonary artery wedge pressure, pulse rate, urine output, and color and temperature of limbs. Titrate infusion rate based on findings and prescriber guidelines.
• Check site frequently for signs and symptoms of extravasation. If they appear, stop infusion immediately and call prescriber. Infiltrate area with 5 to 10 mg phentolamine in 10 to 15 ml of normal saline solution to counteract effect of extravasation. Also, check for blanching along course of infused vein, which may progress to superficial sloughing.
• Protect drug from light. Discard discolored solution or solution that contains precipitate. Solution will deteriorate after 24 hours.
• If prolonged therapy is needed, change injection site frequently.
• Avoid mixing with alkaline solutions, oxidizing drugs, or iron salts. The use of normal saline solution alone isn't recommended because of the lack of oxidation protection.
• **Incompatibilities:** Alkaline-buffered antibiotics, aminophylline, amobarbital, chlorothiazide, chlorpheniramine, insulin, lidocaine, pentobarbital sodium, phenobarbital sodium, phenytoin sodium, ranitidine hydrochloride, sodium bicarbonate, streptomycin, thiopental, whole blood.

ACTION

Stimulates alpha and beta$_1$ receptors in the sympathetic nervous system, causing vasoconstriction and cardiac stimulation.

Route	Onset	Peak	Duration
I.V.	Immediate	Immediate	1–2 min after infusion

Half-life: About 1 minute.

ADVERSE REACTIONS

CNS: *headache,* anxiety, weakness, dizziness, tremor, restlessness, insomnia.
CV: ***bradycardia, severe hypertension, arrhythmias.***
Respiratory: ***asthma attacks,*** respiratory difficulties.
Skin: irritation with extravasation, necrosis and gangrene secondary to extravasation.
Other: ***anaphylaxis.***

INTERACTIONS

Drug-drug. *Alpha blockers:* May antagonize drug effects. Avoid using together.
Antihistamines, atropine, ergot alkaloids, guanethidine, MAO inhibitors, methyldopa, oxytocics: When given with sympathomimetics, may cause severe hypertension (hypertensive crisis). Avoid using together.
Inhaled anesthetics: May increase risk of arrhythmias. Monitor ECG.
Tricyclic antidepressants: May potentiate the pressor response and cause arrhythmias. Use together cautiously.

EFFECTS ON LAB TEST RESULTS

None reported.

CONTRAINDICATIONS & CAUTIONS

• Contraindicated in patients with mesenteric or peripheral vascular thrombosis, profound hypoxia, hypercarbia, or hypotension resulting from blood volume deficit.
• Contraindicated during cyclopropane and halothane anesthesia.
• Use cautiously in patients taking MAO inhibitors or tricyclic or imipramine-type antidepressants.
• Use cautiously in patients with sulfite sensitivity.

NURSING CONSIDERATIONS

• Drug isn't a substitute for blood or fluid replacement therapy. If patient has volume deficit, replace fluids before giving vasopressors.
• Keep emergency drugs on hand to reverse effects of drug: atropine for reflex bradycardia, phentolamine to decrease vasopressor effects, and propranolol for arrhythmias.
• Notify prescriber immediately of decreased urine output.

• When stopping drug, gradually slow infusion rate. Continue monitoring vital signs, watching for possible severe drop in blood pressure.
• ***Look alike–sound alike:*** Don't confuse norepinephrine with epinephrine.

PATIENT TEACHING
• Tell patient to report adverse reactions promptly.
• Advise patient to report discomfort at I.V. insertion site.

olmesartan medoxomil
ol-ma-SAR-tan

Benicar

Pharmacologic class: angiotensin II receptor antagonist
Pregnancy risk category C; D in 2nd and 3rd trimesters

AVAILABLE FORMS
Tablets: 5 mg, 20 mg, 40 mg

INDICATIONS & DOSAGES
➤ **Hypertension**
Adults: 20 mg P.O. once daily if patient has no volume depletion. May increase dosage to 40 mg P.O. once daily if blood pressure isn't reduced after 2 weeks of therapy.
Adjust-a-dose: In patients with possible depletion of intravascular volume (those with impaired renal function who are taking diuretics), consider using lower starting dose.

ADMINISTRATION
P.O.
• Give drug without regard for food.

ACTION
Blocks vasoconstrictor and aldosterone-secreting effects of angiotensin II by selectively blocking the binding of angiotensin II to the angiotensin I, or AT_1, receptor in the vascular smooth muscle.

Route	Onset	Peak	Duration
P.O.	Rapid	1–2 hr	24 hr

Half-life: 13 hours.

ADVERSE REACTIONS
CNS: headache.
EENT: pharyngitis, rhinitis, sinusitis.
GI: diarrhea.
GU: hematuria.
Metabolic: hyperglycemia, hypertriglyceridemia.
Musculoskeletal: back pain.
Respiratory: bronchitis, upper respiratory tract infection.
Other: flulike symptoms, accidental injury.

INTERACTIONS
Drug-herb. *Ma huang:* May decrease antihypertensive effects. Discourage use together.

EFFECTS ON LAB TEST RESULTS
• May increase glucose, triglyceride, uric acid, liver enzyme, bilirubin, and CK levels. May decrease hemoglobin level and hematocrit.

CONTRAINDICATIONS & CAUTIONS
• Contraindicated in patients hypersensitive to the drug or any of its components and in patients who are pregnant.
• Use cautiously in patients who are volume- or sodium-depleted, those whose renal function depends on the renin-angiotensin-aldosterone system (such as patients with severe heart failure), and those with unilateral and bilateral renal artery stenosis.
• It's unknown if drug appears in breast milk. Patient should stop either breast-feeding or using drug.
• Safety and efficacy in children haven't been established.

NURSING CONSIDERATIONS
• Symptomatic hypotension may occur in patients who are volume- or sodium-depleted, especially those being treated with high doses of a diuretic. If hypotension occurs, place patient supine and treat supportively. Treatment may continue once blood pressure is stabilized.
• If blood pressure isn't adequately controlled, a diuretic or other antihypertensive drugs also may be prescribed.
• Overdose may cause hypotension and tachycardia, along with bradycardia from

parasympathetic (vagal) stimulation. Treatment should be supportive.
- Closely monitor patients with heart failure for oliguria, azotemia, and acute renal failure.
- Monitor BUN and creatinine level in patients with unilateral or bilateral renal artery stenosis.
- Drugs that act on the renin-angiotensin system may cause fetal and neonatal complications and death when given to pregnant women after the first trimester. If patient taking drug becomes pregnant, stop drug immediately.

PATIENT TEACHING

- Tell patient to take drug exactly as prescribed and not to stop taking it, even if he feels better.
- Tell patient to take drug without regard to meals.
- Tell patient to report to health care provider any adverse reactions promptly, especially light-headedness and fainting.
- Advise woman of childbearing age to immediately report pregnancy to health care provider.
- Inform diabetic patients that glucose readings may rise and that the dosage of their diabetes drugs may need adjustment.
- Warn patients that inadequate fluid intake, excessive perspiration, diarrhea, or vomiting may lead to an excessive drop in blood pressure, light-headedness, and possibly fainting.
- Instruct patients that other antihypertensives can have additive effects. Patient should inform his prescriber of all medications he's taking, including OTC drugs.

omega-3–acid ethyl esters

oh-may-gah-three-ASS-id

Omacor

Pharmacologic class: ethyl ester
Pregnancy risk category C

AVAILABLE FORMS

Capsules: 1 g

INDICATIONS & DOSAGES

➤ **Adjunct to diet to reduce triglyceride levels 500 mg/dl or higher**
Adults: 4 g P.O. once daily or divided as 2 g b.i.d.

ADMINISTRATION

P.O.
- Give drug without regard for meals.

ACTION

May reduce hepatic formation of triglycerides because two components of drug are poor substrates for the necessary enzymes. These components also block formation of other fatty acids.

Route	Onset	Peak	Duration
P.O.	Unknown	Unknown	Unknown

Half-life: Unknown.

ADVERSE REACTIONS

CNS: pain.
CV: angina pectoris.
GI: altered taste, belching, dyspepsia.
Musculoskeletal: back pain.
Skin: rash.
Other: flulike syndrome, infection.

INTERACTIONS

Drug-drug. *Anticoagulants:* May prolong bleeding time. Monitor patient.

EFFECTS ON LAB TEST RESULTS

- May increase ALT and LDL cholesterol levels.

CONTRAINDICATIONS & CAUTIONS

- Contraindicated in patients hypersensitive to drug or its components.
- Use cautiously in patients sensitive to fish.

NURSING CONSIDERATIONS

- Assess patient for conditions that contribute to increased triglycerides, such as diabetes and hypothyroidism, before treatment.
- Evaluate patient's current drug regimen for any drugs known to sharply increase triglyceride levels, including estrogen therapy, thiazide diuretics, and beta blockers.

Stopping these drugs, if appropriate, may negate the need for drug.
- Continue diet and lifestyle modifications during treatment.
- Obtain baseline triglyceride levels to confirm that they're consistently abnormal before therapy; then recheck periodically during treatment. If patient has an inadequate response after 2 months, stop drug.
- Monitor LDL level to make sure it doesn't increase excessively during treatment.
- ***Look alike–sound alike:*** Don't confuse Omacor with Amicar.

PATIENT TEACHING
- Explain that taking drug doesn't reduce the importance of following the recommended diet and exercise plan.
- Remind patient of the need for follow-up blood work to evaluate progress.
- Advise patient to notify prescriber about bothersome side effects.
- Tell patient to report planned or suspected pregnancy.

orlistat
ORE-lah-stat

Alli ◊, Xenical

Pharmacologic class: lipase inhibitor
Pregnancy risk category B

AVAILABLE FORMS
Capsules: 60 mg ◊, 120 mg

INDICATIONS & DOSAGES
➤ **To manage obesity, including weight loss and weight maintenance with a reduced-calorie diet; to reduce risk of weight gain after previous weight loss**
Adults and children ages 12 to 16: Give 120 mg P.O. t.i.d. with or up to 1 hour after each main meal containing fat.
➤ **Weight loss (OTC)**
Adults age 18 and older: One 60-mg capsule with each meal containing fat. Dosage shouldn't exceed 3 capsules a day.

ADMINISTRATION
P.O.
- Give drug with each main meal containing fat (during or up to 1 hour after the meal).

ACTION
Forms a bond with active site of gastric and pancreatic lipases, inactivating them. As a result, enzymes can't hydrolyze dietary triglycerides into absorbable free fatty acids and monoglycerides. The undigested triglycerides are not absorbed, resulting in caloric deficit.

Route	Onset	Peak	Duration
P.O.	Unknown	Unknown	Unknown

Half-life: 1 to 2 hours.

ADVERSE REACTIONS
CNS: *headache,* dizziness, fatigue, sleep disorder, anxiety, depression.
CV: pedal edema.
EENT: otitis.
GI: *flatus with discharge, fecal urgency, fatty or oily stool, oily spotting, increased defecation, abdominal pain,* fecal incontinence, nausea, infectious diarrhea, rectal pain, vomiting.
GU: menstrual irregularity, vaginitis, UTI.
Musculoskeletal: *back pain, leg pain,* arthritis, myalgia, joint disorder, tendinitis.
Respiratory: *influenza, upper respiratory tract infection,* lower respiratory tract infection.
Skin: rash, dry skin.
Other: tooth and gingival disorders.

INTERACTIONS
Drug-drug. *Cyclosporine:* May decrease cyclosporine levels, risking organ rejection in transplant patients. Avoid using together.
Fat-soluble vitamins (such as vitamins A and E and beta-carotene): May decrease absorption of vitamins. Separate doses by 2 hours.
Pravastatin: May slightly increase pravastatin levels and lipid-lowering effects of drug. Monitor patient.
Warfarin: May change coagulation values. Monitor INR.

EFFECTS ON LAB TEST RESULTS
None reported.

CONTRAINDICATIONS & CAUTIONS
- Contraindicated in patients hypersensitive to drug or its components and in those with chronic malabsorption syndrome or cholestasis.
- Use cautiously in patients with history of hyperoxaluria or calcium oxalate nephrolithiasis or those at risk for anorexia nervosa or bulimia.
- Use cautiously in patients receiving cyclosporine therapy because of potential changes in cyclosporine absorption related to variations in dietary intake.

NURSING CONSIDERATIONS
- Exclude organic causes of obesity, such as hypothyroidism, before starting drug therapy.
- Drug is recommended for use in patients with an initial body mass index (BMI) of 30 or more or those with a BMI of 27 or more and other risk factors (such as hypertension, diabetes, or dyslipidemia).
- ***Alert:*** Drug may cause pancreatitis. Monitor the patient closely.
- In diabetic patients, dosage of oral antidiabetic or insulin may need to be reduced because improved metabolic control may accompany weight loss.
- As with other weight-loss drugs, potential for misuse exists in certain patients (such as those with anorexia nervosa or bulimia).
- ***Look alike–sound alike:*** Don't confuse Xenical with Xeloda.

PATIENT TEACHING
- Advise patient to follow a nutritionally balanced, reduced-calorie diet that derives only 30% of its calories from fat. Tell him to distribute daily intake of fat, carbohydrate, and protein over three main meals. If a meal is occasionally missed or contains no fat, tell patient that dose of drug can be omitted.
- Advise patient to adhere to dietary guidelines. GI effects may increase when patient takes drug with high-fat foods, specifically when more than 30% of total daily calories come from fat.
- Drug reduces absorption of some fat-soluble vitamins and beta-carotene.
- Tell patient with diabetes that weight loss may improve his glycemic control, so dosage of his oral antidiabetic (such as a sulfonylurea or metformin) or insulin may need to be reduced during drug therapy.
- Tell woman of childbearing age to inform prescriber if pregnancy or breast-feeding is planned during therapy.

penicillin G benzathine (benzathine benzylpenicillin)
pen-i-SILL-in

Bicillin L-A, Permapen

Pharmacologic class: natural penicillin
Pregnancy risk category B

AVAILABLE FORMS
Injection: 600,000 units/ml; 1.2 million units/2 ml; 2.4 million units/4 ml

INDICATIONS & DOSAGES
➤ Congenital syphilis
Children younger than age 2: 50,000 units/kg (up to 2.4 million units) I.M. as a single dose.

➤ Group A streptococcal upper respiratory tract infections
Adults: 1.2 million units I.M. as a single injection.
Children who weigh 27 kg (59.5 lb) or more: 900,000 units I.M. as a single injection.
Children who weigh less than 27 kg: 300,000 to 600,000 units I.M. as a single injection.

➤ To prevent poststreptococcal rheumatic fever
Adults and children: 1.2 million units I.M. once monthly or 600,000 units I.M. every 2 weeks.

➤ Syphilis of less than 1 year duration
Adults: 2.4 million units I.M. as a single dose.
Children: 50,000 units/kg I.M. as a single dose. Don't exceed adult dosage.

➤ **Syphilis of more than 1 year duration**
Adults: 2.4 million units I.M. weekly for 3 weeks.
Children: 50,000 units/kg I.M. weekly for 3 weeks. Don't exceed adult dosage.

ADMINISTRATION

I.M.

- Before giving drug, ask patient about allergic reactions to penicillin.
- Obtain specimen for culture and sensitivity tests before giving first dose. Begin therapy while awaiting results.
- Shake well before injecting.
- Give drug at least 1 hour before a bacteriostatic antibiotic.
- Inject deep into upper outer quadrant of buttocks in adults and in midlateral thigh in infants and small children. Rotate injection sites. Avoid injection into or near major nerves or blood vessels to prevent permanent neurovascular damage.
- Injection may be painful, but ice applied to the site may ease discomfort.

ACTION

Inhibits cell-wall synthesis during bacterial multiplication.

Route	Onset	Peak	Duration
I.M.	Unknown	13–24 hr	1–4 wk

Half-life: 30 to 60 minutes.

ADVERSE REACTIONS

CNS: ***seizures,*** agitation, anxiety, confusion, depression, dizziness, fatigue, hallucinations, lethargy, neuropathy, pain.
GI: ***pseudomembranous colitis,*** enterocolitis, nausea, vomiting.
GU: interstitial nephritis, nephropathy.
Hematologic: ***agranulocytosis, leukopenia, thrombocytopenia,*** anemia, eosinophilia, hemolytic anemia.
Skin: exfoliative dermatitis, maculopapular rash.
Other: ***anaphylaxis,*** hypersensitivity reactions, sterile abscess at injection site.

INTERACTIONS

Drug-drug. *Aminoglycosides:* Physical and chemical incompatibility. Give separately.
Colestipol: May decrease penicillin G benzathine level. Give penicillin G benzathine 1 hour before or 4 hours after colestipol.
Hormonal contraceptives: May decrease hormonal contraceptive effectiveness. Advise use of additional form of contraception during therapy.
Probenecid: May increase penicillin level. Probenecid may be used for this purpose.
Tetracycline: May antagonize penicillin G benzathine effects. Avoid using together.

EFFECTS ON LAB TEST RESULTS

- May decrease hemoglobin level.
- May increase eosinophil count. May decrease platelet, WBC, and granulocyte counts. May cause positive Coombs' test results.
- May falsely decrease aminoglycoside level. May cause false-positive CSF protein test results. May alter urine glucose testing using cupric sulfate (Benedict's reagent).

CONTRAINDICATIONS & CAUTIONS

- Contraindicated in patients hypersensitive to drug or other penicillins.
- Use cautiously in patients allergic to other drugs, especially to cephalosporins, because of possible cross-sensitivity.

NURSING CONSIDERATIONS

- ***Alert:*** Bicillin L-A is the only penicillin G benzathine product indicated for sexually transmitted infections. Don't substitute Bicillin C-R because it may not be effective.
- ***Alert:*** Inadvertent I.V. use may cause cardiac arrest and death. Never give I.V.
- Drug's extremely slow absorption time makes allergic reactions difficult to treat.
- If large doses are given or if therapy is prolonged, bacterial or fungal superinfection may occur, especially in elderly, debilitated, or immunosuppressed patients.
- ***Look alike–sound alike:*** Don't confuse drug with Polycillin, penicillamine, or the various types of penicillin.

PATIENT TEACHING

- Tell patient to report adverse reactions promptly.

• Inform patient that fever and increased WBC count are the most common reactions.
• Warn patient that I.M. injection may be painful but that ice applied to the site may ease discomfort.

penicillin V potassium (phenoxymethyl penicillin potassium)
pen-i-SILL-in

Apo-Pen VK†, Novo-Pen-VK†, Nu-Pen-VK†, Penicillin VK, Veetids

Pharmacologic class: natural penicillin
Pregnancy risk category B

AVAILABLE FORMS
Oral suspension: 125 mg/5 ml, 250 mg/5 ml (after reconstitution)
Tablets: 250 mg, 500 mg
Tablets (film-coated): 250 mg, 500 mg

INDICATIONS & DOSAGES
➤ Mild to moderate systemic infections
Adults and children age 12 and older: 125 to 500 mg or P.O. every 6 hours.
Children younger than age 12: 15 to 62.5 mg/kg P.O. daily in divided doses every 6 to 8 hours.
➤ To prevent recurrent rheumatic fever
Adults and children: 250 mg P.O. b.i.d.
➤ Erythema migrans in Lyme disease ♦
Adults: 500 mg P.O. q.i.d. for 10 to 20 days.
Children younger than age 2: 50 mg/kg/day (up to 2 g/day) P.O. in four divided doses for 10 to 20 days.
➤ To prevent inhalation anthrax after possible exposure ♦
Adults: 7.5 mg/kg P.O. q.i.d. Continue treatment until exposure is ruled out. If exposure is confirmed, anthrax vaccine may be indicated. Continue treatment for 60 days.
Children younger than age 9: 50 mg/kg P.O. daily given in four divided doses. Continue treatment until exposure is ruled out. If exposure is confirmed, anthrax vaccine may be indicated. Continue treatment for 60 days.

ADMINISTRATION
P.O.
• Before giving drug, ask patient about allergic reactions to penicillins.
• Obtain specimen for culture and sensitivity tests before giving first dose. Begin therapy while awaiting results.
• Give drug with food if patient has stomach upset.

ACTION
Inhibits cell-wall synthesis during bacterial multiplication.

Route	Onset	Peak	Duration
P.O.	Unknown	30–60 min	Unknown

Half-life: 30 minutes.

ADVERSE REACTIONS
CNS: neuropathy.
GI: *epigastric distress, nausea,* diarrhea, black hairy tongue, vomiting.
GU: nephropathy.
Hematologic: ***leukopenia, thrombocytopenia,*** eosinophilia, hemolytic anemia.
Other: ***anaphylaxis,*** hypersensitivity reactions, overgrowth of nonsusceptible organisms.

INTERACTIONS
Drug-drug. *Hormonal contraceptives:* May decrease hormonal contraceptive effectiveness. Advise use of another form of contraception during therapy.
Probenecid: May increase penicillin level. Probenecid may be used for this purpose.

EFFECTS ON LAB TEST RESULTS
• May decrease hemoglobin level.
• May increase eosinophil count. May decrease platelet, WBC, and granulocyte counts.
• May alter results of turbidimetric test methods using sulfosalicylic acid, acetic acid, trichloroacetic acid, and nitric acid.

CONTRAINDICATIONS & CAUTIONS
- Contraindicated in patients hypersensitive to drug or other penicillins.
- Use cautiously in patients with GI disturbances and in those with other drug allergies, especially to cephalosporins, because of possible cross-sensitivity.

NURSING CONSIDERATIONS
- Periodically assess renal and hematopoietic function in patients receiving long-term therapy.
- If large doses are given or if therapy is prolonged, bacterial or fungal superinfection may occur, especially in elderly, debilitated, or immunosuppressed patients.
- Amoxicillin is the preferred drug to prevent endocarditis because GI absorption is better and drug levels are sustained longer. Penicillin V is considered an alternate drug.
- ***Look alike–sound alike:*** Don't confuse drug with Polycillin, penicillamine, or the various types of penicillin.

PATIENT TEACHING
- Instruct patient to take entire quantity of drug exactly as prescribed, even after he feels better.
- Tell patient to take drug with food if stomach upset occurs.
- Advise patient to notify prescriber if rash, fever, or chills develop. A rash is the most common allergic reaction.

pentoxifylline
pen-tox-IH-fi-leen

Trental

Pharmacologic class: xanthine derivative
Pregnancy risk category C

AVAILABLE FORMS
Tablets (extended-release): 400 mg

INDICATIONS & DOSAGES
➤ **Intermittent claudication from chronic occlusive vascular disease**
Adults: 400 mg P.O. t.i.d. with meals. May decrease to 400 mg b.i.d. if GI and CNS adverse effects occur.

ADMINISTRATION
P.O.
- Give drug whole; don't crush or split tablet.
- Give drug with meals to minimize GI upset.

ACTION
Unknown. Improves capillary blood flow, probably by increasing RBC flexibility and lowering blood viscosity.

Route	Onset	Peak	Duration
P.O.	Unknown	1 hr	Unknown

Half-life: About 30 to 45 minutes.

ADVERSE REACTIONS
CNS: dizziness, headache.
GI: dyspepsia, nausea, vomiting.

INTERACTIONS
Drug-drug. *Anticoagulants:* May increase anticoagulant effect. Monitor PT.
Antihypertensives: May increase hypotensive effect. May need to adjust dosage.
Theophylline: May increase theophylline level. Monitor patient closely.
Drug-lifestyle. *Smoking:* May cause vasoconstriction. Advise patient to avoid smoking.

EFFECTS ON LAB TEST RESULTS
None reported.

CONTRAINDICATIONS & CAUTIONS
- Contraindicated in patients intolerant to this drug or to methylxanthines, such as caffeine, theophylline, and theobromine, and in those with recent cerebral or retinal hemorrhage.

NURSING CONSIDERATIONS
- Drug is useful in patients who aren't good surgical candidates.
- Elderly patients may be more sensitive to drug's effects.
- ***Look alike–sound alike:*** Don't confuse Trental with Trandate.

PATIENT TEACHING
- Advise patient to take drug with meals to minimize GI upset.

• Instruct patient to swallow tablet whole, without breaking, crushing, or chewing.
• Tell patient to report GI or CNS adverse reactions; prescriber may reduce dosage.
• Urge patient not to stop drug during the first 8 weeks of therapy unless directed by prescriber.

perindopril erbumine
pur-IN-doh-pril

Aceon, Coversyl†

Pharmacologic class: ACE inhibitor
Pregnancy risk category C; D in second and third trimesters

AVAILABLE FORMS
Tablets: 2 mg, 4 mg, 8 mg

INDICATIONS & DOSAGES
➤ **To reduce the risk of CV death or nonfatal MI in patients with stable coronary artery disease**
Adults age 70 or younger: 4 mg P.O. once daily for 2 weeks; then, increase as tolerated to 8 mg once daily.
Elderly adults older than age 70: Initially, 2 mg P.O. once daily for the first week; then, 4 mg once daily for the second week and 8 mg once daily after that, if tolerated.
➤ **Essential hypertension**
Adults: Initially, 4 mg P.O. once daily. Increase dosage until blood pressure is controlled or to maximum of 16 mg/day; usual maintenance dosage is 4 to 8 mg once daily; may be given in two divided doses.
Patients older than age 65: Initially, 4 mg P.O. daily as one dose or in two divided doses. Dosage may be increased by more than 8 mg/day only under close medical supervision.
Adjust-a-dose: For renally insufficient patients with creatinine clearance 30 ml/minute or greater, initially 2 mg P.O. daily. Maximum daily maintenance dose is 8 mg. In patients taking diuretics, initially 2 to 4 mg P.O. daily as single dose or in two divided doses, with close medical supervision for several hours and until blood pressure has stabilized. Adjust dosage based on patient's blood pressure response.

ADMINISTRATION
P.O.
• Give drug without regard for food.

ACTION
Prevents conversion of angiotensin I to angiotensin II, a potent vasoconstrictor. Less angiotensin II decreases peripheral arterial resistance, decreasing aldosterone secretion, which reduces sodium and water retention and lowers blood pressure.

Route	Onset	Peak	Duration
P.O.	Unknown	1 hr	Unknown

Half-life: About 1 hour for perindopril; mean half-life, 3 to 10 hours, and terminal elimination half-life, 30 to 120 hours for perindoprilat.

ADVERSE REACTIONS
CNS: *headache,* dizziness, asthenia, sleep disorder, paresthesia, depression, somnolence, nervousness, fever.
CV: palpitations, edema, chest pain, hypotension, abnormal ECG.
EENT: rhinitis, sinusitis, ear infection, pharyngitis, tinnitus.
GI: dyspepsia, diarrhea, abdominal pain, nausea, vomiting, flatulence.
GU: proteinuria, UTI, male sexual dysfunction, menstrual disorder.
Metabolic: ***hyperkalemia.***
Musculoskeletal: back pain, hypertonia, neck pain, joint pain, myalgia, arthritis, arm or leg pain.
Respiratory: *cough,* upper respiratory tract infection.
Skin: rash.
Other: viral infection, injury, seasonal allergy.

INTERACTIONS
Drug-drug. *Diuretics:* May increase hypotensive effect. Monitor patient closely.
Lithium: May increase lithium level and risk of lithium toxicity. Use together cautiously; monitor lithium level.
NSAIDs: May decrease antihypertensive effects. Monitor blood pressure.

Potassium-sparing diuretics (amiloride, spironolactone, triamterene), potassium supplements, other drugs capable of increasing potassium level (cyclosporine, heparin, indomethacin): May increase hyperkalemic effect. Use together cautiously; monitor potassium level.
Drug-herb. *Capsaicin:* May cause cough. Discourage use together.
Drug-food. *Salt substitutes containing potassium:* May cause hyperkalemia. Discourage use together.

EFFECTS ON LAB TEST RESULTS

- May increase ALT, alkaline phosphatase, uric acid, cholesterol, and creatinine levels. May increase potassium level.

CONTRAINDICATIONS & CAUTIONS

- Contraindicated in patients hypersensitive to drug or other ACE inhibitors and in those with a history of angioedema caused by ACE inhibitor use.
- Use cautiously in patients with a history of angioedema unrelated to ACE inhibitor use.
- Use cautiously in patients with renal impairment, heart failure, ischemic heart disease, cerebrovascular disease, or renal artery stenosis and in those with collagen vascular disease, such as systemic lupus erythematosus or scleroderma.

NURSING CONSIDERATIONS

- When used alone in black patients, drug affects blood pressure less than in other patients. Monitor blood pressure closely.
- Patients with a history of angioedema unrelated to ACE inhibitor use may be at increased risk for angioedema during therapy. Black patients are at a higher risk for angioedema regardless of prior ACE inhibitor use.
- ***Alert:*** If angioedema occurs, stop drug and observe patient until swelling disappears. Antihistamines may relieve swelling of the face and lips. Swelling of the tongue, glottis, or throat may cause life-threatening airway obstruction. Give prompt treatment, such as epinephrine.
- Monitor CBC with differential for agranulocytosis and neutropenia before therapy, especially in renally impaired patients with lupus or scleroderma.
- Monitor patient for hypotension when starting therapy and when adjusting dosage. If severe hypotension occurs, place patient in supine position and treat symptomatically.
- Severe hypotension can occur when drug is given with diuretics. If possible, stop diuretic 2 to 3 days before starting this drug. If impossible, use lower doses of either drug.
- In patient who is volume- or sodium-depleted from prolonged diuretic therapy, dietary sodium restriction, dialysis, diarrhea, or vomiting, correct fluid and sodium deficits before starting drug.
- Monitor renal function before and periodically throughout therapy.
- Monitor potassium level closely.

PATIENT TEACHING

- Inform patient that throat and facial swelling, including swelling of the throat, can occur during therapy, especially with the first dose. Advise patient to stop taking drug and immediately report any signs or symptoms of swelling of face, extremities, eyes, lips, or tongue; hoarseness; or difficulty in swallowing or breathing.
- Advise patient to report promptly any sign or symptom of infection (sore throat, fever) or jaundice (yellowing of eyes or skin).
- Advise patient to avoid salt substitutes containing potassium unless instructed otherwise by prescriber.
- Caution patient that light-headedness may occur, especially during first few days of therapy. Advise patient to report light-headedness and, if fainting occurs, to stop drug and consult prescriber promptly.
- Caution patient that inadequate fluid intake or excessive perspiration, diarrhea, or vomiting can lead to an excessive drop in blood pressure.
- Advise woman of childbearing age of the consequences of second- and third-trimester exposure to drug. Advise her to notify prescriber immediately if she suspects pregnancy.

phentermine hydrochloride
FEN-ter-meen

Adipex-P

Pharmacologic class: sympathomimetic amine
Pregnancy risk category NR
Controlled substance schedule IV

AVAILABLE FORMS
Capsules: 18.75 mg, 30 mg, 37.5 mg
Capsules (resin complex, sustained-release): 15 mg, 30 mg
Tablets: 8 mg, 30 mg, 37.5 mg

INDICATIONS & DOSAGES
➤ **Short-term adjunct in exogenous obesity**
Adults: 8 mg P.O. t.i.d. 30 minutes before meals. Or, 15 to 37.5 mg or 15 to 30 mg (as resin complex) P.O. daily as a single dose in the morning. Give Adipex-P before breakfast or 1 to 2 hours after breakfast.

ADMINISTRATION
P.O.
- Give sustained-release capsule whole, at least 10 hours before bedtime.
- Give last dose of immediate-release capsule or tablet at least 4 to 6 hours before bedtime.

ACTION
Unknown. Probably promotes nerve impulse transmission by releasing stored norepinephrine from nerve terminals in the brain, especially in the cerebral cortex and reticular activating system.

Route	Onset	Peak	Duration
P.O.	Unknown	Unknown	12–14 hr

Half-life: 19 to 24 hours.

ADVERSE REACTIONS
CNS: *insomnia,* overstimulation, headache, euphoria, dysphoria, dizziness.
CV: *palpitations, tachycardia,* increased blood pressure.
GI: dry mouth, dysgeusia, constipation, diarrhea, unpleasant taste, other GI disturbances.
GU: impotence.
Skin: urticaria.
Other: altered libido.

INTERACTIONS
Drug-drug. *Acetazolamide, antacids, sodium bicarbonate:* May increase renal reabsorption. Monitor patient for enhanced effects.
Ammonium chloride, ascorbic acid: May decrease level and increase renal excretion of phentermine. Monitor patient for decreased phentermine effects.
Insulin, oral antidiabetics: May alter antidiabetic requirements. Monitor glucose level.
MAO inhibitors: May cause severe hypertension or hypertensive crisis. Avoid using within 14 days of MAO inhibitor therapy.
Drug-food. *Caffeine:* May increase CNS stimulation. Discourage use together.

EFFECTS ON LAB TEST RESULTS
None reported.

CONTRAINDICATIONS & CAUTIONS
- Contraindicated in patients hypersensitive to sympathomimetic amines, in those with idiosyncratic reactions to them, in agitated patients, and in those with hyperthyroidism, moderate-to-severe hypertension, advanced arteriosclerosis, symptomatic CV disease, or glaucoma.
- Contraindicated within 14 days of MAO inhibitor therapy.
- Use cautiously in patients with mild hypertension.

NURSING CONSIDERATIONS
- Use drug with a weight-reduction program.
- Monitor patient for tolerance or dependence.
- ***Look alike–sound alike:*** Don't confuse phentermine with phentolamine.

PATIENT TEACHING
- Tell patient to take sustained-release drug at least 10 hours before bedtime or last dose of immediate-release drug at least 4 to 6 hours before bedtime to avoid sleep interference.

• Advise patient to avoid products that contain caffeine. Tell him to report evidence of excessive stimulation.
• Warn patient that fatigue may result as drug effects wear off and that he'll need more rest.
• Warn patient that drug may lose its effectiveness over time.
• Tell patient to take sustained-release capsule whole and not to chew, crush, or open it.

phentolamine mesylate
fen-TOLE-a-meen

Rogitine†

Pharmacologic class: alpha blocker
Pregnancy risk category C

AVAILABLE FORMS
Injection: 5 mg/ml, 10 mg/ml†

INDICATIONS & DOSAGES
➤ **To aid in diagnosis of pheochromocytoma, to control or prevent hypertension before or during pheochromocytomectomy**
Adults: I.V. or I.M. diagnostic dose is 5 mg with close monitoring of blood pressure. Give 5 mg I.V. or I.M. 1 to 2 hours before surgical removal of tumor. During surgery, patient may need an additional 5 mg I.V.
Children: I.V. diagnostic dose is 1 mg, and I.M. diagnostic dose is 3 mg with close monitoring of blood pressure. Give 1 mg I.V. or I.M. 1 to 2 hours before surgical removal of tumor. During surgery, patient may need an additional 1 mg I.V.
➤ **To prevent dermal necrosis from norepinephrine extravasation**
Adults: Add 10 mg of phentolamine to each liter of solution containing norepinephrine; the pressor effect of norepinephrine is unaffected.
➤ **Dermal necrosis and sloughing after I.V. extravasation of norepinephrine or dopamine**
Adults: Infiltrate area with 5 to 10 mg phentolamine in 10 to 15 ml of normal saline solution. Must be done within 12 hours of extravasation.
Children: Inject 0.1 to 0.2 mg/kg up to a maximum of 10 mg in the extravasation area.

ADMINISTRATION
I.V.
• Reconstitute drug by adding 1 ml of sterile water for injection to vial containing 5 mg of drug; resulting solution contains 5 mg/ml of drug.
• Delay injection until effect of venipuncture on blood pressure has passed, then inject drug rapidly.
• For pheochromocytoma diagnosis, inject drug rapidly. Test result is positive if severe hypotension develops.
• **Incompatibilities:** None reported.
I.M.
• Reconstitute drug by adding 1 ml of sterile water for injection to vial containing 5 mg of drug.
• Document injection site.

ACTION
Competitively blocks the effects of catecholamines on alpha-adrenergic receptors.

Route	Onset	Peak	Duration
I.V.	Immediate	< 2 min	15–30 min
I.M.	Unknown	< 20 min	30–45 min

Half-life: 19 minutes (I.V.).

ADVERSE REACTIONS
CNS: *dizziness, weakness, flushing,* ***cerebrovascular occlusion,*** cerebrovascular spasm.
CV: *hypotension, tachycardia,* ***shock, arrhythmias, MI.***
EENT: *nasal congestion.*
GI: *diarrhea, nausea, vomiting.*

INTERACTIONS
Drug-drug. *Ephedrine, epinephrine:* May cause excessive hypotension. Don't use together.

EFFECTS ON LAB TEST RESULTS
None reported.

CONTRAINDICATIONS & CAUTIONS
• Contraindicated in patients with hypersensitivity to drug and in those with

angina, coronary artery disease, or MI or history of MI.
- Use cautiously in patients with gastritis or peptic ulcer.

NURSING CONSIDERATIONS

- When drug is given as a diagnostic test for pheochromocytoma, check patient's blood pressure first; monitor blood pressure frequently during administration.
- ***Alert:*** Don't give epinephrine to treat phentolamine-induced hypotension because it may cause additional fall in blood pressure ("epinephrine reversal"). Use norepinephrine instead.
- ***Look alike–sound alike:*** Don't confuse phentolamine with phentermine.

PATIENT TEACHING

- Explain use and administration of drug.
- Tell patient to report adverse reactions promptly.

SAFETY ALERT!

phenylephrine hydrochloride

fen-ill-EF-rin

Neo-Synephrine

Pharmacologic class: adrenergic
Pregnancy risk category C

AVAILABLE FORMS

Injection: 10 mg/ml (1%)

INDICATIONS & DOSAGES

➤ Hypotensive emergencies during spinal anesthesia
Adults: 0.2 mg I.V.; subsequent doses should be no more than 0.1 to 0.2 mg over the previous dose; don't exceed 0.5 mg in a single dose.
Children: 0.044 to 0.088 mg/kg I.M. or subcutaneously.

➤ Prevention of hypotension during spinal anesthesia
Adults: 2 to 3 mg I.M. or subcutaneously 3 to 4 minutes before injection of spinal anesthesia.

➤ To prolong spinal anesthesia
Adults: 2 to 5 mg added to anesthetic solution.

➤ Vasoconstrictor for regional anesthesia
Adults: 1 mg phenylephrine added to each 20 ml local anesthetic.

➤ Mild to moderate hypotension
Adults: 2 to 5 mg I.M. (dose ranges from 1 to 10 mg) or subcutaneously; repeat in 1 or 2 hours as needed and tolerated. First dose shouldn't exceed 5 mg. Or, 0.1 to 0.5 mg slow I.V., not to be repeated more often than 10 to 15 minutes.
Children: 0.1 mg/kg or 3 mg/m^2 I.M. or subcutaneously; repeat in 1 or 2 hours as needed and tolerated.

➤ Severe hypotension and shock (including drug-induced)
Adults: 10 mg in 250 to 500 ml of D_5W or normal saline solution for injection. I.V. infusion started at 100 to 180 mcg/minute; then decrease to maintenance infusion of 40 to 60 mcg/minute when blood pressure stabilizes.

➤ Paroxysmal supraventricular tachycardia
Adults: Initially, 0.5 mg rapid I.V.; increase in increments of 0.1 to 0.2 mg. Use cautiously. Maximum single dose is 1 mg.

ADMINISTRATION

I.V.
- For direct injection, dilute 10 mg (1 ml) with 9 ml sterile water for injection to provide 1 mg/ml. Infusions are usually prepared by adding 10 mg of drug to 500 ml of D_5W or normal saline solution for injection. The first I.V. infusion rate is usually 100 to 180 mcg/minute; maintenance rate is usually 40 to 60 mcg/minute.
- Use a central venous catheter or large vein, as in the antecubital fossa, to minimize risk of extravasation. Use a continuous infusion pump to regulate infusion flow rate.
- During infusion, frequently monitor ECG, blood pressure, cardiac output, central venous pressure, pulmonary artery wedge pressure, pulse rate, urine output, and color and temperature of limbs. Titrate infusion rate according to findings and prescriber guidelines. Maintain blood pressure slightly below patient's normal level. In previously normotensive patients, maintain systolic blood pressure at 80 to 100 mm Hg; in previously hypertensive

patients, maintain systolic blood pressure at 30 to 40 mm Hg below usual level.
• Avoid abrupt withdrawal after prolonged I.V. infusions.
• To treat extravasation, infiltrate site promptly with 10 to 15 ml of normal saline solution for injection containing 5 to 10 mg phentolamine. Use a fine needle.
• **Incompatibilities:** Alkaline solutions, iron salts, other metals, phenytoin sodium, thiopental sodium.

I.M.
• Don't give drug if solution is discolored or has particulate matter.
• Document injection site.
• Discard unused solution.

Subcutaneous
• Don't give drug if solution is discolored or has particulate matter.
• Document injection site.
• Discard unused solution.

ACTION
Stimulates alpha receptors in the sympathetic nervous system, causing vasoconstriction.

Route	Onset	Peak	Duration
I.V.	Immediate	Unknown	15–20 min
I.M.	10–15 min	Unknown	30–120 min
Subcut.	10–15 min	Unknown	50–60 min

Half-life: 2 to 3 hours.

ADVERSE REACTIONS
CNS: *headache,* excitability, restlessness, anxiety, nervousness, dizziness, weakness.
CV: ***bradycardia, arrhythmias,*** hypertension.
Respiratory: ***asthmatic episodes.***
Skin: tissue sloughing with extravasation.
Other: ***anaphylaxis,*** tachyphylaxis and decreased organ perfusion with continued use.

INTERACTIONS
Drug-drug. *Alpha blockers, phenothiazines:* May decrease pressor response. Monitor patient closely.
Atropine, guanethidine, oxytocics: May increase pressor response. Monitor patient.
Beta blockers: May block cardiostimulation. Monitor patient closely.
Halogenated hydrocarbon anesthetics, sympathomimetics: May cause serious arrhythmias. Use together with caution.
MAO inhibitors (phenelzine, tranylcypromine): May cause severe headache, hypertension, fever, and hypertensive crisis. Avoid using together.
Tricyclic antidepressants: May potentiate pressor response and cause arrhythmias. Use together cautiously.

EFFECTS ON LAB TEST RESULTS
• May cause false-normal tonometry reading.

CONTRAINDICATIONS & CAUTIONS
• Contraindicated in patients hypersensitive to drug and in those with severe hypertension or ventricular tachycardia.
• Use with caution in elderly patients and in patients with heart disease, hyperthyroidism, severe atherosclerosis, bradycardia, partial heart block, myocardial disease, or sulfite sensitivity.

NURSING CONSIDERATIONS
• Drug causes little or no CNS stimulation.
• Drug may lower intraocular pressure in normal eyes or in open-angle glaucoma.
• Drug is used in OTC eyedrops and cold preparations for decongestant effects.

PATIENT TEACHING
• Tell patient to report adverse reactions promptly.
• Instruct patient to report discomfort at I.V. insertion site.

SAFETY ALERT!

potassium chloride
Apo-K†*, Cena-K, K 10†, Kaon-Cl, Kaon-Cl-10, Kay Ciel, K-Dur 20, K-Lor, Klor-Con, Klor-Con 8, Klor-Con 10, Klor-Con/25, Klor-Con M10, Klor-Con M15, Klor-Con M20, Klotrix, K-Lyte/Cl, K-Tab, Micro-K, Micro-K 10, Micro-K LS, Potasalan

Pharmacologic class: potassium salt
Pregnancy risk category C

AVAILABLE FORMS
Capsules (controlled-release): 8 mEq, 10 mEq

Injection concentrate: 1.5 mEq/ml, 2 mEq/ml
Injection for I.V. infusion: 0.1 mEq/ml, 0.2 mEq/ml, 0.3 mEq/ml, 0.4 mEq/ml
Oral liquid: 20 mEq/15 ml, 30 mEq/15 ml, 40 mEq/15 ml
Powder for oral administration: 15 mEq/packet, 20 mEq/packet, 25 mEq/packet
Tablets (controlled-release): 6.7 mEq, 8 mEq, 10 mEq, 20 mEq
Tablets (extended-release): 8 mEq, 10 mEq, 15 mEq, 20 mEq

INDICATIONS & DOSAGES

➤ To prevent hypokalemia
Adults and children: Initially, 20 mEq of potassium supplement P.O. daily, in divided doses. Adjust dosage, as needed, based on potassium levels.

➤ Hypokalemia
Adults and children: 40 to 100 mEq P.O. in two to four divided doses daily. Maximum dose of diluted I.V. potassium chloride is 40 mEq/L at 10 mEq/hour. Don't exceed 150 mEq daily in adults and 3 mEq/kg daily in children. Further doses are based on potassium levels and blood pH. Give I.V. potassium replacement only with monitoring of ECG and potassium level.

➤ Severe hypokalemia
Adults and children: Dilute potassium chloride in a suitable I.V. solution of less than 80 mEq/L, and give at no more than 40 mEq/hour.

Further doses are based on potassium level. Don't exceed 150 mEq I.V. daily in adults and 3 mEq/kg I.V. daily or 40 mEq/m^2 daily in children. Give I.V. potassium replacement only with monitoring of ECG and potassium level.

➤ Acute MI ♦
Adults: For high dose, 80 mEq/L at 1.5 ml/kg/hour for 24 hours with an I.V. infusion of 25% dextrose and 50 units/L regular insulin. For low dose, 40 mEq/L at 1 ml/kg/hour for 24 hours, with an I.V. infusion of 10% dextrose and 20 units/L regular insulin.

ADMINISTRATION

P.O.

- Make sure powders are completely dissolved before giving.
- Enteric-coated tablets are not recommended because of increased risk of GI bleeding and small-bowel ulcerations.
- Tablets in wax matrix may lodge in the esophagus and cause ulceration in cardiac patients with esophageal compression from an enlarged left atrium. Use sugar-free liquid form in these patients and in those with esophageal stasis or obstruction. Have patient sip slowly to minimize GI irritation.
- Don't crush sustained-release forms.

I.V.

- Use only when oral replacement isn't feasible or when hypokalemia is life-threatening.
- Give by infusion only, never I.V. push or I.M. Give slowly as dilute solution; rapid infusion may cause fatal hyperkalemia.
- If burning occurs during infusion, decrease rate.
- **Incompatibilities:** Amikacin, amoxicillin, amphotericin B, azithromycin, diazepam, dobutamine, ergotamine, etoposide with cisplatin and mannitol, fat emulsion 10%, methylprednisolone, penicillin G, phenytoin, promethazine.

ACTION

Replaces potassium and maintains potassium level.

Route	Onset	Peak	Duration
P.O.	Unknown	Unknown	Unknown
I.V.	Immediate	Immediate	Unknown

Half-life: Unknown.

ADVERSE REACTIONS

CNS: paresthesia of limbs, listlessness, confusion, weakness or heaviness of limbs, flaccid paralysis.
CV: *postinfusion phlebitis,* ***arrhythmias, heart block, cardiac arrest,*** ECG changes, hypotension.
GI: nausea, vomiting, abdominal pain, diarrhea.
Metabolic: ***hyperkalemia.***
Respiratory: ***respiratory paralysis.***

INTERACTIONS

Drug-drug. *ACE inhibitors, digoxin, potassium-sparing diuretics:* May cause hyperkalemia. Use together with extreme caution. Monitor potassium level.

EFFECTS ON LAB TEST RESULTS

- May increase potassium level.

CONTRAINDICATIONS & CAUTIONS

- Contraindicated in patients with severe renal impairment with oliguria, anuria, or azotemia; with untreated Addison's disease; or with acute dehydration, heat cramps, hyperkalemia, hyperkalemic form of familial periodic paralysis, or other conditions linked to extensive tissue breakdown.
- Use cautiously in patients with cardiac disease or renal impairment.

NURSING CONSIDERATIONS

- Patients at an increased risk of GI lesions include those with scleroderma, diabetes, mitral valve replacement, cardiomegaly, or esophageal strictures, and in elderly or immobile patients.
- Drug is commonly used orally with potassium-wasting diuretics to maintain potassium levels.
- Monitor ECG and electrolyte levels during therapy.
- Monitor renal function. After surgery, don't give drug until urine flow is established.
- Many adverse reactions may reflect hyperkalemia.
- Patient may be sensitive to tartrazine in some of these products.
- ***Look alike–sound alike:*** Potassium preparations aren't interchangeable; verify preparation before use and don't switch products.

PATIENT TEACHING

- Teach patient how to prepare powders and how to take drug. Tell patient to take with or after meals with full glass of water or fruit juice to lessen GI distress.
- Teach patient signs and symptoms of hyperkalemia, and tell patient to notify prescriber if they occur.
- Tell patient to report discomfort at I.V. insertion site.
- Warn patient not to use salt substitutes concurrently, except with prescriber's permission.
- Tell patient not to be concerned if wax matrix appears in stool because the drug has already been absorbed.

pravastatin sodium (eptastatin)

prah-va-STA-tin

Pravachol

Pharmacologic class: HMG-CoA reductase inhibitor
Pregnancy risk category X

AVAILABLE FORMS

Tablets: 10 mg, 20 mg, 40 mg, 80 mg

INDICATIONS & DOSAGES

➤ **Primary and secondary prevention of coronary events; hyperlipidemia**

Adults: Initially, 40 mg P.O. once daily at the same time each day, with or without food. Adjust dosage every 4 weeks, based on patient tolerance and response; maximum daily dose is 80 mg.

➤ **Heterozygous familial hypercholesterolemia**

Adolescents ages 14 to 18: Give 40 mg P.O. once daily.
Children ages 8 to 13: Give 20 mg P.O. once daily.
Adjust-a-dose: In patients with renal or hepatic dysfunction, start with 10 mg P.O. daily. In patients taking immunosuppressants, begin with 10 mg P.O. at bedtime and adjust to higher dosages with caution. Most patients treated with the combination of immunosuppressants and pravastatin receive up to 20 mg pravastatin daily.

ADMINISTRATION

P.O.

- Give drug without regard for meals.

ACTION

Inhibits HMG-CoA reductase, an early (and rate-limiting) step in cholesterol biosynthesis.

Route	Onset	Peak	Duration
P.O.	Unknown	60–90 min	Unknown

Half-life: 1¼ to 2¼ hours.

ADVERSE REACTIONS

CNS: dizziness, fatigue, headache.
CV: chest pain.
EENT: rhinitis.
GI: *nausea,* abdominal pain, constipation, diarrhea, flatulence, heartburn, vomiting.
GU: ***renal failure caused by myoglobinuria,*** urinary abnormality.
Musculoskeletal: *localized muscle pain,* ***rhabdomyolysis,*** myalgia, myopathy, myositis.
Respiratory: common cold, cough.
Skin: rash.
Other: flulike symptoms, influenza.

INTERACTIONS

Drug-drug. *Cholestyramine, colestipol:* May decrease pravastatin level. Give pravastatin 1 hour before or 4 hours after these drugs.
Cyclosporine: May decrease metabolism of HMG-CoA reductase inhibitor, increasing toxicity. Monitor patient for adverse effects and report unexplained muscle pain.
Erythromycin, fibric acid derivatives (such as clofibrate, gemfibrozil), immunosuppressants, high doses (1 g or more daily) of niacin (nicotinic acid): May cause rhabdomyolysis. Avoid using together; if unavoidable, monitor patient closely.
Fluconazole, itraconazole, ketoconazole: May increase pravastatin level and adverse effects. Avoid using together; if unavoidable, reduce dose of pravastatin.
Gemfibrozil: May decrease protein-binding and urinary clearance of pravastatin. Avoid using together.
Hepatotoxic drugs: May increase risk of hepatotoxicity. Avoid using together.
Drug-herb. *Eucalyptus, jin bu huan, kava:* May increase the risk of hepatotoxicity. Discourage use together.
Red yeast rice: May increase risk of adverse reactions because herb contains compounds similar to those in drug. Discourage use together.
Drug-lifestyle. *Alcohol use:* May increase risk of hepatotoxicity. Discourage use together.

EFFECTS ON LAB TEST RESULTS

- May increase ALT, AST, CK, alkaline phosphatase, and bilirubin levels.
- May alter thyroid function test values.

CONTRAINDICATIONS & CAUTIONS

- Contraindicated in patients hypersensitive to drug and in those with active liver disease or conditions that cause unexplained, persistent elevations of transaminase levels.
- Contraindicated in pregnant and breast-feeding women and in women of childbearing age.
- Use cautiously in patients who consume large quantities of alcohol or have history of liver disease.
- Safety and efficacy in children younger than age 8 haven't been established.

NURSING CONSIDERATIONS

- Patient should follow a diet restricted in saturated fat and cholesterol during therapy.
- Use in children with heterozygous familial hypercholesterolemia if LDL cholesterol level is at least 190 mg/dl, or if LDL cholesterol is at least 160 mg/dl and patient has either a positive family history of premature CV disease or two or more other CV disease risk factors.
- Obtain liver function test results at start of therapy and then periodically. A liver biopsy may be performed if elevated liver enzyme levels persist.
- ***Look alike–sound alike:*** Don't confuse Pravachol with Prevacid or propranolol.

PATIENT TEACHING

- Advise patient who is also taking a bile-acid resin such as cholestyramine to take pravastatin at least 1 hour before or 4 hours after taking resin.
- Tell patient to notify prescriber of adverse reactions, particularly muscle aches and pains.
- Teach patient about proper dietary management of cholesterol and triglycerides. When appropriate, recommend weight control, exercise, and smoking cessation programs.
- Inform patient that it will take up to 4 weeks to achieve full therapeutic effect.

• *Alert:* Tell woman of childbearing age to stop drug and notify prescriber immediately if she is or may be pregnant or if she's breast-feeding.

prazosin hydrochloride
PRA-zo-sin

Minipress

Pharmacologic class: alpha blocker
Pregnancy risk category C

AVAILABLE FORMS
Capsules: 1 mg, 2 mg, 5 mg

INDICATIONS & DOSAGES
➤ Mild to moderate hypertension
Adults: Test dose is 1 mg P.O. at bedtime to prevent first-dose syncope (severe syncope with loss of consciousness). First dosage is 1 mg P.O. b.i.d. or t.i.d. Dosage may be increased slowly. Maximum daily dose is 20 mg. Maintenance dosage is 6 to 15 mg daily in divided doses. Some patients need larger dosages (up to 40 mg daily).

If other antihypertensives or diuretics are added to therapy, decrease prazosin dosage to 1 to 2 mg t.i.d. and readjust to maintenance dosage.

➤ Benign prostatic hyperplasia ♦
Adults: 2 mg P.O. b.i.d. Dose range is 1 to 9 mg P.O. daily.

ADMINISTRATION
P.O.
• Give drug without regard for meals.

ACTION
Unknown. Thought to act by blocking alpha-adrenergic receptors.

Route	Onset	Peak	Duration
P.O.	30–90 min	2–4 hr	7–10 hr

Half-life: 2 to 4 hours.

ADVERSE REACTIONS
CNS: *dizziness, first-dose syncope,* headache, drowsiness, nervousness, paresthesia, weakness, depression, fever.
CV: orthostatic hypotension, palpitations, edema.
EENT: blurred vision, tinnitus, conjunctivitis, epistaxis, nasal congestion.
GI: vomiting, diarrhea, abdominal cramps, nausea.
GU: priapism, impotence, urinary frequency, incontinence.
Musculoskeletal: arthralgia, myalgia.
Respiratory: dyspnea.
Skin: pruritus.

INTERACTIONS
Drug-drug. *Acebutolol, atenolol, betaxolol, carteolol, esmolol, metoprolol, nadolol, pindolol, propranolol, sotalol, timolol:* May increase the risk of orthostatic hypotension in the early phases of use together. Help patient stand slowly until effects are known.
Diuretics: May increase frequency of syncope with loss of consciousness. Advise patient to sit or lie down if dizziness occurs.
Verapamil: May increase prazosin level. Monitor patient closely.
Drug-herb. *Butcher's broom:* May reduce effect. Discourage use together.
Ma huang: May decrease antihypertensive effects. Discourage use together.

EFFECTS ON LAB TEST RESULTS
• May increase levels of BUN, uric acid, and urinary metabolite of norepinephrine and vanillylmandelic acid.
• May increase liver function test values. May alter results of screening tests for pheochromocytoma.
• May cause positive antinuclear antibody titer.

CONTRAINDICATIONS & CAUTIONS
• Contraindicated in patients hypersensitive to drug or other alpha blockers.
• Use cautiously in patients receiving other antihypertensives.

NURSING CONSIDERATIONS
• Monitor patient's blood pressure and pulse rate frequently.
• Elderly patients may be more sensitive to drug's hypotensive effects.
• Compliance might be improved with twice-daily dosing. Discuss dosing change with prescriber if compliance problems are suspected.

• ***Alert:*** If first dose is more than 1 mg, first-dose syncope may occur.

PATIENT TEACHING

• Warn patient that dizziness may occur with first dose. If he experiences dizziness, tell him to sit or lie down. Reassure him that this effect disappears with continued dosing.
• Caution patient to avoid driving or performing hazardous tasks for the first 24 hours after starting this drug or increasing the dose.
• Tell patient not to suddenly stop taking drug, but to notify prescriber if unpleasant adverse reactions occur.
• Advise patient to minimize low blood pressure and dizziness upon standing by rising slowly and avoiding sudden position changes. Dry mouth can be relieved by chewing gum or sucking on hard candy or ice chips.

procainamide hydrochloride

proe-KANE-a-myed

Pronestyl

Pharmacologic class: procaine derivative
Pregnancy risk category C

AVAILABLE FORMS

Capsules: 250 mg, 375 mg, 500 mg
Injection: 100 mg/ml, 500 mg/ml
Tablets: 250 mg, 375 mg, 500 mg
Tablets (extended-release): 250 mg, 500 mg, 750 mg, 1,000 mg

INDICATIONS & DOSAGES

➤ Symptomatic PVCs, life-threatening ventricular tachycardia
For oral therapy, start at 50 mg/kg/day of P.O. of conventional tablets or capsules in divided doses every 3 hours until therapeutic level is reached. For maintenance, substitute extended-release form to deliver the total daily dose divided every 6 hours or extended-release form (Procanbid) at a dose of 50 mg/kg P.O. in two divided doses every 12 hours.
Adults: 100 mg every 5 minutes by slow I.V. push, no faster than 25 to 50 mg/minute, until arrhythmias disappear, adverse effects develop, or 500 mg has been given. Usual effective loading dose is 500 to 600 mg. Or, give a loading dose of 500 to 600 mg I.V. infusion over 25 to 30 minutes. Maximum total dose is 1 g. When arrhythmias disappear, give continuous infusion of 2 to 6 mg/minute. If arrhythmias recur, repeat bolus as above and increase infusion rate.

For I.M. administration, give 50 mg/kg divided every 3 to 6 hours; if arrhythmias occur during surgery, give 100 to 500 mg I.M.
Children ♦: Dosage not established. Recommendations include 2 to 5 mg/kg I.V., not exceeding 100 mg, repeated as needed at 5- to 10-minute intervals, not exceeding 15 mg/kg in 24 hours or 500 mg in 30 minutes. Or, 15 mg/kg infused over 30 to 60 minutes; then maintenance infusion of 0.02 to 0.08 mg/kg/minute.

➤ To convert atrial fibrillation or paroxysmal atrial tachycardia ♦
Adults: 1.25 g P.O. of conventional tablets or capsules. If arrhythmias persist after 1 hour, give additional 750 mg. If no change occurs, give 500 mg to 1 g P.O. every 2 hours until arrhythmias disappear or adverse effects occur. Maintenance dose is 1 g extended-release every 6 hours.
Children ♦: 15 to 50 mg/kg/day P.O. divided every 3 to 6 hours. Maximum dose 4 g daily. Or, 20 to 30 mg/kg/day I.M. Or, loading dose of 3 to 6 mg/kg I.V. over 5 minutes, up to 100 mg/dose; then maintenance dose 20 to 80 mcg/kg/minute as continuous I.V. infusion. Maximum daily dose is 2 g.

➤ To maintain normal sinus rhythm after conversion of atrial flutter ♦
Adults: 0.5 to 1 g P.O. of conventional tablets or capsules every 4 to 6 hours.

➤ Malignant hyperthermia ♦
Adults: 200 to 900 mg I.V., followed by maintenance infusion.
Adjust-a-dose: For patients with renal or hepatic dysfunction, decrease dose or increase dosing interval, as needed.

ADMINISTRATION

P.O.
• ***Alert:*** Don't crush the extended-release tablets.

• A wax-matrix "ghost" from the tablet may be passed in stools. Drug is completely absorbed before this occurs.

I.V.

• Vials for I.V. injection contain 1 g of drug: 100 mg/ml (10 ml) or 500 mg/ml (2 ml).

• Dilute with compatible I.V. solution, such as D_5W injection, and give with the patient supine at a rate not exceeding 25 to 50 mg/minute. Keep patient supine during I.V. administration.

• Attend patient receiving infusion at all times. Use an infusion-control device to give infusion precisely.

• Monitor blood pressure and ECG continuously during I.V. administration. Watch for prolonged QTc intervals and QRS complexes, heart block, or increased arrhythmias. If such reactions occur, withhold drug, obtain rhythm strip, and notify prescriber immediately. If drug is given too rapidly, hypotension can occur. Watch closely for adverse reactions during infusion, and notify prescriber if they occur.

• **Incompatibilities:** Bretylium, esmolol, ethacrynate, milrinone, phenytoin sodium.

I.M.

• I.M. injections are a substitute for oral administration in patients who are not allowed anything by mouth. Oral dosing should be resumed as soon as possible.

ACTION

Decreases excitability, conduction velocity, automaticity, and membrane responsiveness with prolonged refractory period. Larger than usual doses may induce AV block.

Route	Onset	Peak	Duration
P.O.	Unknown	90–120 min	Unknown
I.V.	Immediate	Immediate	Unknown
I.M.	10–30 min	15–60 min	Unknown

Half-life: About 2½ to 4¾ hours.

ADVERSE REACTIONS

CNS: *fever, **seizures,*** hallucinations, psychosis, giddiness, confusion, depression, dizziness.

CV: *hypotension, **bradycardia, AV block, ventricular fibrillation, ventricular asystole.***

GI: abdominal pain, nausea, vomiting, anorexia, diarrhea, bitter taste.

Skin: *maculopapular rash, urticaria, pruritus, flushing.*

Other: *lupuslike syndrome,* **ANGIONEUROTIC EDEMA.**

INTERACTIONS

Drug-drug. *Amiodarone:* May increase procainamide level and toxicity and have additive effects on QTc interval and QRS complex. Avoid using together.

Anticholinergics: May increase antivagal effects. Monitor patient closely.

Anticholinesterases: May decrease effect of anticholinesterases. Anticholinesterase dosage may need to be increased.

Beta blockers, ranitidine, trimethoprim: May increase procainamide level. Watch for toxicity.

Cimetidine: May increase procainamide level. Avoid using together if possible. Monitor procainamide level closely and adjust the dosage as necessary.

Macrolides and related antibiotics (azithromycin, clarithromycin, erythromycin, telithromycin): May prolong the QT interval. Use with caution. Avoid use with telithromycin.

Neuromuscular blockers: May increase skeletal muscle relaxant effect. Monitor patient closely.

Quinidine, disopyramide: May enhance antiarrhythmic and hypotensive effects. Avoid using together.

Quinolones: Life-threatening arrhythmias, including torsades de pointes, can occur. Avoid using together; sparfloxacin is contraindicated.

Thioridazine, ziprasidone: May prolong QTc interval. Avoid using together.

Drug-herb. *Jimsonweed:* May adversely affect CV function. Discourage use together.

Licorice: May prolong QTc interval. Urge caution.

Drug-lifestyle. *Alcohol use:* May reduce drug level. Discourage use together.

EFFECTS ON LAB TEST RESULTS

• May increase ALT, AST, alkaline phosphatase, LDH, and bilirubin levels.

• May cause positive antinuclear antibody (ANA) titers and positive direct antiglobulin (Coombs) tests.

CONTRAINDICATIONS & CAUTIONS
• Contraindicated in patients hypersensitive to this drug and related drugs.
• Contraindicated in those with complete, second- or third-degree heart block in the absence of an artificial pacemaker. Also contraindicated in those with myasthenia gravis, systemic lupus erythematosus, or atypical ventricular tachycardia (torsades de pointes).
• Use with extreme caution in patients with ventricular tachycardia during coronary occlusion.
• Use cautiously in patients with heart failure or other conduction disturbances, such as bundle-branch heart block, sinus bradycardia, or digoxin intoxication; in those with hepatic or renal insufficiency; and in those with blood dyscrasias or bone marrow suppression.

NURSING CONSIDERATIONS
• Digitalize or cardiovert patients with atrial flutter or fibrillation before therapy with procainamide to prevent ventricular rate acceleration in patient.
• Monitor level of drug and its active metabolite N-acetylprocainamide (NAPA). To suppress ventricular arrhythmias, therapeutic levels of procainamide are 4 to 8 mcg/ml; therapeutic levels of NAPA are 10 to 30 mcg/ml.
• Monitor ECG closely. If QRS widens more than 25% or marked prolongation of the QTc interval occurs, check for overdosage.
• Hypokalemia predisposes patient to arrhythmias. Monitor electrolytes, especially potassium level.
• Elderly patients may be more likely to develop hypotension. Monitor blood pressure carefully.
• Monitor CBC frequently during first 3 months of therapy.
• Positive ANA titer is common in about 60% of patients who don't have symptoms of lupuslike syndrome. This response seems to be related to prolonged use, not dosage. May progress to systemic lupus erythematosus if drug isn't stopped.
• ***Look alike–sound alike:*** Don't confuse Procanbid with probenecid.

PATIENT TEACHING
• Stress importance of taking drug exactly as prescribed. This may require use of an alarm clock for nighttime doses.
• Instruct patient to report fever, rash, muscle pain, diarrhea, bleeding, bruises, or pleuritic chest pain.
• Tell patient not to crush or break extended-release tablets.
• Reassure patient who is taking extended-release form that a wax-matrix "ghost" from the tablet may be passed in stools. Drug is completely absorbed before this occurs.

propafenone hydrochloride
proe-PAF-a-non

Rythmol, Rythmol SR

Pharmacologic class: sodium channel antagonist
Pregnancy risk category C

AVAILABLE FORMS
Capsules (extended-release): 225 mg, 325 mg, 425 mg
Tablets (immediate-release): 150 mg, 225 mg, 300 mg

INDICATIONS & DOSAGES
➤ **To suppress life-threatening ventricular arrhythmias such as sustained ventricular tachycardia; to prevent paroxysmal supraventricular tachycardia (PSVT) and paroxysmal atrial fibrillation or flutter**
Adults: Initially, 150 mg immediate-release tablet P.O. every 8 hours. May increase dosage every 3 or 4 days to 225 mg every 8 hours. If needed, increase dosage to 300 mg every 8 hours. Maximum daily dose, 900 mg.
➤ **To prolong time until recurrence of symptomatic atrial fibrillation**
Adults: Initially, 225 mg extended-release capsule P.O. every 12 hours. May increase dose after 5 days to 325 mg P.O. every 12 hours. May increase dose to 425 mg every 12 hours.

Adjust-a-dose: For patients with hepatic impairment,reduce initial dose of immediate-release tablets by 70% to 80%.

ADMINISTRATION

P.O.

- Give drug with food, to minimize adverse GI reactions.
- Don't crush or open the extended-release capsules.

ACTION

Reduces inward sodium current in cardiac cells, prolongs refractory period in AV node, and decreases excitability, conduction velocity, and automaticity in cardiac tissue.

Route	Onset	Peak	Duration
P.O. (immediate-release)	Unknown	3½ hr	Unknown
P.O. (extended-release)	Unknown	3–8 hr	Unknown

Half-life: Estimated at 10 to 32 hours.

ADVERSE REACTIONS

CNS: *dizziness,* anxiety, ataxia, drowsiness, fatigue, headache, insomnia, syncope, tremor, weakness.
CV: ***heart failure, bradycardia, arrhythmias, ventricular tachycardia, premature ventricular contractions, ventricular fibrillation,*** atrial fibrillation, bundle-branch block, angina, chest pain, edema, first-degree AV block, hypotension, increased QRS complex, intraventricular conduction delay, palpitations.
EENT: blurred vision.
GI: *nausea, vomiting,* abdominal pain or cramps, constipation, diarrhea, dyspepsia, anorexia, flatulence, dry mouth, unusual taste.
Musculoskeletal: arthralgia.
Respiratory: dyspnea.
Skin: rash, diaphoresis.

INTERACTIONS

Drug-drug. *Antiarrhythmics:* May increase risk of prolonged QTc interval. Monitor patient closely.
Beta blockers (metoprolol, propranolol): May decrease metabolism of these drugs. Adjust dosage of beta blocker as needed.
Cimetidine: May increase propafenone levels. Monitor patient for adverse effects and toxicity.
Cyclosporine, ***digoxin:*** May increase levels of these drugs, causing toxicity. Monitor patient closely; dosage adjustment may be necessary.
Desipramine: May decrease desipramine metabolism. Monitor patient closely.
Lidocaine: May decrease lidocaine metabolism. Monitor patient for increased CNS adverse effects and lidocaine toxicity.
Local anesthetics: May increase risk of CNS toxicity. Monitor patient closely.
Mexiletine: May decrease mexiletine metabolism, increasing level and adverse reactions. Monitor mexiletine level and patient closely.
Phenobarbital, rifampin: May increase propafenone clearance. Watch for decreased antiarrhythmic effect.
Quinidine: May decrease propafenone metabolism; may be useful in certain patients refractory to propafenone and quinidine monotherapy. Monitor patient closely.
Ritonavir: May increase propafenone level, causing life-threatening arrhythmias. Avoid using together.
Theophylline: May decrease theophylline metabolism. Monitor theophylline level and ECG closely.
Warfarin: May increase warfarin level. Monitor PT and INR closely, and adjust warfarin dose as needed.

EFFECTS ON LAB TEST RESULTS

- May increase alkaline phosphatase, ALT, and AST levels.
- May cause positive ANA titers.

CONTRAINDICATIONS & CAUTIONS

- Contraindicated in patients hypersensitive to drug and in those with severe or uncontrolled heart failure; cardiogenic shock; SA, AV, or intraventricular disorders of impulse conduction without a pacemaker; bradycardia; marked hypotension; bronchospastic disorders; or electrolyte imbalances.
- Use cautiously in patients with a history of heart failure because drug may weaken the contraction of the heart.

• Use cautiously in patients taking other cardiac depressants and in those with hepatic or renal impairment.
• Use cautiously in patients with myasthenia gravis; may cause exacerbation.

NURSING CONSIDERATIONS

• *Alert:* Perform continuous cardiac monitoring at start of therapy and during dosage adjustments. If PR interval or QRS complex increases by more than 25%, reduce dosage.
• If using with digoxin, frequently monitor ECG and digoxin level.
• Pacing and sensing thresholds of artificial pacemakers may change; monitor pacemaker function.
• Agranulocytosis may develop during the first 2 to 3 months of therapy. If patient has an unexplained fever, monitor leukocyte count.

PATIENT TEACHING

• Stress importance of taking drug exactly as prescribed.
• Tell patient not to double the dose if he misses one, but to take the next dose at the usual time.
• Tell patient to report adverse reactions promptly, including fever, sore throat, chills, and other signs and symptoms of infection.
• Instruct patient to notify prescriber if prolonged diarrhea, sweating, vomiting, or loss of appetite or thirst occurs; these may cause an electrolyte imbalance.
• Tell patient not to crush, chew, or open the extended-release capsules.

SAFETY ALERT!

propranolol hydrochloride

proe-PRAN-oh-lol

Inderal, Inderal LA, InnoPran XL, Novopranol†

Pharmacologic class: beta blocker
Pregnancy risk category C

AVAILABLE FORMS

Capsules (extended-release): 60 mg, 80 mg, 120 mg, 160 mg
Injection: 1 mg/ml
Oral solution: 4 mg/ml, 8 mg/ml, 80 mg/ml (concentrate)
Tablets: 10 mg, 20 mg, 40 mg, 60 mg, 80 mg, 90 mg

INDICATIONS & DOSAGES

➤ Angina pectoris
Adults: Total daily doses of 80 to 320 mg P.O. when given b.i.d., t.i.d., or q.i.d. Or, one 80-mg extended-release capsule daily. Dosage increased at 3- to 7-day intervals.

➤ To decrease risk of death after MI
Adults: 180 to 240 mg P.O. daily in divided doses beginning 5 to 21 days after MI has occurred. Usually given t.i.d. or q.i.d.

➤ Supraventricular, ventricular, and atrial arrhythmias; tachyarrhythmias caused by excessive catecholamine action during anesthesia, hyperthyroidism, or pheochromocytoma
Adults: 1 to 3 mg by slow I.V. push, not to exceed 1 mg/minute. After 3 mg have been given, another dose may be given in 2 minutes; subsequent doses, no sooner than every 4 hours. Usual maintenance dose is 10 to 30 mg P.O. t.i.d. or q.i.d.

➤ Hypertension
Adults: Initially, 80 mg P.O. daily in two divided doses or extended-release form once daily. Increase at 3- to 7-day intervals to maximum daily dose of 640 mg. Usual maintenance dose is 120 to 240 mg daily or 120 to 160 mg daily as extended-release. For InnoPran XL, dose is 80 mg P.O. once daily at bedtime. Give consistently with or without food. Adjust to maximum of 120 mg daily if needed. Full effects are seen in about 2 to 3 weeks.
Children: 0.5 mg/kg (conventional tablets) P.O. b.i.d. Increase every 3 to 5 days to a maximum dose of 16 mg/kg daily. Usual dose is 2 to 4 mg/kg daily in two equally divided doses.

➤ To prevent frequent, severe, uncontrollable, or disabling migraine or vascular headache
Adults: Initially, 80 mg P.O. daily in divided doses or 1 extended-release capsule daily. Usual maintenance dose is 160 to 240 mg daily, t.i.d. or q.i.d.

➤ **Essential tremor**
Adults: 40 mg (tablets or oral solution) P.O. b.i.d. Usual maintenance dose is 120 to 320 mg daily in three divided doses.
➤ **Hypertrophic subaortic stenosis**
Adults: 20 to 40 mg P.O. t.i.d. or q.i.d.; or 80 to 160 mg extended-release capsules once daily.
➤ **Adjunct therapy in pheochromocytoma**
Adults: 60 mg P.O. daily in divided doses with an alpha blocker 3 days before surgery.

ADMINISTRATION

P.O.
• Give drug consistently with meals. Food may increase absorption of propranolol.
• Compliance may be improved by giving drug twice daily or as extended-release capsules. Check with prescriber.
• Check blood pressure and apical pulse before giving drug. If hypotension or extremes in pulse rate occur, withhold drug and notify prescriber.
I.V.
• For direct injection, give into a large vessel or into the tubing of a free-flowing, compatible I.V. solution; don't give by continuous I.V. infusion.
• Drug is compatible with D_5W, half-normal saline solution, normal saline solution, and lactated Ringer solution.
• Infusion rate shouldn't exceed 1 mg/minute.
• Double-check dose and route. I.V. doses are much smaller than oral doses.
• Monitor blood pressure, ECG, central venous pressure, and heart rate and rhythm frequently, especially during I.V. administration. If patient develops severe hypotension, notify prescriber; a vasopressor may be prescribed.
• For overdose, give I.V. isoproterenol, I.V. atropine, or glucagon; refractory cases may require a pacemaker.
• **Incompatibilities:** Amphotericin B, diazoxide.

ACTION

Reduces cardiac oxygen demand by blocking catecholamine-induced increases in heart rate, blood pressure, and force of myocardial contraction. Drug depresses renin secretion and prevents vasodilation of cerebral arteries.

Route	Onset	Peak	Duration
P.O.	30 min	60–90 min	12 hr
P.O. (extended)	Unknown	6–14 hr	24 hr
I.V.	Immediate	1 min	5 min

Half-life: About 4 hours; 8 hours for InnoPran XL.

ADVERSE REACTIONS

CNS: *fatigue, lethargy,* fever, vivid dreams, hallucinations, mental depression, light-headedness, dizziness, insomnia.
CV: *hypotension,* ***bradycardia, heart failure, intensification of AV block,*** intermittent claudication.
GI: abdominal cramping, constipation, diarrhea, nausea, vomiting.
Hematologic: ***agranulocytosis.***
Respiratory: ***bronchospasm.***
Skin: rash.

INTERACTIONS

Drug-drug. *Aminophylline:* May antagonize beta-blocking effects of propranolol. Use together cautiously.
Cardiac glycosides: May reduce the positive inotrope effect of the glycoside. Monitor patient for clinical effect.
Cimetidine: May inhibit metabolism of propranolol. Watch for increased beta-blocking effect.
Diltiazem, verapamil: May cause hypotension, bradycardia, and increased depressant effect on myocardium. Use together cautiously.
Epinephrine: May cause severe vasoconstriction. Monitor blood pressure and observe patient carefully.
Glucagon, isoproterenol: May antagonize propranolol effect. May be used therapeutically and in emergencies.
Haloperidol: May cause cardiac arrest. Avoid using together.
Insulin, oral antidiabetics: May alter requirements for these drugs in previously stabilized diabetics. Monitor patient for hypoglycemia.
Phenothiazines (chlorpromazine, thioridazine): May increase risk of serious adverse reactions of either drug. Use with

thioridazine is contraindicated. If chlorpromazine must be used, monitor patient's pulse and blood pressure; decrease propranolol dose as needed.
Propafenone: May increase propranolol level. Monitor cardiac function, and adjust propranolol dose as needed.
Drug-herb. *Betel palm:* May decrease temperature-elevating effects and enhanced CNS effects. Discourage use together.
Ma huang: May decrease antihypertensive effects. Discourage use together.
Drug-lifestyle. *Alcohol:* May increase propranolol level. Discourage alcohol use.
Cocaine use: May increase angina-inducing potential of cocaine. Inform patient of this interaction.

EFFECTS ON LAB TEST RESULTS

- May increase BUN, transaminase, alkaline phosphatase, potassium, and LDH levels.
- May decrease granulocyte count.

CONTRAINDICATIONS & CAUTIONS

- Contraindicated in patients with bronchial asthma, sinus bradycardia and heart block greater than first-degree, cardiogenic shock, and overt and decompensated heart failure (unless failure is secondary to a tachyarrhythmia that can be treated with propranolol).
- Use cautiously in patients with hepatic or renal impairment, nonallergic bronchospastic diseases, or hepatic disease and in those taking other antihypertensives.
- Use cautiously in patients who have diabetes mellitus because drug masks some symptoms of hypoglycemia.
- In patients with thyrotoxicosis, use drug cautiously because it may mask the signs and symptoms.
- Elderly patients may experience enhanced adverse reactions and may need dosage adjustment.
- Use cautiously in pregnant women because drug may be associated with small placenta and congenital anomalies.

NURSING CONSIDERATIONS

- Drug masks common signs and symptoms of shock and hypoglycemia.
- ***Alert:*** Don't stop drug before surgery for pheochromocytoma. Before any surgical procedure, tell anesthesiologist that patient is receiving propranolol.
- ***Look alike–sound alike:*** Don't confuse propranolol with Pravachol. Don't confuse Inderal with Inderide, Isordil, Adderall, or Imuran.

PATIENT TEACHING

- Caution patient to continue taking this drug as prescribed, even when he's feeling well.
- Instruct patient to take drug with food.
- ***Alert:*** Tell patient not to stop drug suddenly because this can worsen chest pain and trigger a heart attack.

---

protamine sulfate

PROE-ta-meen

Pharmacologic class: heparin antagonist
Pregnancy risk category C

AVAILABLE FORMS

Injection: 10 mg/ml

INDICATIONS & DOSAGES

➤ **Heparin overdose**
Adults: Base dosage on venous blood coagulation studies, usually 1 mg for each 90 to 115 units of heparin. Give by slow I.V. injection over 10 minutes in doses not to exceed 50 mg.

ADMINISTRATION

I.V.

- Have emergency equipment available to treat anaphylaxis or severe hypotension.
- Give slowly by direct injection. Excessively rapid administration may cause acute hypotension, bradycardia, pulmonary hypertension, dyspnea, transient flushing, and a feeling of warmth.
- **Incompatibilities:** Cephalosporins, diatrizoate meglumine 52% and diatrizoate sodium 8%, diatrizoate sodium 60%, ioxaglate meglumine 39.3% and ioxaglate sodium 19.6%, penicillins.

ACTION

Forms a physiologically inert complex with heparin sodium.

Route	Onset	Peak	Duration
I.V.	30–60 sec	Unknown	2 hr

Half-life: Unknown.

ADVERSE REACTIONS

CNS: lassitude.
CV: ***bradycardia, circulatory collapse,*** hypotension, transient flushing.
GI: nausea, vomiting.
Respiratory: ***acute pulmonary hypertension,*** dyspnea, ***pulmonary edema.***
Other: ***anaphylaxis, anaphylactoid reactions,*** feeling of warmth.

INTERACTIONS

None significant.

EFFECTS ON LAB TEST RESULTS

None reported.

CONTRAINDICATIONS & CAUTIONS

- Contraindicated in patients hypersensitive to drug.

NURSING CONSIDERATIONS

- Base postoperative dose on coagulation studies, and repeat activated PTT time 15 minutes after administration.
- Calculate dosage carefully. One milligram neutralizes 90 to 115 units of heparin, depending on salt (heparin calcium or heparin sodium) and source of heparin (beef or pork).
- Risk of hypersensitivity reaction increases in patients hypersensitive to fish, in vasectomized or infertile men, and in patients taking protamine-insulin products.
- Monitor patient continually.
- Watch for spontaneous bleeding (heparin rebound), especially in dialysis patients and in those who have undergone cardiac surgery.
- Drug may act as an anticoagulant in very high doses.
- ***Look alike–sound alike:*** Don't confuse protamine with Protopam.

PATIENT TEACHING

- Explain use and administration of drug to patient and family.
- Tell patient to report adverse effects.

quinapril hydrochloride

KWIN-ah-pril

Accupril

Pharmacologic class: ACE inhibitor
Pregnancy risk category C; D in 2nd and 3rd trimesters

AVAILABLE FORMS

Tablets: 5 mg, 10 mg, 20 mg, 40 mg

INDICATIONS & DOSAGES

➤ Hypertension

Adults: Initially, 10 to 20 mg P.O. daily. Dosage may be adjusted based on patient response at intervals of about 2 weeks. Most patients are controlled at 20, 40, or 80 mg daily as a single dose or in two divided doses. If patient is taking a diuretic, start therapy with 5 mg daily.
Elderly patients: For patients older than age 65, start therapy at 10 mg P.O. daily.
Adjust-a-dose: For adults with creatinine clearance over 60 ml/minute, initially, 10 mg maximum daily; for clearance of 30 to 60 ml/minute, 5 mg; for clearance of 10 to 30 ml/minute, 2.5 mg.

➤ Heart failure

Adults: If patient is taking a diuretic, give 5 mg P.O. b.i.d. initially. If patient isn't taking a diuretic, give 10 to 20 mg P.O. b.i.d. Dosage may be increased at weekly intervals. Usual effective dose is 20 to 40 mg daily in two equally divided doses.
Adjust-a-dose: For patients with creatinine clearance over 30 ml/minute, first dose is 5 mg daily; if clearance is 10 to 30 ml/minute, 2.5 mg.

ADMINISTRATION

P.O.

- Give drug 1 hour before or 2 hours after meals, or with a light meal.
- Don't give drug with a high-fat meal because this may decrease absorption of drug.

ACTION

Prevents conversion of angiotensin I to angiotensin II, a potent vasoconstrictor. Less angiotensin II decreases peripheral arterial resistance, decreasing aldosterone secretion, which reduces sodium and water retention and lowers blood pressure.

Route	Onset	Peak	Duration
P.O.	1 hr	2–6 hr	24 hr

Half-life: 25 hours.

ADVERSE REACTIONS

CNS: somnolence, vertigo, nervousness, headache, dizziness, fatigue, depression.
CV: ***hypertensive crisis,*** palpitations, tachycardia, angina pectoris, orthostatic hypotension, rhythm disturbances.
GI: ***hemorrhage,*** dry mouth, abdominal pain, constipation, vomiting, nausea, diarrhea.
Metabolic: ***hyperkalemia.***
Respiratory: dry, persistent, tickling, nonproductive cough.
Skin: pruritus, photosensitivity reactions, diaphoresis.

INTERACTIONS

Drug-drug. *Diuretics, other antihypertensives:* May cause excessive hypotension. Stop diuretic or reduce dose of quinapril, as needed.
Lithium: May increase lithium level and lithium toxicity. Monitor lithium level.
NSAIDs: May decrease antihypertensive effects. Monitor blood pressure.
Potassium-sparing diuretics, potassium supplements: May cause hyperkalemia. Monitor patient closely.
Tetracycline: May decrease absorption if taken with quinapril. Avoid using together.
Drug-herb. *Capsaicin:* May cause cough. Discourage use together.
Ma huang: May decrease antihypertensive effects. Discourage use together.
Drug-food. *Salt substitutes containing potassium:* May cause hyperkalemia. Discourage use together.

EFFECTS ON LAB TEST RESULTS

- May increase potassium, BUN, and creatinine levels.
- May increase liver function test values.

CONTRAINDICATIONS & CAUTIONS

- Contraindicated in patients hypersensitive to ACE inhibitors and in those with a history of angioedema related to treatment with an ACE inhibitor.
- Use cautiously in patients with impaired renal function.

NURSING CONSIDERATIONS

- Assess renal and hepatic function before and periodically throughout therapy.
- Monitor blood pressure for effectiveness of therapy.
- Monitor potassium level. Risk factors for the development of hyperkalemia include renal insufficiency, diabetes, and concomitant use of drugs that raise potassium level.
- Although ACE inhibitors reduce blood pressure in all races, they reduce it less in blacks taking the ACE inhibitor alone. Black patients should take drug with a thiazide diuretic for a better response.
- ACE inhibitors appear to increase risk of angioedema in black patients.
- Other ACE inhibitors have caused agranulocytosis and neutropenia. Monitor CBC with differential counts before therapy and periodically thereafter.

PATIENT TEACHING

- Advise patient to report signs of infection, such as fever and sore throat.
- ***Alert:*** Facial and throat swelling (including swelling of the larynx) may occur, especially after first dose. Advise patient to report signs or symptoms of breathing difficulty or swelling of face, eyes, lips, or tongue.
- Light-headedness can occur, especially during first few days of therapy. Tell patient to rise slowly to minimize effect and to report signs and symptoms to prescriber. If he faints, patient should stop taking drug and call prescriber immediately.
- Inform patient that inadequate fluid intake, vomiting, diarrhea, and excessive perspiration can lead to light-headedness and fainting. Tell him to use caution in hot weather and during exercise.
- Tell patient to avoid salt substitutes. These products may contain potassium, which can cause high potassium level in patients taking quinapril.
- Advise woman of childbearing age to notify prescriber if pregnancy occurs. Drug will need to be stopped.

• Tell patient to avoid taking with a high-fat meal because this may decrease absorption of drug.

quinidine gluconate
KWIN-i-deen

quinidine sulfate
Biquin Durules†

Pharmacologic class: cinchona alkaloid
Pregnancy risk category C

AVAILABLE FORMS
quinidine gluconate (62% quinidine base)
Injection: 80 mg/ml
Tablets (extended-release): 324 mg, 325 mg†
quinidine sulfate (83% quinidine base)
Injection: 200 mg/ml†
Tablets: 200 mg, 250 mg†, 300 mg
Tablets (extended-release): 300 mg

INDICATIONS & DOSAGES
➤ **Atrial flutter or fibrillation**
Adults: 300 to 400 mg quinidine sulfate or equivalent base P.O. every 6 hours. Or, 200 mg P.O. every 2 to 3 hours for five to eight doses, increased daily until sinus rhythm is restored or toxic effects develop. Maximum, 3 to 4 g daily.
Children ♦: 30 mg/kg or 900 mg/m^2 P.O. (sulfate) or I.V. or I.M. (gluconate) daily in five divided doses.
➤ **Paroxysmal supraventricular tachycardia**
Adults: 400 to 600 mg P.O. gluconate every 2 to 3 hours until toxic adverse reactions develop or arrhythmia subsides.
Children ♦: 30 mg/kg or 900 mg/m^2 P.O. (sulfate) or I.V. or I.M. (gluconate) daily in five divided doses.
➤ **Premature atrial and ventricular contractions, paroxysmal AV junctional rhythm, paroxysmal atrial tachycardia, paroxysmal ventricular tachycardia, maintenance after cardioversion of atrial fibrillation or flutter**
Adults: Test dose is 200 mg P.O. or I.M. Quinidine sulfate or equivalent base 200 to 400 mg P.O. every 4 to 6 hours or 600 mg quinidine sulfate extended-release every 8 to 12 hours; or 324 mg quinidine gluconate extended-release tablets every 8 to 12 hours; or quinidine gluconate 800 mg (10 ml of commercially available solution) added to 40 ml of D_5W, infused I.V. at 0.25 mg/kg/minute.
Children ♦: 30 mg/kg or 900 mg/m^2 P.O. (sulfate) or I.V. or I.M. (gluconate) daily in five divided doses.
➤ **Severe *Plasmodium falciparum* malaria**
Adults: 10 mg/kg gluconate I.V. diluted in 250 ml normal saline solution and infused over 1 to 2 hours; then begin a continuous infusion of 0.02 mg/kg/minute for at least 24 hours, and until parasitemia is reduced to less than 1% and oral therapy can be started. Or, give a loading dose of 24 mg/kg of quinidine gluconate I.V. diluted in 250 ml of normal saline and infused over 4 hours; then 4 hours later, give maintenance dose of 12 mg/kg of quinidine gluconate given by I.V. infusion over 4 hours at 8-hour intervals until three maintenance doses have been given and parasitemia is reduced to less than 1% and oral quinidine sulfate can be initiated.
Children ♦: 10 mg/kg gluconate I.V. over 1 to 2 hours; then continuous infusion of 0.02 mg/kg/minute.
Adjust-a-dose: In patients with hepatic impairment or heart failure, reduce dosage.

ADMINISTRATION
P.O.
• Give drug with food to avoid adverse GI reactions.
• Don't crush or open extended-release tablets. If necessary, scored tablets may be broken in half to adjust quinidine dose.
• Don't give drug with grapefruit juice.
I.V.
• For quinidine gluconate infusion to treat atrial fibrillation or flutter in adults, dilute 800 mg (10 ml of injection) with 40 ml D_5W and infuse at up to 0.25 mg/kg/minute.
• For quinidine gluconate infusion to treat malaria, dilute in 5 ml/kg (usually 250 ml) normal saline solution and infuse

over 1 to 2 hours, followed by a continuous maintenance infusion.
- During infusion, continuously monitor patient's blood pressure and ECG.
- Adjust rate so that the arrhythmia is corrected without disturbing the normal mechanism of the heartbeat.
- Never use discolored (brownish) quinidine solution.
- Store drug away from heat and direct light.
- **Incompatibilities:** Alkalies, amiodarone, atracurium besylate, furosemide, heparin sodium, iodides.

I.M.
- Never use discolored (brownish) quinidine solution.
- Quinidine gluconate I.M. is no longer recommended for arrhythmias because of erratic absorption.
- Store drug away from heat and direct light.

ACTION
A class IA antiarrhythmic with direct and indirect (anticholinergic) effects on cardiac tissue. Decreases automaticity, conduction velocity, and membrane responsiveness; prolongs effective refractory period; and reduces vagal tone.

Route	Onset	Peak	Duration
P.O.	1–3 hr	1–6 hr	6–8 hr
I.V.	Immediate	Immediate	Unknown
I.M.	Unknown	30–90 min	Unknown

Half-life: 5 to 12 hours.

ADVERSE REACTIONS
CNS: *vertigo, fever, headache, lightheadedness,* ataxia, confusion, depression, dementia.
CV: *ECG changes, tachycardia,* ***PVCs, ventricular tachycardia, atypical ventricular tachycardia, complete AV block, aggravated heart failure,*** hypotension.
EENT: *tinnitus,* blurred vision, diplopia, photophobia.
GI: *diarrhea, nausea, vomiting,* anorexia, excessive salivation, abdominal pain.
Hematologic: ***thrombocytopenia, agranulocytosis,*** hemolytic anemia.
Hepatic: ***hepatotoxicity.***
Respiratory: ***acute asthmatic attack, respiratory arrest.***
Skin: rash, petechial hemorrhage of buccal mucosa, pruritus, urticaria, photosensitivity reactions.
Other: *cinchonism,* ***angioedema,*** lupus erythematosus.

INTERACTIONS
Drug-drug. *Antacids, sodium bicarbonate:* May increase quinidine level. Monitor patient for increased effect.
Amiloride: May increase the risk of arrhythmias. If use together can't be avoided, monitor ECG closely.
Amiodarone: May increase quinidine level, producing life-threatening cardiac arrhythmias. Monitor quinidine level closely if use together can't be avoided. Adjust quinidine as needed.
Azole antifungals: May increase the risk of cardiovascular events. Use together is contraindicated.
Barbiturates, phenytoin, rifampin: May decrease quinidine level. Monitor patient for decreased effect.
Cimetidine: May increase quinidine level. Monitor patient for increased arrhythmias.
Digoxin: May increase digoxin level after starting quinidine therapy. Monitor digoxin level.
Drugs that prolong the QT interval (antipsychotics, disopyramide, procainamide, tricyclic antidepressants, sotalol): May have additive effect with quinidine and cause life-threatening cardiac arrhythmias. Avoid using together when possible.
Fluvoxamine, nefazodone, tricyclic antidepressants: May increase antidepressant level, thus increasing its effect. Monitor patient for adverse reactions.
Macrolides and related antibiotics (azithromycin, clarithromycin, erythromycin, telithromycin): May cause additive effects or prolongation of the QT interval. Use with caution. Avoid use with telithromycin.
Neuromuscular blockers: May potentiate effects of these drugs. Avoid use of quinidine immediately after surgery.
Nifedipine: May decrease quinidine level. May need to adjust dosage.
Other antiarrhythmics (such as lidocaine, procainamide, propranolol): May increase risk of toxicity. Use together cautiously.

Protease inhibitors (nelfinavir, ritonavir): May significantly increase quinidine levels and toxicity. Use together is contraindicated.
Quinolones: Life-threatening arrhythmias, including torsades de pointes, can occur. Avoid using together.
Verapamil: May decrease quinidine clearance and cause hypotension, bradycardia, AV block, or pulmonary edema. Monitor blood pressure and heart rate.
Warfarin: May increase anticoagulant effect. Monitor patient closely.
Drug-herb. *Jimsonweed:* May adversely affect CV function. Discourage use together.
Licorice: May have additive effect and prolong QT interval. Urge caution.
Drug-food. *Grapefruit:* May delay absorption and onset of action of drug. Discourage use together.

EFFECTS ON LAB TEST RESULTS

- May decrease hemoglobin level.
- May decrease platelet and granulocyte counts.

CONTRAINDICATIONS & CAUTIONS

- Contraindicated in patients with idiosyncrasy or hypersensitivity to quinidine or related cinchona derivatives.
- Contraindicated in those with myasthenia gravis, intraventricular conduction defects, digoxin toxicity when AV conduction is grossly impaired, abnormal rhythms caused by escape mechanisms, complete AV block, history of drug-induced torsades de pointes, and history of prolonged QT interval syndrome.
- Contraindicated in patients who developed thrombocytopenia after exposure to quinidine or quinine.
- Use cautiously in patients with asthma, muscle weakness, or infection accompanied by fever because hypersensitivity reactions to drug may be masked.
- Use cautiously in patients with hepatic or renal impairment because systemic accumulation may occur.

NURSING CONSIDERATIONS

- Check apical pulse rate and blood pressure before therapy. If extremes in pulse rate are detected, withhold drug and notify prescriber at once.
- ***Alert:*** For atrial fibrillation or flutter, give quinidine only after AV node has been blocked with a beta blocker, digoxin, or a calcium channel blocker to avoid increasing AV conduction.
- Anticoagulant therapy is commonly advised before quinidine therapy in long-standing atrial fibrillation because restoration of normal sinus rhythm may result in thromboembolism caused by dislodgment of thrombi from atrial wall.
- Monitor patient for atypical ventricular tachycardia, such as torsades de pointes and ECG changes, particularly widening of QRS complex, widened QT and PR intervals.
- ***Alert:*** When changing route of administration or oral salt form, prescriber should alter dosage to compensate for variations in quinidine base content.
- ***Alert:*** Hospitalize patients with severe malaria in an intensive care setting, with continuous monitoring. Decrease infusion rate if quinidine level exceeds 6 mcg/ml, uncorrected QT interval exceeds 0.6 seconds, or QRS complex widening exceeds 25% of baseline.
- Monitor liver function test results during first 4 to 8 weeks of therapy.
- Monitor quinidine level. Therapeutic levels for antiarrhythmic effects are 4 to 8 mcg/ml.
- Monitor patient response carefully. If adverse GI reactions occur, especially diarrhea, notify prescriber. Check quinidine level, which is increasingly toxic when greater than 10 mcg/ml. GI symptoms may be decreased by giving drug with meals or aluminum hydroxide antacids.
- ***Look alike–sound alike:*** Don't confuse quinidine with quinine or clonidine.

PATIENT TEACHING

- Stress importance of taking drug exactly as prescribed and taking it with food if adverse GI reactions occur.
- ***Alert:*** Instruct patient not to crush or chew extended-release tablets. If necessary, he may break scored tablets in half to adjust quinidine dose.

• Tell patient to avoid grapefruit juice because it may delay drug absorption and inhibit drug metabolism.
• Advise patient to report persistent or serious adverse reactions promptly, especially signs and symptoms of quinidine toxicity (ringing in the ears, visual disturbances, dizziness, headache, nausea).

ramipril

ra-MI-pril

Altace

Pharmacologic class: ACE inhibitor
Pregnancy risk category C; D in 2nd and 3rd trimesters

AVAILABLE FORMS

Capsules: 1.25 mg, 2.5 mg, 5 mg, 10 mg
Tablets: 1.25 mg, 2.5 mg, 5 mg, 10 mg

INDICATIONS & DOSAGES

➤ Hypertension
Adults: Initially, 2.5 mg P.O. once daily for patients not taking a diuretic, and 1.25 mg P.O. once daily for patients taking a diuretic. Increase dosage, if needed, based on patient response. Maintenance dose is 2.5 to 20 mg daily as a single dose or in divided doses.
Adjust-a-dose: For patients with creatinine clearance less than 40 ml/minute, give 1.25 mg P.O. daily. Adjust dosage gradually based on response. Maximum daily dose is 5 mg.

➤ Heart failure after an MI
Adults: Initially, 2.5 mg P.O. b.i.d. If hypotension occurs; decrease dosage to 1.25 mg P.O. b.i.d. Adjust as tolerated to target dosage of 5 mg P.O. b.i.d.
Adjust-a-dose: For patients with creatinine clearance less than 40 ml/minute, give 1.25 mg P.O. daily. Adjust dosage gradually based on response. Maximum dosage is 2.5 mg b.i.d.

➤ To reduce risk of MI, stroke, and death from CV causes
Adults age 55 and older: 2.5 mg P.O. once daily for 1 week, then 5 mg P.O. once daily for 3 weeks. Increase as tolerated to a maintenance dose of 10 mg P.O. once daily.
Adjust-a-dose: In patients who are hypertensive or who have recently had an MI, daily dose may be divided.

ADMINISTRATION

P.O.
• Give drug without regard for meals.
• Open capsule and sprinkle contents on a small amount of applesauce or mix with 4 oz of water or apple juice. Give to patient immediately.

ACTION

Prevents conversion of angiotensin I to angiotensin II, a potent vasoconstrictor. Less angiotensin II decreases peripheral arterial resistance, decreasing aldosterone secretion, which reduces sodium and water retention and lowers blood pressure.

Route	Onset	Peak	Duration
P.O.	1–2 hr	1–3 hr	24 hr

Half-life: 13 to 17 hours.

ADVERSE REACTIONS

CNS: headache, dizziness, fatigue, asthenia, malaise, light-headedness, anxiety, amnesia, depression, insomnia, nervousness, neuralgia, neuropathy, paresthesia, somnolence, tremor, vertigo, syncope.
CV: *hypotension,* ***heart failure, MI,*** postural hypotension, angina pectoris, chest pain, palpitations, edema.
EENT: epistaxis, tinnitus.
GI: nausea, vomiting, abdominal pain, anorexia, constipation, diarrhea, dyspepsia, dry mouth, gastroenteritis.
GU: impotence.
Metabolic: ***hyperkalemia,*** hyperglycemia, weight gain.
Musculoskeletal: arthralgia, arthritis, myalgia.
Respiratory: dyspnea, dry, persistent, tickling, nonproductive cough.
Skin: rash, dermatitis, pruritus, photosensitivity reactions, increased diaphoresis.
Other: hypersensitivity reactions.

INTERACTIONS

Drug-drug. *Diuretics:* May cause excessive hypotension, especially at start of therapy. Stop diuretic at least 3 days before

therapy begins, increase sodium intake, or reduce starting dose of ramipril.
Insulin, oral antidiabetics: May cause hypoglycemia, especially at start of ramipril therapy. Monitor glucose level closely.
Lithium: May increase lithium level. Use together cautiously and monitor lithium level.
Nesiritide: May increase hypotensive effects. Monitor blood pressure.
NSAIDs: May decrease antihypertensive effects. Monitor blood pressure.
Potassium-sparing diuretics, potassium supplements: May cause hyperkalemia; ramipril attenuates potassium loss. Monitor potassium level closely.
Drug-herb. *Capsaicin:* May cause cough. Discourage use together.
Ma huang: May decrease antihypertensive effects. Discourage use together.
Drug-food. *Salt substitutes containing potassium:* May cause hyperkalemia; ramipril attenuates potassium loss. Discourage use of salt substitutes during therapy.

EFFECTS ON LAB TEST RESULTS

• May increase BUN, creatinine, bilirubin, liver enzymes, glucose, and potassium levels. May decrease hemoglobin level and hematocrit.
• May decrease RBC and platelet counts.

CONTRAINDICATIONS & CAUTIONS

• Contraindicated in patients hypersensitive to ACE inhibitors and in those with a history of angioedema related to treatment with an ACE inhibitor.
• Use cautiously in patients with renal impairment.

NURSING CONSIDERATIONS

• Monitor blood pressure regularly for drug effectiveness.
• Closely assess renal function in patients during first few weeks of therapy. Regular assessment of renal function is advisable. Patients with severe heart failure whose renal function depends on the renin-angiotensin-aldosterone system have experienced acute renal failure during ACE inhibitor therapy. Hypertensive patients with unilateral or bilateral renal artery stenosis also may show signs of worsening renal function during first few days of therapy. Dose reduction or drug stoppage may be necessary.
• Although ACE inhibitors reduce blood pressure in all races, they reduce it less in blacks taking the ACE inhibitor alone. Black patients should take drug with a thiazide diuretic for a more favorable response.
• ACE inhibitors appear to increase risk of angioedema in black patients.
• Monitor CBC with differential counts before therapy and periodically thereafter.
• Drug may reduce hemoglobin and WBC, RBC, and platelet counts, especially in patients with impaired renal function or collagen vascular diseases (systemic lupus erythematosus or scleroderma).
• Monitor potassium level. Risk factors for the development of hyperkalemia include renal insufficiency, diabetes, and concomitant use of drugs that raise potassium level.

PATIENT TEACHING

• Tell patient to notify prescriber if any adverse reactions occur. Dosage adjustment or stoppage of drug may be needed.
• ***Alert:*** Rarely, swelling of the face and throat (including swelling of the larynx) may occur, especially after first dose. Advise patient to report signs or symptoms of breathing difficulty or swelling of face, eyes, lips, or tongue.
• Inform patient that light-headedness can occur, especially during the first few days of therapy. Tell him to rise slowly to minimize this effect and to report signs and symptoms to prescriber. If he faints, patient should stop taking drug and call prescriber immediately.
• Tell patient that if he has difficulty swallowing capsules, he can open drug and sprinkle contents on a small amount of applesauce.
• Advise patient to report signs and symptoms of infection, such as fever and sore throat.
• Tell patient to avoid salt substitutes. These products may contain potassium, which can cause high potassium level in patients taking ramipril.

• Tell woman of childbearing age to notify prescriber if pregnancy occurs. Drug will need to be stopped.

ranolazine

ran-OH-lah-zeen

Ranexa

Pharmacologic class: cardiovascular drug
Pregnancy risk category C

AVAILABLE FORMS

Tablets (extended-release): 500 mg

INDICATIONS & DOSAGES

➤ **Chronic angina, given with amlodipine, beta blockers, or nitrates, in patients who haven't achieved an adequate response with other antianginals**

Adults: Initially, 500 mg P.O. b.i.d. Increase, if needed, to maximum of 1,000 mg b.i.d.

ADMINISTRATION

P.O.

• Give drug without regard for meals.
• Give drug whole; don't crush or cut tablets.
• Don't give drug with grapefruit juice.

ACTION

May result from increased efficiency of myocardial oxygen use when myocardial metabolism is shifted away from fatty acid oxidation toward glucose oxidation. Antianginal and anti-ischemic properties don't decrease heart rate or blood pressure and don't increase myocardial work.

Route	Onset	Peak	Duration
P.O.	Rapid	2–5 hr	Unknown

Half-life: 7 hours.

ADVERSE REACTIONS

CNS: dizziness, headache.
CV: palpitations, peripheral edema, syncope.
EENT: tinnitus, vertigo.
GI: abdominal pain, constipation, dry mouth, nausea, vomiting.
Respiratory: dyspnea.

INTERACTIONS

Drug-drug. *Antipsychotics or tricyclic antidepressants metabolized by CYP2D6:* May increase levels of these drugs. Dosage reduction may be needed.
Cyclosporine, paroxetine, ritonavir: May increase ranolazine level. Use cautiously together, and monitor patient for increased adverse effects.
Digoxin: May increase digoxin level. Monitor digoxin level periodically; digoxin dosage may need to be reduced.
Diltiazem, HIV protease inhibitors, macrolide antibiotics (azithromycin, erythromycin), verapamil: May increase ranolazine level and prolong QT interval. Avoid using together.
Drugs that prolong the QT interval (antiarrhythmics, such as dofetilide, quinidine, and sotalol), antipsychotics, such as thorazine and ziprasidone: May increase the risk of prolonged QT interval. Avoid using together.
Potent CYP3A inhibitors such as ketoconazole: May increase ranolazine level. Use together is contraindicated.
Simvastatin: May increase simvastatin level. Monitor patient for adverse effects, and decrease simvastatin dosage as needed.
Drug-food. *Grapefruit:* May increase drug level and prolong QT interval. Discourage use together.

EFFECTS ON LAB TEST RESULTS

• May increase creatinine and BUN levels. May decrease hemoglobin level and hematocrit.
• May decrease eosinophil count.

CONTRAINDICATIONS & CAUTIONS

• Contraindicated in patients taking QT interval–prolonging drugs or CYP3A inhibitors (including diltiazem), and in patients with ventricular tachycardia, hepatic impairment, or a prolonged QT interval.
• Use cautiously in patients with renal impairment.
• It isn't known whether drug appears in breast milk. Patient should either stop breast-feeding or stop the drug.

NURSING CONSIDERATIONS
• *Alert:* Drug prolongs the QT interval according to the dose. If drug is given with other drugs that prolong the QTc interval, torsades de pointes or sudden death may occur. Don't exceed maximum dosage.
• Monitor ECG for prolonged QT interval and measure the QTc interval regularly.
• If patient has renal insufficiency, monitor blood pressure closely.

PATIENT TEACHING
• Teach patient about this drug's potential to affect the heart's rhythm. Advise patient to immediately report palpitations or fainting.
• Urge patient to tell prescriber about all other prescription or OTC drugs or herbal supplements he takes.
• Tell patient that he should keep taking other drugs prescribed for angina.
• Tell patient that drug may be taken with or without food.
• Advise patient to avoid grapefruit juice while taking this drug.
• *Alert:* Warn patient that tablets must be swallowed whole and not crushed, broken, or chewed.
• Explain that drug won't stop a sudden anginal attack; advise him to keep other treatments, such as S.L. nitroglycerin, readily available.
• Tell patient to avoid activities that require mental alertness until effects of the drug are known.

SAFETY ALERT!

reteplase, recombinant
RET-ah-place

Retavase

Pharmacologic class: tissue plasminogen activator
Pregnancy risk category C

AVAILABLE FORMS
Injection: 10.4 units (18.1 mg)/vial. Supplied in a kit with components for reconstitution for two single-use vials

INDICATIONS & DOSAGES
➤ To manage acute MI
Adults: Double-bolus injection of 10 + 10 units. Give each bolus I.V. over 2 minutes. If complications, such as serious bleeding or anaphylactoid reaction, don't occur after first bolus, give second bolus 30 minutes after start of first.

ADMINISTRATION
I.V.
• Reconstitute drug according to manufacturer's instructions using items provided in kit and sterile water for injection, without preservatives. Make sure reconstituted solution is colorless; resulting concentration is 1 unit/ml. If foaming occurs, let vial stand for several minutes. Inspect for precipitation. Use within 4 hours of reconstitution; discard unused portions.
• Give as a double-bolus injection. If bleeding or anaphylactoid reaction occurs after first bolus, notify prescriber; second bolus may be withheld.
• **Incompatibilities:** Other I.V. drugs.

ACTION
Enhances cleavage of plasminogen to generate plasmin, which leads to fibrinolysis.

Route	Onset	Peak	Duration
I.V.	Unknown	Unknown	Unknown

Half-life: 13 to 16 minutes.

ADVERSE REACTIONS
CNS: ***intracranial hemorrhage.***
CV: ***arrhythmias, cholesterol embolization, hemorrhage.***
GI: ***hemorrhage.***
GU: hematuria.
Hematologic: ***bleeding tendency,*** anemia.
Other: bleeding at puncture sites, hypersensitivity reactions.

INTERACTIONS
Drug-drug. *Heparin, oral anticoagulants, platelet inhibitors (abciximab, aspirin, dipyridamole, eptifibatide, tirofiban):* May increase risk of bleeding. Use together cautiously.

EFFECTS ON LAB TEST RESULTS

- May increase PT, PTT, and INR.
- May alter coagulation study results.

CONTRAINDICATIONS & CAUTIONS

- Contraindicated in patients with active internal bleeding, known bleeding diathesis, history of stroke, recent intracranial or intraspinal surgery or trauma, severe uncontrolled hypertension, intracranial neoplasm, arteriovenous malformation, or aneurysm.
- Use cautiously in patients with previous puncture of noncompressible vessels; in those with recent (within 10 days) major surgery, obstetric delivery, organ biopsy, GI or GU bleeding, or trauma; in those with cerebrovascular disease, systolic blood pressure 180 mm Hg or higher or diastolic pressure 110 mm Hg or higher, and conditions that may lead to left heart thrombus, including mitral stenosis, acute pericarditis, subacute bacterial endocarditis, and hemostatic defects.
- Use cautiously in those with diabetic hemorrhagic retinopathy, septic thrombophlebitis, and other conditions in which bleeding would be difficult to manage.
- Use cautiously in patients age 75 and older and in breast-feeding women.

NURSING CONSIDERATIONS

- Drug remains active in vitro and can lead to degradation of fibrinogen in sample, changing coagulation study results. Collect blood samples with chloromethylketone at 2-micromolar concentrations.
- Drug may be given to menstruating women.
- Carefully monitor ECG during treatment. Coronary thrombolysis may cause arrhythmias linked with reperfusion. Be prepared to treat bradycardia or ventricular irritability.
- Closely monitor patient for bleeding. Avoid I.M. injections, invasive procedures, and nonessential handling of patient. Bleeding is the most common adverse reaction and may occur internally or at external puncture sites. If local measures don't control serious bleeding, stop anticoagulant and notify prescriber. Withhold second bolus of reteplase.
- Potency is expressed in units specific to reteplase and isn't comparable with other thrombolytics.
- Avoid use of noncompressible puncture sites during therapy. If an arterial puncture is needed, use an arm vessel that can be compressed manually. Apply pressure for at least 30 minutes; then apply a pressure dressing. Check site frequently.

PATIENT TEACHING

- Explain use and administration of drug to patient and family.
- Tell patient to report adverse reactions immediately.

---

rosuvastatin calcium

row-SUE-va-sta-tin

Crestor

Pharmacologic class: HMG-CoA reductase inhibitor
Pregnancy risk category X

AVAILABLE FORMS

Tablets: 5 mg, 10 mg, 20 mg, 40 mg

INDICATIONS & DOSAGES

➤ **Adjunct to diet to reduce LDL cholesterol, total cholesterol, apolipoprotein B, non-HDL cholesterol, and triglyceride (TG) levels and to increase HDL cholesterol level in patients with primary hypercholesterolemia (heterozygous familial and nonfamilial) and mixed dyslipidemia (Fredrickson types IIa and IIb); adjunct to diet to treat elevated TG level (Fredrickson type IV)**

Adults: Initially, 10 mg P.O. once daily; 5 mg P.O. once daily in patients needing less aggressive LDL cholesterol level reduction or those predisposed to myopathy. For aggressive lipid lowering, initially, 20 mg P.O. once daily. Increase as needed to maximum of 40 mg P.O. daily. Dosage may be increased every 2 to 4 weeks, based on lipid levels.

✷***NEW INDICATION:*** **Adjunct to diet to slow atherosclerosis progression in patients with elevated cholesterol**

Adults: Initially, 10 mg P.O. daily. Increase as needed every 2 to 4 weeks based on lipid levels, to maximum of 40 mg daily.

➤ **Adjunct to lipid-lowering therapies; to reduce LDL cholesterol, apolipoprotein B, and total cholesterol levels in homozygous familial hypercholesterolemia**

Adults: Initially, 20 mg P.O. once daily. Maximum, 40 mg once daily.

Adjust-a-dose: If creatinine clearance is less than 30 ml/minute, initially, 5 mg once daily; don't exceed 10 mg once daily. For patients requiring less aggressive treatment, those at risk for myopathy, Asian patients, and patients also taking cyclosporine, initial dose is 5 mg.

ADMINISTRATION

P.O.

- Give drug without regard for meals.
- Wait 2 hours after giving dose to give aluminum- or magnesium-containing antacid.

ACTION

Inhibits HMG-CoA reductase, increases LDL receptors on liver cells, and inhibits hepatic synthesis of very–low-density lipoprotein.

Route	Onset	Peak	Duration
P.O.	Unknown	3–5 hr	Unknown

Half-life: About 19 hours.

ADVERSE REACTIONS

CNS: anxiety, asthenia, depression, dizziness, headache, insomnia, neuralgia, paresthesia, vertigo.
CV: angina pectoris, chest pain, hypertension, palpitations, peripheral edema, vasodilation.
EENT: pharyngitis, rhinitis, sinusitis.
GI: abdominal pain, constipation, diarrhea, dyspepsia, flatulence, gastritis, gastroenteritis, nausea, periodontal abscess, vomiting.
GU: UTI.
Hematologic: anemia, ecchymosis.
Metabolic: diabetes mellitus.
Musculoskeletal: arthralgia, arthritis, back pain, hypertonia, myalgia, neck pain, pain, pathologic fracture, pelvic pain.
Respiratory: asthma, bronchitis, dyspnea, increased cough, pneumonia.
Skin: pruritus, rash.
Other: accidental injury, flulike syndrome, infection.

INTERACTIONS

Drug-drug. *Antacids:* May decrease rosuvastatin level. Give antacids at least 2 hours after rosuvastatin.
Cimetidine, ketoconazole, spironolactone: May decrease level or effect of endogenous steroid hormones. Use together cautiously.
Cyclosporine: May increase rosuvastatin level and risk of myopathy or rhabdomyolysis. Don't exceed 5 mg of rosuvastatin daily. Watch for evidence of toxicity.
Gemfibrozil: May increase rosuvastatin level and risk of myopathy or rhabdomyolysis. Don't exceed 10 mg of rosuvastatin once daily. Watch for evidence of toxicity.
Hormonal contraceptives: May increase ethinyl estradiol and norgestrel levels. Watch for adverse effects.
Warfarin: May increase INR and risk of bleeding. Monitor INR, and watch for evidence of increased bleeding.
Drug-lifestyle. *Alcohol use:* May increase risk of hepatotoxicity. Discourage use together.

EFFECTS ON LAB TEST RESULTS

- May increase CK, transaminase, glucose, glutamyl transpeptidase, alkaline phosphatase, and bilirubin levels. May decrease hemoglobin level and hematocrit.
- May cause thyroid function abnormalities, dipstick-positive proteinuria, and microscopic hematuria.

CONTRAINDICATIONS & CAUTIONS

- Contraindicated in patients hypersensitive to rosuvastatin or its components, pregnant patients, patients with active liver disease, and those with unexplained persistently increased transaminases.
- Use cautiously in patients who drink substantial amounts of alcohol or have a history of liver disease and in those at increased risk for myopathies, such as those with renal impairment, advanced age, or hypothyroidism.

• Use cautiously in Asian patients because they have a greater risk of elevated drug levels.

NURSING CONSIDERATIONS

• Before therapy starts, assess patient for underlying causes of hypercholesterolemia, including poorly controlled diabetes, hypothyroidism, nephrotic syndrome, dyslipoproteinemias, obstructive liver disease, drug interaction, and alcoholism.
• Before therapy starts, advise patient to control hypercholesterolemia with diet, exercise, and weight reduction.
• Test liver function before therapy starts, 12 weeks afterward, 12 weeks after any increase in dosage, and twice a year routinely. If AST or ALT level persists at more than three times the upper limit of normal, decrease dose or stop drug.
• ***Alert:*** Rarely, rhabdomyolysis with acute renal failure has developed in patients taking drugs in this class, including rosuvastatin.
• Patients who are 65 or older, have hypothyroidism, or have renal insufficiency may be at a greater risk for developing myopathy while receiving a statin.
• Notify prescriber if CK level becomes markedly elevated or myopathy is suspected, or if routine urinalysis shows persistent proteinuria and patient is taking 40 mg daily.
• Withhold drug temporarily if patient becomes predisposed to myopathy or rhabdomyolysis because of sepsis, hypotension, major surgery, trauma, uncontrolled seizures, or severe metabolic, endocrine, or electrolyte disorders.

PATIENT TEACHING

• Instruct patient to take drug exactly as prescribed.
• Teach patient about diet, exercise, and weight control.
• Tell patient to immediately report unexplained muscle pain, tenderness, or weakness, especially if accompanied by malaise or fever.
• Instruct patient to take drug at least 2 hours before taking aluminum- or magnesium-containing antacids.

sibutramine hydrochloride monohydrate

sih-BUH-trah-meen

Meridia

Pharmacologic class: norepinephrine, serotonin, and dopamine reuptake inhibitor
Pregnancy risk category C
Controlled substance schedule IV

AVAILABLE FORMS

Capsules: 5 mg, 10 mg, 15 mg

INDICATIONS & DOSAGES

➤ **To manage obesity**
Adults: 10 mg P.O. given once daily. May increase to 15 mg P.O. daily after 4 weeks if weight loss is inadequate. Patients who don't tolerate 10 mg daily may receive 5 mg P.O. daily. Don't exceed 15 mg daily.

ADMINISTRATION

P.O.
• Give drug without regard for food.

ACTION

Inhibits reuptake of norepinephrine and, to a lesser extent, serotonin and dopamine.

Route	Onset	Peak	Duration
P.O.	Unknown	3–4 hr	Unknown

Half-life: About 15 hours.

ADVERSE REACTIONS

CNS: *headache, insomnia,* dizziness, nervousness, anxiety, depression, paresthesia, somnolence, CNS stimulation, emotional lability, asthenia, migraine.
CV: tachycardia, vasodilation, hypertension, palpitations, chest pain, generalized edema.
EENT: *rhinitis, pharyngitis,* sinusitis, ear disorder, ear pain.
GI: *anorexia, constipation, dry mouth,* thirst, increased appetite, nausea, dyspepsia, gastritis, vomiting, taste perversion, abdominal pain, rectal disorder.
GU: dysmenorrhea, UTI, vaginal candidiasis, metrorrhagia.

Musculoskeletal: arthralgia, myalgia, tenosynovitis, joint disorder, neck or back pain.
Respiratory: increased cough, laryngitis.
Skin: rash, sweating, acne.
Other: herpes simplex, flulike syndrome, accidental injury, allergic reaction.

INTERACTIONS

Drug-drug. *CNS depressants:* May enhance CNS depression. Use together cautiously.
Dextromethorphan, dihydroergotamine, fentanyl, fluoxetine, fluvoxamine, lithium, MAO inhibitors, meperidine, paroxetine, pentazocine, sertraline, sumatriptan, tryptophan, venlafaxine: May cause hyperthermia, tachycardia, and loss of consciousness. Avoid using together.
Ephedrine, pseudoephedrine: May increase blood pressure or heart rate. Use together cautiously.
Drug-lifestyle. *Alcohol use:* May enhance CNS depression. Discourage use together.

EFFECTS ON LAB TEST RESULTS

- May increase ALT, AST, GGT, LDH, alkaline phosphatase, and bilirubin levels.

CONTRAINDICATIONS & CAUTIONS

- Contraindicated in patients hypersensitive to drug or its active ingredients, in those taking MAO inhibitors or other centrally acting appetite suppressants, and in those with anorexia nervosa.
- Contraindicated in patients with severe renal or hepatic dysfunction, history of hypertension, coronary artery disease, heart failure, arrhythmias, or stroke.
- Contraindicated in elderly patients.
- Use cautiously in patients with history of seizures or angle-closure glaucoma.

NURSING CONSIDERATIONS

- Measure blood pressure and pulse before starting therapy, with dosage changes, and at regular intervals during therapy.
- Use drug in obese patients with a body mass index of 30 or more (27 or more if patient has other risk factors, such as hypertension, diabetes, or dyslipidemia).
- Avoid using drug within 2 weeks of MAO inhibitor.
- *Alert:* Combining this drug with triptans, SSRIs, or SSNRIs may cause serotonin syndrome. Symptoms include restlessness, hallucinations, loss of coordination, fast heartbeat, rapid changes in blood pressure, increased body temperature, hyperreflexia, nausea, vomiting, and diarrhea. The syndrome is more likely to occur when starting or increasing the dose of the triptan, SSRI, or SSNRI.

PATIENT TEACHING

- Advise patient to report rash, hives, or other allergic reactions immediately.
- Instruct patient to notify prescriber before taking other prescription or OTC drugs.
- Advise patient to have blood pressure and pulse monitored at regular intervals. Stress importance of regular follow-up visits with prescriber.
- Advise patient to follow a reduced-calorie diet.
- Tell patient that weight loss can cause gallstones. Teach signs and symptoms, and tell patient to notify prescriber promptly if they occur.
- Tell patient to take drug daily in the morning to avoid sleep disturbances.

sildenafil citrate

sill-DEN-ah-fill

Revatio

Pharmacologic class: cyclic guanosine monophosphate (cGMP)-specific phosphodiesterase type-5, or PDE5, inhibitor
Pregnancy risk category B

AVAILABLE FORMS

Tablets: 20 mg

INDICATIONS & DOSAGES

➤ To improve exercise ability in patients with World Health Organization group I pulmonary arterial hypertension (PAH)
Adults: 20 mg P.O. t.i.d., 4 to 6 hours apart.

ADMINISTRATION

P.O.

- Give drug without regard for food.
- Don't give to patients taking nitrates.

ACTION

Increases cGMP level by preventing its breakdown by phosphodiesterase, prolonging smooth muscle relaxation of the pulmonary vasculature, which leads to vasodilation.

Route	Onset	Peak	Duration
P.O.	15–30 min	30–120 min	4 hr

Half-life: 4 hours.

ADVERSE REACTIONS

CNS: *headache,* dizziness, fever.
CV: *flushing,* hypotension.
EENT: blurred vision, burning, epistaxis, impaired color discrimination, photophobia, rhinitis, sinusitis.
GI: *dyspepsia,* diarrhea, gastritis.
Musculoskeletal: myalgia.
Skin: erythema.

INTERACTIONS

Drug-drug. *Alpha blockers:* May cause symptomatic hypotension. Consider dosage reduction.
Amlodipine: May further reduce blood pressure. Monitor blood pressure closely.
Bosentan: May decrease sildenafil level. Monitor patient.
Cytochrome P-450 inducers, rifampin: May reduce sildenafil level. Monitor effect.
Hepatic isoenzyme inhibitors (such as cimetidine, erythromycin, itraconazole, ketoconazole): May increase sildenafil level. Avoid using together.
Isosorbide, nitroglycerin: May cause severe hypotension. Use of nitrates in any form is contraindicated during therapy.
Protease inhibitors (ritonavir): May significantly increase sildenafil level. Don't use together.
Vitamin K antagonists: May increase risk of bleeding (primarily epistaxis). Monitor patient.
Drug-food. *Grapefruit:* May increase drug level, while delaying absorption. Discourage use together.

EFFECTS ON LAB TEST RESULTS

None reported.

CONTRAINDICATIONS & CAUTIONS

- Contraindicated in patients hypersensitive to drug or its components and in those taking organic nitrates.
- Don't use in patients with pulmonary veno-occlusive disease.
- Use cautiously in patients with resting hypotension, severe left ventricular outflow obstruction, autonomic dysfunction, and volume depletion.
- Use cautiously in elderly patients; in patients with hepatic or severe renal impairment, retinitis pigmentosa, bleeding disorders, or active peptic ulcer disease; in those who have suffered an MI, stroke, or life-threatening arrhythmia in last 6 months; in those with history of coronary artery disease causing unstable angina or of uncontrolled high or low blood pressure; in those with deformation of the penis or with conditions that may cause priapism (such as sickle cell anemia, multiple myeloma, or leukemia); and in those taking bosentan.
- It's unknown if drug appears in breast milk. Use cautiously in breast-feeding women.
- Safety and efficacy in children haven't been established.

NURSING CONSIDERATIONS

- The serious CV events linked to this drug's use in erectile dysfunction mainly involve patients with underlying CV disease who are at increased risk for cardiac effects related to sexual activity.
- Patients with PAH caused by connective tissue disease are more prone to epistaxis during therapy than those with primary pulmonary hypertension.
- ***Alert:*** Don't substitute Viagra for Revatio because there isn't an equivalent dose.

PATIENT TEACHING

- Warn patient that drug should never be used with nitrates.
- Advise patient to rise slowly from lying down.
- Inform patient that drug can be taken with or without food.

• Warn patient that discrimination between colors, such as blue and green, may become impaired during therapy; warn him to avoid hazardous activities that rely on color discrimination.
• Instruct patient to notify prescriber of visual changes, dizziness, or fainting.
• Caution patient to take drug only as prescribed.

simvastatin (synvinolin)
sim-va-STAH-tin

Zocor

Pharmacologic class: HMG-CoA reductase inhibitor
Pregnancy risk category X

AVAILABLE FORMS
Tablets: 5 mg, 10 mg, 20 mg, 40 mg, 80 mg

INDICATIONS & DOSAGES
➤ **To reduce risk of death from CV disease and CV events in patients at high risk for coronary events**
Adults: Initially, 20 to 40 mg P.O. daily in evening. In patients at high risk for a coronary heart disease event due to existing coronary heart disease, diabetes, peripheral vascular disease, or history of stroke, the recommended initial dose is 40 mg P.O. daily. Adjust dosage every 4 weeks based on patient tolerance and response. Maximum, 80 mg daily.
➤ **To reduce total and LDL cholesterol levels in patients with homozygous familial hypercholesterolemia**
Adults: 40 mg daily in evening; or, 80 mg daily in three divided doses of 20 mg in morning, 20 mg in afternoon, and 40 mg in evening.
➤ **Heterozygous familial hypercholesterolemia**
Children ages 10 to 17: Give 10 mg P.O. once daily in the evening. Maximum, 40 mg daily.
Adjust-a-dose: For patients taking cyclosporine, begin with 5 mg P.O. simvastatin daily; don't exceed 10 mg P.O. simvastatin daily. In patients taking fibrates or niacin, maximum is 10 mg P.O. simvastatin daily. In patients taking amiodarone or verapamil, maximum is 20 mg P.O. simvastatin daily. In patients with severe renal insufficiency, start with 5 mg P.O. daily.

ADMINISTRATION
P.O.
• Give drug in the evening.

ACTION
Inhibits HMG-CoA reductase, an early (and rate-limiting) step in cholesterol biosynthesis.

Route	Onset	Peak	Duration
P.O.	Unknown	1–2 hr	Unknown

Half-life: 3 hours.

ADVERSE REACTIONS
CNS: asthenia, headache.
GI: abdominal pain, constipation, diarrhea, dyspepsia, flatulence, *nausea, vomiting.*
Respiratory: upper respiratory tract infection.

INTERACTIONS
Drug-drug. *Amiodarone,* ***verapamil:*** May increase risk of myopathy and rhabdomyolysis. Don't exceed 20 mg simvastatin daily.
Cyclosporine, *fibrates, niacin:* May increase risk of myopathy and rhabdomyolysis. Avoid using together; if unavoidable, monitor patient closely and don't exceed 10 mg simvastatin daily.
Digoxin: May slightly increase digoxin level. Closely monitor digoxin levels at the start of simvastatin therapy.
Diltiazem, macrolides (azithromycin, clarithromycin, erythromycin, telithromycin), nefazodone: May decrease metabolism of HMG-CoA reductase inhibitor, increasing toxicity. Monitor patient for adverse effects and report unexplained muscle pain.
Fluconazole, itraconazole, ketoconazole: May increase simvastatin level and adverse effects. Avoid using together or, if it can't be avoided, reduce dose of simvastatin.
Hepatotoxic drugs: May increase risk for hepatotoxicity. Avoid using together.
Protease inhibitors (amprenavir, atazanavir, indinavir, lopinavir and ritonavir, nelfinavir,

ritonavir, saquinavir): May inhibit metabolism of simvastatin and increase the risk of adverse effects, including rhabdomyolysis. Avoid using together.
Warfarin: May slightly enhance anticoagulant effect. Monitor PT and INR when therapy starts or dose is adjusted.
Drug-herb. *Eucalyptus, jin bu huan, kava:* May increase risk of hepatotoxicity. Discourage use together.
Red yeast rice: May increase risk of adverse events or toxicity because it contains similar components to those in drugs. Discourage use together.
Drug-food. *Grapefruit juice:* May increase drug levels, increasing risk of adverse effects including myopathy and rhabdomyolysis. Discourage use together.
Drug-lifestyle. *Alcohol use:* May increase risk of hepatotoxicity. Discourage use together.

EFFECTS ON LAB TEST RESULTS
- May increase ALT, AST, and CK levels.

CONTRAINDICATIONS & CAUTIONS
- Contraindicated in patients hypersensitive to drug and in those with active liver disease or conditions that cause unexplained persistent elevations of transaminase levels.
- Contraindicated in pregnant and breast-feeding women and in women of childbearing age.
- Use cautiously in patients who consume large amounts of alcohol or have a history of liver disease.

NURSING CONSIDERATIONS
- Patient should follow a diet restricted in saturated fat and cholesterol during therapy.
- Obtain liver function test results at start of therapy and then periodically. A liver biopsy may be performed if enzyme elevations persist.
- A daily dose of 40 mg significantly reduces risk of death from coronary heart disease, nonfatal MIs, stroke, and revascularization procedures.
- ***Look alike–sound alike:*** Don't confuse Zocor with Cozaar.

PATIENT TEACHING
- Instruct patient to take drug in the evening.
- Teach patient about proper dietary management of cholesterol and triglycerides. When appropriate, recommend weight control, exercise, and smoking cessation programs.
- Tell patient to inform prescriber if adverse reactions occur, particularly muscle aches and pains.
- ***Alert:*** Tell woman to stop drug and notify prescriber immediately if she is or may be pregnant or if she's breast-feeding.

sotalol hydrochloride
SOH-ta-lol

Betapace, Betapace AF, Rylosol†

Pharmacologic class: nonselective beta blocker
Pregnancy risk category B

AVAILABLE FORMS
Betapace
Tablets: 80 mg, 120 mg, 160 mg, 240 mg
Betapace AF
Tablets: 80 mg, 120 mg, 160 mg

INDICATIONS & DOSAGES
➤ Documented, life-threatening ventricular arrhythmias
Adults: Initially, 80 mg Betapace P.O. b.i.d. Increase dosage every 3 days as needed and tolerated. Most patients respond to 160 to 320 mg/day, although some patients with refractory arrhythmias need up to 640 mg/day.
Adjust-a-dose: If creatinine clearance is 30 to 60 ml/minute, increase dosage interval to every 24 hours; if clearance is 10 to 29 ml/minute, increase interval to every 36 to 48 hours; and if clearance is less than 10 ml/minute, individualize dosage.
➤ To maintain normal sinus rhythm or to delay recurrence of atrial fibrillation or atrial flutter in patients with symptomatic atrial fibrillation or flutter who are currently in sinus rhythm

Adults: 80 mg Betapace AF P.O. b.i.d. Increase dosage as needed to 120 mg P.O. b.i.d. after 3 days if the QTc interval is less than 500 msec. Maximum dose is 160 mg P.O. b.i.d.
Adjust-a-dose: If creatinine clearance is 40 to 60 ml/minute, increase dosage interval to every 24 hours. If clearance is less than 40 ml/minute, Betapace AF is contraindicated.

ADMINISTRATION

P.O.

- Give 1 hour before or 2 hours after meals or antacids.

ACTION

Depresses sinus heart rate, slows AV conduction, decreases cardiac output, and lowers systolic and diastolic blood pressure. Drug also has class III antiarrhythmic action potential's duration and prolongation.

Route	Onset	Peak	Duration
P.O.	Unknown	2½–4 hr	Unknown

Half-life: 12 hours.

ADVERSE REACTIONS

CNS: *asthenia, headache, dizziness, weakness, fatigue, light-headedness,* sleep problems.
CV: *chest pain, palpitations,* ***bradycardia, arrhythmias, heart failure, AV block, proarrhythmic events (including polymorphic ventricular tachycardia, PVCs, ventricular fibrillation),*** edema, ECG abnormalities, hypotension.
GI: *nausea, vomiting,* diarrhea, dyspepsia.
Metabolic: hyperglycemia.
Respiratory: *dyspnea,* ***bronchospasm.***

INTERACTIONS

Drug-drug. *Antiarrhythmics:* May increase drug effects. Avoid using together.
Antihypertensives, catecholamine-depleting drugs (such as guanethidine, reserpine): May increase hypotensive effects or cause marked bradycardia. Monitor blood pressure and pulse closely.
Calcium channel blockers: May increase myocardial depression. Avoid using together.
Clonidine: May enhance rebound effect after withdrawal of clonidine. Stop sotalol several days before withdrawing clonidine.
Drugs that prolong the QT interval (Class I and III antiarrhythmics, bepridil, phenothiazines, tricyclics): May cause excessive QT prolongation. Monitor QT interval.
General anesthetics: May increase myocardial depression. Monitor patient closely.
Insulin, oral antidiabetics: May cause hyperglycemia and may mask signs and symptoms of hypoglycemia. Adjust dosage accordingly.
Macrolides and related antibiotics (azithromycin, clarithromycin, erythromycin, telithromycin): May cause additive effects or prolong the QT interval. Use with caution. Avoid use with telithromycin.
Prazosin: May increase the risk of orthostatic hypotension. Assist patient to stand slowly until effects are known.
Quinolones: May cause life-threatening arrhythmias, including torsades de pointes. Avoid using together.
Drug-food. *Any food:* May decrease absorption by 20%. Advise patient to take on empty stomach.

EFFECTS ON LAB TEST RESULTS

- May increase glucose level.
- May cause false-positive catecholamine level.

CONTRAINDICATIONS & CAUTIONS

- Contraindicated in patients hypersensitive to drug.
- Contraindicated in those with severe sinus node dysfunction, sinus bradycardia, second- and third-degree AV block unless patient has a pacemaker, congenital or acquired long QT-interval syndrome, cardiogenic shock, uncontrolled heart failure, and bronchial asthma.
- Use cautiously in patients with renal impairment or diabetes mellitus (beta blockers may mask signs and symptoms of hypoglycemia).

NURSING CONSIDERATIONS

- Because proarrhythmic events may occur at start of therapy and during dosage adjustments, hospitalize patient for a minimum of 3 days. Facilities and personnel

should be available for cardiac rhythm monitoring and interpretation of ECG.
- The baseline QTc interval must be less than or equal to 450 msec before starting Betapace AF.
- Assess patient for new or worsened symptoms of heart failure.
- Although patients receiving I.V. lidocaine may start sotalol therapy without ill effects, withdraw other antiarrhythmics before therapy begins. Sotalol therapy typically is delayed until two or three half-lives of the withdrawn drug have elapsed. After withdrawing amiodarone, give sotalol only after QT interval normalizes.
- Adjust dosage slowly, allowing 3 days between dosage increments for adequate monitoring of QT intervals and for drug levels to reach a steady-state level.
- ***Alert:*** Don't substitute Betapace for Betapace AF.
- Monitor electrolytes regularly, especially if patient is receiving diuretics. Electrolyte imbalances, such as hypokalemia or hypomagnesemia, may enhance QT-interval prolongation and increase the risk of serious arrhythmias such as torsades de pointes.
- ***Look alike–sound alike:*** Don't confuse sotalol with Stadol.

PATIENT TEACHING

- Explain to patient that he will need to be hospitalized for initiation of drug therapy.
- Stress need to take drug as prescribed, even when he is feeling well. Caution patient against stopping drug suddenly.
- Caution patient against using OTC drugs and decongestants while taking drug.
- Because food and antacids can interfere with absorption, tell patient to take drug on an empty stomach, 1 hour before or 2 hours after meals or antacids.

spironolactone

speer-on-oh-LAK-tone

Aldactone, Novospiroton†

Pharmacologic class: potassium-sparing diuretic; aldosterone receptor antagonist
Pregnancy risk category C

AVAILABLE FORMS

Tablets: 25 mg, 50 mg, 100 mg

INDICATIONS & DOSAGES

➤ Edema
Adults: Initially, 100 mg P.O. daily given as a single dose or in divided doses. Usual range is 25 to 200 mg P.O. daily.
Children: Give 3.3 mg/kg P.O. daily or in divided doses.

➤ Hypertension
Adults: 50 to 100 mg P.O. daily or in divided doses. Some practitioners use a lower dose range of 25 to 50 mg daily and add another antihypertensive to the regimen, rather than continually increasing this drug.
Children ♦: Give 1 to 3.3 mg/kg P.O. (up to 100 mg daily) as a single dose or divided b.i.d.

➤ Diuretic-induced hypokalemia
Adults: 25 to 100 mg P.O. daily.

➤ To detect primary hyperaldosteronism
Adults: 400 mg P.O. daily for 4 days (short test) or 3 to 4 weeks (long test). If hypokalemia and hypertension are corrected, a presumptive diagnosis of primary hyperaldosteronism is made.

➤ To manage primary hyperaldosteronism
Adults: 100 to 400 mg P.O. daily. Use lowest effective dose.

➤ Heart failure, as adjunct to ACE inhibitor or loop diuretic, with or without cardiac glycoside ♦
Adults: 12.5 to 25 mg P.O. daily. May increase to 50 mg daily after 8 weeks.

➤ Hirsutism ♦
Women: 50 to 200 mg P.O. daily. Or, 50 mg P.O. b.i.d. days 4 to 21 of menstrual cycle.

➤ **Premenstrual syndrome ♦**
Adults: 25 mg P.O. q.i.d. starting on day 14 of the menstrual cycle.
➤ **Acne vulgaris ♦**
Adults: 100 mg P.O. daily.
➤ **Familial male precocious puberty ♦**
Boys: 2 mg/kg P.O. daily with 20 to 40 mg/kg testolactone P.O. daily for at least 6 months.

ADMINISTRATION

P.O.

- To enhance absorption, give drug with meals.
- Give drug in morning to prevent nocturia. If second dose is needed, give it with food in early afternoon.
- Protect tablets from light.

ACTION

Antagonizes aldosterone in the distal tubules, increasing sodium and water excretion.

Route	Onset	Peak	Duration
P.O.	1–2 days	2–3 days	2–3 days

Half-life: 1¼ to 2 hours.

ADVERSE REACTIONS

CNS: headache, drowsiness, lethargy, confusion, ataxia.
GI: diarrhea, gastric bleeding, ulceration, cramping, gastritis, vomiting.
GU: inability to maintain erection, menstrual disturbances.
Hematologic: ***agranulocytosis.***
Metabolic: ***hyperkalemia,*** dehydration, hyponatremia, mild acidosis.
Skin: urticaria, hirsutism, maculopapular eruptions.
Other: ***anaphylaxis,*** gynecomastia, breast soreness, drug fever.

INTERACTIONS

Drug-drug. *ACE inhibitors, indomethacin, other potassium-sparing diuretics, potassium supplements:* May increase risk of hyperkalemia. Use together cautiously, especially in patients with renal impairment. Monitor potassium level.
Anticoagulants: May decrease anticoagulant effects. Monitor PT and INR.
Aspirin and other salicylates: May block diuretic effect of spironolactone. Watch for diminished spironolactone response.
Digoxin: May alter digoxin clearance, increasing risk of toxicity. Monitor digoxin level.
Drug-herb. *Licorice:* May block ulcer-healing and aldosterone-like effects of herb; may increase risk of hypokalemia. Discourage use together.
Drug-food. *Potassium-rich foods, such as citrus fruits and tomatoes, salt substitutes containing potassium:* May increase risk of hyperkalemia. Urge caution.

EFFECTS ON LAB TEST RESULTS

- May increase BUN and potassium levels. May decrease sodium level.
- May decrease granulocyte count.
- May alter fluorometric determinations of plasma and urinary 17-hydroxycorticosteroid levels.

CONTRAINDICATIONS & CAUTIONS

- Contraindicated in patients hypersensitive to drug and in those with anuria, acute or progressive renal insufficiency, or hyperkalemia.
- Use cautiously in patients with fluid or electrolyte imbalances, impaired renal function, or hepatic disease, or in pregnant women.

NURSING CONSIDERATIONS

- Monitor electrolyte levels, fluid intake and output, weight, and blood pressure.
- Monitor elderly patients closely, who are more susceptible to excessive diuresis.
- Inform laboratory that patient is taking spironolactone because drug may interfere with tests that measure digoxin level.
- Drug is less potent than thiazide and loop diuretics and is useful as an adjunct to other diuretic therapy. Diuretic effect is delayed 2 to 3 days when used alone.
- Maximum antihypertensive response may be delayed for up to 2 weeks.
- Watch for hyperchloremic metabolic acidosis, especially in patients with hepatic cirrhosis.
- ***Look alike–sound alike:*** Don't confuse Aldactone with Aldactazide.

PATIENT TEACHING

- Instruct patient to take drug in morning to prevent need to urinate at night. If second dose is needed, tell him to take it with food in early afternoon.
- ***Alert:*** To prevent serious hyperkalemia, warn patient to avoid excessive ingestion of potassium-rich foods (such as citrus fruits, tomatoes, bananas, dates, and apricots), salt substitutes containing potassium, and potassium supplements.
- Caution patient not to perform hazardous activities if adverse CNS reactions occur.
- Advise men about possible breast tenderness or enlargement.

SAFETY ALERT!

streptokinase

strep-to-KIN-ase

Streptase

Pharmacologic class: plasminogen activator
Pregnancy risk category C

AVAILABLE FORMS

Injection: 250,000 international units; 750,000 international units; 1.5 million international units in vials for reconstitution

INDICATIONS & DOSAGES

➤ Arteriovenous-cannula occlusion
Adults: 250,000 international units in 2 ml I.V. solution by I.V. pump infusion into each occluded limb of the cannula over 25 to 35 minutes. Clamp off cannula for 2 hours. Then aspirate contents of cannula, flush with normal saline solution, and reconnect.

➤ Venous thrombosis, pulmonary embolism, arterial thrombosis, and embolism
Adults: Loading dose is 250,000 international units by I.V. infusion over 30 minutes. Sustaining dose is 100,000 international units/hour I.V. infusion for 72 hours for deep vein thrombosis and 100,000 international units/hour over 24 to 72 hours by I.V. infusion pump for pulmonary embolism and arterial thrombosis or embolism.

➤ Lysis of coronary artery thrombi following acute MI
Adults: Infuse 1.5 million international units I.V. over 30 to 60 minutes.

ADMINISTRATION

I.V.

- Reconstitute drug in each vial with 5 ml of normal saline solution for injection or D_5W solution. Further dilute to 45 ml (if needed, total volume may be increased to 500 ml in a glass or 50 ml in a plastic container). Don't shake; roll gently to mix. Solution may precipitate after reconstituting; discard if large amounts are present.
- Filter solution with 0.8-micron or larger filter.
- Use immediately after reconstitution. If refrigerated, solution can be used for direct I.V. administration within 8 hours.
- Use an infusion pump to start a continuous infusion of heparin 1 to 4 hours after stopping streptokinase. Starting heparin 12 hours after intracoronary streptokinase may minimize bleeding risk.
- Store powder at room temperature.
- **Incompatibilities:** Dextrans. Don't mix with other drugs or give other drugs through the same I.V. line.

ACTION

Converts plasminogen to plasmin by directly cleaving peptide bonds at two sites, causing fibrinolysis.

Route	Onset	Peak	Duration
I.V.	Immediate	20 min–2 hr	4–24 hr

Half-life: First phase, 18 minutes; second phase, 83 minutes.

ADVERSE REACTIONS

CNS: polyradiculoneuropathy, headache, *fever.*
CV: ***reperfusion arrhythmias,*** *hypotension,* vasculitis, flushing.
EENT: periorbital edema.
GI: nausea.
Hematologic: ***bleeding,*** moderately decreased hematocrit.
Respiratory: minor breathing difficulty, ***bronchospasm, pulmonary edema.***
Skin: urticaria, pruritus.

Other: phlebitis at injection site, hypersensitivity reactions, ***anaphylaxis,*** delayed hypersensitivity reactions, ***angioedema,*** shivering.

INTERACTIONS

Drug-drug. *Anticoagulants:* May increase risk of bleeding. Monitor patient closely.
Antifibrinolytic drugs (such as aminocaproic acid): May inhibit and reverse streptokinase activity. Avoid using together.
Aspirin, dipyridamole, drugs affecting platelet activity (abciximab, eptifibatide, tirofiban), indomethacin, NSAIDs, phenylbutazone: May increase risk of bleeding. Monitor patient closely.

EFFECTS ON LAB TEST RESULTS

- May decrease hematocrit, plasminogen, and fibrinogen levels.
- May increase PT, PTT, and INR.

CONTRAINDICATIONS & CAUTIONS

- Contraindicated in patients with active internal bleeding; recent (within 2 months) cerebrovascular accident, or intracranial or intraspinal surgery; intracranial neoplasm; severe uncontrolled hypertension, or any patient with a history of an allergic reaction to the drug.
- Contraindicated with I.M. injections and other invasive procedures.
- Use cautiously in patients with recent (within 10 days) major surgery, obstetric delivery, organ biopsy, previous puncture of noncompressible vessels, serious GI bleeding, or trauma including cardiopulmonary resuscitation.
- Use cautiously in patients with a systolic blood pressure of 180 mm Hg or greater or a diastolic blood pressure of 110 mm Hg or greater, a high likelihood of left heart thrombus (mitral stenosis with atrial fibrillation), subacute bacterial endocarditis, hemostatic defects including those secondary to severe hepatic or renal disease, age older than 75 years, pregnancy, cerebrovascular disease, diabetic hemorrhagic retinopathy, septic thrombophlebitis or occluded AV cannula at seriously infected site, or any other condition in which bleeding constitutes a significant hazard or would be particularly difficult to manage because of its location.

NURSING CONSIDERATIONS

- For acute MI, give as soon as possible after symptom onset. The greatest benefit in mortality reduction was observed when streptokinase was given within 4 hours, but significant benefit has been reported up to 24 hours.
- For pulmonary embolism, deep vein thrombosis, arterial thrombosis, or embolism, institute treatment as soon as possible after thrombotic event onset, preferably within 7 days.
- Drug may be given to menstruating women.
- Only prescribers with experience managing thrombotic disease should give drug and only where clinical and laboratory monitoring can be performed.
- Before using drug to clear an occluded AV cannula, try flushing with heparinized saline solution.
- Keep aminocaproic acid available to treat bleeding and corticosteroids to treat allergic reactions.
- Before starting therapy, draw blood for coagulation studies, hematocrit, platelet count, and type and crossmatching. Rate of infusion depends on thrombin time and drug resistance.
- To check for hypersensitivity in acutely ill patients or patients with known allergies, give 100 international units I.D.; a wheal-and-flare response within 20 minutes means patient is probably allergic. Monitor vital signs frequently.
- For patient who has had a streptococcal infection or has been treated with streptokinase or anistreplase in the last 2 years, use a different thrombolytic.
- Combined therapy with low-dose aspirin (162.5 mg) or dipyridamole has improved short- and long-term results.
- Monitor patient for excessive bleeding every 15 minutes for first hour, every 30 minutes for second through eighth hours, and then every 4 hours. If bleeding is evident, stop therapy and notify prescriber. Pretreatment with heparin or drugs that affect platelets causes high risk of bleeding but may improve long-term results.

• Monitor pulse, color, and sensation of arms and legs every hour.
• Keep involved limb in straight alignment to prevent bleeding from infusion site.
• Monitor blood pressure closely.
• Avoid unnecessary handling of patient; pad side rails. Bruising is more likely during therapy.
• Keep a laboratory flow sheet on patient's chart to monitor PTT, PT, thrombin time, hemoglobin level, and hematocrit. Monitor vital signs and neurologic status.
• Avoid I.M. injection. Keep venipuncture sites to a minimum; use pressure dressing on puncture sites for at least 15 minutes.
• ***Alert:*** Watch for signs of hypersensitivity and notify prescriber immediately if any occur. Antihistamines or corticosteroids may be used for mild allergic reactions. If a severe reaction occurs, stop infusion immediately and notify prescriber.

PATIENT TEACHING
• Explain use and administration of drug to patient and family.
• Tell patient to promptly report adverse reactions, such as bleeding and bruising.

telmisartan

tell-mah-SAR-tan

Micardis

Pharmacologic class: angiotensin II receptor antagonist
Pregnancy risk category C; D in 2nd and 3rd trimesters

AVAILABLE FORMS
Tablets: 20 mg, 40 mg, 80 mg

INDICATIONS & DOSAGES
➤ **Hypertension (used alone or with other antihypertensives)**
Adults: 40 mg P.O. daily. Blood pressure response is dose-related over a range of 20 to 80 mg daily.

ADMINISTRATION
P.O.
• Give drug without regard to meals.

ACTION
Blocks vasoconstricting and aldosterone-secreting effects of angiotensin II by preventing angiotensin II from binding to the angiotensin I receptor.

Route	Onset	Peak	Duration
P.O.	Unknown	30–60 min	24 hr

Half-life: 24 hours.

ADVERSE REACTIONS
CNS: dizziness, pain, fatigue, headache.
CV: chest pain, hypertension, peripheral edema.
EENT: pharyngitis, sinusitis.
GI: *nausea,* abdominal pain, diarrhea, dyspepsia.
GU: UTI.
Musculoskeletal: back pain, myalgia.
Respiratory: cough, upper respiratory tract infection.
Other: flulike symptoms.

INTERACTIONS
Drug-drug. *Digoxin:* May increase digoxin level. Monitor digoxin level closely.
Warfarin: May decrease warfarin level. Monitor INR.
Drug-herb. *Ma huang:* May decrease antihypertensive effects. Discourage use together.
Drug-food. *Salt substitutes containing potassium:* May cause hyperkalemia. Discourage use together.

EFFECTS ON LAB TEST RESULTS
• May increase liver enzyme levels.

CONTRAINDICATIONS & CAUTIONS
• Contraindicated in patients hypersensitive to drug or its components.
• Use cautiously in patients with biliary obstruction disorders or renal and hepatic insufficiency and in those with an activated renin-angiotensin system, such as volume- or sodium-depleted patients (for example, those being treated with high doses of diuretics).
• Drug may cause fetal and neonatal death when given to pregnant women after the first trimester. If pregnancy is suspected, notify prescriber to stop drug.

NURSING CONSIDERATIONS

- Monitor patient for hypotension after starting drug. Place patient supine if hypotension occurs, and give I.V. normal saline, if needed.
- Most of the antihypertensive effect occurs within 2 weeks. Maximal blood pressure reduction is usually reached after 4 weeks. Diuretic may be added if blood pressure isn't controlled by drug alone.
- ***Alert:*** In patients whose renal function may depend on the activity of the renin-angiotensin-aldosterone system (such as those with severe heart failure), drug may cause oliguria or progressive azotemia and (rarely) acute renal failure or death.
- Drug isn't removed by hemodialysis. Patients undergoing dialysis may develop orthostatic hypotension. Closely monitor blood pressure.

PATIENT TEACHING

- Instruct patient to report suspected pregnancy to prescriber immediately.
- Inform woman of childbearing age of the consequences of second and third trimester exposure to drug.
- Advise breast-feeding woman about risk of adverse drug effects in infants and the need to stop either drug or breast-feeding.
- Tell patient that if he feels dizzy or has low blood pressure on standing, he should lie down, rise slowly from a lying to standing position, and climb stairs slowly.
- Tell patient that drug may be taken without regard to meals.
- Tell patient not to remove drug from blister-sealed packet until immediately before use.

SAFETY ALERT!

tenecteplase

teh-NEK-ti-plaze

TNKase

Pharmacologic class: recombinant tissue plasminogen activator
Pregnancy risk category C

AVAILABLE FORMS

Injection: 50 mg

INDICATIONS & DOSAGES

➤ To reduce risk of death from an acute MI

Adults who weigh 90 kg (198 lb) or more: 50 mg (10 ml) by I.V. bolus over 5 seconds.
Adults who weigh 80 to 90 kg (176 to 198 lb): 45 mg (9 ml) by I.V. bolus over 5 seconds.
Adults who weigh 70 to just under 80 kg (154 to 176 lb): 40 mg (8 ml) by I.V. bolus over 5 seconds.
Adults who weigh 60 to just under 70 kg (132 to 154 lb): 35 mg (7 ml) by I.V. bolus over 5 seconds.
Adults who weigh less than 60 kg (132 lb): 30 mg (6 ml) by I.V. bolus over 5 seconds.
Maximum dose is 50 mg.

ADMINISTRATION

I.V.

- Use syringe prefilled with sterile water for injection, and inject the entire contents into drug vial. Gently swirl solution once mixed. Don't shake. Visually inspect product for particulate matter before administration.
- Draw up the appropriate dose needed from the reconstituted vial with the syringe and discard any unused portion. Give drug immediately, or refrigerate and use within 8 hours.
- Give drug in a designated line. Flush dextrose-containing lines with normal saline solution before administration.
- Give the drug rapidly over 5 seconds.
- **Incompatibilities:** Solutions containing dextrose, other I.V. drugs.

ACTION

Binds to fibrin and converts plasminogen to plasmin. The specificity to fibrin decreases systemic activation of plasminogen and the resulting breakdown of circulating fibrinogen.

Route	Onset	Peak	Duration
I.V.	Immediate	Immediate	Unknown

Half-life: 20 minutes to 2 hours.

ADVERSE REACTIONS

CNS: ***stroke, intracranial hemorrhage,*** fever.

CV: ***arrhythmias, cardiogenic shock, myocardial reinfarction, thrombosis, embolism,*** hypotension.
EENT: pharyngeal bleeding, epistaxis.
GI: ***GI bleeding,*** nausea, vomiting.
GU: hematuria.
Respiratory: ***pulmonary edema.***
Skin: *hematoma.*
Other: bleeding at puncture site, hypersensitivity reactions.

INTERACTIONS

Drug-drug. *Anticoagulants (heparin, vitamin K antagonists), drugs that alter platelet function (acetylsalicylic acid, dipyridamole, glycoprotein IIb/IIIa inhibitors, NSAIDs):* May increase risk of bleeding when used before, during, or after tenecteplase use. Use together cautiously.

EFFECTS ON LAB TEST RESULTS

- May increase PT, PTT, and INR.

CONTRAINDICATIONS & CAUTIONS

- Contraindicated in patients with active internal bleeding; history of stroke; intracranial or intraspinal surgery or trauma during previous 2 months; intracranial neoplasm, aneurysm, or arteriovenous malformation; severe uncontrolled hypertension; or bleeding diathesis.
- Use cautiously in patients who have had recent major surgery (such as coronary artery bypass graft), organ biopsy, obstetric delivery, or previous puncture of noncompressible vessels.
- Use cautiously in pregnant women, patients age 75 and older, and patients with recent trauma, recent GI or GU bleeding, high risk of left ventricular thrombus, acute pericarditis, systolic blood pressure 180 mm Hg or higher or diastolic pressure 110 mm Hg or higher, severe hepatic dysfunction, hemostatic defects, subacute bacterial endocarditis, septic thrombophlebitis, diabetic hemorrhagic retinopathy, or cerebrovascular disease.

NURSING CONSIDERATIONS

- Begin therapy as soon as possible after onset of MI symptoms.
- Avoid noncompressible arterial punctures and internal jugular and subclavian venous punctures. Minimize all arterial and venous punctures during treatment.
- Avoid I.M. use.
- Give heparin but not in the same I.V. line.
- Monitor patient for bleeding. If serious bleeding occurs, stop heparin and antiplatelet drugs immediately.
- ***Alert:*** Use exact patient weight for dosage. An overestimation in patient weight can lead to significant increase in bleeding or intracerebral hemorrhage.
- Monitor ECG for reperfusion arrhythmias.
- A life-threatening cholesterol embolism is rarely caused by thrombolytics. Signs and symptoms may include livedo reticularis (blue toe syndrome), acute renal failure, gangrenous digits, hypertension, pancreatitis, MI, cerebral infarction, spinal cord infarction, retinal artery occlusion, bowel infarction, and rhabdomyolysis.

PATIENT TEACHING

- Advise patient about proper dental care to avoid excessive gum bleeding.
- Tell patient to report any adverse effects or excessive bleeding immediately.
- Explain use of drug to patient and family.

terazosin hydrochloride

ter-AY-zoe-sin

Hytrin

Pharmacologic class: alpha blocker
Pregnancy risk category C

AVAILABLE FORMS

Capsules: 1 mg, 2 mg, 5 mg, 10 mg
Tablets: 1 mg, 2 mg, 5 mg, 10 mg

INDICATIONS & DOSAGES

➤ **Hypertension**

Adults: Initially, 1 mg P.O. at bedtime. Dosage may be increased gradually based on response. Usual dosage range is 1 to 5 mg daily. Maximum recommended dose is 20 mg daily.

➤ **Symptomatic BPH**

Adults: Initially, 1 mg P.O. at bedtime. Dosage may be titrated to 2, 5, or 10 mg once daily to achieve optimal response.

Most patients need 10 mg daily for optimal response.

ADMINISTRATION
P.O.
• Give drug without regard for meals.

ACTION
Improves urine flow in patients with BPH by blocking alpha-adrenergic receptors in the bladder neck and prostate, relieving urethral pressure. Drug also reduces peripheral vascular resistance and blood pressure via arterial and venous dilation.

Route	Onset	Peak	Duration
P.O.	15 min	2–3 hr	24 hr

Half-life: About 12 hours.

ADVERSE REACTIONS
CNS: *headache, dizziness,* asthenia, first-dose syncope, nervousness, paresthesia, somnolence.
CV: *peripheral edema,* palpitations, orthostatic hypotension, tachycardia, atrial fibrillation.
EENT: *nasal congestion,* sinusitis, blurred vision.
GI: nausea.
GU: impotence, priapism.
Hematologic: ***thrombocytopenia.***
Musculoskeletal: back pain, muscle pain.
Respiratory: dyspnea.

INTERACTIONS
Drug-drug. *Antihypertensives:* May cause excessive hypotension. Use together cautiously.
Drug-herb. *Butcher's broom:* May decrease drug effect. Discourage use together.
Ma huang: May decrease antihypertensive effects. Discourage use together.

EFFECTS ON LAB TEST RESULTS
• May decrease total protein and albumin levels. May decrease hemoglobin level and hematocrit.
• May decrease WBC and platelet counts.

CONTRAINDICATIONS & CAUTIONS
• Contraindicated in patients hypersensitive to drug.

NURSING CONSIDERATIONS
• Monitor blood pressure frequently.
• ***Alert:*** If terazosin is stopped for several days, readjust dosage using first dosing regimen (1 mg P.O. at bedtime).

PATIENT TEACHING
• Tell patient not to stop drug suddenly, but to notify prescriber if adverse reactions occur.
• Warn patient to avoid hazardous activities that require mental alertness, such as driving or operating heavy machinery, for 12 hours after first dose.
• Tell patient that light-headedness can occur, especially during the first few days of therapy. Advise him to rise slowly to minimize this effect and to report signs and symptoms to prescriber.

ticlopidine hydrochloride
tye-KLOH-pih-deen

Ticlid

Pharmacologic class: platelet aggregation inhibitor
Pregnancy risk category B

AVAILABLE FORMS
Tablets: 250 mg

INDICATIONS & DOSAGES
➤ **To reduce risk of thrombotic stroke in patients who have had a stroke or stroke precursors**
Adults: 250 mg P.O. b.i.d. with meals.
➤ **Adjunct to aspirin to prevent subacute stent thrombosis in patients having coronary stent placement**
Adults: 250 mg P.O. b.i.d., combined with antiplatelet doses of aspirin. Start therapy after stent placement and continue for up to 30 days. If prescribed longer than 30 days, use is off-label.

ADMINISTRATION
P.O.
• Give drug with meals.

ACTION
Unknown. An antiplatelet that probably blocks adenosine diphosphate–induced

platelet-to-fibrinogen and platelet-to-platelet binding.

Route	Onset	Peak	Duration
P.O.	Unknown	2 hr	Unknown

Half-life: 1½ hours after single dose; 4 to 5 days after multiple doses.

ADVERSE REACTIONS

CNS: ***intracranial bleeding,*** dizziness, peripheral neuropathy.
CV: vasculitis.
EENT: conjunctival hemorrhage.
GI: *diarrhea,* abdominal pain, anorexia, bleeding, dyspepsia, flatulence, nausea, vomiting.
GU: dark urine, hematuria.
Hematologic: ***agranulocytosis, aplastic anemia, immune thrombocytopenia, neutropenia, pancytopenia.***
Musculoskeletal: arthropathy, myositis.
Respiratory: *allergic pneumonitis.*
Skin: ***thrombocytopenic purpura,*** ecchymoses, maculopapular rash, pruritus, rash, urticaria.
Other: hypersensitivity reactions, postoperative bleeding.

INTERACTIONS

Drug-drug. *Antacids:* May decrease ticlopidine level. Separate doses by at least 2 hours.
Aspirin: May increase effect of aspirin on platelets. Use together cautiously.
Cimetidine: May decrease clearance of ticlopidine and increase risk of toxicity. Avoid using together.
Digoxin: May decrease digoxin level. Monitor digoxin level.
Phenytoin: May increase phenytoin level. Monitor patient closely.
Theophylline: May decrease theophylline clearance and risk of toxicity. Monitor patient closely and adjust theophylline dosage.
Drug-herb. *Red clover:* May cause bleeding. Discourage use together.

EFFECTS ON LAB TEST RESULTS

- May increase ALT, AST, alkaline phosphatase, cholesterol, and triglyceride levels.
- May decrease neutrophil, WBC, RBC, platelet, and granulocyte counts.

CONTRAINDICATIONS & CAUTIONS

- Contraindicated in patients hypersensitive to drug and in those with severe hepatic impairment, hematopoietic disorders, active pathologic bleeding from peptic ulceration, or active intracranial bleeding.
- Use cautiously and with close monitoring of CBC and WBC differentials, watching for signs and symptoms of neutropenia and agranulocytosis.

NURSING CONSIDERATIONS

- Because of life-threatening adverse reactions, use drug only in patients who are allergic to, can't tolerate, or have failed aspirin therapy.
- Obtain baseline liver function test results before therapy.
- Determine CBC and WBC differentials at second week of therapy and repeat every 2 weeks until end of third month.
- Monitor liver function test results and repeat if dysfunction is suspected.
- Thrombocytopenia has occurred rarely. Stop drug in patients with platelet count of 80,000/mm^3 or less. If needed, give methylprednisolone 20 mg I.V. to normalize bleeding time within 2 hours.
- When used preoperatively, drug may decrease risk of graft occlusion in patients receiving coronary artery bypass grafts and reduce severity of drop in platelet count in patients receiving extracorporeal hemoperfusion during open heart surgery.

PATIENT TEACHING

- Tell patient to take drug with meals.
- Warn patient to avoid aspirin and aspirin-containing products unless directed to by prescriber and to check with prescriber or pharmacist before taking OTC drugs.
- Explain that drug will prolong bleeding time and that patient should report unusual or prolonged bleeding. Advise patient to tell dentists and other health care providers that he takes ticlopidine.
- Stress importance of regular blood tests. Because neutropenia can result with increased risk of infection, tell patient to immediately report signs and symptoms

of infection, such as fever, chills, or sore throat.
• If drug is being substituted for a fibrinolytic or anticoagulant, tell patient to stop those drugs before starting ticlopidine therapy.
• Advise patient to stop drug 10 to 14 days before undergoing elective surgery.
• Tell patient to immediately report to prescriber yellow skin or sclera, severe or persistent diarrhea, rashes, bleeding under the skin, light-colored stools, or dark urine.

SAFETY ALERT!

tirofiban hydrochloride
tye-row-FYE-ban

Aggrastat

Pharmacologic class: glycoprotein (GP) IIb/IIIa receptor antagonist
Pregnancy risk category B

AVAILABLE FORMS
Injection: 25-ml and 50-ml vials (250 mcg/ml), 250-ml and 500-ml premixed vials (50 mcg/ml)

INDICATIONS & DOSAGES
➤ Acute coronary syndrome, with heparin or aspirin, including patients who are to be managed medically and those undergoing percutaneous transluminal coronary angioplasty (PTCA) or atherectomy
Adults: I.V. loading dose of 0.4 mcg/kg/minute for 30 minutes; then continuous I.V. infusion of 0.1 mcg/kg/minute. Continue infusion through angiography and for 12 to 24 hours after PTCA or atherectomy.
Adjust-a-dose: If creatinine clearance is less than 30 ml/minute, use a loading dose of 0.2 mcg/kg/minute for 30 minutes; then continuous infusion of 0.05 mcg/kg/minute. Continue infusion through angiography and for 12 to 24 hours after PTCA or atherectomy.

ADMINISTRATION
I.V.
• Dilute injections of 250 mcg/ml to same strength as 500-ml premixed vials (50 mcg/ml) as follows: Withdraw and discard 100 ml from a 500-ml bag of sterile normal saline solution or D_5W and replace this volume with 100 ml of tirofiban injection (from four 25-ml vials or two 50-ml vials); or withdraw 50 ml from a 250-ml bag of sterile normal saline solution or D_5W and replace this volume with 50 ml of tirofiban injection (from two 25-ml vials or one 50-ml vial), to yield 50 mcg/ml.
• Inspect solution for particulate matter before giving, and check for leaks by squeezing the inner bag firmly. If bag leaks or particles are visible, discard solution.
• Avoid use of noncompressible sites (such as subclavian or jugular veins).
• Heparin and tirofiban may be given through the same I.V. catheter. Tirofiban may be given through the same I.V. line as dopamine, lidocaine, potassium chloride, and famotidine.
• Discard unused solution 24 hours after the start of infusion.
• Store drug at room temperature. Protect from light.
• **Incompatibilities:** Diazepam.

ACTION
Reversibly binds to the GP IIb/IIIa receptor on human platelets and inhibits platelet aggregation.

Route	Onset	Peak	Duration
I.V.	Immediate	Immediate	4–6 hr

Half-life: About 2 hours.

ADVERSE REACTIONS
CNS: dizziness, fever, headache.
CV: ***bradycardia, coronary artery dissection,*** edema, vasovagal reaction.
GI: *occult bleeding,* nausea.
Hematologic: *bleeding,* ***thrombocytopenia.***
Musculoskeletal: leg pain.
Skin: sweating.
Other: *bleeding at arterial access site,* pelvic pain.

INTERACTIONS

Drug-drug. *Anticoagulants such as warfarin, aspirin, clopidogrel, dipyridamole, heparin, NSAIDs, thrombolytics, ticlopidine:* May increase risk of bleeding. Monitor patient closely.
Levothyroxine, omeprazole: May increase tirofiban renal clearance. Monitor patient.

EFFECTS ON LAB TEST RESULTS

- May decrease hemoglobin level and hematocrit.
- May decrease platelet count.

CONTRAINDICATIONS & CAUTIONS

- Contraindicated in patients hypersensitive to drug or its components.
- Contraindicated in those with active internal bleeding or history of bleeding diathesis within the previous 30 days and in those with history of intracranial hemorrhage, intracranial neoplasm, arteriovenous malformation, aneurysm, thrombocytopenia after previous exposure to drug, stroke within 30 days, or hemorrhagic stroke.
- Contraindicated in those with history, symptoms, or findings suggestive of aortic dissection; severe hypertension (systolic blood pressure higher than 180 mm Hg or diastolic blood pressure higher than 110 mm Hg); acute pericarditis; major surgical procedure or severe physical trauma within previous month; or concomitant use of another parenteral GP IIb/IIIa inhibitor.
- Use cautiously in patients with increased risk of bleeding, including those with hemorrhagic retinopathy or platelet count less than 150,000/mm^3.
- Safety and efficacy of drug haven't been studied in patients younger than age 18.

NURSING CONSIDERATIONS

- Monitor hemoglobin level, hematocrit, and platelet count before starting therapy, 6 hours after loading dose, and at least daily during therapy. If thrombocytopenia occurs, notify prescriber.
- Give drug with aspirin and heparin.
- Monitor patient for bleeding.
- ***Alert:*** The most common adverse effect is bleeding at the arterial access site for cardiac catheterization.
- The risk of bleeding may decrease with early sheath removal and by keeping the access site immobile. The sheath may be removed during infusion, but only after heparin has been stopped and its effects largely reversed.
- Minimize use of arterial and venous punctures, I.M. injections, urinary catheters, and nasotracheal and nasogastric tubes.
- Elderly patients have a higher risk of bleeding complications.
- ***Look alike–sound alike:*** Don't confuse Aggrastat with argatroban.

PATIENT TEACHING

- Explain that drug is a blood thinner used to prevent chest pain and heart attack.
- Explain that risk of serious bleeding is far outweighed by the benefits of drug.
- Instruct patient to report chest discomfort or other adverse effects immediately.
- Tell patient that frequent blood sampling may be needed to evaluate therapy.

---

tobramycin sulfate

toe-bra-MYE-sin

TOBI

Pharmacologic class: aminoglycoside
Pregnancy risk category D

AVAILABLE FORMS

Multidose vials (pediatric): 10 mg/ml, 40 mg/ml
Nebulizer solution (for inhalation): 300 mg/5 ml
Prefilled syringe (pediatric): 40 mg/ml
Premixed parenteral injection for infusion: 60 mg or 80 mg in normal saline solution

INDICATIONS & DOSAGES

➤ **Serious infection by sensitive strains of *Escherichia coli, Proteus, Klebsiella, Enterobacter, Serratia, Morganella morganii, Staphylococcus aureus, Citrobacter, Pseudomonas*, or *Providencia***

Adults: 3 mg/kg/day I.M. or I.V. in divided doses. For life-threatening infections, give up to 5 mg/kg/day in divided doses every 6 to 8 hours; reduce to 3 mg/kg daily as soon as clinically indicated.

Children: 6 to 7.5 mg/kg/day I.M. or I.V., divided t.i.d. or q.i.d.
Neonates younger than age 1 week or premature infants: Up to 4 mg/kg/day I.V. or I.M. in two equal doses every 12 hours.
Adjust-a-dose: For patients with renal impairment, give loading dose of 1 mg/kg; then give decreased doses at 8-hour intervals or same dose at prolonged intervals. For patients with severe cystic fibrosis, initial dose is 10 mg/kg/day I.V. or I.M., divided q.i.d.

➤ **To manage cystic fibrosis patients with *Pseudomonas aeruginosa***
Adults and children age 6 and older: 300 mg via nebulizer every 12 hours for 28 days. Continue cycle of 28 days on drug and 28 days off.

ADMINISTRATION

I.V.

- Obtain specimen for culture and sensitivity tests before giving. Begin therapy while awaiting results.
- For adults, dilute in 50 to 100 ml of normal saline solution or D_5W; use a smaller volume for children.
- Infuse over 20 to 60 minutes.
- After infusion, flush line with normal saline solution or D_5W.
- Obtain blood for peak level 30 minutes after infusion stops; draw blood for trough level just before next dose. Don't collect blood in a heparinized tube because of incompatibility.
- **Incompatibilities:** Allopurinol; amphotericin B; azithromycin; beta lactam antibiotics; cefepime; clindamycin; dextrose 5% in Isolyte E, M, or P; heparin sodium; hetastarch; indomethacin; propofol; sargramostim; solutions containing alcohol.

I.M.

- Obtain specimen for culture and sensitivity tests before giving. Begin therapy while awaiting results.
- Obtain blood for peak level 1 hour after I.M. injection; draw blood for trough level just before next dose. Don't collect blood in a heparinized tube because of incompatibility.

Inhalational

- Obtain specimen for culture and sensitivity tests before giving. Begin therapy while awaiting results.
- Give nebulizer solution over 10 to 15 minutes using handheld Pari LC Plus reusable nebulizer with DeVilbiss Pulmo-Aide compressor.

ACTION

Generally bactericidal. Inhibits protein synthesis by binding directly to the 30S ribosomal subunit.

Route	Onset	Peak	Duration
I.V.	Immediate	30 min	8 hr
I.M.	Unknown	30–60 min	8 hr
Inhalation	Unknown	Unknown	Unknown

Half-life: 2 to 3 hours.

ADVERSE REACTIONS

CNS: ***seizures,*** headache, lethargy, confusion, disorientation, fever.
EENT: *ototoxicity, hoarseness, pharyngitis.*
GI: vomiting, nausea, diarrhea.
GU: ***nephrotoxicity,*** possible increase in urinary excretion of casts.
Hematologic: anemia, eosinophilia, ***leukopenia, thrombocytopenia, agranulocytosis.***
Metabolic: electrolyte imbalances.
Musculoskeletal: muscle twitching.
Respiratory: ***bronchospasm.***
Skin: rash, urticaria, pruritus.

INTERACTIONS

Drug-drug. *Acyclovir, amphotericin B, cephalosporins, cidofovir, cisplatin, methoxyflurane, vancomycin, other aminoglycosides:* May increase nephrotoxicity. Monitor renal function test results.
Atracurium, pancuronium, rocuronium, vecuronium: May increase effects of nondepolarizing muscle relaxants, including prolonged respiratory depression. Use together only when necessary, and expect to reduce dosage of nondepolarizing muscle relaxant.
Dimenhydrinate: May mask symptoms of ototoxicity. Monitor patient's hearing.
General anesthetics: May increase neuromuscular blockade. Monitor patient for increased clinical effects.
I.V. loop diuretics such as furosemide: May increase ototoxicity. Monitor patient's hearing.

Parenteral penicillins: May inactivate tobramycin in vitro. Don't mix together.

EFFECTS ON LAB TEST RESULTS

- May increase BUN, creatinine, nonprotein nitrogen, and urine urea levels. May decrease calcium, magnesium, and potassium levels.
- May increase eosinophil count. May decrease WBC, platelet, and granulocyte counts.

CONTRAINDICATIONS & CAUTIONS

- Contraindicated in patients hypersensitive to drug or other aminoglycosides.
- Use cautiously in patients with impaired renal function or neuromuscular disorders and in elderly patients.

NURSING CONSIDERATIONS

- Weigh patient and review renal function studies before therapy.
- ***Alert:*** Evaluate patient's hearing before and during therapy. If patient complains of tinnitus, vertigo, or hearing loss, notify prescriber.
- Don't dilute or mix with dornase alpha in a nebulizer.
- Unrefrigerated drug, which is normally slightly yellow, may darken with age. This change doesn't indicate a change in product quality.
- Avoid exposing ampules to intense light.
- ***Alert:*** Peak levels over 12 mcg/ml and trough levels over 2 mcg/ml may increase the risk of toxicity. Reserve higher peak levels for cystic fibrosis patients, who need a greater lung penetration.
- ***Alert:*** Monitor renal function: urine output, specific gravity, urinalysis, creatinine clearance, and BUN and creatinine levels. Notify prescriber about signs and symptoms of decreasing renal function.
- Watch for signs and symptoms of superinfection, such as continued fever, chills, and increased pulse rate.
- If no response occurs in 3 to 5 days, therapy may be stopped and new specimens obtained for culture and sensitivity testing.
- ***Look alike–sound alike:*** Don't confuse tobramycin with Trobicin.

PATIENT TEACHING

- Instruct patient to report adverse reactions promptly.
- Caution patient not to perform hazardous activities if adverse CNS reactions occur.
- Encourage patient to maintain adequate fluid intake.
- Teach patient how to use and maintain nebulizer.
- Tell patient using several inhaled therapies to use this drug last.
- Instruct patient not to use if the solution is cloudy or contains particles or if it has been stored at room temperature for longer than 28 days.

---

torsemide

TOR-seh-mide

Demadex

Pharmacologic class: loop diuretic
Pregnancy risk category B

AVAILABLE FORMS

Injection: 10 mg/ml
Tablets: 5 mg, 10 mg, 20 mg, 100 mg

INDICATIONS & DOSAGES

➤ **Diuresis in patients with heart failure**

Adults: Initially, 10 to 20 mg P.O. or I.V. once daily. If response is inadequate, double dose until desired effect is achieved. Maximum, 200 mg daily.

➤ **Diuresis in patients with chronic renal failure**

Adults: Initially, 20 mg P.O. or I.V. once daily. If response is inadequate, double dose until response is obtained. Maximum, 200 mg daily.

➤ **Diuresis in patients with hepatic cirrhosis**

Adults: Initially, 5 to 10 mg P.O. or I.V. once daily with an aldosterone antagonist or a potassium-sparing diuretic. If response is inadequate, double dose until desired effect is achieved. Maximum, 40 mg daily.

➤ **Hypertension**

Adults: Initially, 5 mg P.O. daily. Increased to 10 mg if needed and tolerated. Add another antihypertensive if response is still inadequate.

ADMINISTRATION

P.O.

- To prevent nocturia, give drug in the morning.

I.V.

- Inspect ampules for precipitate or discoloration before use.
- Give by direct injection over at least 2 minutes. Rapid injection may cause ototoxicity. Don't give more than 200 mg at a time.
- Drug may be given as a continuous infusion.
- Drug remains stable for 24 hours at room temperature when mixed in D_5W, normal saline solution, or half-normal saline solution.
- **Incompatibilities:** Solutions with pH below 8.3. Flush line with normal saline before and after administration to avoid incompatibility.

ACTION

Enhances excretion of sodium, chloride, and water by acting on the ascending loop of Henle.

Route	Onset	Peak	Duration
P.O.	1 hr	1–2 hr	6–8 hr
I.V.	10 min	1 hr	6–8 hr

Half-life: 3½ hours.

ADVERSE REACTIONS

CNS: asthenia, dizziness, headache, nervousness, insomnia, syncope.
CV: ECG abnormalities, chest pain, edema, orthostatic hypotension.
EENT: rhinitis, sore throat.
GI: *excessive thirst,* ***hemorrhage,*** diarrhea, constipation, nausea, dyspepsia.
GU: excessive urination, impotence.
Metabolic: *electrolyte imbalances including hypokalemia and,* ***hypomagnesemia, dehydration,*** hypochloremic alkalosis, hyperuricemia, hypercholesterolemia.
Musculoskeletal: arthralgia, myalgia.
Respiratory: cough.
Skin: rash.

INTERACTIONS

Drug-drug. *Aminoglycoside antibiotics, cisplatin:* May increase ototoxicity. Use together cautiously.
Amphotericin B, corticosteroids, metolazone: May increase risk of hypokalemia. Monitor potassium level.
Anticoagulants: May enhance anticoagulant activity. Use together cautiously.
Antidiabetics: May decrease hypoglycemic effect, resulting in higher glucose level. Monitor glucose level.
Chlorothiazide, chlorthalidone, hydrochlorothiazide, indapamide, metolazone: May cause excessive diuretic response, resulting in serious electrolyte abnormalities or dehydration. Adjust doses carefully, and monitor patient closely for signs and symptoms of excessive diuretic response.
Cholestyramine: May decrease absorption of torsemide. Separate doses by at least 3 hours.
Digoxin: Electrolyte imbalance caused by diuretic may lead to digoxin-induced arrhythmia. Use together cautiously.
Lithium: May increase lithium level and cause toxicity. Use together cautiously and monitor lithium level.
NSAIDs: May decrease effects of loop diuretics. Use together cautiously.
Probenecid: May decrease diuretic effect. Avoid using together.
Salicylates: May decrease excretion, possibly leading to salicylate toxicity. Avoid using together.
Spironolactone: May decrease renal clearance of spironolactone. Use together cautiously.
Drug-herb. *Dandelion:* May interfere with drug activity. Discourage use together.
Licorice: May cause unexpected rapid potassium loss. Discourage use together.
Drug-lifestyle. *Sun exposure:* May cause photosensitivity. Advise patient to take precautions.

EFFECTS ON LAB TEST RESULTS

- May increase BUN, creatinine, cholesterol, glucose, and uric acid levels. May decrease potassium and magnesium levels.

CONTRAINDICATIONS & CAUTIONS

- Contraindicated in patients hypersensitive to drug or other sulfonamide derivatives and in those with anuria.
- Use cautiously in patients with hepatic disease and related cirrhosis and ascites; sudden changes in fluid and electrolyte balance may precipitate hepatic coma in these patients.

NURSING CONSIDERATIONS

- Monitor fluid intake and output, electrolyte levels, blood pressure, weight, and pulse rate during rapid diuresis and routinely with long-term use. Drug can cause profound diuresis and water and electrolyte depletion.
- Watch for signs of hypokalemia, such as muscle weakness and cramps.
- Consult prescriber and dietitian about providing a high-potassium diet or potassium supplement. Foods rich in potassium include citrus fruits, tomatoes, bananas, dates, and apricots.
- Monitor elderly patients, who are especially susceptible to excessive diuresis with potential for circulatory collapse and thromboembolic complications.
- ***Look alike–sound alike:*** Don't confuse torsemide with furosemide.

PATIENT TEACHING

- Tell patient to take drug in morning to prevent the need to urinate at night.
- Advise patient to change positions slowly to prevent dizziness and to limit alcohol intake and strenuous exercise in hot weather to prevent dizziness.
- Advise patient to immediately report ringing in ears because it may indicate toxicity.
- Tell patient to report weakness, cramping, nausea, and dizziness.
- Tell patient to check with prescriber or pharmacist before taking OTC drugs.
- Advise patient that drug may cause photosensitivity, and tell him to take precautions with sun exposure.

trandolapril

tran-DOLE-ah-pril

Mavik

Pharmacologic class: ACE inhibitor
Pregnancy risk category C; D in 2nd and 3rd trimesters

AVAILABLE FORMS

Tablets: 1 mg, 2 mg, 4 mg

INDICATIONS & DOSAGES

➤ Hypertension

Adults: For patients not taking a diuretic, initially 2 mg P.O. for a black patient and 1 mg P.O. for all other races, once daily. If control isn't adequate, increase dosage at intervals of at least 1 week. Maintenance doses for most patients range from 2 to 4 mg daily. Some patients taking once-daily doses of 4 mg may need b.i.d. doses. For patients also taking a diuretic, initially, 0.5 mg P.O. once daily. Subsequent dosage adjustment is based on blood pressure response.

➤ Heart failure or ventricular dysfunction after MI

Adults: Initially, 1 mg P.O. daily, adjusted to 4 mg P.O. daily. If patient can't tolerate 4 mg, continue at highest tolerated dose.
Adjust-a-dose: If creatinine clearance is below 30 ml/minute, first dose is 0.5 mg daily.

ADMINISTRATION

P.O.

- Give drug without regard for food.
- Don't give antacid 1 hour before or up to 2 hours after dose.

ACTION

Thought to inhibit ACE, reducing angiotensin II formation, which decreases peripheral arterial resistance, decreases aldosterone secretion, reduces sodium and water retention, and lowers blood pressure. Drug is converted in the liver to the prodrug, trandolaprilat.

Route	Onset	Peak	Duration
P.O.	4 hr	1–10 hr	24 hr

Half-life: 5 to 10 hours; longer in patients with renal impairment.

ADVERSE REACTIONS

CNS: *dizziness,* headache, fatigue, drowsiness, insomnia, paresthesia, vertigo, anxiety.
CV: *hypotension,* ***bradycardia,*** chest pain, first-degree AV block, edema, flushing, palpitations.
EENT: epistaxis, throat irritation.
GI: ***pancreatitis,*** diarrhea, dyspepsia, abdominal distention, abdominal pain or cramps, constipation, vomiting.
GU: urinary frequency, impotence.
Hematologic: ***neutropenia, leukopenia.***
Metabolic: ***hyperkalemia,*** hyponatremia.
Respiratory: *persistent, nonproductive cough,* dyspnea, upper respiratory tract infection.
Skin: rash, pruritus, pemphigus.
Other: decreased libido.

INTERACTIONS

Drug-drug. *Azathioprine:* May increase risk of anemia or leukopenia. Monitor hematologic studies.
Diuretics: May cause excessive hypotension. Stop diuretic or reduce first dosage of trandolapril.
Lithium: May increase lithium level and lithium toxicity. Avoid using together; monitor lithium level.
NSAIDs: May decrease antihypertensive effects. Monitor blood pressure.
Potassium-sparing diuretics, potassium supplements: May cause hyperkalemia. Monitor potassium level closely.
Drug-herb. *Capsaicin:* May cause cough. Discourage use together.
Ma huang: May decrease antihypertensive effects. Discourage use together.
Drug-food. *Salt substitutes containing potassium:* May cause hyperkalemia. Discourage use of salt substitutes.

EFFECTS ON LAB TEST RESULTS

- May increase BUN, creatinine, potassium, and liver enzyme levels. May decrease sodium level.
- May decrease neutrophil and WBC counts.

CONTRAINDICATIONS & CAUTIONS

- Contraindicated in patients hypersensitive to drug and in those with a history of angioedema related to previous treatment with an ACE inhibitor. Also contraindicated in pregnant patients.
- Use cautiously in patients with impaired renal function, heart failure, or renal artery stenosis.
- Safety and effectiveness of drug in children haven't been established.
- Don't use drug in breast-feeding women.

NURSING CONSIDERATIONS

- Monitor potassium level closely.
- Watch for hypotension. Excessive hypotension can occur when drug is given with diuretics. If possible, stop diuretic therapy 2 to 3 days before starting trandolapril to decrease potential for excessive hypotension response. If drug doesn't adequately control blood pressure, diuretic therapy may be started again cautiously.
- Assess patient's renal function before and periodically throughout therapy.
- Other ACE inhibitors have been reported to cause agranulocytosis and neutropenia. Monitor CBC with differential before therapy, especially in patients with collagen vascular disease and impaired renal function.
- Although drug reduces blood pressure in patients of all races, drug reduces pressure less in blacks taking this drug alone. Blacks should take drug with a thiazide diuretic for a more favorable response.
- ***Alert:*** Angioedema involving the tongue, glottis, or larynx may be fatal because of airway obstruction. Give appropriate therapy, including epinephrine 1:1,000 (0.3 to 0.5 ml) subcutaneously; have resuscitation equipment for maintaining a patent airway readily available. The risk of angioedema is higher in blacks.
- If patient develops jaundice, stop drug under prescriber's advice because, although rare, ACE inhibitors have been linked to a syndrome of cholestatic jaundice, fulminant hepatic necrosis, and death.

PATIENT TEACHING

- Instruct patient to report yellowing of skin or eyes.
- Advise patient to report fever and sore throat (signs of infection), easy bruising or bleeding; swelling of the tongue, lips, face, eyes, mucous membranes, or extremities; difficulty swallowing or breathing; hoarseness; and nonproductive, persistent cough.
- Tell patient to avoid salt substitutes during drug therapy. These products may contain potassium, which can cause high potassium level in patients taking drug.
- Tell patient that light-headedness can occur, especially during first few days of therapy. Advise him to rise slowly to minimize this effect and to report it immediately.
- Advise patient to use caution in hot weather and during exercise. Inadequate fluid intake, vomiting, diarrhea, and excessive perspiration can lead to light-headedness and fainting.
- Tell woman of childbearing age to report suspected pregnancy immediately. Drug will need to be stopped.
- Advise patient planning to undergo surgery or receive anesthesia to inform prescriber that he is taking this drug.
- Tell patient drug may be taken with or without food.
- Instruct patient not to take an antacid 1 hour before or up to 2 hours after dose.

treprostinil sodium

tra-PROS-tin-ill

Remodulin

Pharmacologic class: vasodilator
Pregnancy risk category B

AVAILABLE FORMS

Injection: 1 mg/ml, 2.5 mg/ml, 5 mg/ml, 10 mg/ml in 20-ml vials

INDICATIONS & DOSAGES

➤ To reduce symptoms caused by exercise in patients with New York Heart Association class II to IV pulmonary arterial hypertension (PAH)

Adults: Initially, 1.25 nanogram/kg/minute by continuous subcutaneous infusion. If patient doesn't tolerate initial dose, reduce infusion rate to 0.625 nanogram/kg/minute. Increase by 1.25 nanogram/kg/minute each week for the first 4 weeks and then by no more than 2.5 nanogram/kg/minute each week for the remaining duration of infusion. Maximum infusion rate is 40 nanogram/kg/minute. May be given I.V. through a central catheter if subcutaneous route isn't tolerated.

Adjust-a-dose: In patients with mild or moderate hepatic insufficiency, initially, 0.625 nanogram/kg ideal body weight per minute, and increase cautiously.

➤ To decrease the rate of clinical deterioration in patients requiring transition from epoprostenol sodium (Flolan)

Adults: Start treprostinil at 10% of the current epoprostenol dose; increase dose as the epoprostenol dose is reduced. Decrease epoprostenol dose in 20% increments and increase treprostinil in 20% increments, always maintaining a total dose of 110% of epoprostenol starting dose. Once epoprostenol is at 20% of starting dose and treprostinil is at 90%, decrease epoprostenol to 5% and increase treprostinil to 110%. Finally, stop epoprostenol and maintain treprostinil dose at 110% of epoprostenol starting dose plus an additional 5% to 10% as needed. Change rate based on individual patient response. Treat worsening of PAH symptoms with increases in treprostinil dose. Treat adverse effects associated with prostacyclin and prostacyclin analogs with decreases in epoprostenol dose.

ADMINISTRATION

I.V.

- Give I.V. through a central venous catheter only if subcutaneous route isn't tolerated.
- Dilute with either sterile water for injection or normal saline solution.
- Inspect for particulate matter and discoloration before giving.
- Give by continuous infusion through a surgically placed indwelling central venous

catheter, using an infusion pump designed for I.V. drug delivery.
• To avoid potential interruptions in drug delivery, make sure patient has immediate access to a backup infusion pump and infusion sets.
• Diluted drug is stable at room temperature for up to 48 hours.
• **Incompatibilities:** Other I.V. drugs.

Subcutaneous
• Preferred route is continuous subcutaneous infusion via a self-inserted subcutaneous catheter, using an infusion pump designed for subcutaneous drug delivery.
• The infusion pump should be small and lightweight; adjustable to about 0.002 ml/hour; have occlusion/no delivery, low-battery, programming-error, and motor-malfunction alarms; have delivery accuracy of ± 6% or better; and be positive-pressure driven.
• The reservoir should be made of polyvinyl chloride, polypropylene, or glass.

ACTION
Directly vasodilates pulmonary and systemic arterial vascular beds and inhibits platelet aggregation.

Route	Onset	Peak	Duration
I.V.	Unknown	Unknown	Unknown
Subcut.	Rapid	Unknown	Unknown

Half-life: 2 to 4 hours.

ADVERSE REACTIONS
CNS: dizziness, fatigue, *headache.*
CV: *vasodilation,* ***right ventricular heart failure,*** chest pain, edema, hypotension.
GI: *diarrhea, nausea.*
Musculoskeletal: *jaw pain.*
Respiratory: dyspnea.
Skin: *infusion site pain, infusion site reaction, rash,* pallor, pruritus.

INTERACTIONS
Drug-drug. *Anticoagulants:* May increase risk of bleeding. Monitor patient closely for bleeding.
Antihypertensives, diuretics, vasodilators: May worsen reduction in blood pressure. Monitor blood pressure.

EFFECTS ON LAB TEST RESULTS
None reported.

CONTRAINDICATIONS & CAUTIONS
• Contraindicated in patients hypersensitive to drug or structurally related compounds.
• Use cautiously in patients with hepatic or renal impairment and in elderly patients.

NURSING CONSIDERATIONS
• Assess the patient's ability to accept, place, and care for a subcutaneous catheter and to use an infusion pump.
• During use, a single reservoir syringe can be given for up to 72 hours at 98.6° F (37° C).
• Don't use a single vial longer than 14 days after the initial introduction to the vial.
• Start treatment in setting where adequate monitoring and emergency care are available.
• Increase dose if patient doesn't improve or symptoms worsen, and decrease if drug effects become excessive or unacceptable infusion site symptoms develop.
• Avoid abrupt withdrawal or sudden large dose reductions because PAH symptoms may worsen.

PATIENT TEACHING
• Inform patient that he'll need to continue therapy for a prolonged period, possibly years.
• Tell patient that subsequent disease management may require I.V. therapy.
• Inform patient that many side effects, such as labored breathing, fatigue, and chest pain, may be related to the underlying disease.
• Tell patient that the most common local reactions are pain, redness, tissue hardening, and rash at the infusion site.
• Tell patient that a backup infusion pump must be available to avoid interruption in therapy.

triamterene

try-AM-ter-een

Dyrenium

Pharmacologic class: potassium-sparing diuretic
Pregnancy risk category C

AVAILABLE FORMS

Capsules: 50 mg, 100 mg

INDICATIONS & DOSAGES

➤ Edema

Adults: Initially, 100 mg P.O. b.i.d. after meals. Maximum, 300 mg daily.

ADMINISTRATION

P.O.

- Give drug after meals to minimize nausea.
- If a single daily dose is prescribed, give it in the morning to prevent nocturia.

ACTION

Inhibits sodium reabsorption and potassium and hydrogen excretion by direct action on the distal tubules.

Route	Onset	Peak	Duration
P.O.	2–4 hr	6–8 hr	12–16 hr

Half-life: 3 hours.

ADVERSE REACTIONS

CNS: dizziness, weakness, fatigue, headache.
GI: dry mouth, nausea, vomiting, diarrhea.
GU: interstitial nephritis, nephrolithiasis.
Hematologic: ***thrombocytopenia, agranulocytosis,*** megaloblastic anemia from low folic acid level.
Hepatic: jaundice.
Metabolic: ***hyperkalemia,*** azotemia, hypokalemia, hyponatremia, hyperglycemia, acidosis.
Musculoskeletal: muscle cramps.
Skin: photosensitivity reactions, rash.
Other: ***anaphylaxis.***

INTERACTIONS

Drug-drug. *ACE inhibitors, potassium supplements:* May increase risk of hyperkalemia. If used together, monitor potassium level.
Amantadine: May increase risk of amantadine toxicity. Avoid using together.
Chlorpropamide: May increase risk of hyponatremia. Monitor sodium level.
Cimetidine: May increase bioavailability and decrease renal clearance of triamterene. Monitor potassium level and blood pressure closely.
Lithium: May decrease lithium clearance, increasing risk of lithium toxicity. Monitor lithium level.
NSAIDs: May enhance risk of nephrotoxicity. Use together cautiously.
Quinidine: May interfere with some laboratory tests that measure quinidine level. Inform laboratory that patient is taking triamterene.
Drug-herb. *Licorice:* May increase risk of hypokalemia. Discourage use together.
Drug-food. *Potassium-containing salt substitutes, potassium-rich foods:* May increase risk of hyperkalemia. Urge caution, and monitor potassium level.
Drug-lifestyle. *Sun exposure:* May increase risk for photosensitivity reactions. Advise patient to avoid excessive sunlight exposure.

EFFECTS ON LAB TEST RESULTS

- May increase BUN, creatinine, glucose, and uric acid levels. May decrease sodium and hemoglobin levels. May increase or decrease potassium level.
- May decrease granulocyte and platelet counts. May increase liver function test values.
- May interfere with enzyme assays that use fluorometry, such as quinidine determinations.

CONTRAINDICATIONS & CAUTIONS

- Contraindicated in patients hypersensitive to drug and in those with anuria, severe or progressive renal disease or dysfunction, severe hepatic disease, or hyperkalemia.
- Use cautiously in elderly or debilitated patients and in those with hepatic impairment or diabetes mellitus.

NURSING CONSIDERATIONS

- Monitor blood pressure, uric acid, CBC, and glucose, BUN, and electrolyte levels.
- Monitor potassium levels frequently, especially with dosage changes or with illness that may affect renal function.
- Obtain an ECG if hyperkalemia is present or suspected.
- Stop potassium supplements when therapy starts.
- Watch for blood dyscrasia.
- To minimize excessive rebound potassium excretion, withdraw drug gradually.
- Drug is less potent than thiazides and loop diuretics and is useful as an adjunct to other diuretic therapy. It's usually used with potassium-wasting diuretics; full effect is delayed 2 to 3 days when used alone.
- ***Look alike–sound alike:*** Don't confuse triamterene with trimipramine.

PATIENT TEACHING

- Tell patient to take drug after meals to minimize nausea.
- If a single daily dose is prescribed, instruct patient to take it in the morning to prevent need to urinate at night.
- ***Alert:*** Warn patient to avoid excessive ingestion of potassium-rich foods (such as citrus fruits, tomatoes, bananas, dates, and apricots), potassium-containing salt substitutes, and potassium supplements to prevent serious hyperkalemia.
- Teach patient to avoid direct sunlight, wear protective clothing, and use sunblock to prevent photosensitivity reactions.
- Tell patient that urine may turn blue.

SAFETY ALERT!

urokinase

yoor-oh-KIN-ase

Abbokinase, Kinlytic

Pharmacologic class: enzyme
Pregnancy risk category B

AVAILABLE FORMS

Injection: 250,000 international units/vial

INDICATIONS & DOSAGES

➤ Lysis of acute massive pulmonary embolism and of pulmonary embolism with unstable hemodynamics

Adults: For I.V. infusion only by constant infusion pump. For priming dose, give 4,400 international units/kg with normal saline solution or D_5W solution, over 10 minutes, followed by 4,400 international units/kg/hour for 12 hours. Then give continuous I.V. infusion of heparin and oral anticoagulants.

➤ Lysis of coronary artery thrombi following an acute MI ♦

Adults: After bolus dose of heparin ranging from 2,500 to 10,000 units, infuse 6,000 international units/minute urokinase into occluded artery for up to 2 hours. Average total dose is 500,000 international units. Start drug within 6 hours after symptoms start.

➤ Venous catheter occlusion ♦

Adults: Instill 5,000 international units into occluded line.

ADMINISTRATION

I.V.

- Reconstitute according to manufacturer's directions using sterile water for injection. Gently roll vial; don't shake. Don't use bacteriostatic water for injection to reconstitute; it contains preservatives. Dilute further with normal saline solution or D_5W solution before infusion. Filter urokinase solutions through a 0.45-micron or smaller cellulose-membrane filter before administration. Discard unused solution. Total volume of fluid given by I.V. infusion shouldn't exceed 200 ml.
- Heparin by continuous infusion may be started concurrently or within 3 to 4 hours after urokinase has been stopped to prevent recurrent thrombosis.
- **Incompatibilities:** Other I.V. drugs.

ACTION

Converts plasminogen to plasmin by directly cleaving peptide bonds at two different sites, causing fibrinolysis.

Route	Onset	Peak	Duration
I.V.	Immediate	20 min–4 hr	12–24 hr

Half-life: 10 to 20 minutes.

ADVERSE REACTIONS

CNS: fever.
CV: ***reperfusion arrhythmias,*** tachycardia, transient hypotension or hypertension.
GI: nausea, vomiting.
Hematologic: ***bleeding.***
Respiratory: ***bronchospasm,*** minor breathing difficulties.
Skin: phlebitis at injection site, rash.
Other: ***anaphylaxis,*** chills.

INTERACTIONS

Drug-drug. *Anticoagulants, aspirin, dipyridamole, indomethacin, NSAIDs, phenylbutazone, other drugs affecting platelet activity:* May increase risk of bleeding. Monitor patient.

EFFECTS ON LAB TEST RESULTS

- May decrease hematocrit.
- May increase PT, PTT, and INR.

CONTRAINDICATIONS & CAUTIONS

- Contraindicated in patients with a history of hypersensitivity to the drug; active internal bleeding; recent (within 2 months) cerebrovascular accident, or intracranial or intraspinal surgery; recent trauma including cardiopulmonary resuscitation; intracranial neoplasm, arteriovenous malformation, or aneurysm; severe uncontrolled hypertension, or known bleeding diatheses.
- Contraindicated with I.M. injections and other invasive procedures.
- Use cautiously in patients with recent (within 10 days) major surgery, obstetric delivery, organ biopsy, previous puncture of noncompressible vessels, or serious GI bleeding. Also use cautiously in patients with a high likelihood of left heart thrombus (mitral stenosis with atrial fibrillation), subacute bacterial endocarditis, hemostatic defects including those secondary to severe hepatic or renal disease, pregnancy, cerebrovascular disease, diabetic hemorrhagic retinopathy, or any other condition in which bleeding constitutes a significant hazard or would be particularly difficult to manage because of its location.

NURSING CONSIDERATIONS

- Give other drugs through separate I.V. line.
- Have aminocaproic acid and cross-matched and crosstyped RBCs, whole blood, plasma expanders (other than dextran) available for bleeding. Keep corticosteroids, epinephrine, and antihistamines available for allergic reactions.
- Drug may be given to menstruating women.
- Only prescribers with extensive experience in thrombotic disease management should use drug and only in facilities where clinical and laboratory monitoring can be performed.
- Monitor patient for excessive bleeding every 15 minutes for first hour; every 30 minutes for second through eighth hours; then once every 4 hours. Pretreatment with drugs affecting platelets places patient at high risk of bleeding.
- Monitor pulse, color, and sensation of arms and legs every hour.
- Although risk of hypersensitivity reactions is low, monitor patient.
- Keep a laboratory flow sheet on patient's chart to monitor PTT, PT, thrombin time, hemoglobin level, and hematocrit.
- Monitor vital signs and neurologic status. Don't take blood pressure in legs because doing so could dislodge a clot.
- Keep venipuncture sites to a minimum; use pressure dressing on puncture sites for at least 15 minutes.
- Avoid I.M. injections.
- Keep involved limb in straight alignment to prevent bleeding from infusion site.
- Because bruising is more likely during therapy, avoid unnecessary handling of patient, and pad side rails.
- Rarely, orolingual edema, urticaria, cholesterol embolization, and infusion reactions causing hypoxia, cyanosis, acidosis, and back pain may occur.

PATIENT TEACHING

- Explain use and administration of drug to patient and family.
- Instruct patient to report adverse reactions promptly.

valsartan

val-SAR-tan

Diovan

Pharmacologic class: angiotensin II receptor antagonist

Pregnancy risk category C; D in 2nd and 3rd trimesters

AVAILABLE FORMS

Tablets: 40 mg, 80 mg, 160 mg, 320 mg

INDICATIONS & DOSAGES

➤ Hypertension (used alone or with other antihypertensives)

Adults: Initially, 80 mg P.O. once daily. Expect to see a reduction in blood pressure in 2 to 4 weeks. If additional antihypertensive effect is needed, dose may be increased to 160 or 320 mg daily, or a diuretic may be added. (Addition of a diuretic has a greater effect than dosage increases beyond 80 mg.) Usual dosage range is 80 to 320 mg daily.

➤ New York Heart Association class II to IV heart failure

Adults: Initially, 40 mg P.O. b.i.d.; increase as tolerated to 80 mg b.i.d., and then to target dose of 160 mg b.i.d.

➤ To reduce CV death in stable post-MI patients with left-ventricular failure or dysfunction

Adults: 20 mg P.O. b.i.d. Initial dose may be given as soon as 12 hours after MI. Increase dose to 40 mg b.i.d. within 7 days. Increase subsequent doses, as tolerated, to target dose of 160 mg b.i.d.

ADMINISTRATION

P.O.

- Give drug without regard for food.

ACTION

Blocks the binding of angiotensin II to receptor sites in vascular smooth muscle and the adrenal gland, which inhibits the pressor effects of the renin-angiotensin-aldosterone system.

Route	Onset	Peak	Duration
P.O.	2 hr	2–4 hr	24 hr

Half-life: 6 hours.

ADVERSE REACTIONS

CNS: *dizziness,* headache, insomnia, fatigue, vertigo.
CV: edema, hypotension, orthostatic hypotension, syncope.
EENT: rhinitis, sinusitis, pharyngitis, blurred vision.
GI: abdominal pain, diarrhea, nausea, dyspepsia.
GU: renal impairment.
Hematologic: ***neutropenia.***
Metabolic: hyperkalemia.
Musculoskeletal: arthralgia, back pain.
Respiratory: upper respiratory tract infection, cough.
Other: ***angioedema,*** viral infection.

INTERACTIONS

Drug-drug. *Lithium:* May increase lithium level. Monitor lithium level and patient for toxicity.
Potassium supplements, potassium-sparing diuretics, other angiotensin II blockers: May increase potassium level. May also increase creatinine level in heart failure patients. Avoid using together.
Drug-herb. *Ma huang:* May decrease antihypertensive effects. Discourage use together.
Drug-food. *Salt substitutes containing potassium:* May increase potassium level. May also increase creatinine level in heart failure patients. Discourage use together.

EFFECTS ON LAB TEST RESULTS

- May increase potassium, BUN, and creatinine levels.
- May decrease neutrophil count.

CONTRAINDICATIONS & CAUTIONS

- Contraindicated in patients hypersensitive to drug.
- Contraindicated in pregnant woman in the second or third trimester and in breast-feeding women.
- Use cautiously in patients with renal or hepatic disease.
- Safety and efficacy of drug in children haven't been established.

NURSING CONSIDERATIONS
- Watch for hypotension. Excessive hypotension can occur when drug is given with high doses of diuretics.
- Correct volume and sodium depletions before starting drug.
- ***Alert:*** Drugs that act directly on the renin-angiotensin system can cause injury and even death to the developing fetus. When pregnancy is detected, stop Diovan as soon as possible.

PATIENT TEACHING
- Tell woman of childbearing age to notify prescriber if pregnancy occurs. Drug will need to be stopped.
- Advise patient that drug may be taken without regard for food.

vancomycin hydrochloride
van-koh-MYE-sin

Vancocin, Vancoled

Pharmacologic class: glycopeptide
Pregnancy risk category C; B for capsules only

AVAILABLE FORMS
Capsules: 125 mg, 250 mg
Powder for injection: 500-mg vials, 1-g vials
Powder for oral solution: 1-g bottles, 10-g bottles

INDICATIONS & DOSAGES
➤ Serious or severe infections when other antibiotics are ineffective or contraindicated, including those caused by methicillin-resistant *Staphylococcus aureus, S. epidermidis,* or diphtheroid organisms
Adults: 500 mg I.V. every 6 hours or 1 g I.V. every 12 hours.
Children: 10 mg/kg I.V. every 6 hours.
Neonates and young infants: 15 mg/kg I.V. loading dose; then 10 mg/kg I.V. every 12 hours if child is younger than age 1 week or 10 mg/kg I.V. every 8 hours if child is older than 1 week but younger than 1 month.
Elderly patients: 15 mg/kg I.V. loading dose. Subsequent doses are based on renal function and drug levels.
➤ Antibiotic-related pseudomembranous *Clostridium difficile* and *S. enterocolitis*
Adults: 125 to 500 mg P.O. every 6 hours for 7 to 10 days.
Children: 40 mg/kg P.O. daily, in divided doses every 6 hours for 7 to 10 days. Maximum daily dose is 2 g.
➤ Endocarditis prophylaxis for dental procedures
Adults: 1 g I.V. slowly over 1 to 2 hours, completing infusion 30 minutes before procedure.
Children: 20 mg/kg I.V. over 1 to 2 hours, completing infusion 30 minutes before procedure.
Adjust-a-dose: In renal insufficiency, adjust dosage based on degree of renal impairment, drug level, severity of infection, and susceptibility of causative organism. Initially, give 15 mg/kg, and adjust subsequent doses as needed. One possible schedule is as follows: If creatinine level is less than 1.5 mg/dl, give 1 g every 12 hours. If creatinine level is 1.5 to 5 mg/dl, give 1 g every 3 to 6 days. If creatinine level is greater than 5 mg/dl, give 1 g every 10 to 14 days. Or, if GFR is 10 to 50 ml/minute, give usual dose every 3 to 10 days, and if GFR is less than 10 ml/minute, give usual dose every 10 days.
➤ Bacterial endocarditis from methicillin-resistant or methicillin-susceptible staphylococci in patients with native cardiac valves
Adults: 30 mg/kg I.V. daily given in two divided doses for 4 to 6 weeks. Doses over 2 g require monitoring of drug level.

ADMINISTRATION
P.O.
- Obtain specimen for culture and sensitivity tests before giving. Because of the emergence of vancomycin-resistant enterococci, reserve use of drug for treatment of serious infections caused by gram-positive bacteria resistant to beta-lactam anti-infectives.
- ***Alert:*** This form is ineffective for systemic infections.

• Solution is stable for 2 weeks if refrigerated.

I.V.

• Obtain specimen for culture and sensitivity tests before giving. Because of the emergence of vancomycin-resistant enterococci, reserve use of drug for treatment of serious infections caused by gram-positive bacteria resistant to beta-lactam anti-infectives.
• This form is ineffective for pseudomembranous (*Clostridium difficile*) diarrhea.
• Reconstitute 500-mg vial with 10 ml or 1-g vial with 20 ml sterile water for injection to provide a solution containing 50 mg/ml.
• For infusion, further dilute 500 mg in 100 ml or 1 g in 200 ml normal saline solution for injection or D_5W, and infuse over 60 minutes; if dose is greater than 1 g, infuse over 90 minutes.
• Check site daily for phlebitis and irritation. Severe irritation and necrosis can result from extravasation.
• Refrigerate solution after reconstitution and use within 14 days.
• **Incompatibilities:** Albumin, alkaline solutions, aminophylline, amobarbital, amphotericin B, aztreonam, cephalosporins, chloramphenicol, chlorothiazide, corticosteroids, dexamethasone sodium phosphate, foscarnet, gatifloxacin, heavy metals, heparin, hydrocortisone, idarubicin, methotrexate, nafcillin, omeprazole, penicillin G potassium, pentobarbital, phenobarbital, phenytoin, piperacillin, piperacillin sodium and tazobactam sodium, sargramostim, sodium bicarbonate, ticarcillin disodium, ticarcillin disodium and clavulanate potassium, vitamin B complex with C, warfarin.

ACTION

Hinders bacterial cell-wall synthesis, damaging the bacterial plasma membrane and making the cell more vulnerable to osmotic pressure. Also interferes with RNA synthesis.

Route	Onset	Peak	Duration
P.O.	Unknown	Unknown	Unknown
I.V.	Immediate	Immediate	Unknown

Half-life: 6 hours.

ADVERSE REACTIONS

CNS: fever, pain.
CV: hypotension, thrombophlebitis at injection site.
EENT: ototoxicity, tinnitus.
GI: ***pseudomembranous colitis,*** nausea.
GU: ***nephrotoxicity.***
Hematologic: ***leukopenia, neutropenia,*** eosinophilia.
Respiratory: dyspnea, wheezing.
Skin: red-man syndrome (with rapid I.V. infusion).
Other: ***anaphylaxis,*** chills, superinfection.

INTERACTIONS

Drug-drug. *Aminoglycosides, amphotericin B, cisplatin, pentamidine:* May increase risk of nephrotoxicity and ototoxicity. Monitor renal function and hearing function tests.
Nondepolarizing muscle relaxants: May enhance neuromuscular blockade. Monitor patient closely.

EFFECTS ON LAB TEST RESULTS

• May increase BUN and creatinine levels.
• May increase eosinophil counts. May decrease neutrophil and WBC counts.

CONTRAINDICATIONS & CAUTIONS

• Contraindicated in patients hypersensitive to drug.
• Use cautiously in patients receiving other neurotoxic, nephrotoxic, or ototoxic drugs; in patients older than age 60; and in those with impaired hepatic or renal function, hearing loss, or allergies to other antibiotics.

NURSING CONSIDERATIONS

• Patients with renal dysfunction need dosage adjustment. Monitor blood levels to adjust I.V. dosage. Normal therapeutic levels of vancomycin are peak, 30 to 40 mg/L (drawn 1 hour after infusion ends), and trough, 5 to 10 mg/L (drawn just before next dose is given).
• Obtain hearing evaluation and renal function studies before therapy.
• Monitor patient's fluid balance and watch for oliguria and cloudy urine.
• Monitor patient carefully for red-man syndrome, which can occur if drug is infused too rapidly. Signs and symptoms

include maculopapular rash on face, neck, trunk, and limbs and pruritus and hypotension caused by histamine release. If wheezing, urticaria, or pain and muscle spasm of the chest and back occur, stop infusion and notify prescriber.
• Don't give drug I.M.
• Monitor renal function (BUN, creatinine and creatinine clearance levels, urinalysis, and urine output) during therapy.
• Monitor patient for signs and symptoms of superinfection.
• Have patient's hearing evaluated during prolonged therapy.
• For staphylococcal endocarditis, give for at least 4 weeks.

PATIENT TEACHING
• Tell patient to take entire amount of drug exactly as directed, even after he feels better.
• Instruct patient receiving drug I.V. to report discomfort at I.V. insertion site.
• Tell patient to report ringing in ears.
• Tell patient to report adverse reactions to prescriber immediately.

verapamil hydrochloride
ver-AP-a-mill

Apo-Verap†, Calan, Calan SR, Covera-HS, Isoptin SR, Novo-Veramil†, Nu-Verap†, Verelan, Verelan PM

Pharmacologic class: calcium channel blocker
Pregnancy risk category C

AVAILABLE FORMS
Capsules (extended-release): 100 mg, 120 mg, 180 mg, 200 mg, 240 mg, 300 mg
Capsules (sustained-release): 120 mg, 180 mg, 240 mg, 360 mg
Injection: 2.5 mg/ml
Tablets: 40 mg, 80 mg, 120 mg
Tablets (extended-release): 120 mg, 180 mg, 240 mg
Tablets (sustained-release): 120 mg, 180 mg, 240 mg

INDICATIONS & DOSAGES
➤ **Vasospastic angina (Prinzmetal's or variant angina); classic chronic, stable angina pectoris; chronic atrial fibrillation**
Adults: Starting dose is 80 to 120 mg P.O. t.i.d. Increase dosage at daily or weekly intervals as needed. Some patients may require up to 480 mg daily.
➤ **To prevent paroxysmal supraventricular tachycardia**
Adults: 80 to 120 mg P.O. t.i.d. or q.i.d.
➤ **Supraventricular arrhythmias**
Adults: 0.075 to 0.15 mg/kg (5 to 10 mg) by I.V. push over 2 minutes with ECG and blood pressure monitoring. Repeat dose of 0.15 mg/kg (10 mg) in 30 minutes if no response occurs.
Children ages 1 to 15: Give 0.1 to 0.3 mg/kg as I.V. bolus over 2 minutes; not to exceed 5 mg. Repeat dose in 30 minutes if response is inadequate.
Children younger than age 1: Give 0.1 to 0.2 mg/kg as I.V. bolus over 2 minutes with continuous ECG monitoring. Repeat dose in 30 minutes if no response occurs.
➤ **Digitalized patients with chronic atrial fibrillation or flutter**
Adults: 240 to 320 mg P.O. daily, divided t.i.d. or q.i.d.
➤ **Hypertension**
Adults: 240 mg extended-release tablet P.O. once daily in the morning. If response isn't adequate, give an additional 120 mg in the evening or 240 mg every 12 hours, or an 80-mg immediate-release tablet t.i.d. If using Verelan PM, 200 mg P.O. daily at bedtime. May increase to 300 mg at bedtime if response is inadequate. Maximum dose is 400 mg. If using Covera-HS, 180 mg P.O. daily at bedtime. May increase to 240 mg daily if response is inadequate. Subsequent dosage adjustments may be made in 120-mg increments up to a maximum of 420 mg at bedtime.

ADMINISTRATION
P.O.
• Pellet-filled capsules may be given by carefully opening the capsule and sprinkling the pellets on a spoonful of applesauce. This should be swallowed immediately without chewing, followed

by a glass of cool water to ensure all the pellets are swallowed.
- Give long-acting forms of the drug whole; don't crush or break tablet.

I.V.
- This form is contraindicated in patients receiving I.V. beta blockers and in those with ventricular tachycardia.
- Inject directly into a vein or into the tubing of a free-flowing, compatible solution, such as D_5W, half-normal saline solution, normal saline solution, Ringer's solution, or lactated Ringer's solution.
- Give doses over at least 2 minutes (3 minutes in elderly patients) to minimize the risk of adverse reactions.
- Monitor ECG and blood pressure continuously.
- **Incompatibilities:** Albumin, aminophylline, amphotericin B, ampicillin sodium, co-trimoxazole, dobutamine, hydralazine, nafcillin, oxacillin, propofol, sodium bicarbonate, solutions with a pH greater than 6.

ACTION
Not clearly defined. A calcium channel blocker that inhibits calcium ion influx across cardiac and smooth-muscle cells, thus decreasing myocardial contractility and oxygen demand; it also dilates coronary arteries and arterioles.

Route	Onset	Peak	Duration
P.O.	30 min	1–2 hr	8–10 hr
P.O. (extended)	30 min	5–9 hr	24 hr
I.V.	Immediate	1–5 min	1–6 hr

Half-life: 6 to 12 hours.

ADVERSE REACTIONS
CNS: dizziness, headache, asthenia, fatigue, sleep disturbances.
CV: *transient hypotension,* ***heart failure, bradycardia, AV block, ventricular asystole, ventricular fibrillation,*** peripheral edema.
GI: *constipation,* nausea, diarrhea, dyspepsia.
Respiratory: dyspnea, pharyngitis, ***pulmonary edema,*** rhinitis, sinusitis, upper respiratory infection.
Skin: rash.

INTERACTIONS
Drug-drug. *Acebutolol, atenolol, betaxolol, carteolol,* ***digoxin,*** *esmolol, metoprolol, nadolol, penbutolol, pindolol, propranolol, timolol:* May increase effects of both drugs. Monitor cardiac function closely and decrease doses as needed.
Amiodarone: May cause bradycardia and decrease cardiac output. Monitor patient closely.
Antihypertensives, quinidine: May cause hypotension. Monitor blood pressure.
Carbamazepine: May increase levels of carbamazepine. Monitor patient for toxicity and adjust dosage as needed.
Cyclosporine: May increase cyclosporine level. Monitor cyclosporine level.
Disopyramide, flecainide: May cause heart failure. Avoid using together.
Dofetilide: May increase dofetilide level. Avoid using together.
Lithium: May decrease or increase lithium level. Monitor lithium level.
Phenytoin: May decrease effects of verapamil. Monitor patient closely and adjust dose as needed.
Rifampin: May decrease oral bioavailability of verapamil. Monitor patient for lack of effect.
Neuromuscular-blocking drugs: May potentiate the activity of these drugs. Monitor neuromuscular function and adjust dosages of either drug as needed.
Sirolimus, tacrolimus: May increase levels of these drugs. Monitor drug levels closely and adjust dosage as needed.
Drug-herb. *Black catechu:* May cause additive effects. Discourage use together.
St. John's wort: May decrease drug level and effect. Discourage use together.
Yerba maté: May decrease clearance of herb's methylxanthines and cause toxicity. Urge caution.
Drug-food. *Grapefruit juice:* May increase drug level. Discourage use together.
Drug-lifestyle. *Alcohol use:* May enhance the effects of alcohol. Discourage use together.

EFFECTS ON LAB TEST RESULTS
- May increase ALT, AST, alkaline phosphatase, and bilirubin levels.

CONTRAINDICATIONS & CAUTIONS

- Contraindicated in patients hypersensitive to drug and in those with severe left ventricular dysfunction, cardiogenic shock, second- or third-degree AV block or sick sinus syndrome except in presence of functioning pacemaker, atrial flutter or fibrillation and accessory bypass tract syndrome, severe heart failure (unless secondary to therapy), and severe hypotension.
- I.V. form is contraindicated in patients receiving I.V. beta blockers and in those with ventricular tachycardia.
- Use cautiously in elderly patients and in those with increased intracranial pressure or hepatic or renal disease.

NURSING CONSIDERATIONS

- Patients receiving beta blockers should receive lower doses of this drug. Monitor these patients closely.
- When clinically advisable, have the patient perform vagal maneuvers before giving drug.
- Monitor blood pressure at the start of therapy and during dosage adjustments. Assist patient with walking because dizziness may occur.
- If signs and symptoms of heart failure occur, such as swelling of hands and feet and shortness of breath, notify prescriber.
- Monitor liver function test results during prolonged treatment.
- ***Look alike–sound alike:*** Don't confuse Verelan with Vivarin, Voltaren, or Virilon.

PATIENT TEACHING

- Instruct patient to take oral form of drug exactly as prescribed.
- Tell patient that long-acting forms shouldn't be crushed or chewed.
- Caution patient against abruptly stopping drug.
- If patient continues nitrate therapy during oral verapamil dosage adjustment, urge continued compliance. S.L. nitroglycerin may be taken, as needed, for acute chest pain.
- Encourage patient to increase fluid and fiber intake to combat constipation. Give a stool softener.
- Drug significantly inhibits alcohol elimination. Advise patient to avoid or severely limit alcohol use.
- Inform patient taking Covera-HS that the outer shell of the drug may be excreted in feces.

SAFETY ALERT!

warfarin sodium

WAR-far-in

Coumadin, Jantoven

Pharmacologic class: coumarin derivative
Pregnancy risk category X

AVAILABLE FORMS

Powder for injection: 2 mg/ml
Tablets: 1 mg, 2 mg, 2.5 mg, 3 mg, 4 mg, 5 mg, 6 mg, 7.5 mg, 10 mg

INDICATIONS & DOSAGES

➤ Pulmonary embolism, deep vein thrombosis, MI, rheumatic heart disease with heart valve damage, prosthetic heart valves, chronic atrial fibrillation

Adults: 2 to 5 mg P.O. or I.V. daily for 2 to 4 days; then dosage based on daily PT and INR. Usual maintenance dosage is 2 to 10 mg P.O. or I.V. daily.

ADMINISTRATION

P.O.

- Draw blood to establish baseline coagulation parameters before therapy. PT and INR determinations are essential for proper control. INR range for chronic atrial fibrillation is usually 2 to 3.
- Give drug at same time daily.

I.V.

- Draw blood to establish baseline coagulation parameters before therapy. PT and INR determinations are essential for proper control. INR range for chronic atrial fibrillation is usually 2 to 3.
- I.V. form may be ordered in rare instances when oral therapy can't be given.

• Reconstitute powder with 2.7 ml sterile water, or as instructed in manufacturer guidelines.
• Give as a slow bolus injection over 1 to 2 minutes into a peripheral vein.
• Because onset of action is delayed, heparin sodium is often given during the first few days of treatment of embolic disease. Blood for PT and INR may be drawn at any time during continuous heparin infusion.
• **Incompatibilities:** Aminophylline, ammonium chloride, bretylium tosylate, ceftazidime, cimetidine, ciprofloxacin, dobutamine, esmolol, gentamicin, heparin sodium, labetalol, lactated Ringer injection, metronidazole, promazine, Ringer injection, vancomycin.

ACTION

Inhibits vitamin K–dependent activation of clotting factors II, VII, IX, and X, formed in the liver.

Route	Onset	Peak	Duration
P.O.	Within 24 hr	4 hr	2–5 days
I.V.	Within 24 hr	< 4 hr	2–5 days

Half-life: 20 to 60 hours.

ADVERSE REACTIONS

CNS: *fever,* headache.
GI: *diarrhea,* anorexia, nausea, vomiting, cramps, mouth ulcerations, sore mouth, melena.
GU: enhanced uric acid excretion, hematuria, excessive menstrual bleeding.
Hematologic: ***hemorrhage.***
Hepatic: ***hepatitis,*** jaundice.
Skin: dermatitis, urticaria, necrosis, gangrene, alopecia, *rash.*

INTERACTIONS

Drug-drug. *Acetaminophen:* May increase bleeding with long-term therapy (more than 2 weeks) at high doses (more than 2 g/day) of acetaminophen. Monitor patient very carefully.
Allopurinol, ***amiodarone, anabolic steroids,*** *antidepressants,* ***azole antifungals,*** *aspirin, celecoxib, cephalosporins, chloramphenicol, cimetidine,* ***danazol,*** *diazoxide, diflunisal, disulfiram, erythromycin, ethacrynic acid,* ***fibric acids, fluoxymesterone, fluoroquinolones,*** *furosemide, glucagon, heparin, influenza virus vaccine, isoniazid,* ***lansoprazole,*** *meclofenamate, methimazole, methyldopa, methylphenidate,* ***methyltestosterone, metronidazole, nalidixic acid,*** *neomycin (oral),* ***NSAIDs,*** *omeprazole,* ***oxandrolone,*** *pentoxifylline, propafenone, propoxyphene, propylthiouracil, quinidine,* ***salicylates,*** *SSRIs,* ***sulfinpyrazone,*** *sulfamethoxazole and trimethoprim,* ***sulfonamides,*** *tamoxifen, tetracyclines, thiazides, thrombolytics,* ***thyroid drugs,*** *ticlopidine, tramadol, vitamin E, valproic acid, zafirlukast:* May increase anticoagulant effect. Monitor patient carefully for bleeding. Reduce anticoagulant dosage as directed.
Anticonvulsants: May increase levels of phenytoin and phenobarbital. Monitor drug levels closely.
Ascorbic acid, ***barbiturates,*** *carbamazepine, clozapine, corticosteroids, corticotropin, cyclosporine, dicloxacillin, ethchlorvynol, griseofulvin, haloperidol, meprobamate, mercaptopurine, nafcillin, oral contraceptives containing estrogen, rifampin, spironolactone, sucralfate, thiazide diuretics, trazodone, vitamin K:* May decrease PT and INR with reduced anticoagulant effect. Monitor PT and INR carefully. Increase warfarin dosage, as needed.
Chloral hydrate, cyclophosphamide, HMG-CoA reductase inhibitors, phenytoin, propylthiouracil, ranitidine: May increase or decrease PT and INR. Monitor PT and INR carefully.
Cholestyramine: May decrease response when given too closely together. Give 6 hours after oral anticoagulants.
Sulfonylureas (oral antidiabetics): May increase hypoglycemic response. Monitor glucose levels.
Drug-herb. *Angelica (dong quai):* May significantly prolong PT and INR. Discourage use together.
Anise, arnica flower, asafoetida, bogbean, bromelain, capsicum, celery, chamomile, clove, dandelion, danshen, devil's claw, dong quai, fenugreek, feverfew, garlic, ginger, ***ginkgo, ginseng,*** *horse chestnut, horseradish, licorice, meadowsweet, motherwort, onion, papain, parsley, passion flower, quassia, red clover, Reishi*

mushroom, rue, sweet clover, turmeric, white willow: May increase risk of bleeding. Discourage use together.
Coenzyme Q10, ginseng, St. John's wort: May reduce action of drug. Ask patient about use of herbal remedies, and advise caution.
Green tea: May decrease anticoagulant effect caused by vitamin K content of green tea. Advise patient to minimize variable consumption of green tea and other foods or nutritional supplements containing vitamin K.
Drug-food. *Foods, multivitamins, and other enteral products containing vitamin K:* May impair anticoagulation. Tell patient to maintain consistent daily intake of foods containing vitamin K.
Cranberry juice: May increase risk of severe bleeding. Discourage use together.
Drug-lifestyle. *Alcohol use:* May enhance anticoagulant effects. Tell patient to avoid large amounts of alcohol.

EFFECTS ON LAB TEST RESULTS

- May increase ALT and AST levels.
- May increase INR, PT, and PTT.
- May falsely decrease theophylline level.

CONTRAINDICATIONS & CAUTIONS

- Contraindicated in patients hypersensitive to drug and in those with bleeding from the GI, GU, or respiratory tract; aneurysm; cerebrovascular hemorrhage; severe or malignant hypertension; severe renal or hepatic disease; subacute bacterial endocarditis, pericarditis, or pericardial effusion; or blood dyscrasias or hemorrhagic tendencies.
- Contraindicated during pregnancy, threatened abortion, eclampsia, or preeclampsia, and after recent surgery involving large open areas, eye, brain, or spinal cord; recent prostatectomy; major regional lumbar block anesthesia, spinal puncture, or diagnostic or therapeutic invasive procedures.
- Avoid using in patients with a history of warfarin-induced necrosis; in unsupervised patients with senility, alcoholism, or psychosis; or in situations in which there are inadequate laboratory facilities for coagulation testing.
- Use cautiously in patients with diverticulitis, colitis, mild or moderate hypertension, or mild or moderate hepatic or renal disease; with drainage tubes in any orifice; with regional or lumbar block anesthesia; with heparin-induced thrombocytopenia and deep venous thrombosis; or in conditions that increase risk of hemorrhage.
- Use cautiously in breast-feeding women.

NURSING CONSIDERATIONS

- Avoid all I.M. injections.
- Regularly inspect patient for bleeding gums, bruises on arms or legs, petechiae, nosebleeds, melena, tarry stools, hematuria, and hematemesis.
- Check for unexpected bleeding in breast-fed children of women who take this drug.
- Monitor patient for purple-toes syndrome, characterized by a dark purple or mottled color of the toes; may occur 3 to 10 weeks, or even later after start of therapy.
- ***Alert:*** Withhold drug and call prescriber at once in the event of fever or rash (signs of severe adverse reactions).
- Effect can be neutralized by oral or parenteral vitamin K.
- Elderly patients and patients with renal or hepatic failure are especially sensitive to drug's effect.

PATIENT TEACHING

- Stress importance of complying with prescribed dosage and follow-up appointments. Tell patient to carry a card that identifies his increased risk of bleeding.
- Tell patient and family to watch for signs of bleeding or abnormal bruising and to call prescriber at once if they occur.
- Warn patient to avoid OTC products containing aspirin, other salicylates, or drugs that may interact with warfarin unless ordered by prescriber.
- Advise patient to consult with prescriber before initiating any herbal therapy; many herbs have anticoagulant, antiplatelet, or fibrinolytic properties.
- Tell patient to consult a prescriber before using miconazole vaginal cream or suppositories. Abnormal bleeding and bruising have occurred.

- Instruct woman to notify prescriber if menstruation is heavier than usual; she may need dosage adjustment.
- Tell patient to use electric razor when shaving and to use a soft toothbrush.
- Tell patient to read food labels. Food, nutritional supplements, and multivitamins that contain vitamin K may impair anticoagulation.
- Tell patient to eat a daily, consistent diet of food and drinks containing vitamin K, because eating varied amounts may alter anticoagulant effects.

Appendices & Index

Preventing miscommunication in drug administration

Nurses carry a great deal of responsibility for administering drugs safely and correctly, for making sure the right patient gets the right drug, in the right dose, at the right time, and by the right route. By staying aware of potential trouble areas, you can minimize your risk of making medication errors and maximize the therapeutic effects of your patient's drug regimens.

Name game

Drugs with similar-sounding names can be easily confused. Even different-sounding names can look similar when written rapidly by hand on a prescription form. An example is Soriatane and Loxitane, which are both capsules. If the patient's drug order doesn't seem right for his diagnosis, call the prescriber to clarify the order.

Allergy alert

Once you've verified your patient's full name, check to see if he's wearing an allergy bracelet. If he is, the allergy bracelet should conspicuously display the name of the allergen. The allergy information should also be labeled on the front of the patient's chart and on his medication record. Whether the patient is wearing an allergy bracelet or not, take the time to double-check and ask the patient whether he has any allergies—even if he is in distress.

A patient who is severely allergic to peanuts could have an anaphylactic reaction to ipratropium bromide (Atrovent) aerosol given by metered-dose inhaler. Ask your patient or his parents whether he's allergic to peanuts before you give this drug. If you find that he's allergic, you need to use the nasal spray and inhalation solution form of the drug. Because it doesn't contain soy lecithin, it's safe for patients allergic to peanuts.

Compound errors

Many medication errors occur because of a compound problem—a mistake or group of mistakes that could have been caught at any of several steps along the way. For a drug to be given correctly, each member of the health care team must fill the appropriate role:

- The prescriber must write the order correctly and legibly.
- The pharmacist must evaluate whether the order is appropriate and fill it correctly.
- The nurse must evaluate whether the order is appropriate and administer it correctly.

A breakdown anywhere along this chain of events can lead to a medication error. That's why it's important for members of the health care team to act as a real team so that they can check each other and catch any problems that might arise before these problems affect the patient's health. Encourage an environment in which professionals double-check each other.

Route trouble

Many drug errors happen, at least in part, from problems related to the route of administration. The risk of error increases when a patient has several I.V. lines running for different purposes.

Risky abbreviations

Abbreviating drug names is risky. Abbreviations may not be commonly known and, in some cases, the same abbreviation may be used for different drugs or compounds. For example, epoetin alfa is commonly abbreviated EPO; however, some use the abbreviation EPO to stand for "evening primrose oil." Ask all prescribers to spell out drug names.

Unclear orders

A patient was supposed to receive one dose of the antineoplastic lomustine to treat brain cancer. (Lomustine is typically given in a single dose once every 6 weeks.) The doctor's order read, "Administer h.s." Because a nurse misinterpreted the order to mean every night, the patient received nine daily doses, developed severe thrombocytopenia and leukopenia, and died.

If you are unfamiliar with a drug, check a drug book before giving it. If a prescriber uses "h.s." and doesn't specify the frequency of administration, ask him to clarify the order. When documenting orders, note "at bedtime nightly" or "at bedtime one dose today."

Color changes

If a familiar drug seems to have an unfamiliar appearance, investigate the cause. If the pharmacist cites a manufacturer change, ask him to double-check whether he has received verification from the manufacturer. Always document the appearance discrepancy, your actions, and the pharmacist's response in the patient record.

Stress levels

Committing a serious error can cause enormous stress and cloud your judgment. If you're involved in a drug error, ask another professional to give the antidote.

Reconciling medications

Medication reconciliation is the process of comparing a patient's medication orders to all of the medications that the patient has been taking. This reconciliation is done to avoid medication errors, such as omissions, duplications, dosing errors, or drug interactions. Medication errors related to medication reconciliation are more likely to occur at admission, upon transfer to another unit, or when discharged from a facility. Studies have shown that a medication reconciliation process can successfully reduce medication errors.

At discharge, it is important to provide both the patient and the next care provider a complete list of current medications, including all prescription and over-the-counter medications, as well as any vitamins, herbal medications, and nutraceuticals.

Be sure to provide a clearly written list that includes:

- the name of each medication and the reason for taking it
- all new medications and pre-hospital medications that the patient is to discontinue
- the correct dose and frequency, highlighting changes from the pre-hospital instructions
- a list of over-the-counter drugs that shouldn't be taken.

In addition to the reconciled list, it's important to ensure the availability of medications upon discharge to the patient and to determine if the patient can read his medication labels correctly, can afford the necessary medications, and is able to get to the pharmacy.

Common combination drugs: Indications and dosages

ANTIDIABETICS

Avandamet

Generic components
Tablets
1 mg rosiglitazone and 500 mg metformin
2 mg rosiglitazone and 500 mg metformin
2 mg rosiglitazone and 1 g metformin
4 mg rosiglitazone and 500 mg metformin
4 mg rosiglitazone and 1 g metformin

Dosages
Adults: 4 mg rosiglitazone with 500 mg metformin, once per day or in divided doses. Not for initial therapy; adjust using individual drugs alone, then switch to the appropriate dosage of the combination product. See package insert for details on adjusting dosage based on use of other drugs and previous dosage levels.

Glucovance

Generic components
Tablets
1.25 mg glyburide and 250 mg metformin
2.5 mg glyburide and 500 mg metformin
5 mg glyburide and 500 mg metformin

Dosages
Adults: 1 tablet P.O. per day usually in the morning. Not for initial therapy; adjust using the individual drugs alone, then switch to the appropriate dosage of the combination product.

Metaglip

Generic components
Tablets
2.5 mg glipizide and 250 mg metformin
2.5 mg glipizide and 500 mg metformin
5 mg glipizide and 500 mg metformin

Dosages
Adults: 1 tablet per day with a meal; adjust dose based on patient response. Maximum dose, 20 mg glipizide with 2,000 mg metformin per day.

ANTIHYPERTENSIVES

Accuretic

Generic components
Tablets
10 mg quinapril and 12.5 mg hydrochlorothiazide
20 mg quinapril and 12.5 mg hydrochlorothiazide
20 mg quinapril and 25 mg hydrochlorothiazide

Dosages
Adults: 1 tablet P.O. per day in the morning. Adjust drug using the individual products, then switch to appropriate dosage of the combination product.

Aldoclor

Generic components
Tablets
250 mg methyldopa and 150 mg chlorothiazide
250 mg methyldopa and 250 mg chlorothiazide

Dosages
Adults: 1 tablet P.O. per day in the morning. Adjust dosage using the individual products, then switch to the combination product when patient's adjustment schedule is stable.

Aldoril
Aldoril D

Generic components
Tablets
250 mg methyldopa and 15 mg hydrochlorothiazide
250 mg methyldopa and 25 mg hydrochlorothiazide
500 mg methyldopa and 30 mg hydrochlorothiazide
500 mg methyldopa and 50 mg hydrochlorothiazide

Dosages
Adults: 1 tablet P.O. per day in the morning. Adjust dosage using the individual products, then switch to the combination product when patient's adjustment schedule is stable.

Atacand HCT

Generic components
Tablets
16 mg candesartan and 12.5 mg hydrochlorothiazide
32 mg candesartan and 12.5 mg hydrochlorothiazide

Dosages
Adults: 1 tablet P.O. per day in the morning. Adjust dosage using the individual products, then switch to appropriate dosage.

Avalide

Generic components
Tablets
150 mg irbesartan and 12.5 mg hydrochlorothiazide
300 mg irbesartan and 12.5 mg hydrochlorothiazide
300 mg irbesartan and 25 mg hydrochlorothiazide

Dosages
Adults: 1 tablet P.O. per day. Adjust dosage using the individual products, then switch to combination product when patient's condition is stabilized. Maximum daily dose, 300 mg irbesartan and 25 mg hydrochlorothiazide.

Benicar HCT

Generic components
Tablets
20 mg olmesartan and 12.5 mg hydrochlorothiazide
40 mg olmesartan and 12.5 mg hydrochlorothiazide
40 mg olmesartan and 25 mg hydrochlorothiazide

Dosages
Adults: 1 tablet P.O. per day in the morning. Adjust dosage using the individual products, then switch to the combination product when patient's adjustment schedule is stable.

Capozide

Generic components
Tablets
25 mg captopril and 15 mg hydrochlorothiazide
50 mg captopril and 15 mg hydrochlorothiazide
25 mg captopril and 25 mg hydrochlorothiazide
50 mg captopril and 25 mg hydrochlorothiazide

Dosages
Adults: 1 to 2 tablets P.O. per day in the morning. Adjust dosage using the individual products, then switch to the combination product when patient's adjustment schedule is stable.

Clorpres

Generic components

Tablets

15 mg chlorthalidone and 0.1 mg clonidine hydrochloride
15 mg chlorthalidone and 0.2 mg clonidine hydrochloride
15 mg chlorthalidone and 0.3 mg clonidine hydrochloride

Dosages

Adults: 1 to 2 tablets P.O. per day in the morning. Adjust dosage using the individual products, then switch to the combination product when patient's adjustment schedule is stable.

Corzide

Generic components

Tablets

40 mg nadolol and 5 mg bendroflumethiazide
80 mg nadolol and 5 mg bendroflumethiazide

Dosages

Adults: 1 tablet P.O. per day in the morning. Adjust dosage using the individual products, then switch to the combination product when patient's adjustment schedule is stable.

Diovan HCT

Generic components

Tablets

80 mg valsartan and 12.5 mg hydrochlorothiazide
160 mg valsartan and 12.5 mg hydrochlorothiazide
160 mg valsartan and 25 mg hydrochlorothiazide
320 mg valsartan and 12.5 mg hydrochlorothiazide
320 mg valsartan and 25 mg hydrochlorothiazide

Dosages

Adults: 1 tablet P.O. per day. Not for initial therapy; adjust dosage using the individual products, then switch to the combination product when patient's adjustment schedule is stable.

Hyzaar

Generic components

Tablets

50 mg losartan and 12.5 mg hydrochlorothiazide
100 mg losartan and 12.5 mg hydrochlorothiazide
100 mg losartan and 25 mg hydrochlorothiazide

Dosages

Adults: 1 tablet P.O. per day in the morning. Not for initial therapy; start using each component and if desired effects are obtained, Hyzaar may be used.

Inderide

Generic components

Tablets

40 mg propranolol hydrochloride and 25 mg hydrochlorothiazide
80 mg propranolol hydrochloride and 25 mg hydrochlorothiazide

Dosages

Adults: 1 tablet P.O. b.i.d. Adjust dosage using the individual products, then switch to the combination product when patient's adjustment schedule is stable. Maximum total daily dose shouldn't exceed 160 mg propranolol and 50 mg hydrochlorothiazide.

Lexxel

Generic components

Extended-release Tablets

5 mg enalapril maleate and 2.5 mg felodipine

5 mg enalapril maleate and 5 mg felodipine

Dosages

Adults: 1 tablet P.O. per day. Adjust dosage using the individual products, then switch to the combination product when patient's adjustment schedule is stable. Make sure that patient swallows tablet whole. Don't cut, crush, or allow him to chew.

Lopressor HCT

Generic components

Tablets
50 mg metoprolol and 25 mg hydrochlorothiazide
100 mg metoprolol and 25 mg hydrochlorothiazide
100 mg metoprolol and 50 mg hydrochlorothiazide

Dosages

Adults: 1 tablet P.O. per day. Adjust dosage using the individual products, then switch to the combination product when patient's adjustment schedule is stable.

Lotensin HCT

Generic components

Tablets
5 mg benazepril and 6.25 mg hydrochlorothiazide
10 mg benazepril and 12.5 mg hydrochlorothiazide
20 mg benazepril and 12.5 mg hydrochlorothiazide
20 mg benazepril and 25 mg hydrochlorothiazide

Dosages

Adults: 1 tablet P.O. per day in the morning. Adjust dosage using the individual products, then switch to the combination product when patient's adjustment schedule is stable.

Lotrel

Generic components

Capsules
2.5 mg amlodipine and 10 mg benazepril
5 mg amlodipine and 10 mg benazepril
5 mg amlodipine and 20 mg benazepril
5 mg amlodipine and 40 mg benazepril
10 mg amlodipine and 20 mg benazepril
10 mg amlodipine and 40 mg benazepril

Dosages

Adults: 1 tablet P.O. per day in the morning. Monitor patient for hypertension and adverse effects closely over first 2 weeks and regularly thereafter.

Micardis HCT

Generic components

Tablets
40 mg telmisartan and 12.5 mg hydrochlorothiazide
80 mg telmisartan and 12.5 mg hydrochlorothiazide
80 mg telmisartan and 25 mg hydrochlorothiazide

Dosages

Adults: 1 tablet P.O. per day; may be adjusted up to 160 mg telmisartan and 25 mg hydrochlorothiazide, based on patient's response.

Monopril-HCT

Generic components

Tablets
10 mg fosinopril and 12.5 mg hydrochlorothiazide
20 mg fosinopril and 12.5 mg hydrochlorothiazide

Dosages

Adults: 1 tablet P.O. per day in the morning. Adjust dosage using the individual products, then switch to appropriate dosage of the combination product.

Prinzide
Zestoretic

Generic components

Tablets

10 mg lisinopril and 12.5 mg hydrochlorothiazide
20 mg lisinopril and 12.5 mg hydrochlorothiazide
20 mg lisinopril and 25 mg hydrochlorothiazide

Dosages

Adults: 1 tablet P.O. per day in the morning. Adjust dosage using the individual products, then switch to the combination product when patient's adjustment schedule is stable.

Tarka

Generic components

Tablets

1 mg trandolapril and 240 mg verapamil
2 mg trandolapril and 180 mg verapamil
2 mg trandolapril and 240 mg verapamil
4 mg trandolapril and 240 mg verapamil

Dosages

Adults: 1 tablet P.O. per day, taken with food. Adjust dosage using the individual products, then switch to the combination product when patient's adjustment schedule is stable. Make sure that patient swallows tablet whole. Don't cut, crush, or allow him to chew.

Teczem

Generic components

Extended-release tablets

5 mg enalapril maleate and 180 mg diltiazem hydrochloride

Dosages

Adults: 1 to 2 tablets P.O. per day in the morning. Adjust dosage using the individual products, then switch to the combination product when patient's adjustment schedule is stable. Make sure that patient swallows tablet whole. Don't cut, crush, or allow him to chew.

Tenoretic

Generic components

Tablets

50 mg atenolol and 25 mg chlorthalidone
100 mg atenolol and 25 mg chlorthalidone

Dosages

Adults: 1 tablet P.O. per day in the morning. Adjust dosage using the individual products, then switch to appropriate dosage of the combination product.

Teveten HCT

Generic components

Tablets

600 mg eprosartan and 12.5 mg hydrochlorothiazide
600 mg eprosartan and 25 mg hydrochlorothiazide

Dosages

Adults: 1 tablet P.O. per day. Adjust dosage using the individual products, then switch to appropriate dosage of the combination product; if blood pressure isn't controlled on 600 mg/25 mg tablet, 300 mg eprosartan may be added each evening.

Uniretic

Generic components

Tablets

7.5 mg moexipril and 12.5 mg hydrochlorothiazide
15 mg moexipril and 12.5 mg hydrochlorothiazide
15 mg moexipril and 25 mg hydrochlorothiazide

Dosages

Adults: Give ½ to 2 tablets per day. Not for initial therapy. Adjust dosage to maintain appropriate blood pressure.

Vaseretic

Generic components
Tablets
5 mg enalapril maleate and 12.5 mg hydrochlorothiazide
10 mg enalapril maleate and 25 mg hydrochlorothiazide

Dosages
Adults: 1 to 2 tablets P.O. per day in the morning. Adjust dosage using the individual products, then switch to the combination product when patient's adjustment schedule is stable.

Ziac

Generic components
Tablets
2.5 mg bisoprolol and 6.25 mg hydrochlorothiazide
5 mg bisoprolol and 6.25 mg hydrochlorothiazide
10 mg bisoprolol and 6.25 mg hydrochlorothiazide

Dosages
Adults: 1 tablet P.O. per day in the morning. Initial dose is 2.5/6.25 mg tablet P.O. per day. Adjust dosage within 1 week; optimal antihypertensive effect may require 2 to 3 weeks.

ANTIPLATELET DRUGS

Aggrenox

Generic components
Capsules
25 mg aspirin and 200 mg dipyridamole

Dosages
Adults: To decrease risk of stroke, 1 capsule P.O. b.i.d. in the morning and evening. Swallow capsule whole; may be taken with or without food.

DIURETICS

Aldactazide

Generic components
Tablets
25 mg spironolactone and 25 mg hydrochlorothiazide
50 mg spironolactone and 50 mg hydrochlorothiazide

Dosages
Adults: One to eight 25-mg spironolactone and 25-mg hydrochlorothiazide tablets per day. Or, one to four 50-mg spironolactone and 50-mg hydrochlorothiazide tablets per day.

Dyazide

Generic components
Capsules
37.5 mg triamterene and 25 mg hydrochlorothiazide

Dosages
Adults: 1 to 2 tablets per day.

Maxzide

Generic components
Tablets
37.5 mg triamterene and 25 mg hydrochlorothiazide
75 mg triamterene and 50 mg hydrochlorothiazide

Dosages
Adults: 1 tablet per day.

Moduretic

Generic components
Tablets
5 mg amiloride and 50 mg hydrochlorothiazide

Dosages
Adults: 1 to 2 tablets per day with meals.

HEART FAILURE DRUGS

BiDil

Generic components
Tablets
20 mg isosorbide dinitrate and 37.5 mg hydralazine

Dosages
Adults: 1 to 2 tablets P.O. t.i.d.

LIPID-LOWERING DRUGS

Advicor

Generic components
Tablets
20 mg lovastatin and 500 mg niacin
20 mg lovastatin and 750 mg niacin
20 mg lovastatin and 1,000 mg niacin
40 mg lovastatin and 1,000 mg niacin

Dosages
Adults: 1 tablet P.O. per day at night.

Pravigard PAC

Generic components
Tablets
20 mg pravastatin packaged with 81 mg buffered aspirin
40 mg pravastatin packaged with 81 mg buffered aspirin
80 mg pravastatin packaged with 81 mg buffered aspirin
20 mg pravastatin packaged with 325 mg buffered aspirin
40 mg pravastatin packaged with 325 mg buffered aspirin
80 mg pravastatin packaged with 325 mg buffered aspirin

Dosages
Adults: Initially, 40 mg pravastatin with 81 or 325 mg buffered aspirin; adjust dose to regulate cholesterol levels.

Vytorin

Generic components
Tablets
10 mg ezetimibe with 10 mg simvastatin
10 mg ezetimibe with 20 mg simvastatin
10 mg ezetimibe with 40 mg simvastatin
10 mg ezetimibe with 80 mg simvastatin

Dosages
Adults: 1 tablet per day, in the evening in combination with a cholesterol-lowering diet and exercise. Dosage of simvastatin in the combination may be adjusted based on patient response. If given with a bile sequestrant, must be given at least 2 hours before or 4 hours after the bile sequestrant.

MISCELLANEOUS CARDIAC DRUGS

Caduet

Generic components
Tablets
2.5 mg amlodipine with 10 mg, 20 mg, or 40 mg atorvastatin
5 mg amlodipine with 10 mg, 20 mg, 40 mg, or 80 mg atorvastatin
10 mg amlodipine with 10 mg, 20 mg, 40 mg, or 80 mg atorvastatin

Dosages
Adults, boys, and postmenarchal girls age 10 and older: Determine the most effective dose for each component, then select the most appropriate combination product.

OPIOID AGONISTS

Suboxone
CSS III

Generic components
Sublingual tablets
2 mg buprenorphine and 0.5 mg naloxone
8 mg buprenorphine and 2 mg naloxone

Dosages
Opioid dependence
Adults: 12 to 16 mg sublingual once per day, after induction with sublingual buprenorphine.

Drugs by therapeutic class

Amebicides, antiprotozoals, and anthelmintics
- Metronidazole

Aminoglycosides
- Amikacin
- Gentamicin
- Tobramycin

Antagonists and antidotes
- Protamine sulfate

Antianginals
- Amlodipine besylate
- Atenolol
- Diltiazem hydrochloride
- Hydrochloride
- Isosorbide dinitrate
- Isosorbide mononitrate
- Metoprolol
- Nadolol
- Nicardipine hydrochloride
- Nifedipine
- Nitroglycerin
- Propranolol hydrochloride
- Ranolazine
- Verapamil hydrychloride

Antiarrhythmics
- Adenosine
- Amiodarone hydrochloride
- Atropine sulfate
- Digoxin
- Disopyramide
- Disopyramide phosphate
- Dofetilide
- Esmolol hydrochloride
- Flecainide acetate
- Ibutilide fumarate
- Isoproterenol hydrochloride
- Lidocaine hydrochloride
- Magnesium sulfate
- Mexiletine hydrochloride
- Procainamide hydrochloride
- Propafenone hydrochloride
- Propranolol hydrochloride (also see Antianginals)
- Quinidine gluconate
- Quinidine sulfate
- Sotalol hydrochloride
- Verapamil hydrochloride (also see Antianginals)

Anticoagulants
- Argatroban
- Bivalirudin
- Dalteparin sodium
- Enoxaparin sodium
- Fondaparinux sodium
- Heparin sodium
- Warfarin sodium

Antihypertensives
- Aliskiren
- Amlodipine
- Atenolol (also see Antianginals)
- Benazepril hydrochloride
- Candesartan cilexetil
- Captopril
- Carvedilol
- Carvedilol phosphate
- Clonidine hydrochloride
- Diltiazem hydrochloride (also see Antianginals)
- Doxazosin mesylate
- Enalaprilat
- Enalapril maleate
- Eplerenone
- Eprosartan mesylate
- Ethacrynate sodium (also see Diuretics)
- Felodipine
- Fosinopril sodium
- Furosemide (also see Diuretics)
- Guanfacine hydrochloride
- Hydralazine hydrochloride
- Hydrochlorothiazide (also see Diuretics)
- Indapamide (also see Diuretics)
- Irbesartan
- Labetalol hydrochloride
- Lisinopril
- Losartan potassium
- Methyldopa
- Methyldopa hydrochloride

- Metolazone (also see Diuretics)
- Metoprolol succinate
- Metoprolol tatrate
- Minoxidil
- Nadolol (also see Antianginals)
- Nicardipine hydrochloride (also see Antianginals)
- Nifedipine (also see Antianginals)
- Nisoldipine
- Nitroglycerin (also see Antianginals)
- Nitroprusside sodium
- Olmesartan medoxomil
- Perindopril erbumine
- Phentolamine mesylate
- Prazosin hydrochloride
- Propranolol hydrochloride (also see Antianginals)
- Quinapril hydrochloride
- Ramipril
- Spironolactone (also see Diuretics)
- Telmisartan
- Terazosin hydrochloride
- Torsemide (also see Diuretics)
- Trandolapril
- Valsartan
- Verapamil hydrochloride (also see Antianginals)

Antilipemics

- Atorvastatin calcium
- Cholestyramine
- Colesevelam hydrochloride
- Ezetimibe
- Fenofibrate
- Fluvastatin sodium
- Gemfibrozil
- Lovastatin
- Niacin
- Omega-3-acid ethyl esters
- Pravastatin sodium
- Rosuvastatin calcium
- Simvastatin

CNS stimulants

- Phentermine hydrochloride
- Sibutramine hydrochloride monohydrate

Diuretics

- Acetazolamide
- Acetazolamide sodium
- Bumetanide
- Ethacrynate sodium
- Ethacrynic acid
- Furosemide
- Hydrochlorothiazide
- Indapamide
- Mannitol
- Metolazone
- Spironolactone
- Torsemide
- Triamterene

Electrolyte balancing drugs

- Potassium chloride

Inotropics

- Dobutamine hydrochloride (also see Vasopressors)
- Dopamine hydrochloride (also see Vasopressors)
- Digoxin
- Ephedrine sulfate (also see Vasopressors)
- Epinephrine
- Inamrinone lactate
- Milrinone lactate

Miscellaneous anti-infectives

- Chloramphenicol
- Clindamycin
- Vancomycin

Miscellaneous cardiovascular drugs

- Alprostadil
- Midodrine hydrochloride
- Pentoxifylline

Nonopioid analgesics and antipyretics

- Aspirin

Nonsteroidal anti-inflammatories

- Indomethacin

Opioid analgesics

- Morphine

Penicillins

- Ampicillin
- Penicillin G benzathine
- Penicillin V potassium

Platelet drugs
• Abciximab
• Cilostazol
• Clopidogrel bisulfate
• Dipyridamole
• Eptifibatide
• Ticlopidine hydrochloride
• Tirofiban hydrochloride

Thrombolytic enzymes
• Alteplase
• Reteplase, recombinant
• Streptokinase
• Tenecteplase
• Urokinase

Uncategorized drugs
• Orlistat

Vasodilators
• Ambrisentan
• Bosentan
• Hydralazine hydrochloride (also see Antihypertensives)
• Iloprost
• Isosorbide dinitrate (also see Antianginals)
• Isosorbide mononitrate (also see Antianginals)
• Minoxidil (also see Antihypertensives)
• Nesiritide
• Nimodipine
• Nitroglycerin (also see Antianginals)
• Nitroprusside sodium (also see Antihypertensives)
• Sildenafil citrate
• Treprostinil sodium

Vasopressors
• Dobutamine hydrochloride
• Dopamine hydrochloride
• Ephedrine sulfate
• Epinephrine
• Norepinephrine bitartrate
• Phenylephrine hydrochloride

Vitamins and minerals
• Vitamin K

Selected references

Diseases, 4th ed. Philadelphia: Lippincott Williams & Wilkins, 2006.

Dracup, K., et al. "Acute Coronary Syndrome: What Do Patients Know?" *Archives of Internal Medicine* 168(10):1049–54, May 2008.

Drake, R., et al. *Gray's Atlas of Anatomy,* St. Louis: W.B. Saunders, 2008.

Fauci, A.S., et al., eds. *Harrison's Principles of Internal Medicine,* 17th ed. New York: McGraw-Hill, 2008.

Gendreau-Webb, R. "Is It a Kidney Stone or Abdominal Aortic Aneurysm?" *Nursing* 36(5 Suppl):22–4, Spring 2006.

Nursing2009 Drug Handbook, Philadelphia: Lippincott Williams & Wilkins, 2009.

Porth, C.M. *Essentials of Pathophysiology: Concepts of Altered Health States,* 2nd ed. Philadelphia: Lippincott Williams & Wilkins, 2007.

Professional Guide to Diseases, 9th ed. Philadelphia: Lippincott Williams & Wilkins, 2009.

Professional Guide to Pathophysiology, 2nd ed. Philadelphia: Lippincott Williams & Wilkins, 2007.

Reckard, D., et al. "Mitral Valve Replacement: A Case Report," *AANA Journal* 76(2):125–9, April 2008.

Seeley, R.R., et. al. *Anatomy and Physiology,* 8th ed. New York: McGraw-Hill, 2007.

Smeltzer, S.C, et. al. *Brunner and Suddarth's Textbook of Medical-Surgical Nursing,* 11th ed. Philadelphia: Lippincott Williams & Wilkins, 2006.

Stephen, S.A., et al. "Symptoms of Acute Coronary Syndrome in Women with Diabetes: An Integrative Review of the Literature," *Heart & Lung* 37(3): 179–89, May-June 2008.

Swart, S., and Tiffen, J. "Acute Pericarditis," *AAOHN Journal* 55(2):44–6, February 2007.

Washburn, S.C., and Hornberger, C.A. "Nurse Educator Guidelines for the Management of Heart Failure," *Journal of Continuing Education in Nursing* 39(6):263–7, June 2008.

Woods, S.L., et al. *Cardiac Nursing*, 5th ed. Philadelphia: Lippincott Williams & Wilkins, 2005.

Wung, S.F., and Kozik, T. "Electrocardiographic Evaluation of Cardiovascular Status," *Journal of Cardiovascular Nursing* 23(2):169–74, March-April 2008.

Yates, G., and Saunders, K. "Pulmonary Hypertension: A Review for Nurses," *Canadian Journal of Cardiovascular Nursing* 18(1):7–14, 2008.

Zeigler, V.L. "Congenital Heart Disease and Genetics," *Critical Care Nursing Clinics of North America* 20(2): 159–69, v., June 2008.

Index

i refers to an illustration; t refers to a table

A

B

D

E

F

G

H

I

N

Q

R

S

V

W

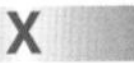

X

Z